Teaching Atlas of Pediatric Imaging

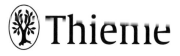

Teaching Atlas of Pediatric Imaging

Paul S. Babyn, M.D., F.R.C.P.C.
Associate Professor
Department of Medical Imaging
University of Toronto
Radiologist in Chief
Department of Diagnostic Imaging
The Hospital for Sick Children
Toronto, Ontario, Canada

Thieme
New York • Stuttgart

Thieme Medical Publishers, Inc.
333 Seventh Ave.
New York, NY 10001

Editor: Timothy Hiscock
Vice President, Production and Electronic Publishing: Anne T. Vinnicombe
Associate Editor: Birgitta Brandenburg
Production Editor: Print Matters, Inc.
Sales Manager: Ross Lumpkin
Chief Financial Officer: Peter van Woerden
President: Brian D. Scanlan
Compositor: Compset
Printer: Edwards Brothers
Cover Painting: Elizabeth Van Wersch Babyn

Library of Congress Cataloging-in-Publication Data

Teaching atlas of pediatric imaging / [edited by] Paul S. Babyn.
    p. ; cm.
  Includes bibliographical references and index.
  ISBN 1-58890-339-7 (US) — ISBN 3-13-141991-1 (GTV)
    1. Pediatric radiology—Atlases. 2. Pediatric diagnostic imaging—Atlases. 3. Children—Diseases—Diagnosis—Atlases.
    [DNLM: 1. Radiography—methods—Child—Atlases. 2. Radiography—methods—Child—Case Reports. 3. Radiography—methods—Infant—Atlases. 4. Radiography—methods—Infant—Case Reports. 5. Diagnostic Imaging—methods—Child—Atlases. 6. Diagnostic Imaging—methods—Child—Case Reports. 7. Diagnostic Imaging—methods—Infant—Atlases. 8. Diagnostic Imaging—methods—Infant—Case Reports. WN 17 T2532 2005] I. Babyn, Paul S.
  RJ51.R3T43 2005
  618.92′00757—dc22

                                                                                                        2005050641

Printed in the United States of America
5 4 3 2 1
TMP ISBN 1-58890-339-7
        978-1-58890-339-6

GTV ISBN 3-13-141991-1
        978-3-13-141001 0

DEDICATION

To my wife Elizabeth and especially my children, Andre, Laura, Michael, and Jonathan.

To my colleagues whose efforts and willingness to share and make pediatric radiology such a fulfilling profession.

To the many trainees who have taught me so much.

To Susan Jewell, Managing Director of Diagnostic Radiology, and the rest of the staff of the diagnostic imaging department at The Hospital for Sick Children, individuals who always strive for excellence, ensuring the utmost for our patients and their families.

CONTENTS

SECTION III
Chest
David Manson, Section Editor

SECTION IV
Cardiac
Shi-Joon Yoo, Section Editor

SECTION V
Abdominal
Kamaldine Oudjhane and Karen E. Thomas, Section Editors

SECTION VI
Genitourinary
Kieran McHugh, Section Editor

SECTION VII
Musculoskeletal
Don Soboleski and Paul S. Babyn, Section Editors

SECTION VIII
Interventional
Peter Chait, Section Editor

SECTION IX
Dysplasias
Stephen F. Miller, Section Editor

FOREWORD

When I was asked to write the foreword for the *Teaching Atlas of Pediatric Radiology* edited by Dr. Paul Babyn and colleagues from The Hospital for Sick Children in Toronto, I enthusiastically agreed since the Department of Radiology at "SickKids" has been a world leader for decades. As I saw the scope of their work emerge—every area of pediatric radiology covered with all modalities utilized—I realized that this book would be unique. It is literally like sitting down with an experienced teacher—whether the reader is a medical student, intern, or pediatric or radiology resident—and going through histories and imaging and reaching a diagnosis with time spent on differential diagnosis.

As such, the atlas serves as much more than a collection of cases. The cases in each section together comprise a short book on that anatomic region. The 125 cases take the reader through solutions to the daily problems in pediatric radiology and also a board review, making this atlas an exceptional reference source. I will use it along with the books on syndromes and the classic multivolume multiauthored texts on pediatric X-ray diagnosis, and I suspect I will use this atlas the most. I commend Dr. Babyn and his colleagues.

Walter E. Berdon, M.D.
Professor
Department of Radiology
College of Physicians and Surgeons
Columbia University
New York, New York

PREFACE

Pediatric patients pose many challenges to the radiologist. As with all areas of radiology, tricks of the trade evolve from experience. Written by experienced pediatric radiologists, this new clinically oriented teaching atlas contains 125 cases illustrating a wide range of pediatric diseases. By presenting clinical cases, we impart a variety of important points that will hopefully guide those involved in pediatric imaging. The clinical cases presented in this book vary in complexity and directly reflect what radiologists will see in practice, as well as provide insight into a few unusual cases offering practical guidelines for accurate diagnoses. We believe that the overall approach of the book and case format is ideal for all those in training (whether in radiology or pediatrics) and preparing for examinations.

Cases are organized into anatomical sections: neuroradiology, head and neck, chest, cardiac, abdominal, genitourinary, musculoskeletal, interventional radiology, and dysplasias. For each case, a clinical presentation, radiological findings, diagnosis, clinical findings, discussion, and suggested readings are provided. Each case also provides a list of differential diagnoses in a format that is tailored for self-testing or quick review. Where applicable, additional information pertaining to etiology, pathology/histology, treatment, and complications is also included. Further, the diagnosis has been deliberately omitted from the first page of each case so that the reader can use the clinical presentation and diagnostic images for self-assessment before reading the correct diagnosis and explanatory discussions.

The book and case format provides valuable up-to-date teaching points for daily practice from the straightforward to the advanced as follows:

- The book is conveniently organized into nine sections based on anatomic region.
- The bullet format makes it a user-friendly clinical reference or review book.
- 125 cases stress real-life clinical problems.
- Each case presents a complete patient workup that is supported by numerous high-quality diagnostic images and illustrations for maximum comprehension.
- Differential diagnoses are thoroughly covered, highlighting similar clinical presentations.
- Pearls and pitfalls target important points and sources of error in image interpretation.
- Reviews of current literature, with short lists of recommended reading, are included.

Teaching Atlas of Pediatric Imaging is useful/ideal at several levels:

- For residents or fellows preparing for the radiology board examinations and rotating through the subspecialty pediatric radiology, this comprehensive compilation of cases should also serve as an excellent resource to review a variety of cases that are seen in daily pediatric radiology practice.

- For fellows and practitioners looking for help in passing the Certificate of Added Qualification (CAQ) in Pediatric Radiology
- For general radiologists and for more experienced radiologists and pediatricians, who will find it to be an excellent text for quick and easy reference in daily practice
- For general radiologists and pediatricians who will find this format useful in daily practice to quickly review practical guidelines

ACKNOWLEDGMENTS

I want to acknowledge the tremendous efforts of Dr. Harpal K. Gahunia, M.Sc., Ph.D., whose assistance in this endeavor made the difficult not only possible but enjoyable.

EDITORS

Editor

Paul S. Babyn, M.D., F.R.C.P.C.
Associate Professor
Department of Medical Imaging
University of Toronto
Radiologist in Chief
Department of Diagnostic Imaging
The Hospital for Sick Children
Toronto, Ontario, Canada

Coordinating Editor

Harpal K. Gahunia, M.Sc., Ph.D.
Department of Diagnostic Imaging
The Hospital for Sick Children
Toronto, Ontario, Canada

Section Editors

Peter Chait, M.B.B.Ch., F.F.R.A.D., F.R.C.R.
Associate Professor
Department of Medical Imaging
University of Toronto
Department of Diagnostic Imaging
The Hospital for Sick Children,
Toronto, Ontario, Canada

David Manson, M.D., F.R.C.P.C, F.A.A.P.
Assistant Professor
Department of Medical Imaging
University of Toronto
Department of Diagnostic Imaging
The Hospital for Sick Children
Toronto, Ontario, Canada

Kieran McHugh, M.B., F.R.C.R., F.R.C.P.I.,
D.C.H.
Pediatric Radiologist
Department of Radiology
Great Ormond Street Hospital for
Children
London, United Kingdom

Stephen F. Miller, M.D., F.R.C.P.C.
Assistant Professor
Department of Medical Imaging
University of Toronto
Department of Diagnostic Imaging
The Hospital for Sick Children
Toronto, Ontario, Canada

Kamaldine Oudjhane, M.Sc., M.D.
Associate Professor
Department of Medical Imaging
University of Toronto
Department of Diagnostic Imaging
The Hospital for Sick Children,
Toronto, Ontario, Canada

Charles Raybaud, M.D. F.R.C.P.C.
Professor
Department of Medical Imaging
University of Toronto
Head, Division of Neuroradiology
Department of Diagnostic Imaging
The Hospital for Sick Children,
Toronto, Ontario, Canada

xvii

Don Soboleski, M.D., F.R.C.P
Assistant Professor
Department of Diagnostic Radiology
Kingston General Hospital
Queen's University
Kingston, Ontario, Canada

Karen E. Thomas, M.D., M.R.C.P., F.R.C.R.
Assistant Professor
Department of Medical Imaging
University of Toronto
Department of Diagnostic Imaging
The Hospital for Sick Children
Toronto, Ontario, Canada

Shi-Joon Yoo, M.D., F.R.C.P.C.
Professor
Department of Medical Imaging
University of Toronto
Department of Diagnostic Imaging
The Hospital for Sick Children
Toronto, Ontario, Canada

CONTRIBUTORS

Paul S. Babyn, M.D., F.R.C.P.C.
Associate Professor
Department of Medical Imaging
University of Toronto
Radiologist in Chief
Department of Diagnostic Imaging
The Hospital for Sick Children
Toronto, Ontario, Canada

Susan Blaser, M.D., F.R.C.P.C.
Associate Professor
Department of Medical Imaging
University of Toronto
Department of Diagnostic Imaging
The Hospital for Sick Children
Toronto, Ontario, Canada

Helen Branson, M.D.
Fellow
Department of Diagnostic Imaging
The Hospital for Sick Children
Toronto, Ontario, Canada

Peter Chait, M.B.B.Ch., F.F.R.A.D., F.R.C.R.
Associate Professor
Department of Medical Imaging
University of Toronto
Department of Diagnostic Imaging
The Hospital for Sick Children
Toronto, Ontario, Canada

Justine Cohen
Medical Student
University of Toronto Medical School
Toronto, Ontario, Canada

Noel Fanning, M.B., F.R.C.S.I.
Fellow
Department of Diagnostic Imaging
The Hospital for Sick Children
Toronto, Ontario, Canada

Katharine Foster, M.B.B.S., M.R.C.P.Ch., F.R.C.R.
Consultant Radiologist
Birmingham's Children Hospital
Birmingham, United Kingdom

Harpal K. Gahunia, M.Sc., Ph.D.
Department of Diagnostic Imaging
The Hospital for Sick Children,
Toronto, Ontario, Canada

Flavia Gasparini, M.D.
Fellow
Department of Diagnostic
    Imaging
The Hospital for Sick Children
Toronto, Ontario, Canada

Mohannad Ibrahim, M.D.
Fellow
Department of Diagnostic Imaging
The Hospital for Sick Children
Toronto, Ontario, Canada

Pierre-Jean Lattanzio, M.D., Ph.D.
Resident
Division of Orthopedics
The Ottawa Hospital General
    Campus
Ottawa, Ontario, Canada

Erika Mann, M.D., F.R.C.P.C.
Fellow
Department of Diagnostic Imaging
The Hospital for Sick Children
Toronto, Ontario, Canada

David Manson, M.D., F.R.C.P.C., F.A.A.P.
Assistant Professor
Department of Medical Imaging
University of Toronto
Department of Diagnostic Imaging
The Hospital for Sick Children
Toronto, Ontario, Canada

Kieran McHugh, M.B., F.R.C.R., F.R.C.P.I., D.C.H.
Pediatric Radiologist
Department of Radiology
Great Ormond Street Hospital for Children
London, United Kingdom

Stephen F. Miller, M.D., F.R.C.P.C.
Assistant Professor
Department of Medical Imaging
University of Toronto
Department of Diagnostic Imaging
The Hospital for Sick Children
Toronto, Ontario, Canada

Kamaldine Oudjhane, M.Sc., M.D.
Associate Professor
Department of Medical Imaging
University of Toronto
Department of Diagnostic Imaging
The Hospital for Sick Children
Toronto, Ontario, Canada

Rodrigo Ozelame, M.D.
Fellow
Department of Diagnostic Imaging
The Hospital for Sick Children
Toronto, Ontario, Canada

Hemant Parmar, M.B.B.S., M.D.
Fellow
Department of Diagnostic Imaging
The Hospital for Sick Children
Toronto, Ontario, Canada

Marilyn Ranson, M.D., F.R.C.P.C.
Assistant Professor
Department of Medical Imaging
University of Toronto
Department of Diagnostic Imaging
The Hospital for Sick Children
Toronto, Ontario, Canada

Charles Raybaud, M.D., F.R.C.P.C.
Professor
Department of Medical Imaging
University of Toronto
Head, Division of Neuroradiology
Department of Diagnostic Imaging
The Hospital for Sick Children
Toronto, Ontario, Canada

Eran Shlomovitz
Senior Medical Student
Schulich School of Medicine
University of Western Ontario
London, Ontario, Canada

Don Soboleski, M.D., F.R.C.P
Assistant Professor
Department of Diagnostic Radiology
Kingston General Hospital
Queen's University
Kingston, Ontario, Canada

Karen E. Thomas, M.D., M.R.C.P.,
   F.R.C.R.
Assistant Professor
Department of Medical Imaging
University of Toronto
Department of Diagnostic Imaging
The Hospital for Sick Children
Toronto, Ontario, Canada

Sheldon Wiebe, M.D., F.R.C.P.C.
Assistant Professor
Department of Medical Imaging
Associated Member
Department of Pediatrics
College of Medicine
University of Saskatchewan
Saskatoon, Saskatchewan, Canada

Jaron A Yau, M.D.
Resident
Department of Medical
   Imaging
Faculty of Medicine
McGill University
Montreal, Quebec, Canada

Shi-Joon Yoo, M.D., F.R.C.P.C.
Professor
Department of Medical Imaging
University of Toronto
Department of Diagnostic Imaging
The Hospital for Sick Children
Toronto, Ontario, Canada

ABBREVIATIONS

Diagnostic Imaging Terminology

CECT	contrast-enhanced computed tomography
CT	computed tomography
DWI	diffusion-weighted imaging
ERCP	endoscopic retrograde cholangiopancreatography
HIDA	hepatic iminodiacetic acid
IVU	intravenous urogram
MRCP	magnetic resonance cholangiopancreatography
MRI	magnetic resonance imaging
NECT	non-enhanced computed tomography
PET	positron-emission tomography
SPGR	spoiled gradient recall echo
T1W	T1-weighted
T2W	T2-weighted
TR	repetition time
US	ultrasound
VCUG	voiding cystourethrography

Anatomic Terminology

AA	aortic arch
Ao	aorta
BCC	branchial cleft complex
CNS	central nervous system
CSF	cerebrospinal fluid
DJJ	duodenojejunal junction
GI	gastrointestinal
IAC	internal auditory canal
IVC	inferior vena cava
LA	left atrium
LCA	left carotid artery
LMB	left main bronchus
LPA	left pulmonary artery

LPV	left portal vein
LSA	left subclavian artery
LV	left ventricle
RA	right atrium
PA	pulmonary artery
PNS	peripheral nerve sheath
PUV	posterior urethral valves
RCA	right carotid artery
RMB	right main bronchus
RPA	right pulmonary artery
RSA	right subclavian artery
RV	right ventricle
RVOT	right ventricular outflow tract
SCM	sternocleidomastoid muscle
SMA	superior mesenteric artery
SSS	superior sagittal sinus
SVC	superior vena cava
UPJ	ureteropelvic junction
UVJ	ureterovesical junction

Other Abbreviations

ADPKD	autosomal dominant polycystic kidney disease
AFP	alpha-fetoprotein
ALL	acute lymphoblastic leukemia
ARDS	acute respiratory distress syndrome
ARPKD	autosomal recessive polycystic kidney disease
ASD	atrial septal defect
ATD	asphyxiating thoracic dystrophy
ATM	acute transverse myelitis
AVN	avascular necrosis
CCAM	congenital cystic adenomatoid malformation

CDH	congenital diaphragmatic hernia	NF	neurofibromatosis
CDP	chondrodysplasia punctata	OI	osteogenesis imperfecta
CF	cystic fibrosis	OM	chronic osteomyelitis
CLE	congenital lobar emphysema	OS	osteosarcoma
CMV	cytomegalovirus	PDA	patent ductus arteriosus
CPA	cerebellopontine angle	PFFD	proximal focal femoral deficiency
CSVT	cerebral sinovenous thrombosis		
DDH	developmental dysplasia of the hip	PHP	pseudohypoparathyroidism
DJJ	duodenojejunal junction	PICC	peripherally inserted central catheter
DIC	disseminated intravascular coagulation		
		RCC	renal cell carcinoma
DIOS	distal intestinal obstruction syndrome	RVT	renal vein thrombosis
		SCFE	slipped capital femoral epiphyses
ECMO	extracorporal membrane oxygenation	SHH	sonic hedgehog
		SLE	systemic lupus erythematosus
FGFR	fibroblast growth factor receptor	SOD	septo-optic dysplasia
FNA	fine-needle aspiration	STIR	short tau inversion recovery
GH	growth hormone	TAPVC	total anomalous pulmonary venous connection
GT	glutamyl transferase		
HFM	hemifacial microsomia	TB	tuberculosis
HMD	hyaline membrane disease	TCOF	Treacher Collins-Fraceschetti syndrome
HPE	holoprosencephaly		
HPS	hypertrophic pyloric stenosis	TCS	Treacher Collins syndrome
HU	Hounsfield units	TD	thanatophoric dysplasia
LCH	Langerhans' cell histiocytosis	TE	echo-time
LCP	Legg-Calvé-Perthes disease	TIPS	transjugular intrahepatic portosystemic shunt
LLD	leg length discrepancy		
MAPCAs	major aortopulmonary collateral arteries	tPA	tissue plasmingen activator
		TPN	total parenteral nutrition
MCDK	multicystic dysplastic kidney	TS	tuberous sclerosis
MDP	methylene diphosphonate	TTN	transient tachypnea of the newborn
MGP	matrix GLA protein		
MHE	multiple hereditary exostoses	UTI	urinary tract infection
MS	multiple sclerosis	VHL	von Hippel-Lindau
MSUD	maple syrup urine disease	VUR	vescicoureteral reflex
MTX	methotrexate	VSD	ventricular septal defect
MVA	motor vehicle accident	WBC	white blood cell count
NEC	necrotizing enterocolitis		

SECTION I

Neuroradiology

CASE 1

Clinical Presentation

A child presents with vomiting, headaches, and, later, personality changes.

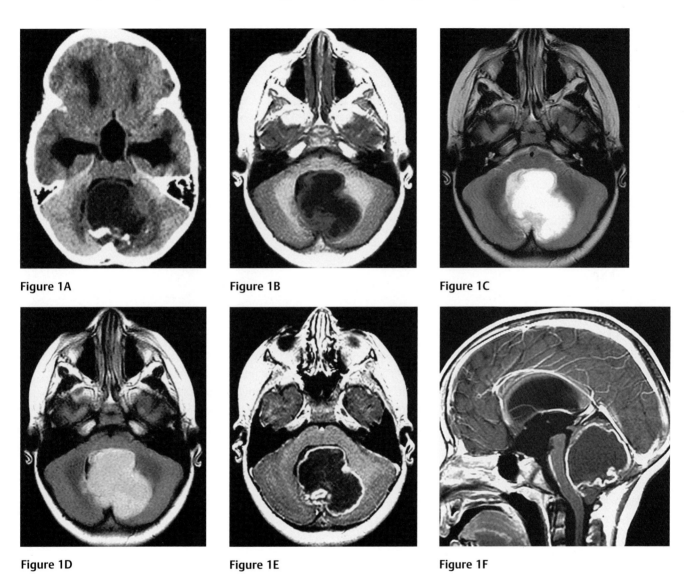

Figure 1A   Figure 1B   Figure 1C

Figure 1D   Figure 1E   Figure 1F

Radiologic Findings

Initial CT without contrast demonstrated dilated third ventricle and temporal horns (with compressed hippocampi) (**Fig. 1A**). A large, rounded hypodense mass is noted behind the fourth ventricle, in the vermis and adjacent portions of the cerebellar hemispheres. This mass appears cystic with two solid mural nodules, one anterior on the left and the other posterior on the right with calcification. Nonenhanced MR images show similar findings with low T1 (**Fig. 1B**) and high T2/FLAIR (**Figs. 1C** and **1D**). The cyst content presents attenuation and signals different from the adjacent CSF. Following contrast, MRI (**Figs. 1E** and **1F**) demonstrates enhancement of the cyst wall and of the solid mural nodules. Note the anterior third ventricle bulging into a large cisternal space (presurgical ventriculocisternotomy possible to alleviate hydrocephalus) and the tonsillar herniation through the foramen magnum (risk of acute compression of the medulla),

Vomiting first led to abdominal investigations before the increase in intracranial pressure was evident.

Diagnosis

Cerebellar juvenile pilocytic astrocytoma (JPA)

Differential Diagnosis

- Cystic masses of the cerebellum: Hemangioblastomas have a similar appearance to JPAs. These are more common in young adults and older children, usually as part of von Hippel-Lindau disease. Other cystic lesions such as parasitic, destructive, dysembryoplastic (dermoids), or inflammatory lesions also have to be considered.
- Others: Medulloblastomas and ependymomas usually have a shorter clinical history. They are typically centered on the lumen of the 4th ventricle, iso- or hyperdense on nonenhanced CT, and characteristically not cystic, but purely solid JPAs do occur. Medulloblastoma also may develop away from the ventricular lumen into the cerebellar hemispheres.
- Anaplastic (malignant) astrocytomas of the cerebellum exist. The gliomatous portion of a cerebellar ganglioglioma may present exactly like a JPA.

Discussion

Background

Astrocytomas are the most common brain tumors of childhood, with 60% occurring in the posterior fossa (40% in the cerebellum, 20% in the brain stem). Most of them are JPAs. JPAs are always benign tumors, whereas fibrillary astrocytomas such as those observed in the pons tend to become anaplastic. JPAs have rather specific locations: cerebellum, dorsal brain stem (with expansion toward the fourth ventricular lumen), medulla, and anterior optic pathways/anterior third ventricle. In neurofibromatosis type 1, JPA of the anterior optic pathways/anterior third ventricle is a common complication in young children.

Clinical Findings

The frequency of cerebellar JPAs is equal in boys and girls, usually occurring between birth and 9 years of age (hence its name). The symptoms (headaches, early morning vomiting, ataxia) develop gradually over several months to become persistent and acute. These symptoms are often misleading and may suggest an abdominal cause.

Pathology

As a rule, JPAs arise from the midline, ~30% extending into the cerebellar hemispheres. Most are large at presentation (>5 cm). The tumor usually consists of a cyst with a solid nodule within the cyst wall. The cyst is most typically adjacent to the tumor (no peripheral enhancement), but in 40%, it may develop within it as a cystlike necrotic center (peripheral enhancement). The cyst may be single or multiple. Ten percent are fully solid tumors without necrosis. Calcification is seen in 20%; hemorrhage is very rare.

Histology

Typically, loose spongy areas alternating with more compact cellular regions characterize JPAs, likely leading to the increased signal intensity seen on T2-weighted MRI. The coalescence of the microcysts is believed to result in the large cysts characteristic of these tumors. The tumor cells have a large cytoplasm with a small nucleus, explaining the low attenuation on CT. Rosenthal fibers and eosinophilic rod-shaped granular bodies are prominent. Nuclear atypia, mitoses, endothelial proliferation, and necrosis can sometimes be found in JPA, but these features do not indicate a worse prognosis. These tumors are not graded histopathologically. Unlike other low-grade astrocytomas, the endothelial cells have open tight junctions and fenestrations, with a high vascularity, which probably explains the marked enhancement of these tumors.

Imaging Findings

CT

- Typically, large predominantly cystic tumor with a solid hypodense mural nodule
- Calcification occurs in 20%.
- Contrast enhancement of the nodule is nearly always present and is usually heterogeneous (different from hemangioblastoma).
- Cyst wall usually does not enhance. In these cases the wall actually represents compressed cerebellar tissue. In the case where the cystic component develops within the solid tumor, the wall may enhance, and there may be extension of enhancement into the surrounding cerebellum.
- Layering of contrast is sometimes observed within the cyst.

MRI

- MRI appearances are variable.
- Solid and cystic portions are identified. The cystic component is of low T1 and high T2 signal intensity.
- Solid nodule has a different signal from the cyst, and multilocular cysts have different signals on T2-weighted images.
- Solid components enhance, as seen on CT.
- A small number of these lesions are purely solid.
- Rarely, cerebellar JPA may present as solid, nonenhancing masses that are diagnosed at histology only.
- MR spectroscopy and MR perfusion studies present paradoxical "malignant" patterns in spite of the strictly benign nature of the lesion.

Treatment

- Total surgical resection is usually curative.
- Surgical resection is possible when the tumor does not extend into the brain stem.
- Appropriate chemotherapies may be effective.
- Often, residual tumors have a very low potential for growth.

Prognosis

- JPA has a better prognosis than most other astrocytomas.
- If gross total resection is possible, which is usual in the cerebellum, the 10-year survival rate is as high as 90%.
- After subtotal resection or biopsy, the 10-year survival rate is still as high as 45%.
- Morbidity is related to the location of the tumor and to the associated complications of tumor resection.
- In spite of its constant benignity, the JPA may exceptionally metastasize to the CSF, and such a finding does not exclude the diagnosis (pilomixoid astrocytoma).

PEARL

- The most common appearances are hydrocephalus revealing a well-defined posterior fossa cyst with mural enhancing or a thick-walled enhancing mass with central necrosis.

PITFALL

- Lesion should not be assumed to be cystic just because it is homogeneously low signal on T1- and high signal on T2-weighted MRI sequences.

Suggested Readings

Campbell JW, Pollack IF. Cerebellar astrocytomas in children. J Neurooncol 1996;28:223–231

Luh GY, Bird CR. Imaging of brain tumors in the pediatric population. Neuroimaging Clin N Am 1999;9:691–716

Rashidi M, DaSilva VR, Minagar A, Rutka JT. Nonmalignant pediatric brain tumors. Curr Neurol Neurosci Rep 2003;3:200–205

CASE 2

Clinical Presentation

A 2-year-old child presents with early morning vomiting, headaches, progressive seclusion, irritability, and recent torticollis.

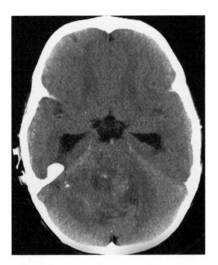

Figure 2A

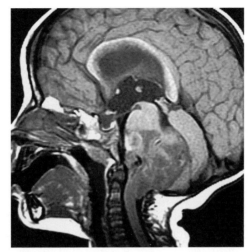

Figure 2B

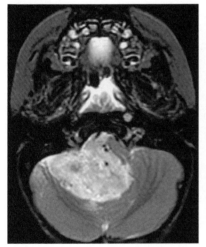

Figure 2C

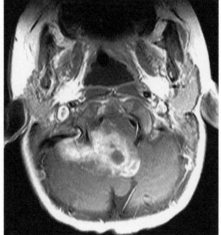

Figure 2D

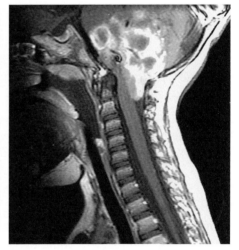

Figure 2E

Radiologic Findings

Nonenhanced CT demonstrates hydrocephalus and a mass in the central posterior fossa. This mass is ill-demarcated and heterogeneous with hypo-, iso-, and hyperdense portions and with punctiform calcifications (**Fig. 2A**). The fourth ventricular lumen is not seen. Sagittal T1- (**Fig. 2B**) and axial T2-weighted MR imaging (**Fig. 2C**) exhibits inhomogeneity with a large infiltration of the brain stem, whereas the vermis appears pushed backward instead. Although centered on the fourth ventricle, the mass shows cisternal extensions through the ventricular foramina into the upper cervical canal and the right cerebellopontine cistern. Contrast enhancement (**Fig. 2D**) is relatively mild and irregular and confirms the poor demarcation of the lesion. Spinal imaging (**Fig. 2E**) is important, as ependymomas tend to generate drop metastases in the CSF spaces.

Diagnosis

Posterior fossa ependymoma

Differential Diagnosis

- Medulloblastoma also develops in the fourth ventricle, but it arises from the vermis to develop within the ventricular lumen, has no cisternal extension, and usually has no brain stem infiltration. Both are rather dense on nonenhanced CT, but medulloblastoma typically is more compact, better demarcated, and less often calcified. Both may be edematous, hemorrhagic, or necrotic. Both may seed into the CSF spaces.
- Choroid plexus papilloma occurs in infants. It is rare, especially in the posterior fossa. Noninvasive, it enhances markedly with contrast agents.
- Choroid plexus carcinoma is a malignant papilloma observed in older children up to 5 years. It looks like a papilloma but is more invasive into the adjacent brain tissue.

Discussion

Background

Of the primary CNS neoplasms in children, 8 to 9% are ependymomas. They can occur within the forebrain or in the posterior fossa (and only very rarely in the cord in children, except in a context of neurofibromatosis type 2). The posterior fossa tumor is described as "plastic" because it extends primarily outside the ventricle to mold the cisterns, surrounding and infiltrating the cranial nerves. This generates specific clinical features, such as swallowing difficulties or torticollis, and makes surgical removal difficult. Drop metastases occur not infrequently.

Etiology

Ependymomas are derived from the ependymal cells lining the ventricles. In the posterior fossa they originate from the lateral-ventral portion of the fourth ventricle and extend to the fourth ventricle and to the cisterns. In the forebrain they tend to develop into the white matter, but they may bulge within the ventricles also.

Clinical Findings

Patients typically are <6 years of age and have a long clinical history. Infiltration of the ventricular floor explains the frequent vomiting; obstruction leads to hydrocephalus and increased intracranial pressure, and the cisternal infiltration of the cranial nerves leads to corresponding deficits, mostly swallowing problems and torticollis with intense neck pain.

Pathology

Posterior fossa ependymomas typically arise from the floor of the fourth ventricle. Most are solid, with calcification seen in 50% and cysts in 20%. They are typically soft, malleable tumors, grayish red in color. They tend to insinuate around blood vessels and nerves, by extending through the lateral recesses and behind the medulla into the cervical canal. They also tend to infiltrate the ventricular wall and adhere to surrounding brain. Therefore, complete resection is often difficult. Higher-grade tumors are more likely to metastasize within the subarachnoid space.

Histology

Classically, ependymomas are well-circumscribed lesions with moderate cellularity and glial and epithelial features. Most form characteristic pseudo-rosettes: cells arranged around a central blood vessel, separated by a nuclear-free zone consisting of cellular processes that are glial fibrillary acidic protein positive. Less commonly, true rosettes are formed: cells arranged circumferentially around a central blood vessel. The World Health Organization (WHO) revised classification lists a grade I, more benign, and a grade II, anaplastic, more invasive lesion showing more incidence of metastasis. Only 10% of ependymomas metastasize to other areas of the neuraxis; these metastases are almost always associated with tumor recurrence at the primary site.

Imaging Findings

CT

- Ependymomas are typically heterogeneously isodense on noncontrast CT, but small lucencies (edema, cysts) and calcification may be seen.
- Hemorrhage occurs in ~10%.

MRI

- Ependymomas vary in signal characteristics, depending on the presence of edema, cysts, necrosis, high vascularity, hemorrhage, and calcification.
- Typically, ependymomas are isointense on T1 and slightly hyperintense on T2 imaging.
- The most important characteristic is the way the tumor insinuates through foramina, into the cisterns, and around blood vessels and nerves.
- Mild to moderate, and often heterogeneous, enhancement is typically seen.
- Spinal screening with MRI is essential before surgery.

Treatment

- The best management of ependymoma is a complete resection, even of a recurring tumor.
- Small-volume residual disease is best managed with localized radiotherapy unless there is metastatic disease, which is then managed by craniospinal irradiation.
- The utility of chemotherapy is uncertain.

Prognosis

- There is a low incidence of recurrence after total resection.
- The risk of disseminated disease is ~70% in patients with subtotal resection.
- Relatively low survival rate in children (~30%)
- Morbidity is related to the location of the tumor and to the associated complications of tumor resection and treatment.

Complications

- Infiltration of the cranial nerves and the brain stem
- Drop metastases along the whole CSF axis
- Postoperative cervical instability

PEARLS_____

- Fourth ventricular mass developing more in the cisterns than toward the ventricle, usually with an extended upper cervical tongue
- Torticollis and swallowing difficulties

Suggested Readings

Fletcher DT, Warner WC, Muhlbauer MS, Merchant TE. Cervical subluxation after surgery and irradiation of childhood ependymoma. Pediatr Neurosurg 2002;36:189–196

Koeller KK, Sandberg GD. (Armed Forces Institute of Pathology, From the archives of the AFIP). Cerebral intraventricular neoplasms: radiologic-pathologic correlation. Radiographics 2002;22: 1473–1505 (Review)

Rezai AR, Woo HH, Lee M, Cohen H, Zagzag D, Epstein FJ. Disseminated ependymomas of the central nervous system. J Neurosurg 1996;85:618–624

Van Veelen-Vincent ML, Pierre-Kahn A, Kalifa C, et al. Ependymoma in childhood: prognostic factors, extent of surgery, and adjuvant therapy. J Neurosurg 2002;97:827–835

CASE 3

Clinical Presentation

The first case shows a 1-week-old premature neonate, born after premature rupture of the membranes. Case 1 presents with severe neonatal sepsis (**Fig. 3A**) and late change is shown in the second case (**Fig. 3B**).

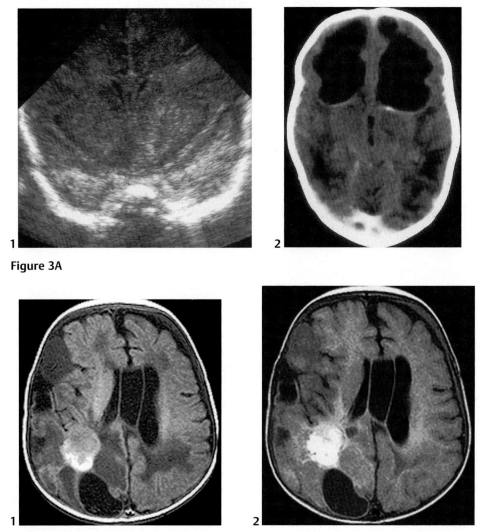

Figure 3A

3B (*Continued on p. 12*)

Radiologic Findings

Figs. 3A1 and **3A2** show a 1-week-old neonate. Ultrasonography performed in the early stage of the disease (**Fig. 3A1**) demonstrates diffuse, increased echogenicity of the anterior part of the brain, especially on the left. Subsequent enhanced CT (**Fig. 3A2**) demonstrates large, necrotic cavitations with no mass effect and little enhancement in the white matter of both frontal lobes. **Figs. 3B1** to **3B4** show the late changes in a 3-month-old child (different from the child pictured in **Figs. 3A1** and **3A2**) who survived the infection; the nonenhanced T1-weighted (**Fig. 3B1**), FLAIR (**Fig. 3B2**), and T2-weighted (**Fig. 3B3**) imaging shows massive and diffuse loss of white matter with multiple cysts of different

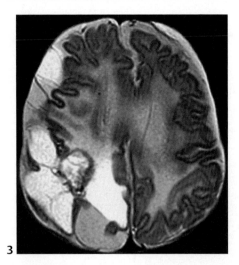
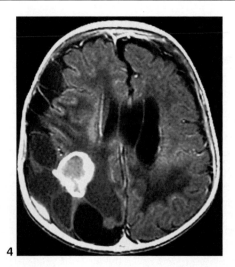

Figure 3B (*Continued*)

signals, of which one in the posterior right hemisphere appears to be hemorrhagic. On the enhanced T1-weighted image (**Fig. 3B4**), the dense, presumably hemorrhagic lesion demonstrated a marked ring enhancement.

Diagnosis

Neonatal *Citrobacter* brain abscesses

Differential Diagnosis

- Sepsis in a neonate is a clinical, laboratory, and therapeutic problem. Diagnostic imaging is needed to confirm the diagnosis of meningocerebral involvement, to stage the brain infection, and to appreciate the complications. Therefore, the differential diagnosis is somewhat theoretical.
- Other bacterial abscesses: At this age, all have a severe prognosis if not treated early and efficiently. The early identification of the germ and the efficacy of treatment depend on laboratory, not on imaging, studies.
- *Citrobacter* infections tend to cavitate: It is important not to mistake these cavitations in the white matter for sequelae of an earlier ischemic or hemorrhagic insult. Contrast-enhanced studies will demonstrate the infection-related enhancement.
- Other mass lesions: Congenital/neonatal tumors are uncommon (choroid plexus papillomas, craniopharyngiomas, teratomas, atypical teratoid/rhabdoid tumors). Even when partly cystic, they present solid, nodular components different from the inflammatory ring of a cerebral infection. Diffusion imaging may help as diffusion is restricted in abscesses.
- Early cerebritis should not be mistaken for normal, immature white matter, nor for cicatricial leukomalacia.

Discussion

Background

Although rare in the neonate, brain abscesses have a high rate of mortality and complications. Neonates are usually left with severe residual permanent damage, the more so as these infections are often insidious. Neonatal abscesses are most often due to various members of the *Citrobacter* genus

or to *Proteus mirabilis*, more rarely to *Escherichia coli* or *Listeria monocytogenes*. Maternal antibodies from the placenta and the colostrum protect normal neonates. However, premature and low-birth-weight infants are immunocompromised. The transmission may be sporadic or vertical from the mother (local vaginal infection, rupture of the membranes), and outbreaks have been reported due to horizontal nosocomial transmission by asymptomatic nursery staff.

Etiology

Citrobacter spp is a group of gram-negative bacteria, members of the Enterobacteriaceae family. Neonates are at increased risk of infection, typically from *C. koseri* (formerly *C. diversus*), *C. freundii*, and *C. sedlakii*. These organisms are prone to cause sepsis, ventriculitis, and cerebritis with frequent multiple brain abscesses. Among the other germs affecting the neonate, they have a unique propensity to penetrate, survive, and replicate into vascular endothelial cells and macrophages. As a consequence, although *Citrobacter* causes only 5% of meningitis in neonates, it causes 80% of brain abscesses.

Clinical Findings

Neonatal *Citrobacter* brain abscesses are rare beyond the first month, and they are more common in premature or low-weight babies. Neonates presents with nonspecific clinical features of sepsis, meningitis, and cerebritis. An increased temperature and neck stiffness are usually lacking. They are usually very sick and may have seizures, apnea, and a bulging fontanelle.

Pathology/Laboratory Findings

- Macroscopic findings include purulent exudates, opaque leptomeninges, pus, and ventriculitis/ependymitis. The lobar white matter is typically affected.
- Biologic documentation of the infection, identification of the germ, especially of the *Citrobacter* subtype (11 distinct subtypes are recognized), and assessment of its response to antibiotics.

Histology

Citrobacter bacteria may be identified in the walls of congested vessels. The cavities resulting from the infection do not develop well-formed fibrotic walls.

Imaging Findings

- Stages of disease
  - In formation of every brain abscess, several stages may be noted; the staging of the infection is as follows: (1) early cerebritis stage (no ring enhancement); (2) late cerebritis stage (inflammatory ring enhancement but no pus); (3) early capsule stage (ring enhancement, central necrosis, and pus collection); and (4) late capsule stage (ring enhancement, well-collected pus).
  - In neonates, the evolution from one stage to the other is faster in the soft, immature neonatal brain tissue, and necrosis is more common.
  - Early and massive tissue necrosis is a specific feature of *Citrobacter* brain infection. Early in the disease, a diffuse cerebritis predominates in the white matter. Later, necrotic cavities develop in multiple locations. They are initially "square" in shape and non-tense. When pus forms and collects in these cavities, they tend to become more rounded in shape.

ULTRASOUND

- Lacks specificity
- At the early stages, the increased echogenicity of the white matter should lead to MRI or at least CT.
- At a later stage, the cavitation, mass effect, developing hydrocephalus, and response to treatment may be assessed.

CT

- **Early stage of cerebritis:** more or less ill-defined; areas of low attenuation may be seen with faint variable enhancement
- **Later stage of necrosis:** multiple large cavities develop, replacing (destroying) the white matter. Septa may be present. The walls and septa enhance with a typical central dotlike focus of enhancement.
- **Pus collection:** more rounded appearance of the lesion with peripheral enhancement
- **Late, cicatricial stage:** long-lasting enhancement of the lesion, due to persisting fibrosis (not to infection), commonly calcified. Or persisting cavity that, associated with septated ventriculitis, may result in multicystic hydrocephalus. Global loss of brain substance

MRI

- **Early cerebritis:** heterogeneous, multi-loculated low signal on T1- and high signal on T2-weighted imaging. There is usually subtle contrast enhancement.
- **Later cavitation stage:** small cavities coalesce to form large cavities, containing septations. There is enhancement of the walls, or septa, and a dotlike enhanced central focus may be observed. This enhancement may be subtle or marked. Because of the white matter necrosis, no significant mass effect is seen.
- **Abscess formation:** more mass effect; the "square cavity" becomes more rounded.
- **Late follow-up:** "contraction" of the cavities; marked, asymmetric white matter losses; calcification and protracted enhancement related to persisting fibrous tissue (**Figs. 2A** to **2D**); common associated hydrocephalus due to the ventriculitis

Treatment

- The major treatment consists of antibiotics, usually two drugs, and is prolonged as late abscesses may occur. A broad spectrum of cephalosporins is often used, given that they have good penetration into the CNS. Like all bacterial infections, determining antibiotic sensitivity is mandatory.
- If the response to medical treatment is poor, the surgical aspiration of the collected pus reduces the mass effect and enhances the efficacy of the antibiotics.

Complications

- Inflammatory cells and bacteria infiltrate and spread along the main vessel walls: This can result in both arterial and venous infarction in addition to the cavitations related to smaller-vessel disease.
- Exudates within the ventricles and ventriculitis may obstruct the ventricular foramina and result in a multicystic hydrocephalus, with consequent long-lasting shunting difficulties.
- Necrotizing meningoencephalitis with pneumocephalus has been reported.

Prognosis

- Twenty-five to 30% of neonates with *Citrobacter* die. Seventy-five percent of survivors have significant neurologic damage (complex hydrocephalus, neurologic deficits, mental delay, epilepsy).

PEARLS_____

- Square cavities ("square abscess") in a newborn, which replace white matter instead of displacing it
- Cavities that become rounded are more likely to represent abscesses.

PITFALLS_____

- As the immature white matter tends to present with high echogenicity, low attenuation and low T1/high T2 signals, it is important not to mistake an early cerebritis for a normal immature white matter, nor for cicatricial leukomalacia.
- Long-lasting, persisting enhancement does not mean persisting infection.
- Abscesses may still occur late in the course of the disease.
- Square cavities may also be necrotic white matter.

Suggested Readings

Badger JL, Stins MF, Kim KS. *Citrobacter freundii* invades and replicates in human brain microvascular endothelial cells. Infect Immun 1999;67:4208–4215

Britt RH, Enzmann DR. Clinical stages of human brain abscesses on serial CT scans after contrast infusion: computerized tomographic, neuropathological and clinical correlations. J Neurosurg 1983;59:972–989

Doran TI. The role of *Citrobacter* in clinical disease of children: review. Clin Infect Dis 1999; 28:384–394

Dyer J, Hayani KC, Janda WM, Schreckenberger PC. *Citrobacter sedlakii* meningitis and brain abscess in a premature infant. J Clin Microbiol 1997;35:2686–2688

Feferbaum R, Diniz EMA, Valente M, et al. Brain abscess by *Citrobacter diversus* in infancy. Arq Neuropsiquiatr 2000;58:736–740

Hedlund GL. Citrobacter meningitis. In: Blaser S, Illner A, Castillo M, Hedlund GL, Osborn AG, eds. Pocket Radiologist Peds Neuro Top 100 Diagnosis. Salt Lake City, UT: Amirsys; 2003:158–160

Pooboni SK, Mathur SK, Dux A, Hewertson J, Nichani S. Pneumocephalus in neonatal meningitis: diffuse, necrotizing meningo-encephalitis in *Citrobacter* meningitis presenting with pneumatosis oculi and pneumocephalus. Pediatr Crit Care Med 2004;5:393–395

Soriano AL, Russel RG, Johnson D, Lagos R, Sechter I. Morris Jg. Pathophysiology of *Citrobacter diversus* neonatal meningitis: comparative studies in an infant mouse model. Infect Immun 1991;59: 1352–1358

Townsend SM, Pollack HA, Gonzalez-Gomez I, Shimada H, Badger JL. *Citrobacter koseri* brain abscess in the neonatal rat: survival and replication within human and rat macrophages. Infect Immun 2003;71:5871–5880

Tung GA, Evangelista P, Rogg JM, Duncan JA. Diffusion-weighted MR imaging of rim-enhanced brain masses: is markedly decreased water diffusion specific for brain abscess? AJR Am J Roentgenol 2001;177:709–712

CASE 4

Clinical Presentation

A 9-year-old child presents with rapidly developing deficit of all four limbs.

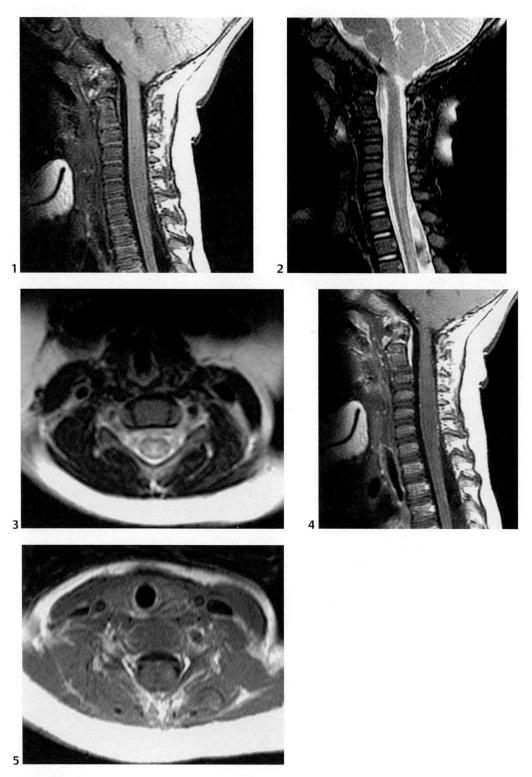

Figure 4A

Radiologic Findings

The sagittal T1-weighted image (**Fig. 4A1**) demonstrates fusiform enlargement of the cervical spinal cord, with patent surrounding CSF spaces, however. The signal of the cord is homogeneous, but with occasional cavitation, necrosis, or hemorrhage. Sagittal T2-weighted imaging (**Fig. 4A2**) demonstrates a homogeneous hypersignal extending from C3 to T1, and the axial cut (**Fig. 4A3**) shows that the abnormality covers both sides of the cord, fitting the anatomic definition of transverse myelitis. Infusion of contrast agent (**Figs. 4A4** and **4A5**) demonstrates a faint enhancement only, in the periphery of the lesion on the left side.

Diagnosis

Acute transverse myelitis (ATM)

Differential Diagnosis

- Spinal cord tumor: more heterogeneous mass, occupying the whole section of the cord often associated with extended edema, cavitation and/or syringomyelia, hemorrhage, disappearance of the perimedullary space with occasional enlargement of the spinal canal, more nodular enhancements
- Spinal cord compression: from spinal, extradural, dural, or intradural infections or tumors
- Guillain-Barré syndrome (GBS, ascending polyradiculoneuritis), featuring an ascending flaccid para- then tetraplegia, with intense muscular pains, and characteristically high protein level but no cellularity in the CSF
- Multiple sclerosis (MS): chronic demyelinating disease. The first attack of the disease may present like ATM. The MRI appearance of the lesions of the spinal cord helps confirm the diagnosis (see **Table 4–1**), together with the laboratory assessment of the CSF (oligoclonal IgG bands present in MS, consistently absent in ATM). The brain as a rule is also affected. Devic's disease (neuromyelitis optica) is assumed to be a variant of MS, affecting both the cord and the optic nerves.
- Necrotizing myelitis: direct infectious necrosis (usually viral) of the cord. Poliomyelitis used to be a major problem in infected areas, but it is disappearing with worldwide vaccination.
- Other myelitis: systemic lupus erythematosus (SLE), antiphospholipids antibody syndrome, other connective tissue diseases, paraneoplastic syndromes
- Rarely: hemorrhage (arteriovenous malformations, cavernomas), ischemia (usually iatrogenic)

Discussion

Background

ATM belongs, together with acute disseminated encephalomyelitis (ADEM) and GBS, to the group of postinfectious, immune-related acute demyelinating disorders. The typical clinical course starts with an acute, often seasonal infection, which is followed after a few days by a sudden neurological impairment due to an acute episode of demyelination of the nervous system. Most commonly, the entire CNS is involved with disseminated areas of demyelination, making up the ADEM. Less frequently, only the spinal cord is involved, and the patient then presents with ATM. Even less frequent, only the nerve roots and distal nerves are affected, usually in an ascending manner, which defines the GBS. Acute demyelination is provoked by the antibodies induced by the initial infection, where the myelin has an antigenicity similar to that of the infectious agent. In *acute* demyelination the axons and the oligodendrocytes are not destroyed, so complete remyelination is possible and the patient may progressively recover normal neurological functions. This is in contrast to the chronic demyelination seen with MS, in which the oligodendrocytes are progressively destroyed, with residual demyelinated plaques. However, permanent sequelae may persist in acute demyelination also.

Table 4–1   Features of Acute Transverse Myelitis (ATM), Multiple Sclerosis (MS), and Spinal Cord (SC) Tumors

	ATM	MS	SC Tumors
Transverse extent	Bilateral central $>^2/_3$ of the cord	Unilateral peripheral $<^1/_2$ of the cord	Depends on tumor type, often involves whole section
Longitudinal extent	>3 vertebral segments	<2 vertebral segments	Variable
Cord swelling	Common, mild	None	Massive, fills CSF spaces; may expand spinal canal
Appearance	High T2, low T1	High T2, low T1	Heterogeneous T2, T1
Central dot	Yes	No	No
Contrast enhancement	Patchy, peripheral	Central	Heterogeneous, multinodular
Number of foci	Commoly unifocal; if not, lesions same age	Multifocal, lesions different ages	Unifocal
Clinical features	Neurological deficit plus backaches, meningeal irritation	Pure neurological deficit	Pain, neurological deficit
Causal context	Idiopathic seasonal, or postinfectious or postimmunization	None	None specific

The distinction between ADEM or ATM, on one hand, and MS, on the other hand, are not always clear. Relapsing forms of ADEM and ATM exist, and MS may sometimes present initially like a true ADEM/ATM.

Clinical Findings

ATM may be considered a strictly spinal form of ADEM. It is unusual before 2 years of age, and it affects children and young adults. In 50% of cases, it is *idiopathic* (no causal agent identified, but then often seasonal between late fall and early spring). In postinfectious cases, a previous history of infection is found, either viral (herpes simplex virus, varicella-zoster virus, cytomegalovirus, Epstein-Barr virus, hepatitis A, echovirus, Coxsackie, measles, rubella, mumps, etc.) or nonviral (tuberculosis, brucellosis, mycoplasma, Lyme disease). *Vaccination* also may induce the disease (rabies, Japanese B encephalitis).

The onset is acute, often with generalized back pain and meningeal irritation, a generalized motor weakness (even flaccid paraplegia), asymmetric sensory deficits with areflexia, or uni- or bilateral hyperreflexia and plantar extension, and a bladder dysfunction. The face is not involved in 80% of cases, the upper limbs in 50%. Respiratory depression may occur in up to 33%. Recovery occurs in days or weeks, the bladder function recovering last, often after months. Rare relapsing forms do exist, with a few attacks occurring over a period of several years.

Pathology

The term *transverse myelitis* applies to an inflammation extending horizontally across most of the cord. Vertically, it affects several segments. It is localized to the thoracic cord in 80% of cases, to the cervical cord in 10% and to the lower cord in 10%. The cord is typically swollen, due to edema and vascular congestion.

Histology

Characteristic perivenous lesions are seen, affecting both gray and white matter. The small veins are engorged, ensheathed by parenchymal infiltrates of reactive microglia (mostly macrophages). Demyelination, restricted to these hypercellular zones, is due to the macrophagic activity. At the early stage of the disease, before the cellular reaction has developed, no demyelination is observed. Demyelination is more conspicuous in the subpial layer of white matter that surrounds the cord. Axons are mostly preserved. All lesions are of the same age (which is not true for MS), the small lesions coalescing to form larger lesions during the course of the disease. Punctate hemorrhages may be associated.

Laboratory Findings

- Normal or slightly elevated CSF protein level, *without* IgG oligoclonal band
- Identification of the causal agent by polymerase chain reaction (PCR)

Imaging Findings

MRI

- MRI is the primary imaging modality in the diagnosis of ATM.
- Plain x-rays and CT are not helpful, even with myelography, as they do not depict the intrinsic cord abnormalities.
- ATM is typically of sudden onset: It is important to remember that MRI may still be normal initially. But, in the context of acute neurological deficit, it rules out other spinal cord disorders, especially those that can be relieved by emergency surgery, including hemorrhage, tumor, or extrinsic compression.
- The typical MRI features of ATM on sagittal cuts are a mild fusiform swelling and a well-demarcated T2 hyperintensity of the cord, typically at the thoracic level (but also seen at the cervical or the terminal levels). This extends longitudinally over more than 3 vertebral segments, commonly 8 to 10, and on occasion over most of the cord. On axial cuts, this lesion extends bilaterally across the midline, occupying typically more than two thirds of the transverse diameter, in both gray and white matter, more anterior than posterior. A small preserved area in the core of the lesion has been described as a "central dot." Although bilateral, the anomalies are usually asymmetrical.
- Contrast enhancement may be more or less extensive, nodular, or diffuse, often patchy along the lesion, typically peripheral. Contrast enhancement may not be present initially or in late stages of the illness. Some enhancement also may appear in the meninges and along the nerve roots.
- The perimedullary CSF spaces are typically patent. No sign of significant bleeding, syrinx, or cyst is seen.
- In pure ATM, the brain is normal. MRI may show other similar lesions of acute demyelination that are not symptomatic: The disease then is a true ADEM with spinal cord symptoms only. An important point when multiple lesions are observed is that they all appear of the same age.
- After a few weeks the signal abnormalities and the swelling recede while the child recovers. If the child does not recover fully, follow-up studies are usually performed at 1 month, which may be normal, or infrequently, which may demonstrate segmental atrophy or even scarring and necrosis of the cord.

Treatment

- The use and the effectiveness of steroids are controversial.
- Antibiotics are needed when the causative agent is sensitive.
- Supportive care to avoid urinary, respiratory, or cutaneous complications

Prognosis

- Contradictory data. Residual paralysis persists in 50% of cases of the most severe, flaccid ATMs. Including all cases, the results are somewhat better but still worrisome: 31 to 44% good, 33 to 44% fair, 23 to 25% poor.
- Whether the prognosis correlates with the severity of the MRI findings or with the age of the patients is controversial, as is the effect of steroids.
- Generally, the prognosis is better in children than in adults.

PEARLS_____

- The lesions of ATM extend to both halves of the cord, whereas MS plaques are unilateral. ATM extends longitudinally over more vertebral segments (at least three) than MS (typically fewer than two).
- Plaques of different ages are observed in MS, whereas all lesions are the same age in ATM.
- Usually idiopathic/seasonal or clearly postinfectious/immunization, ATM also may reveal a systemic disease such as systemic lupus erythematosus.

PITFALL_____

- Mistaking an ATM for a tumor, with subsequent surgery, would significantly worsen the functional prognosis.

Suggested Readings

Al Deeb SM, Yakub BA, Bruyn GW, Biary NM. Acute transverse myelitis: a localized form of postinfectious encephalomyelitis. Brain 1997;120:1115–1122

Andronikou S, Albuquerque-Jonathan G, Wilmhurst J, Hewlett R. MRI findings in acute idiopathic transverse myelopathy in children. Pediatr Radiol 2003;33:624–629

Choi KH, Lee KS, Chung SO, et al. Idiopathic transverse myelitis: MR characteristics. AJNR Am J Neuroradiol 1996;17:1151–1160

Kim KK. Idiopathic recurrent transverse myelitis. Arch Neurol 2003;60:1290–1294

Morris AMS, Elliott EJ, D'Souza RM, Antony J, Kenneth M, Longbottom H. Acute flaccid paralysis in Australian children. J Paediatr Child Health 2003;39:22–26

Prineas JW, McDonald WI, Franklin RJM. Demyelinating diseases. In: Graham DI, Lantos PL eds. Greenfield's Neuropathology. 7th ed. Vol 2. New York: Arnold; 2002:471–550

Shen WC, Lee SK, Ho YJ, Lee KR, Mak SC, Chi CS. MRI of sequela of transverse myelitis. Pediatr Radiol 1992;22:382–383

Tartaglino LM, Croul SE, Flanders AE, et al. Idiopathic acute transverse myelitis: MR imaging findings. Radiology 1996;201:661–669

CASE 5

Clinical Presentation

A neonate presents with convulsions on day 6 of life.

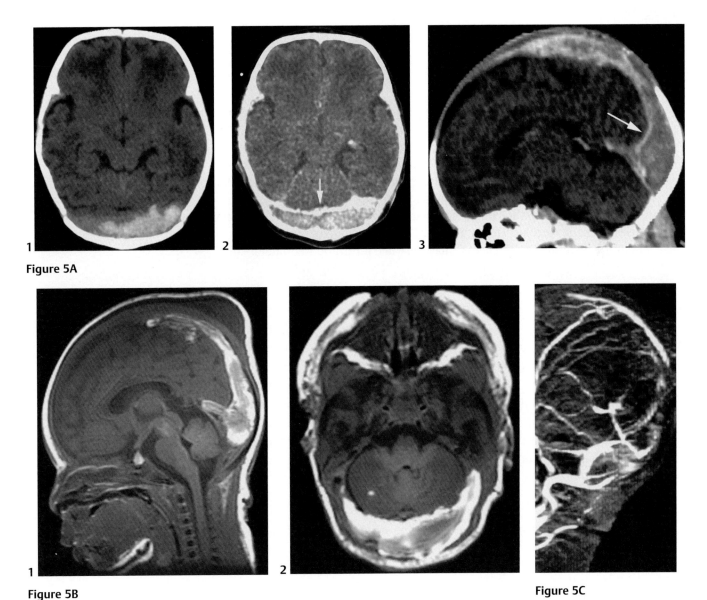

Figure 5A

Figure 5B

Figure 5C

Radiologic Findings

The nonenhanced CT (**Fig. 5A1**) demonstrates a heterogeneous high density within the enlarged lateral sinuses bilaterally, suggestive of intravenous clotting; the brain itself looks normal. Axial contrast-enhanced CT through the same plane shows that the contrast surrounds the clot in the dilated sinuses (**Fig. 5A2**, arrow). A reformatted image along the sagittal plane (**Fig. 5A3**, arrow) confirms clotting and shows that the thrombosis extends into the posterior half of the superior sagittal sinus (SSS). T1-weighted MRI confirms the thrombosis, its extension into the posterior portion of the straight sinus (**Fig. 5B1**), and into the lateral sinuses (**Fig. 5B2**). **Fig. 5B1** also reveals cephalhematoma, which was an incidental finding. Note the dilation of the obstructed venous sinuses. MR time-of-flight (TOF) venography (**Fig. 5C**) shows that the flow is totally interrupted in the posterior part of the SSS and into the torcular, whereas it is somewhat maintained around the clot in the other segments affected with the intraluminal thrombosis.

Diagnosis

Sinovenous thrombosis

Differential Diagnosis

- In neonates, normal blood on nonenhanced CT is hyperdense in relation to the immature brain tissue due to relative increased hematocrit, presence of fetal hemoglobin, slower venous flow, and unmyelinated brain, which can simulate thrombosis.
- The anterior third of the SSS may not form until the fontanel is closed.
- Anatomic variants such as a duplicate sinus, a "high splitting" tentorium, or a congenital hypoplasia/absence of a transverse sinus may mimic a defect.
- In older children, giant arachnoid granulations may appear as defects, mainly in the transverse sinuses near the torcular. This is a normal anatomic variant.
- Subdural hematoma (or empyema) may look like a thrombosed lateral sinus.

Discussion

Background

The clinical presentation of cerebral sinovenous thrombosis (CSVT) in the neonate is subtle and nonspecific, making the clinical diagnosis more difficult than in older children or in adults. However, the disease has been increasingly recognized recently due to improved neuroimaging techniques. Also, the number of children at high risk for CSVT has increased because previously lethal disorders have an increased survival rate now (prematurity, congenital heart disease, leukemia, cancer). Only imaging can establish the diagnosis with certainty, which is needed before therapy because of the potential danger of prolonged anticoagulant treatment.

Risk Factors

- **Neonates** are more prone to have CSVT due to specific physiologic factors such as maternal hypercoagulable state, deformation of the cranial bones during delivery, high hematocrit, slow flow in the dural sinus, and reduced level of protective clotting factors. Other predisposing conditions are:
  - Head and neck disease (10%)
  - Acute systemic disease (84%): perinatal complications (infections, gestational diabetes, prolonged rupture of membranes, abruptio placenta, hypoxic/ischemic encephalopathy), dehydration
  - Abnormal prothrombic state (20%)
- **Older infants and children** have essentially similar risk factors as adults, often multiple:
  - Head and neck diseases (38%), mostly infections
  - Acute systemic diseases with dehydration
  - Chronic systemic diseases (60%) such as connective-tissue diseases, nephrotic syndromes, inflammatory bowel disease, hematologic disorders and iron deficiency anemia, or cancer
  - Abnormal prothrombic states (54%): anticardiolipin antibody, defects in Protein S, Protein C, antithrombin, etc,
  - In-dwelling catheters

Pathophysiology

Whatever the primary cause of the clotting, the clot obstructs venous drainage. The blood circulation is interrupted upstream: This prevents normal arterial perfusion of the affected territory, and it leads to ischemia, intracellular edema, and eventually tissue necrosis. The increased venous pressure causes parenchymal swelling, interstitial edema, and hemorrhage. The local venous hematocrit increases as the blood loses water, and this, together with the absence of flow and the release of thrombotic factors by the clot, generates progressive extension of the thrombus. The venous pressure increase may be such as to compromise normal CSF resorption.

Preventing clot extension and thrombus dissolution is the primary aim of the treatment. In contrast with arterial occlusion (in which the flow restoration might cause further damage to the brain if done after the first few hours), venous flow restoration will be beneficial any time after occlusion.

Clinical Findings

- **Neonates:** Seizures (72%) are the main presentation, followed by diffuse neurologic signs (59%), including lethargy and jitteriness. Focal neurologic deficits are rare. Late signs of increased intracranial pressure (tense fontanels, splaying of the cranial sutures, dilated scalp veins, and swelling of the eyelids) may develop.
- **Older infants and children:** Half of them present with seizures. Signs of increased intracranial pressure predominate, including headache (59%), papilledema (22%), and decreased level of consciousness (49%). Visual defects such as diplopia or central scotoma may occur (18%).

Imaging Findings

- Above all, imaging should recognize the clot: only then can a quick, efficient treatment be applied.
- In most cases (80%) the thrombosis affects the superficial venous drainage system (superior sagittal and lateral sinuses mostly, less frequently the cortical veins), but the galenic system (straight sinus mostly, internal cerebral veins/vein of Galen) and the jugular veins are commonly involved (35–40%).
- Thrombosis without an apparent brain lesion is enough to start the treatment. Parenchymal lesions are not the disease but complications.

CRANIAL CT

- The "cord sign" (dense cortical vein) and the dense sinus on nonenhanced CT and the empty "delta sign" (clot surrounded by the enhanced dural wall of the sinus) on enhanced CT are pathognomonic.
- The vein/sinus also may be dilated.
- CT venography is considered an excellent diagnostic tool: It demonstrates the interruption of the sinus or the clot surrounded by contrast. However, hazards related to radiation and, in the neonate, to iodinated contrast agents should be considered.
- Parenchymal involvement includes focal or diffuse brain swelling/edema, venous infarction (anatomic territory), hemorrhage (common, especially in neonates), gyral enhancement, and evidence of venous stasis (tentorial or falcine enhancement).

MRI

- At 1 to 5 days, the thrombus appears as a loss of the normal flow void, with normal or hyperintense T1 signal and hypointense T2 signal.
- At 6 to 15 days, the thrombus becomes hyperintense on both T1- and T2-weighted sequences.
- After 2 to 3 weeks, there may be evidence of recanalization (flow voids) and/or collateral circulation.

- MRI venography can be done either with 3D TOF or phase-contrast (PC) sequences. The 3D gadolinium-enhanced technique is preferred as it is less prone to artifacts.
- The parenchymal complications (edema, necrosis, hemorrhage, enhancement) are optimally depicted on MRI. Early diffusion weighted imaging may demonstrate cellular ("cytotoxic") edema before the subsequent interstitial ("vasogenic") edema: The anoxic neuronal injury seems to antecede the mechanical effect of venous engorgement.

CEREBRAL ANGIOGRAPHY

- Classically considered the "gold standard," cerebral angiography is now only performed as part of local thrombolysis.

Treatment

- Anticoagulant therapy prevents the extension of the thrombus and favors the recanalization of the sinus.
- Thrombolysis may be considered; in contrast with arterial strokes, it is not limited to the early stage of the disease. But catheterization of the sinuses may release thrombotic factors.
- Anticonvulsant as needed
- Hydration, treatment of the causal disease when applicable

Prognosis

- Death may occur in 8% of patients. In half, it is related to the causal disease and in half to the sinovenous thrombosis itself.
- Complete recovery is observed in 54%.
- Residual disabilities include neurologic deficits in 38% (mostly motor defect but also cognitive defects, mental delay, speech or visual disorders, etc.) and epilepsy in 20% of neonates, 11% of older children.
- Recurrent venous thrombosis, cerebral or not, may concern 8% of neonates and 17% of nonneonates.
- The best predictors of bad outcome are seizures in the nonneonate and infarction in all.

PEARLS

- Because neurologic symptoms in neonates are nonspecific, brain imaging is the only available way to recognize or rule out cerebral sinovenous thrombosis.
- Occluded veins and sinuses are often dilated.

PITFALLS

- Sinovenous thrombosis in neonates should not be mistaken for the normal blood hyperdensity or for the common postdelivery subdural hemorrhage.
- Missing a thrombosis may lead to cerebral necrosis, and even death. Conversely, overdiagnosing a thrombosis exposes to a useless, long-lasting, and risky anticoagulant therapy.

Suggested Readings

Barnes C, Newall F, Furmedge J, Mackay M, Monagle P. Cerebral sinus venous thrombosis in children. J Paediatr Child Health 2004;40:53–55

De Schryver EL, Blom I, Kapelle LJ, Rinkel GJ, Peters AC, Jennekens-Schinkel A. Long-term prognosis of cerebral venous sinus thrombosis in childhood. Dev Med Child Neurol 2004;46:514–519

deVeber G, Andrew M, Adams C, et al, for the Canadian Pediatric Ischemic Stroke Study Group. Cerebral sinovenous thrombosis in children. N Engl J Med 2001;345:417–423

Osborn AG. Venous occlusion. In Blaser S, Illner A, Castillo M, Hedlund GL, Osborn AG. Pocket Radiologist—Peds Neuro. Salt Lake City, UT: Amirsys; 2003:196–198

Renowden S. Cerebral venous sinus thrombosis. Eur Radiol 2004;14:215–226

Shroff M, deVeber G. Sinovenous thrombosis in children. Neuroimaging Clin N Am 2003;13:115–138

CASE 6

Clinical Presentation

A neonate presents with an acute severe encephalopathy and odor of maple syrup (or burnt sugar).

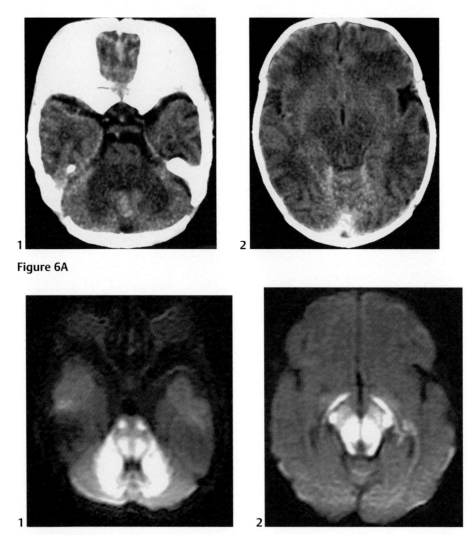

Figure 6A

Figure 6B (*Continued on page 27*)

Radiologic Findings

CT of the posterior fossa displays low attenuation of the cerebellar white matter, brachium pontis, and tegmentum pontis, as well as of the corticospinal fascicles of the anterior pons, with effacement of the fourth ventricle (**Fig. 6A1**). The midbrain and the cerebral hemispheres appear swollen also with diffusely low attenuation (**Fig. 6A2**). Diffusion-weighted MRI (DWI) of the posterior fossa shows a marked increase of signal of the cerebellar white matter, brachium pontis, tegmentum pontis, and corticospinal tracts (**Fig. 6B1**). The midbrain is swollen, with increased DWI signal of the superior cerebellar peduncles, of the central midbrain including the red nuclei, and of the lateral part of the

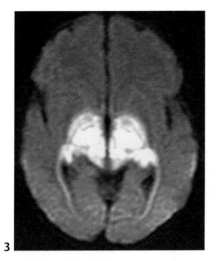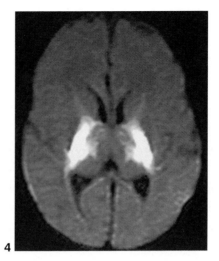

3   4

Figure 6B (*Continued*)

pes pedunculi, as well as of the optic tracts (**Fig. 6B2**). The level above illustrates the involvement of the lateral geniculate bodies (**Fig. 6B3**), whereas the cut passing through the basal ganglia demonstrates involvement of the posterior limbs of the internal capsules bilaterally, as well as of the adjacent globi pallidi, and to some degree, of the anterior-lateral thalamic nuclei (**Fig. 6B4**).

Diagnosis

Maple syrup urine disease (MSUD; also called leucinosis)

Differential Diagnosis

- Hypoxic-ischemic encephalopathy (HIE): cerebellum and brain stem usually not swollen, characteristic appearances, positive history usual
- Sepsis: lack of typical MSUD pattern
- Other metabolic disease of the newborn: lack of typical MSUD pattern

Discussion

Background

MSUD, also referred to as leucinosis, is a disorder that was first reported in 1954 in a family that lost four infants within the first 3 months of their lives because of a neurodegenerative disorder. The urine of these infants had an odor resembling that of maple syrup.

MSUD is a branched-chain amino-acidopathy caused by a decreased activity of branched-chain a-ketoacid (BCKA) dehydrogenase, the second enzyme in the pathway for the degradation of leucine, isoleucine, and valine. The disease is mostly due to the increased concentration of leucine, as isoleucine and valine present little toxicity. This defect is rare in the general population (1/850,000) but may be common in some closed communities such as Mennonite settlements (up to 1/170).

There are two forms of the disease. Both may be expressed in the same family. The *classic form* is characterized by an acute neonatal presentation, a low leucine tolerance, and a very low enzyme activity (<2.5% of controls). The *variant phenotypes* are less severe with a late onset, a reasonable leucine tolerance, and a fair enzyme activity (from 7 to 20% of controls), but variant forms also may develop acute deterioration

Etiology

MSUD is an autosomal recessive disorder. There are now more than 50 different mutations known in genes, which govern the enzyme components of branched-chain amino acids (BCAAs) and BCKA dehydrogenase complex.

Pathophysiology

Endogenous protein catabolism releases significant amounts of BCAAs and BCKA. Acute deterioration occurs in physiologic stress that increases the catabolism: postpartum for the neonate; fasting, infection, heavy exercise, injury, or surgery for older children. High leucine concentration impairs the normal mechanisms of cell volume regulation. It causes decreased serum sodium concentration and further abnormal redistribution of water into the intracellular space.

Leucine is a strong competitor of other amino acids for access into the cells. High leucine levels generate deficiencies of other amino acids; tyrosine deficiency contributes to acute dystonia and choreoathetosis.

Clinical Findings

In the classic form at birth, the infant is clinically normal, except for the maple syrup smell of the cerumen (but not yet of the urine). Only the biologic tests (with the familial context) can make the diagnosis. The physiologic endogenous catabolism of the postpartum period leads to an increase of the three BCAAs. At 2 days, there is an increase in ketonuria, irritability, dystonia, poor feeding, and lethargy. By 4 days, the dystonia increases, with seizures, apneic episodes, and signs of cerebral edema (specific feature of the MSUD). The child needs emergency therapy and may even require dialysis when diagnosed late. The outcome is then poorer.

In older children under treatment, or in children with variant phenotypes (intermediate, intermittent, thiamine-responsive, and E3-deficient leucinosis), the decompensation appears in situations with high endogenous protein catabolism. The presenting symptoms include muscle fatigue, epigastric pain and vomiting, decreased cognitive functions with hyperactivity, sleep disturbances, anorexia, hallucination, dystonia, and then stupor. Death results from massive cerebral edema.

Laboratory Findings

Neonatal MSUD is a therapeutic emergency and requires early diagnosis.

- The increasing level of leucine in the newborn with MSUD (compared with the decreasing level of leucine in the unaffected newborn) is diagnostic by 12 hours of age. As alanine decreases concomitantly in the newborn with MSUD, the leucine:alanine ratio is more sensitive. Rapid methods of amino acid chromatography are available and diagnostic before any clinical sign (other than the maple syrup smell in cerumen) is apparent.
- Elevated levels of the three amino acids leucine, isoleucine, and valine in urine and plasma. Documentation of alloisoleucine in plasma is diagnostic. Molecular testing is available.
- Ketosis or ketoacidosis, and hyperammonemia

Pathology

Brain stem edema and spongy degeneration of white matter and basal ganglia are characteristic of MSUD. The early myelinated areas are most affected.

Histology

Histologic features of MSUD include spongy degeneration of white matter, basal ganglia, and brain stem. Also, loss of oligodendrocytes and astrocytes is observed, as well as abnormal neuronal migration and orientation with abnormal dendrites and dendritic spines.

Imaging Findings

CT

- CT is negative in the first 24 hours, then demonstrates a generalized brain edema with compression of the ventricular lumen and the pericerebral fluid-filled spaces.

MRI

- In the early phase, diffuse brain swelling with gyral effacement not sparing the brain stem and cerebellum. Later, it shows the typical MSUD edema pattern characterized by high T2, and low T1 signal of the deep cerebellar white matter, peduncles, and dentate, of the tegmentum pontis, the midbrain tegmentum (reticular formation), and red nucleus, of the globus pallidus, hypothalamus, septal nuclei, and amygdala, as well as of the hemispheric white matter and posterior limb of the internal capsule. This edema seems to be related to the hyponatremia. It is absent or milder in patients with normonatremia. Later, the edema resolves but leaves a "pallor" of the involved areas and some loss of brain substance.
- Because the neonatal brain is immature, the anomalies are much better depicted by DWI than by conventional T1- or T2-weighted images. Diffusion demonstrates restricted motion of the protons [increased DWI signal, decreased apparent diffusion coefficient (ADC)], as well as decreased anisotropy in the affected, partly myelinated white matter, suggesting a cellular, and especially an intramyelinic, edema. In contrast, increased ADC has been found in the nonmyelinated areas, suggesting an associated interstitial edema. Follow-up studies during treatment have shown improvement in the areas with cellular and intramyelinic edema but loss of substance in the areas with interstitial edema.
- Proton magnetic resonance spectroscopy during acute metabolic deterioration shows elevation of the lactate peak that correlates with the presence of brain edema and an abnormal peak at 0.9 to 1 ppm that expresses the accumulation of BCAAs and BCKA. This peak disappears when the concentration of BCAAs in the blood and CSF goes back to normal.

Treatment

- Acutely ill neonate: Parenteral nutritional solutions with MSUD-specific elemental amino acid formulas applied before 72 hours considerably decreases morbidity, morbidity, and eventual medical care costs.
- The mainstay of treatment for MSUD is continuous dietary control of BCAAs. Careful follow-up planning is needed to avoid acute deterioration.
- Acute deterioration spells need osmotherapy with correction of the hyponatremia.

Prognosis

- If treated early and subsequently well controlled, the patient may survive to adulthood, with excellent development.

Complications

- Metabolic deterioration can occur any time with any physiologic stress.
- Excessive dietary restrictions may result in poor growth, anemia, and immunodeficiency; the

brain may show dysmyelination, poor neuronal arrangement, and dendritic branching, with neurodevelopmental delay.

PEARL

- Infratentorial edema is a diagnostic clue.

PITFALLS

- Missed or delayed diagnosis: MSUD prognosis depends on whether immediate care is taken in the first hours/days of life.
- With a known familial history, a biologic test is used at birth. In other contexts, the diagnosis depends more on radiology (typical pattern, DWI).

Suggested Readings

Blaser S. Maple syrup urine disease. In Blaser S, Illner A, Castillo M, Hedlund GL, Osborn AG, eds. Pocket Radiologist—Peds Neuro. Salt Lake City, UT: Amirsys; 2003:229–231

Cavalleri F, Berardi A, Burlina AB, Ferrari F, Mavilla L. Diffusion-weighted MRI of maple syrup urine disease encephalopathy. Neuroradiology 2002;44:499–502

Felber SR, Sperl W, Chemelli A, Murr C, Wendel U. Maple syrup urine disease: metabolic decompensation monitored by proton magnetic resonance imaging and spectroscopy. Ann Neurol 1993;33:396–401

Ha JS, Kim TK, Eun BL, et al. Maple syrup urine disease encephalopathy: a follow up study in the acute stage using diffusion-weighted MRI. Pediatr Radiol 2004;34:163–166

Jan W, Zimmerman RA, Wang ZJ, Berry GT, Kaplan PB, Kaye EM. MR diffusion imaging and MR spectroscopy of maple syrup disease during acute metabolic decompensation. Neuroradiology 2003;45:393–399

Kamei A, Takashima S, Chan F, Becker LE. Abnormal dendrite development in maple syrup urine disease. Pediatr Neurol 1992;8:145–147

Morton DH, Strauss KA, Robinson DL, Puffenberger EG, Kelley RI. Diagnosis and treatment of maple syrup urine disease: a study of 36 patients. Pediatrics 2002;109:999–1008

Parmar H, Sitoh YY, Ho L. Maple syrup urine disease: diffusion-weighted and diffusion-tensor magnetic resonance imaging findings. J Comput Assist Tomogr 2004;28:93–97

Righini A, Ramenghi LA, Parini R, Triulzi F, Mosca F. Water apparent diffusion coefficient and T2 changes in the acute stage of maple syrup urine disease: evidence of intramyelinic and vasogenic-interstitial edema. J Neuroimaging 2003;13:162–165

Saudubray JM, Amedee-Manesme O, Munnich A, et al. Heterogeneity of leucinosis: correlations between clinical manifestations, protein tolerance and enzyme deficiency [in French]. Arch Fr Pediatr 1982;39(Suppl 2):735–740

CASE 7

Clinical Presentation

A 12-year-old child presents with bilateral deafness.

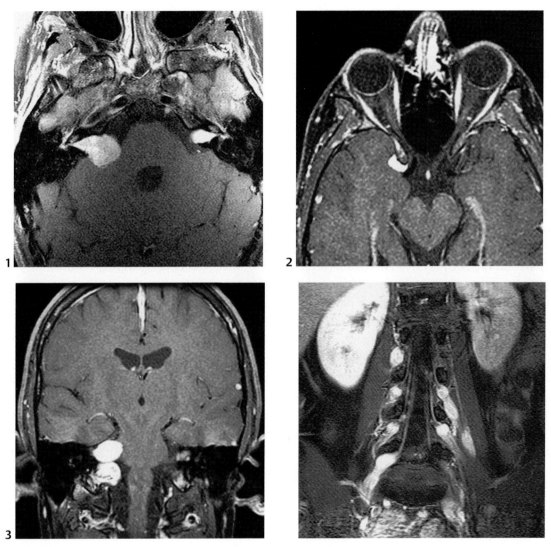

Figure 7A   Figure 7B

Radiologic Findings

The contrast-enhanced T1-weighted images of the head with fat saturation exhibit numerous lesions. On the axial plane through the internal auditory canals (IACs; **Fig. 7A1**), three schwannomas were identified. The largest one has developed from the right vestibular nerve; it occupies the whole IAC (flared) and the cerebellopontine angle (CPA) cistern, and encroaches on the middle cerebellar peduncle. On the left, another schwannoma is noted within the IAC. Two such lesions are sufficient for the diagnosis of neurofibromatosis type 2 (NF2). A smaller, third lesion is seen on the cisternal segment of the left abducens nerve. On the axial plane, through the temporal fossae

31

and orbits (**Fig. 7A2**), another lesion is seen curving around the right clinoid, with a large inser-tion on the dura typical for a meningioma. On the coronal plane passing through the CPA cisterns (**Fig. 7A3**), the two vestibular schwannomas are seen again in the IACs, as well as a broad-based meningioma inserted on the dura of the right foramen lacerum. Another, thinner meningioma is seen on the falx cerebri.

Imaging of the spine in patients with NF2 is mandatory. On the coronal T1-weighted, fat-saturated image of the lumbar spine (**Fig. 7B**), schwannomas are seen at nearly every level in the intervertebral foramina, extending toward the periphery.

Diagnosis

Neurofibromatosis type 2 (NF2)

Differential Diagnosis

Neurofibromatosis type 1 (NF1) for decades has been confused with NF2, although the expression of the two diseases is quite different (**Table 7–1**) with clearly identified different genetic defects. Both are tumor-producing diseases. NF1 is the most common genetic disease. It is characterized clinically by multiple, large, conspicuous "café au lait" spots, and by the presence of ocular Lisch nodules. Tumors in NF1 appear early in life. The most typical CNS tumors are the juvenile pilocytic astrocy-toma (JPA) and the peripheral nerve sheath (PNS) neurofibroma. JPAs develop mostly on the anterior optic pathways, the tuber cinereum, and the basal ganglia/thalami. They are less aggressive than the sporadic ones, may enhance or not, or only partially, and tend to become dormant over the years. Neurofibromas may be proximal, paraspinal, peripheral, or cutaneous. As opposed to schwannomas, neurofibromas develop not from the sensory root but from the nerve. A strikingly complex form of neurofibroma is the plexiform neurofibroma that extends inextricably along the network of nerves into the soft tissues. On MRI and CT, neurofibromas enhance following contrast administration, but large masses may remain nonenhanced centrally. Rarely, neurofibromas may degenerate into neurofibrosarcomas, especially after radiation therapy. Other hallmarks of the disease are the bright signal spots (so-called hamartomas) that may be observed asymmetrically in the basal ganglia, posterior thalami, brain stem, and central cerebellum. These usually disappear at adulthood. Other brain tumors may rarely occur, as well as aqueductal stenosis. The last feature of NF1 that is never observed

Table 7–1   Comparison of Features of Neurofibromatosis Type 1 (NF1) and Type 2 (NF2)

Features	NF1	NF2
Incidence	1/3000	1/50,000
Chromosomal anomaly	Long arm 17	22q11
Age at first symptoms	Early years	2nd decade
Optic/hypothalamic JPA	Common	None
"Unidentified" bright spots	Common	None
Neurofibromas, paraspinal	Common	None
Neurofibromas, peripheral	Common	Rare
Bone, dural, arterial dysplasia	Common	None
Multiple schwannomas	None	Common
Multiple meningiomas	None	Common
Spinal cord low-grade tumors	None	Common

in NF2 is the mesenchymal dysplasia that affects the base of the skull (dysplasia or agenesis of the greater wing of the sphenoid, often associated with an adjacent plexiform neurofibroma), the spine (vertebral scalloping), the long bones, the dura (multiple lateral meningoceles), and the arteries (dysplastic giant aneurysms, moyamoya disease).

Sporadic schwannomas and meningiomas are rare tumors in children. Therefore, any child presenting with either of these tumors should be screened clinically, radiologically, and genetically for NF2.

Discussion

Background

NF2 is a rare autosomal dominant disorder characterized by the development of multiple nervous system tumors. Although often considered to be an adult-onset disease, in 18% of patients the disease presents before the age of 15 years. About half the cases have no family history. Symptomatic cranial nerve dysfunction is less common in children at presentation than in adults. In children, the presentation is more protean, perhaps contributing to the lack of recognition of the disease. Skin tumors in children are an especially important clue to diagnosis because they are frequently present months to years before the diagnosis. They are an early marker of severe NF2 in ~25% of the patients. Cataract also is present early.

Etiology

NF2 is associated with an abnormality of chromosome 22 (critical region of approximately six megabases within 22q12). The product of *NF2*, a tumor repressor gene inhibited by the mutation, is *merlin*, a protein involved in the regulation of cell motility and proliferation. NF2 is a separate entity from NF1 (or von Recklinghausen's disease), a frequent (1 of every 3000) autosomal dominant disease, which has its locus on chromosome 17. Although NF2 is also autosomal dominant, it is much less frequent than NF1, with an estimated incidence of 1 of every 50,000 people in the population.

Clinical Findings

Clinical presentation is usually in the second, third, or fourth decade of life. Patients may present with auditory/vestibular symptoms (43%, less than in the adult population), symptoms of other cerebral tumors; that is, meningiomas (31%), or of spinal tumors (11%) or cutaneous tumor (9%). Pre-symptomatic lesions often are found with familial screening when NF2 is diagnosed in one family member. Children with schwannomas and/or meningiomas should be suspected of having NF2, and children of affected patients should be screened, as they are at 50% risk of NF2.

The criteria for diagnosis of NF2 are met by an individual who has:

- Bilateral vestibular schwannoma seen with appropriate imaging technique (CT or MRI); or
- A first-degree relative with NF2 and either:
  - A unilateral vestibular schwannoma or
  - With two of the following:
    - Neurofibroma
    - Meningioma
    - Glioma
    - Schwannoma
    - Juvenile posterior subcapsular lenticular opacity, or
    - Cerebral calcification

- Or, two of the following:
  - Unilateral vestibular schwannoma
  - Multiple meningiomas
  - Features listed above (except for meningioma)
- In addition to the previously described skin and ocular lesions and tumors, mononeuropathy and a more widespread peripheral neuropathy (cutaneous schwannomas) also are well-recognized features of NF2.

Imaging Findings

- **Intracranial manifestations** are mainly schwannomas of the vestibular and other cranial nerves, and meningiomas (usually multiple).
  - Bilateral vestibular schwannomas are considered to be the hallmark of the disease, but the roots of other cranial nerves also may be involved. Schwannomas are hypo- to isointense on NECT and occasionally calcify. Central necrosis can occur in large lesions. On CECT, there is homogeneous enhancement of the solid portion of the tumor, although inhomogeneity due to necrosis and cyst formation occurs. They are more often in the multilocular than sporadic form. Intracanalicular lesions usually enlarge the canals by pressure necrosis. Enlarged cranial nerves course through enlarged nerve foramina (i.e., the foramen ovale and the foramen rotundum in trigeminal schwannomas and the internal auditory canal in vestibular schwannomas). On MRI, large tumors show heterogeneity with areas of mixed signal intensity on long TR sequences; the areas of T2 shortening are most likely caused by the by-products of intratumoral hemorrhage, whereas the areas of long T2 are usually regions of cystic necrosis. Presentation with acute intratumoral hemorrhage is extremely rare. MRI has the potential of demonstrating small-size tumors (1 or 2 mm), and extreme care should be taken when assessing these patients as the multiplicity of tumors makes the difference between the sporadic vestibular schwannoma (rare in children but of good prognosis) and the much more severe NF2 disease.
  - Meningiomas are typically isodense on CT and isointense T1 and T2 on MRI, and they are densely enhanced by the contrast agents. They are typically multiple and are distributed over the calvarium, falx, skull base (especially the suprasellar/supracavernous region), and optic nerve sheaths, and in the posterior fossa. They may extend outside the skull cavity through the foramina, especially through the foramen lacerum toward the parapharyngeal space. They frequently form "en plaque" tumors and tend to grow rapidly in children. They are significant predictors of poor prognosis.
- **Spinal manifestations** include multiple spinal schwannomas, dural meningiomas, and spinal cord ependymomas. These lesions are more often symptomatic (cord compression) than the more paraspinal lesions seen in NF1 (neurofibromas).
  - Schwannomas develop typically on the preganglionic segment of the sensory nerve roots. They are therefore intraspinal. But they may involve both intra- and extraspinal compartments with involvement of the intervening neural foramen. They are extremely numerous in the spine, but most are dormant. They are isointense to neural tissue on short TR sequences, hyperintense (usually) on long TR sequences, and enhance uniformly. Neurofibromas are uncommon in NF2 but may occur and are typically paraspinal and cutaneous.
  - Intradural extramedullary meningiomas are common, especially in the thoracic region. They are dura-based masses, which compress the cord or cause pressure erosion of adjacent bone. Meningiomas are usually isointense with cord on both short TR/TE and long TR/TE images, and uniformly enhance after contrast infusion.
  - Ependymomas and astrocytomas of the spinal cord have a high incidence in NF2. They may be indistinguishable on MRI. The most common is the ependymoma, but ependymomas and

astrocytomas may occur in different segments of the cord in the same patient. The cervical segment is most frequently involved in children. The MRI features are variable, from a faint central enhancement of the cord to a well-demarcated, compact, and/or cystic mass enlarging the cord. They tend to be rather dormant in NF2, but their development is more conspicuous in children, as it is the age when they appear.

Treatment

- Treatment is primarily surgical resection of the tumors. However, surgery is delayed when it is bound to result in a loss of function, as the multiplicity of the lesions (schwannomas) and their common recurrence (meningiomas) will result in extensive cumulative deficits (complete deafness, bilateral facial palsy, paraparesis, and radicular defects).
- Radiosurgery, hearing preservation surgery, and rehabilitation with auditory brain stem implants are also possible.

Complications

- Progressive dysfunction of the cranial and spinal nerves
- Optic nerves, brain stem, spinal cord compressions
- Intracranial hypertension

Prognosis

- The heavy burden of tumors leads to neurologic disability and early mortality.
- The disease is more severe in children than it is in adults.
- It has been reported that the risk of mortality increases with decreasing age at diagnosis and is greater in patients with intracranial meningiomas.

PEARLS

- Children presenting with schwannomas or meningiomas should be suspected of having NF2.
- Schwannomas as small as 1 to 2 mm are sufficient to make the diagnosis.
- Ninety percent of NF2 patients develop some kind of spinal tumor, but only 25 to 30% of these become symptomatic.

PITFALL

- Not recognizing the multiplicity of the tumors

Suggested Readings

Aoki S, Barkovich AJ, Nishimura K, et al. Neurofibromatosis types 1 and 2: cranial MR findings. Radiology 1989;172:527–536

Barkovich AJ. Pediatric Neuroimaging. 3rd ed. Philadelphia: Lippincott Williams and Wilkins; 2000:400–404

Baser ME, Friedman JM, Aeschliman D, et al. Predictors of the risk of mortality in neurofibromatosis 2. Am J Hum Genet 2002;71:715–723

Evans DGR, Birch JM, Ramsden RT. Paediatric presentation of type 2 neurofibromatosis. Arch Dis Child 1999;81:496–499

Evans DGR, Sainio M, Baser ME. Neurofibromatosis type 2. J Med Genet 2000;37:897–904

Mautner VF, Lintenau M, Baser ME, et al. The neuroimaging and clinical spectrum of neurofibromatosis 2. Neurosurgery 1996;38:880–885

Mautner VF, Tatagiba M, Guthoff R, Samii M, Pulst SM. Neurofibromatosis 2 in the pediatric age group. Neurosurgery 1993;33:92–96

Nunes F, McCollin M. Neurofibromatosis 2 in the pediatric population. J Child Neurol 2003; 18:718–724

Otsuka G, Saito K, Nagatani T, Yoshida J. Age of symptom onset and long-term survival in patients with neurofibromatosis type 2. J Neurosurg 2003;99:480–483

Patronas NJ, Courcoutsakis N, Bromley CM, Katzman GL, MacCollin M, Parry DM. Intramedullary and spinal canal tumors in patients with neurofibromatosis 2: MR imaging findings and correlation with genotype. Radiology 2001;218:434–442

Xiao GH, Chernoff J, Testa JR. NF2: the wizardry of Merlin. Genes Chromosomes Cancer 2003;38:389–399

CASE 8

Clinical Presentation

A child presents to the hospital with recurrent nausea and vomiting. Abdominal assessment leads to abdominal MRI and subsequent CNS evaluation.

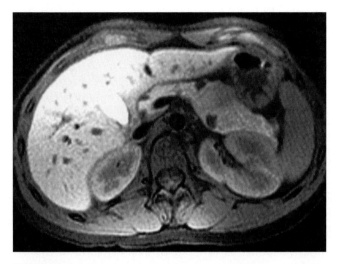

Figure 8A

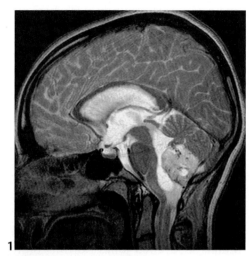

Figure 8B

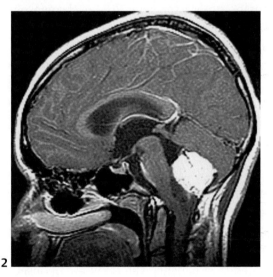

Figure 8B

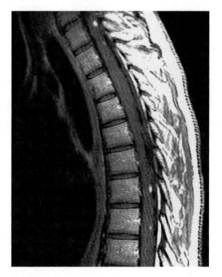

Figure 8C

Radiologic Findings

Fat-saturated axial T1-weighted image depicts multiple low T1 signal pancreatic cysts (**Fig. 8A**). This prompts the CNS assessment, which demonstrates on the sagittal T2-weighted image (**Fig. 8B1**) mild hydrocephalus and a hyperintense, well-demarcated mass of the lower vermis. A large anterior cyst obstructs the fourth ventricle, and multiple signal voids indicate high vascularity and fast flow.

37

Contrast-enhanced sagittal T1-weighted image (**Fig. 8B2**) shows the marked homogeneous enhancement of a vascular tumor, specific for hemangioblastoma, and the anterior cyst. Note that the signal of the cyst is slightly different from that of the CSF on both T1- and T2-weighted sequences. Imaging of the spine (T1-weighted sagittal with contrast, **Fig. 8C**) completes the CNS investigation and demonstrates multiple, small hemangioblastoma nodules.

Diagnosis

Pancreatic cysts, multiple CNS hemangioblastomas. This association is pathognomonic for von Hippel-Lindau disease (VHL).

Differential Diagnosis

Pilocytic astrocytoma (cerebellum), but the patient is usually younger, and enhancement is less.

Discussion

Background

Von Hippel-Lindau (VHL) disease is a rare, autosomal dominant inherited cancer syndrome predisposing to a variety of malignant or benign neoplasms, more frequently retinal, cerebellar, and spinal hemangioblastoma; renal cell carcinoma (RCC); pheochromocytoma; and pancreatic tumors (OMIM, 1966–2005 Johns Hopkins University). Its incidence is low, ~1 of every 40,000 births. Its expression is variable but with a striking tendency for familial clustering of particular features. Both sexes are affected equally. The cause is a defective tumor suppressor gene *VHL* at chromosome 3p25–p26. Another defect on 11q13 is found in pheochromocytoma-associated VHL.

Posterior fossa hemangioblastomas are present in about half of patients with VHL. They may occur in the cerebellum or brain stem and are the second most common cause of initial symptoms. They often recur after surgical resection. Spinal cord hemangioblastomas were previously thought to be uncommon because they are usually asymptomatic in patients with VHL. However, spinal MRI shows that these lesions are fairly common.

Clinical Findings

The onset of VHL is typically in adulthood (third or fourth decades), but symptoms occasionally appear in the first 2 decades. Early diagnoses often follow screening of affected families, as this allows timely detection of lesions requiring treatment. Diagnosis is usually established when either the cerebellar or retinal tumors are recognized (**Table 8–1**).

- Visual symptoms due to retinal hemangiomas occur in 40% of patients. The mean age of onset is 25 years. Clinical findings include reactive retinal inflammation with exudates and hemorrhage, followed by retinal detachment, glaucoma, cataract, and uveitis. The visual function deteriorates with age.
- Cerebellar hemangioblastomas develop in 60% of the patients, as the presenting lesion in 35%. It is the most common feature of the disease and the cause of death in nearly 50%. The mean age of onset is 30 years, with signs of obstructive hydrocephalus (headache, vomiting), dysmetria, and vertigo. One peculiar hematologic feature of hemangioblastoma of the cerebellum is polycythemia.
- Spinal cord hemangioblastomas are less common (15% of cases), often multiple and small, and commonly not symptomatic or with sensory deficits only. However, this vascular tumor may result in hemodynamic complications, either hydrosyringomyelia (sensory defects) or progressive myelopathy (typically with progressive asymmetry).

Table 8–1 Diagnostic Criteria of von Hippel-Lindau disease (VHL)

Family history positive	Any one of the typical VHL tumors:
	    Retinal hemangioma
	    Cerebellar, spinal cord hemangioblastoma
	    RCC
	    Pheochromocytoma
	    ELST
	    Multiple pancreatic cysts
	
	(Renal cysts and epididymal cysts are too common in the general population to be reliable criteria of the disease)

Family history negative	Two hemangioblastomas, or
	One hemangioblastoma, with:
	    Pheochromocytoma, or
	    RCC, or
	    Multiple pancreatic cysts

- Endolymphatic sac tumor (ELST) occurs in 11% of cases. The nearly constant symptoms are hearing loss, tinnitus, and vertigo.
- Abdominal malignancies include RCC (25% of patients) and pheochromocytoma. Pheochromocytomas occur in 15% of cases, but they do not occur in families that present with renal or pancreatic cysts. They commonly produce arterial hypertension.
- *Cysts* may be seen in the pancreas, kidneys, and epididymis. Pancreatic cysts are usually asymptomatic but may cause pain when large and tense or biliary obstruction.

Classification

VHL is classified as follows:
- VHL type 1
  - Without pheochromocytoma
- VHL type 2
  - Type 2A with pheochromocytoma
  - Type 2B with pheochromocytoma and RCC
  - Type 2C with isolated pheochromocytoma

Pathophysiology and Genetics

The cause of the disease is a recently identified defective tumor suppressor gene on chromosome 3p25–p26. This gene is involved in cell cycle regulation and in angiogenesis. There are different mutations, which explain the varying clinical features. For example, inactivating mutations (nonsense mutations/deletions) predispose to VHL type 1, and missense mutations predispose to VHL types 2A and 2B. The VHL gatekeeper tumor suppressor gene is inactivated in most sporadic clear cell RCCs. In cases with pheochromocytomas, a terminal deletion 11q13 is also observed.

Pathology

Hemangioblastoma: well-circumscribed, vascular nodule, often associated with a cyst in the cerebellum, and not uncommonly with a syrinx in the cord

Histology

Hemangioblastomas contain trabeculae of large vacuolated, lipid-laden stromal cells with clear cytoplasm, distributed within a rich, well-defined often telangiectatic capillary network.

Laboratory Findings

- Polycythemia in cerebellar hemangioblastoma
- Elevated urinary catecholamines in association with pheochromocytomas

Imaging Findings

- **In the CNS:**
  - Hemangioblastoma is in the cerebellum (75%) or the cord (25%), rarely the meninges, the cranial and spinal nerve roots, or the pituitary stalk.
  - Cerebellar hemangioblastomas are cystic in 75% of cases, with a peripheral solid vascular nodule that is often small, isodense on CT, hypointense T1 and hyperintense T2 on MRI, and often with vascular flow voids and without calcification.
  - Contrast administration is essential because the lesion is often too small to appear otherwise. The enhancement is intense on CT and MRI.
  - The full cord and cauda equina should be investigated, as multiple lesions make the diagnosis of VHL very likely. In the cord, a syringomyelia is not infrequently observed, which may cause the first symptoms of the disease. In any syringomyelia without obvious explanation, a contrast-enhanced MRI should be performed to specifically look for hemangioblastomas.
  - Conventional angiography is useful as a first step of presurgical embolization. It shows a very densely opacified nodule, often associated with a prominent early filling vein.
- **The ELST:**
  - The destructive lesion of the posterior wall of the petrous pyramid at the site of the vestibular aqueduct is apparent on CT.
  - On MRI, heterogeneous solid mass predominantly isointense to the brain on T1-weighted images, hyperintense on T2-weighted images, diffusely enhanced with contrast agent
- **In the kidneys:**
  - Fifty to seventy percent of patients will develop renal cysts, but renal impairment is rare in VHL.
  - Cysts are easily detected by US or CT, except if hemorrhagic.
  - RCC is often multicentric and bilateral in VHL. It should be diagnosed early to preserve renal parenchyma, and therefore imaging surveillance is needed.
- **In the pancreas:**
  - Involved in more than 50% of patients
  - The spectrum of lesions includes simple cysts, cystosis, cystadenomas, islet tumors, and rare adenocarcinomas.
  - Islet cell tumors occur in ~5 to 17% of VHL patients. They are small, asymptomatic, and slow growing, with a low frequency of malignancy. On US they are typically hypoechoic with increased flow on color Doppler but are best detected with contrast-enhanced CT and MRI.
- **Pheochromocytoma:**
  - Twenty percent of these tumors are associated with VHL.
  - They tend to appear in younger patients and are often bilateral and extra-adrenal.
  - On US and CT, they appear as either solid/cystic or complex masses with areas of hemorrhage or necrosis.
  - On CT the lesion enhances markedly (the patient has to be a-blocked before the study to prevent a hypertensive crisis).

Table 8–2 Recommended Planning for Imaging Surveillance (in Association with Yearly Clinical Exam)

	Start	Frequency	Modality
CNS hemangioblastoma	15 years	1–3 years	MRI
ELST	15 years	1–3 year	CT or MRI
Renal disease	10–15 years	1 year	US or CT or MRI
Pancreatic disease	10–15 years	1 year	US or CT or MRI
Pheochromocytoma	2 years	1 year	US or CT or MRI (with urinary catecholamines)

  ○ MRI is the procedure of choice: lesions iso- or slightly hypointense to the liver on T1-weighted image, extremely hyperintense on T2-weighted image, markedly enhanced after contrast administration.

Treatment

- Surgical resection of symptomatic cerebellar/spinal hemangioblastomas
- Stereotactic radiosurgery may control smaller lesions, tumor residues, or recurrences.
- Laser treatment of retinal angiomata

Complications

- The most serious is the malignant degeneration of renal cysts.
- Renal cysts are seldom clinically significant; however, they have an appreciable rate of malignant transformation.
- Retinal hemangioblastomas, although not malignant, can result in considerable morbidity through retinal detachment or visual loss, which results directly from an enlarging lesion.

Prognosis

- The mean age of death is 41 years (for 31 years as the mean age of diagnosis and 26 years as the mean age at onset of symptoms).
- Depends on early ophthalmoscopy and neurologic examination; regular imaging for screening/surveillance (**Table 8–2**)

PEARLS_____

- The occurrence of any VHL-associated tumor in a patient of age younger than is usually encountered should prompt a complete cerebrospinal, renal, pancreatic, and retroperitoneal evaluation.
- The discovery of a cerebellar hemangioblastoma should prompt the evaluation of the entire cerebrospinal axis.
- Systematic screening of patients at risk may allow earlier, and less mutilating, removal of dangerous tumors.

PITFALL_____

- Not realizing that a tumor is part of VHL

Suggested Readings

Chu BC, Terae S, Hida K, Furukawa M, Abe S, Miyasaka K. MR findings in spinal hemangioblastoma: correlation with symptoms and with angiographic and surgical findings. AJNR Am J Neuroradiol 2001;22:206–217

Colombo N, Kucharczyk W, Brandt-Zawadzki M, Norman D, Scotti G, Newton TH. Magnetic resonance imaging of spinal cord hemangioblastoma. Acta Radiol Suppl 1986;369:734–737

Hes FJ, Hoppener JW, Lips CJ. Clinical review 155: pheochromocytoma in von Hippel-Lindau disease. J Clin Endocrinol Metab 2003;88:969–974

Keeler LL, III, Klauber GT. Von Hippel-Lindau disease and renal cell carcinoma in a 16-year-old boy. J Urol 1992;147:1588–1591

Maddock IR, Moran A, Maher ER, et al. A genetic register for von Hippel-Lindau disease. J Med Genet 1996;33:120–127

Manski TJ, Heffner DK, Glenn GM, et al. Endolymphatic sac tumors: a source of morbid hearing loss in von Hippel-Lindau disease. JAMA 1997;277:1461–1466

OMIM (Online Mendelian Inheritance in Man). Von Hippel-Lindau VHL. Baltimore: Johns Hopkins University, 2005

Torreggiani WC, Keogh C, Al-Ismail K, Munk PL, Nicolaou S. Von Hippel-Lindau disease: a radiological essay. Clin Radiol 2002;57:670–680

CASE 9

Clinical Presentation

A 2-year-old child presents with partial-onset seizures, microcephaly, severe developmental delay, and quadriparesis.

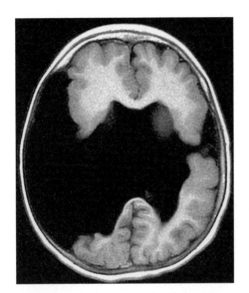

Figure 9A

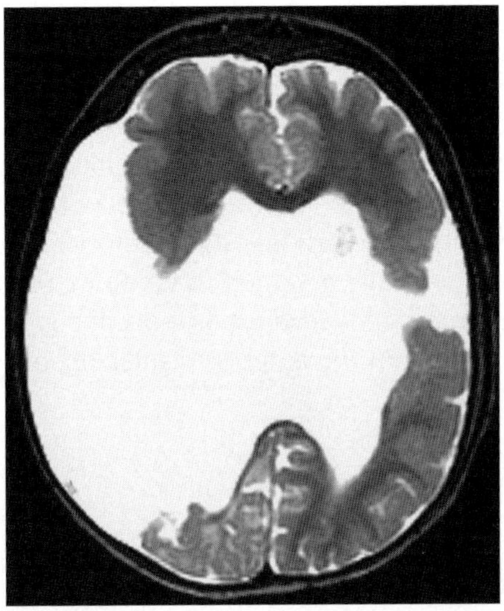

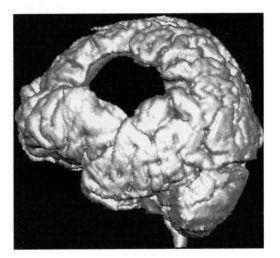

Figure 9B

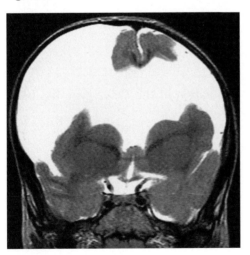

Figure 9C

Figure 9D

Radiologic Findings

Axial T1- (**Fig. 9A**), axial T2- (**Fig. 9B**), and coronal T2-weighted (**Fig. 9C**) images show bilateral, asymmetrical, large open clefts in both hemispheres. The surface opening is well depicted on the surface rendering of the left hemisphere (**Fig. 9D**). The septum pellucidum is absent. The clefts are lined with a somewhat thick, irregular, polymicrogyric cortex that extends to the lateral ventricles. The cortex surrounding the clefts also looks polymicrogyric. Surface rendering shows the cortical sulci converging toward the defect. The corpus callosum is thin posteriorly, presumably by lack of corresponding cortex with which to connect. Over the fluid-filled cavity of the large cleft on the right, the vault is thinned and expanded.

Diagnosis

Bilateral schizencephaly, open-lipped type

Differential Diagnosis

- Destructive porencephalic cysts, either posthemorrhagic (juxtaventricular) or ischemic (fitting an arterial, usually middle cerebral, territory). Schizencephaly is thought to develop early in gestation, whereas destructive porencephalic cysts develop in the last trimester. The walls of destructive porencephalic cysts are made of white matter, without any cortical covering.
- Hydranencephaly with some residual supratentorial tissue in distribution of anterior and posterior cerebral arteries is generally assumed to be an extreme form of bilateral porencephaly, but it is difficult to differentiate from severe schizencephaly.
- Arachnoid cysts, usually in the anterior insular region, are strictly extracerebral.

Discussion

Background

Schizencephaly is defined as a congenital brain cleft, which extends from the pial to ventricular surface (transmantle defect) and is lined by dysplastic cortex joining the lateral ventricles.

Etiology

The etiology is usually unknown.
- Most cases are idiopathic.
- Rare familial cases have been observed, and a germline mutation in the *EMX2* gene has been detected in one.
- Observed as an occasional complication of intrauterine cytomegalovirus (CMV) infection.
- Trauma in early pregnancy has been postulated in some instances.

Clinical Findings

The clinical finding of schizencephaly is cerebral palsy in which the psychomotor defect is related to the location of the lesion. Epilepsy develops in ~50% of cases. The severity of clinical presentation is dependent on the extent of the abnormality.

Pathology

If the transmantle cleft is bilateral, then it is typically symmetric in location but asymmetric in size. These clefts may be unilateral or bilateral, open, cystic, or with fused lips. In this case, the ventricular opening of the cleft is funnel-like, described as a "kissing ventricle." The cleft is lined with polymicrogyric cortex covered with pia that joins the ependyma (pial-ependymal seam). The cortex surrounding the superficial opening of the cleft is usually polymicrogyric, to a variable extent, and the sulci are converging toward the umbilication ("diving gyri"). An arachnoid cyst may overlie the cleft. When the cleft, uni- or bilateral, is located in the frontal, central, or parieto-opercular region, the septum pellucidum is defective or absent.

Histology

Beyond the gross brain abnormalities, microscopic dysplasias are observed in the cortex (poor organization) and the white matter (macroscopic or microscopic gray matter heterotopias). Other abnormalities may be related to specific etiologies such as a CMV infection.

Embryology

The cerebral cortex develops from the migration of differentiating neuronal cells from the subventricular germinal zone to the external surface along the guiding filament of the radial glia. This migration process begins about the seventh week and is essentially completed by mid-pregnancy (20 weeks). The white matter forms as a second step from the accumulation of the numerous axons extending from the cortical neurons into the subcortical intermediate zone to connect cortical areas together or cortical areas with subcortical gray matter (basal ganglia, brain stem, spinal cord), and from the thalamic axons toward connecting with the cortex.

Pathophysiology

The pathophysiology of schizencephaly is unknown. Because the cerebral mantle is focally absent, the primary defect must occur early, likely by the third month. Two theoretical models have been postulated.

- The defect is constitutional: In one portion of the cerebral mantle, uni- or bilaterally, the proliferation of the neural cells fails, this portion does not expand, and the surrounding cerebral mantle becomes umbilicated around the defect. This defect could be "segmental," explaining why the lesion is often bilateral, and involves the septum pellucidum when this is topographically consistent. This would fit the occasional occurrence of familial cases. The *EMX2* gene homologue in the mouse controls the proliferation of neuroblasts.
- The defect is acquired: This was initially deduced from the common perisylvian location of the clefts, suggesting an arterial ischemia. For various reasons, especially the normality of the arterial tree when angiography used to be performed, the arterial ischemic hypothesis has been abandoned. But an early focal lesion (infectious, hemorrhagic, etc.) in the germinal matrix might, by impeding the radial growth of the corresponding cerebral mantle, cause the focal growth defect with the ensuing umbilication of the surrounding gray matter.

These two theories are not exclusive. In the early developing brain, diverse causes—genetic, destructive, neurochemical—may result in similar defects.

Associated Conditions

The associated conditions include abnormal white matter, especially focal callosal defects, abnormalities of the hippocampus, defects of the anterior visual pathways, subcortical heterotopias, and agenesis of the pituitary stalk. In as much as 33% of the cases, anomalies are such that it may be difficult to decide between schizencephaly and variants of septo-optic dysplasia.

Imaging Findings

CT

- Although CT may be used to diagnose schizencephaly, MRI brings more complete and detailed information
- Open-lipped schizencephaly: The walls of the cleft are widely separated, the cleft appearing as a cyst-like, fluid-filled space extending from the surface of the brain to the ventricular lumen.

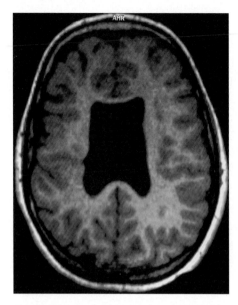 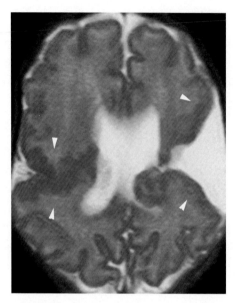

Figure 9E T1-weighted image of closed-lip schizencephaly with kissing ventricle.

Figure 9F T2-weighted image of a neonate with bilateral schizencephaly, closed lipped on the right, open lipped on the left with extensive polymicrogyrii (arrowheads).

- Closed-lipped schizencephaly: The walls of the cleft are apposed so that no fluid is seen in it. The ventricular opening usually forms a funnel-like dimple, giving the appearance of the "kissing ventricle" on slice imaging (**Fig. 9E**).
- In both instances the cleft is lined with polymicrogyric cortex, which may extend and cover a variable area over the surface of the brain (**Fig. 9F**).
- Fronto-centro-operculo-parietal clefts are accompanied by a defect of the septum pellucidum.
- The cleft is unilateral in ~50% of the cases. In these, a focal area of polymicrogyria, or a subcortical heterotopia, is sometimes observed facing the contralateral cleft. This finding suggests a possible pathogenetic continuity between the three conditions.
- In widely open clefts, the vault is thinned and expanded over the fluid-filled cavity, with a paradoxical unilateral macrocrania.
- An arachnoid cyst is not infrequently observed overlying the cystic cleft.
- In cases of CMV infection, characteristic features are found: microcephaly, calcifications, abnormal myelination/gliosis, and diffuse cortical dysplasia.
- Associated anomalies of the hippocampi, anterior optic pathways, and pituitary stalk may be seen.
- Surface rendering is useful in exhibiting the cortical abnormalities better.

ULTRASOUND

- Ultrasonography is most helpful during pregnancy.

MRI

- MRI diagnosis of the lesion is possible in the fetus also in the second half of the pregnancy.
- Better-detailed evaluation is seen with similar findings to those described for CT above.

Treatment

- Control of the epilepsy
- Supportive management in the case of hemiparesis and developmental delay

Prognosis

The prognosis of schizencephaly is dependent on the size and location of the clefts. Some rules can apply:

- A medium or large cleft increases the likelihood of a contralateral hemiparesis.
- Bilateral schizencephaly or a medium or large cleft is associated with moderate or severe developmental delay.
- Small clefts, especially not involving the frontal lobes, have a better functional prognosis.
- Epilepsy may become worse as the child becomes older.

PEARLS_____

- The salient feature is the cortex lining the cleft.
- Look for "diving gyri" on 3D reconstructions.
- Look for the "kissing ventricle" in case of closed cleft schizencephaly.

PITFALLS_____

- Severe bilateral postnatal middle cerebral artery infarctions may simulate schizencephaly.
- Look for the gray matter lining of the cleft to confirm schizencephaly.
- Fronto-temporo-sylvian arachnoid cysts are extracerebral.

Suggested Readings

Barkovich AJ, Kjos BO. Schizencephaly: correlation of clinical findings with MR characteristics. AJNR Am J Neuroradiol 1992;13:85–94

Barth PG. Schizencephaly and nonlissencephalic cortical dysplasias. AJNR Am J Neuroradiol 1992;13:104–106

Blaser SL. Schizencephaly. In Blaser SI, Illner A, Castillo M, Hedlund GL, Osborn A, eds. Pocket Radiologist—Peds Neuro: Top 100 Diagnoses. Salt Lake City, UT: Amirsys; 2003:51–53

Ceccherini AF, Twining P, Variend S. Schizencephaly: antenatal detection using ultrasound. Clin Radiol 1999;54:620–622

Denis D, Chateil J-F, Brun M, et al. Schizencephaly: clinical and imaging features of 30 infantile cases. Brain Dev 2000;22:475–483

Guerrini R, Carrozzo R. Epilepsy and genetic malformations of the cerebral cortex. Am J Med Genet (Semin Med Genet) 2001;106:160–173

Hayashi N, Tsutsumi Y, Barkovich AJ. Morphological features and associated anomalies of schizencephaly in the clinical population: detailed analysis of MR images. Neuroradiology 2002;44:418–427

Raybaud C, Girard N, Levrier O, et al. Schizencephaly: correlation between the lobar topography of the cleft(s) and absence of the septum pellucidum. Childs Nerv Syst 2001;17:217–222

Raybaud C, Levrier O, Brunel H, Girard N, Farnarier P. MR Imaging of fetal brain malformations. Childs Nerv Syst 2003;19:455–470

CASE 10

Clinical Presentation

Antenatal US diagnosis of a brain anomaly included absent septum pellucidum and microcephaly. Early neonatal MRI study was performed for better malformation depiction and identification.

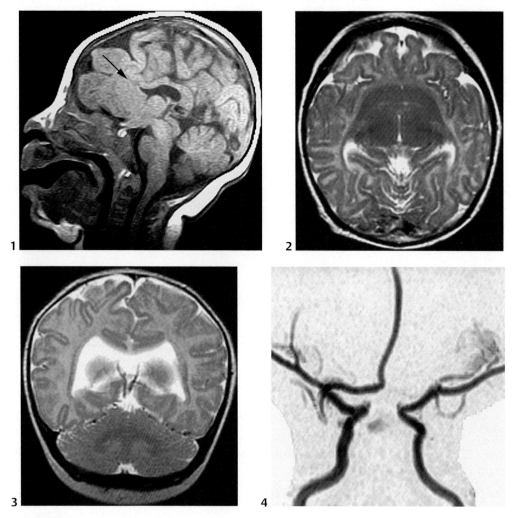

Figure 10A

Radiologic Findings

On the sagittal T1-weighted image (**Fig. 10A1**), fusion of cortical gray matter (arrow) across the expected location of the genu of the corpus callosum was noted. The callosal body and splenium are present but no fornices. The axial T2-weighted image (**Fig. 10A2**) illustrates the fused anterior basal ganglia (heads of caudate nuclei) and frontal white matter across the midline. The thalami are not fused in this case. Note the fairly well developed cortical pattern. The posterior coronal T2-weighted image (**Fig. 10A3**) demonstrates the lack of the normal structures of the midline (septum pellucidum, fornices) and single ventricular cavity. An azygous anterior cerebral artery is depicted by MR angiography (**Fig. 10A4**).

Diagnosis

Holoprosencephaly (HPE), semilobar

Differential Diagnosis

- **Septo-optic dysplasia (SOD)** is characterized by the absence of the septum pellucidum and abnormal anterior optic pathways. However, the two hemispheres are clearly separated, and the corpus callosum, fornix, and hippocampal commissure are fully developed. It has sometimes been postulated that SOD could be a milder form or subset of HPE, but this is controversial.
- **Extreme forms of hydrocephalus,** especially those that arise antenatally, may be mistaken for HPE, as the septum pellucidum may be ruptured and the sulcation poorly developed. Yet the hemispheres are clearly separated, and children with hydrocephalus are macrocephalic, whereas children with HPE are either micro- or normocephalic.
- **Schizencephaly** is another malformation in which the septum pellucidum is commonly absent. However, separate hemispheres are clearly identified along with characteristic cleft(s) of schizencephaly.
- **Arhinencephaly** (absence of the olfactory bulbs) has been used in the literature as a synonym for HPE. Although the lack or hypoplasia of the olfactory bulbs is a common feature of HPE, it is a distinct entity, often found incidentally at autopsy, especially when isolated.

Discussion

Background

HPE represents a spectrum of brain malformations characterized by the failure of the prosencephalon to form two lateral telencephalic vesicles, or more simply, failure of the front part of the brain to develop into separate halves. The incidence is variable but is said to occur in ~5 to 12/100,000 live births. There is equal sex incidence.

Classically, there are four described types:

- **Alobar:** It is the most severe form (**Fig. 10B**). Complete failure of cleavage, so the falx and interhemispheric fissure are absent, and the thalami and basal ganglia are fused with a holoventricle. This can communicate with a dorsal cyst (expanded tela choroidea). The sulcation/gyration is extremely poor. There are severe facial anomalies ("the face predicts the brain") with various degrees of midline structural defects, the extreme form being cyclopia.
- **Semilobar:** There is a single ventricular cavity, with anterior single frontal lobe, whereas the posterior/dorsal portion of the brain (temporo-occipital lobes) is better divided into distinct hemispheres with an intervening fissure and falx. The basal ganglia and thalami are still partially fused. Posteriorly, fibers cross the midline to form an apparent splenium of the corpus callosum. The hippocampi are poorly formed.
- **Lobar:** There is cortical continuity of the frontal lobes across the midline, with the most anterior part of the interhemispheric fissure present, with a falx. The septum pellucidum is absent with variable formation of the anterior corpus callosum. The face is normal, but in some genetic disorders, there may be a single midline incisor.
- **Syntelencephaly:** Many intermediate degrees of the malformation may be observed, with various degrees of cortical disorganization. In the mildest form, described as the "middle interhemispheric (MIH) variant" or syntelencephaly, there is failure of separation between the posterior frontal and parietal lobes with interhemispheric continuity of the gray matter, whereas the occipital and frontal lobes are well separated. The septum pellucidum remains absent.

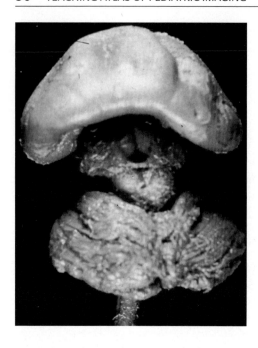

Figure 10B Alobar holoprosencephaly. A single "pancakelike" cerebral vesicle is observed, with almost no sulcation. The basal structures are seen through what was a large dorsal cyst (torn at autopsy). Grossly normal looking cerebellum.

Etiology

Causes of HPE are either genetic or teratogenic (*Veratrum californicum*), with maternal diabetes being a major risk factor. Mutations in the sonic hedgehog signaling (SHH) pathway, *ZIC2*, *SIX3*, and transforming growth factor have been implicated. The spectrum of HPE abnormalities depends on the gene involved and on the timing of SHH signal blockade.

Clinical Findings

Alobar HPE is characteristically associated with facial abnormalities, including cyclopia, ethmocephaly (hypotelorism and central proboscis), cebocephaly (hypotelorism and single nostril), midline facial cleft, hypo/hypertelorism, and isolated agenesis of the medial incisors. Patients with alobar HPE often have seizures, increased muscle tone, and a dysfunctional pituitary gland. Behavior fluctuates between calmness and irritability. Their cry is often high-pitched, and they have choking and gagging during feeding. They all have anosmia. Failure to thrive and death in a few weeks or months are the rule. Up to ~25% of patients may have a syndrome, which may include pseudo-trisomy 13, Smith-Lemli-Opitz (disorder of the cholesterol metabolism), or Pallister-Hall (hypothalamic hamartoblastoma).

On the contrary, in the lobar forms, the patients may be nearly normal and are able to have affected children.

Pathology

The cerebral hemispheres are more or less undivided, the basal ganglia and thalami are fused, and the septum pellucidum is absent. The corpus callosum and anterior commissure are often absent. A disorganized cluster of vessels called "rete mirabile" extends anteriorly from the internal carotid arteries, and there may be a single anterior cerebral artery.

Histology

Cortical organization is commonly disrupted predominantly in the anterior part of the hemisphere where frontal cortical differentiation is typically absent, with periventricular and white matter glioneuronal heterotopia. The hippocampus may show abnormal development. The basal ganglia have a disorganized architecture and are fused along the midline by lack of the floor plate. The cerebellum may also show cortical dysplasia and heterotopia. The corticobulbar and corticospinal tracts may be hypoplastic. The olfactory bulbs and tracts are absent, and the optic nerves are often hypoplastic.

Embryology

There is defective development of the anterior neural plate from which the midface and the forebrain (prosencephalon: telencephalon and diencephalons) develop. The floor plate fails to develop, with fusion of the anterobasal structures and absent or only partial division of the dorsal plate.

Associated Conditions

Facial anomalies are found in 80%. HPE can be seen in several syndromes such as Patau's syndrome (trisomy 13) and Edwards' syndrome (trisomy 18). Approximately 20 to 40% of cases of HPE have chromosomal anomalies. Of these, 55 to 75% have trisomy 13, with trisomy 18 being the next most common.

Evolution

This is a stable, nonprogressive, congenital malformation.

Pathophysiology and Pathogenetic Mechanisms

Either there is failure of cleavage of the neural tube or the hemisphere does not grow out of the neural tube. This may be due to growth failure or increased apoptosis. There may be a primary defect of induction and patterning of the rostral neural tube, which should occur in the first 4 weeks. Some studies postulate that the dorsal cyst seen in the alobar type is due to noncleavage of the thalamus, which blocks outflow from the third ventricle.

Classic HPE is thought to be due to lack of induction of the embryonic floor plate. The MIH variant is thought to be due to impaired induction or expression of genetic factors that influence the embryonic roof plate and is associated with ZIC2 mutation.

Imaging Findings

The specific morphologic features of the malformation should be looked for, with a tentative classification as a major, intermediate, or milder form, recognizing that the morphologic phenotypes do not correlate with the causal defect.

CT

- Absent septum pellucidum with a holoventricle and dorsal cyst in the alobar variety
- Variable separation of the hemispheres, basal ganglia, and thalami depending on the type
- Best depiction of the facial defects, from a mild hypotelorism to the midline fusion of the lateral hemiorbits (cyclopia)

MRI

- MRI is the best modality for accurate assessment
- Above findings with absent or hypoplastic olfactory nerves
- Delay in myelin maturation

- Anteriorly placed sylvian fissures
- Absent or partial corpus callosum
- Variable hypothalamic and caudate noncleavage
- The abnormalities, whichever the type, always predominate anteriorly.

Treatment

- Is supportive. Pituitary function should be assessed, and patients may need hormone replacement.

Prognosis

- Prognosis is dependent on the severity.
- Patients with the alobar variety and those with cyclopia, ethmocephaly, and cebocephaly virtually all die within 1 week.
- Prognosis is worse for those who have a cytogenetic abnormality, with ~2% surviving >2 years versus 30 to 54% for those without.
- The degree of mental retardation correlates with the degree of brain severity.

Complications

- Failure to thrive
- Hypopituitarism

PEARLS_____

- Absence of septum pellucidum and interhemispheric fissure is the clue.
- The lack of facial midline structures (hypotelorism or more) is pathognomonic.
- "The face predicts the brain, the brain predicts the outcome."

PITFALLS_____

- May be difficult to differentiate from agenesis of the corpus callosum and interhemispheric cyst antenatally
- The presence of a falx bordering the cyst is the salient feature of commissural agenesis.

Suggested Readings

Barkovich AJ. Magnetic resonance imaging: role in understanding of cerebral malformations. Brain Dev 2002;24:2–12

Barr M Jr, Cohen MM Jr. Holoprosencephaly survival and performance. Am J Med Genet 1999;89:116–120

Blaser SI, Illner A, Castillo M, Hedlund G L, Osborn A, eds. Pocket Radiologist—Peds Neuro: Top 100 Diagnoses. Salt Lake City, UT: Amirsys and WB Saunders; 2003

Cordero D, Marcucio R, Hu D, Gaffield W, Tapadia M, Helms JA. Temporal perturbations in sonic hedgehog signaling elicit the spectrum of holoprosencephaly phenotypes. J Clin Invest 2004; 114:485–494

Encha-Razavi F. Identification of brain malformations: neuropathological approach. Childs Nerv Syst 2003;19;448–454

Golden JA. Towards a greater understanding of the pathogenesis of holoprosencephaly. Brain Dev 1999;21:513–521

Hahn JS, Plawner LL. Evaluation and management of children with holoprosencephaly. Pediatr Neurol 2004;31:79–88

Kinsman SL, Plawner LL, Hahn JS. Holoprosencephaly: recent advances and new insights. Curr Opin Neurol 2000;13:127–132

Norman MG, McGillivray BC, Kalousek DK, Hill A, Poskitt KJ. Congenital Malformations of the Brain: Pathological, Embryological, Clinical, Radiological and Genetic Aspects. New York and Oxford: Oxford University Press; 1995

Simon EM, Hevner RF, Pinter JD, et al. Assessment of deep gray nuclei in holoprosencephaly. AJNR Am J Neuroradiol 2000;21:1955–1961

Simon EM, Hevner RF, Pinter JD, et al. The dorsal cyst in holoprosencephaly and the role of the thalamus in its formation. Neuroradiology 2001;43:787–791

Simon EM, Hevner RF, Pinter JD, et al. The middle interhemispheric variant of holoprosencephaly. AJNR Am J Neuroradiol 2002;23:151–155

CASE 11

Clinical Presentation

Fetal MRI was requested following abnormal prenatal ultrasound in two different patients.

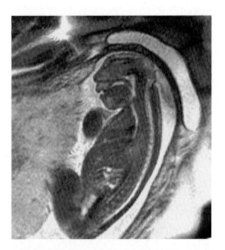

Figure 11A

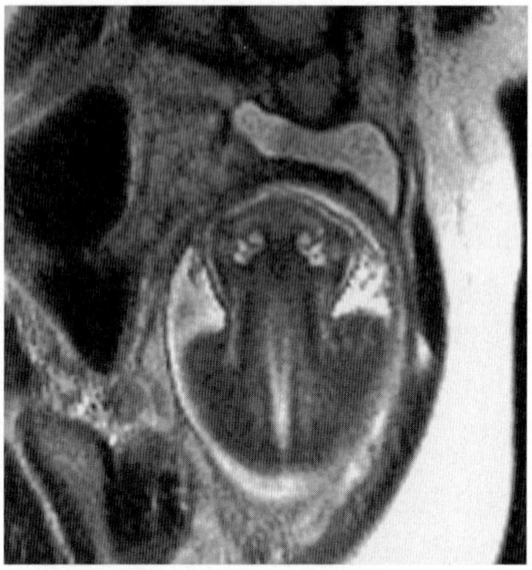

Figure 11B

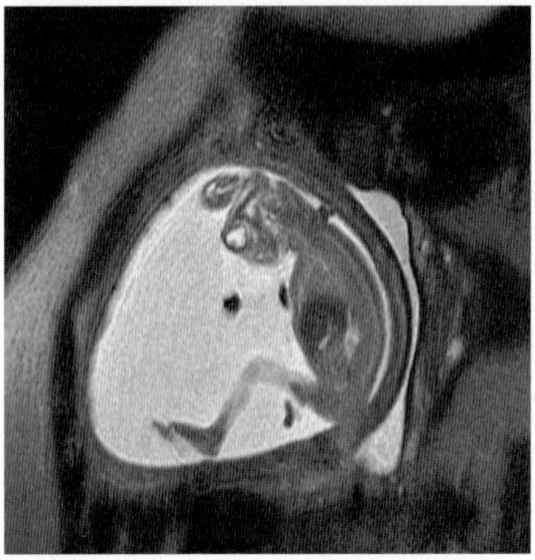

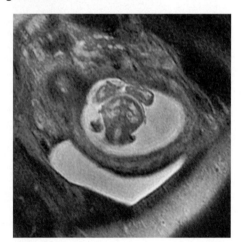

Figure 11C

Figure 11D

Radiologic Findings

Anencephaly and exencephaly are primarily morphologic diagnoses, typically recognized by fetal ultrasonography and better depicted by fetal MRI. A series of views from prenatal MRI study shows the typical features of anencephaly. There is total absence of the cerebrum and calvarium superior to the orbits and the misshaped skull base (**Figs. 11A** and **11B**). The fetal MRI of exencephaly (**Figs. 11C** and **11D**) demonstrates that the hemispheres are extruded from the open skull and floating into the amniotic fluid.

Diagnosis

Exencephaly/anencephaly sequence

Differential Diagnosis

- Severe microcephaly: No defect observed on the skin, scalp, or calvarium; exceedingly small but complete brain.
- Encephalocele: Basically a lesser degree of exencephaly, compatible with life. Brain-containing meningeal sac herniated through a skull defect, affecting more commonly the occipital lobes, the posterior fossa content (Chiari III), or the basal structures (frontal, nasal, sphenoidal encephaloceles).
- Hydranencephaly: Secondary, presumably ischemic destruction of most of the forebrain, within a normal skull, whereas anencephaly is the destruction of an unprotected extruded brain tissue.
- Amniotic band syndrome: Often associated with acrania, but secondary to entrapment by the fibrous bands. Other parts of the body are affected as well.
- Cutis aplasia is a defect of skin, scalp, and skull, usually without any subjacent brain necrosis.

Discussion

Background

Anencephaly/exencephaly sequence is a type of neural tube defect related to myelomeningocele (Chiari II). A high serum a-feto protein may be the first clue during early pregnancy. Fetal ultrasound is confirmatory. There is a variable reported frequency of 0.5 to 10 per 1000 live births, with a strong female predominance. The incidence of anencephalic births is decreasing due to maternal folate administration and prenatal recognition.

Etiology

Anencephaly has been linked with folate deficiency and the methylene tetrahydrofolate reductase (MTHFR) unfavorable genotype or folate antagonists. Clomiphene citrate ovulation induction is another possible factor. Familial cases have been reported. Chromosomal abnormalities (aneuploidy) are present in ~2%, in particular trisomy 2p.

Embryology

Anencephaly is thought to result from failure of closure of the first part of the caudal rhomben-cephalon (cranial to spinal cord). Normal closure is by coordinated interaction of at least four waves of discontinuous neural tube closure. Anencephaly is thought to result from failure of wave 2. Progressive destruction from acrania (absent calvarium) to exencephaly, and finally to anencephaly, has been reported.

Clinical Findings

A large full-thickness scalp, skull, and meningeal defect exposes deformed and membrane-covered rudimentary brain tissue. The cerebrum and cerebellum are absent, and the defect may extend to include the cervical spinal cord. The globes protrude as the bony orbital roof is deficient.

Pathology/Laboratory Findings

Anencephaly is characterized by absence of skin, cranium, cerebrum, and leptomeninges. There is a disorganized mass of neuronal elements and glia, which is red and amorphous, called the "area cerebrovasculosa," encircled by temporal and occipital skin. The frontal bones (above the supraciliary ridge), the parietal bones, and portions of the occipital bones are absent. The skull base is poorly formed with a shallow sella turcica.

Histology

There is a conglomeration of prominent blood vessels, mesenchymal tissue, neuroglial tissue, and choroid plexus. There may be a thin covering of squamous epithelium.

Associated Conditions

Occasional additional deformities are facial clefts, nasal teeth, clubfoot, and omphalocele. The adrenals are hypoplastic due to premature involution of the fetal zone of the cortex, as the fetus does not take over placental chorionic gonadotropin after the placenta ceases production. Anencephaly can be associated with open spinal defects.

Evolution

Stages of disease: lethal abnormality, progressive in utero

Pathophysiology and Pathogenetic Mechanism

Anencephaly involves neural tube defect with progressive destruction of incompletely covered brain. Exencephaly may lead to anencephaly due to progressive destruction of uncovered brain tissue. The previously existing brain tissue is proved by the remaining eyeballs, developed from the diencephalon.

Imaging Findings

RADIOGRAPHY

- Absent cranium except skull base and orbits; flat sella turcica

PRENATAL ULTRASOUND

- Amniotic fluid has increased echogenicity in first trimester.
- Polyhydramnios is usual.
- Exencephaly in the first trimester may show "Mickey Mouse" appearance of free-floating cerebral hemispheres.
- Progressive destruction of cerebral tissue leads to characteristic appearance of anencephaly in second trimester.
- Prenatal ultrasound demonstrates absence of the brain with a collapsed skull in the second trimester and "frog-eyes" or "bug-eyes" appearance.
- Diagnosis is more difficult in the second trimester, but look for Mickey Mouse ears due to cerebral hemispheres free-floating in amniotic fluid.
- The amniotic fluid also may be echogenic, and the crown–rump length is reduced.

CT

CT is no longer suggested, although it shows:

- Varying remnants of frontal bone (mostly absent above the supraciliary ridge), temporal squama, and occipital bones. The parietal bones are usually absent.
- Facial bones are shortened transversely.
- Skull base shows a stunted and laterally narrowed sphenoid bone with thickened greater wings resulting in a "folded bat-wing appearance." There are rudimentary lesser wings, and the pterygoids are lengthened and anteriorly deviated.
- A downward rotation of the petrous bone is noted, and the inner ear may be affected with a spectrum from Mondini malformation to cochlea hypoplasia. The middle ear/external ear canal and ossicles may be absent or hypoplastic. The vestibule and semicircular canals are usually normal.

MRI FETAL

- MRI may be performed antenatally to confirm or clarify the diagnosis on ultrasound.

MRI POSTNATAL

- MRI confirms severity and extent of cranial and cerebral deficiency.
- Absent cranial vault
- Normal skin ceases at the skull base and encircles the "area cerebrovasculosa."
- There is a rudimentary brain stem and primordium of cerebellum.
- The eyes may be normal or demonstrate globe and optic nerve atrophy.
- Possible inner ear congenital anomalies
- The pituitary gland may be absent.

Treatment

- None

Prognosis

- Universally fatal, may be stillborn or survive a few hours
- Those without a functional hypothalamo-hypophyseal system die within a few hours of birth.
- If they have a functional hypothalamo-hypophyseal system, they may survive for up to 3 days or longer.
- Longer survival is dependent on amount of residual cerebral tissue.

Complications

- Post-term delivery is common due to pituitary/hypothalamic deficiency leading to failure of spontaneously induced birth.
- Survival is usually only hours to days.
- There are rare reports of somewhat longer survival, which is dependent on the amount of residual brain tissue.

PEARLS

- Encephaly is a lethal abnormality requiring extensive parental counseling.
- There is a risk of recurrence of anencephaly of 5%, which doubles after the second affected fetus.
- Belongs to the group of neural tube defects/open dysraphism

PITFALL

- Very early imaging may be inconclusive due to the variable presence of brain tissue.

Suggested Readings

Becker LE. The nervous system. In: Stocker TJ, Dehner LD, eds. Pediatric Pathology. Vol 1. Philadelphia: Lippincott Williams and Wilkins; 2001

Cafici D, Sepulveda W. First-trimester echogenic amniotic fluid in the acrania-anencephaly sequence. J Ultrasound Med 2003;22:1075–1079

Calzolari F, Gambi B, Garani G, Tamisari L. Anencephaly: MRI findings and pathogenetic theories. Pediatr Radiol 2004;34:1012–1016

Chatzipapas IK, Whitlow BJ, Economides DL. The "Mickey Mouse" sign and the diagnosis of anencephaly in early pregnancy. Ultrasound Obstet Gynecol 1999;13:196–199

Cincore V, Ninios A, Pavlik J, Hsu C. Prenatal diagnosis of acrania associated with amniotic band syndrome. Obstet Gynecol 2003;102:1176–1178

Dias MS, Partington M. Embryology of myelomeningocele and anencephaly. Neurosurg Focus 2004;16:E1

Thomas JA, Markovac J, Ganong WF. Anencephaly and other neural tube defects. Front Neuroendocrinol 1994;15:197–201

Timor-Tritsch IE, Greenebaum E, Monteagudo A, Baxi L. Exencephaly-anencephaly sequence: proof by ultrasound imaging and amniotic fluid cytology. J Matern Fetal Med 1996;5:182–185

Virapongse C, Sarwar M, Bhimani S, Crelin ES. Computed tomography in the study of the development of the skull base, II: Anencephaly, the aberrant skull form. J Comput Assist Tomogr 1985;9:95–102

Weissman A, Diukman R, Auslender R. Fetal acrania: five new cases and review of the literature. J Clin Ultrasound 1997;25:511–514

CASE 12

Clinical Presentation

Infant girl presents with dysfunction of the lower cranial nerves, a large, posterior soft mass of the neck present since birth, and microcephaly.

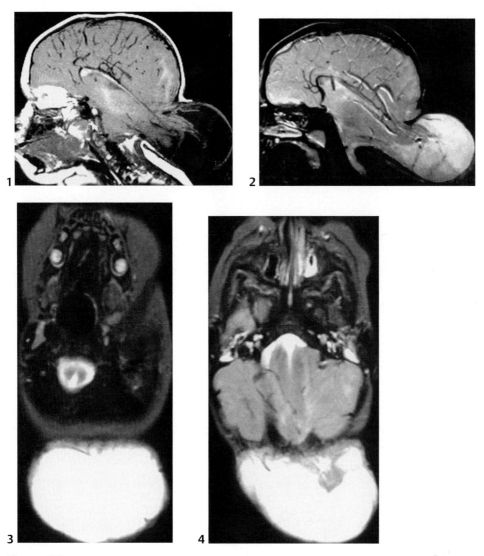

Figure 12A

Radiologic Findings

Sagittal MRI T1-weighted image (**Fig. 12A1**) shows a large posterior herniated sac filled with cerebrospinal fluid and cerebellum as well as posterior parts of the cerebral hemispheres. No subcutaneous fat is seen over it. The bony defect involves the infratentorial and supratentorial occipital bone, and therefore the posterior falx and tentorium as well. This implies that the dural venous sinuses are abnormal. Sagittal MRI T1-weighted image (**Fig. 12A2**) confirms the same anomalies, together with deformation of the course of the cerebral arteries. The axial T2-weighted images reveal the posterior split in the medulla (**Fig. 12A3**) and disorganization of the cerebellum (**Fig. 12A4**). The "heart-shaped" midbrain is tethered posteriorly to the sac (**Fig. 12A4**).

Diagnosis

Chiari III malformation

Differential Diagnosis

- Simple occipital meningocele: exceedingly rare, and more usually found at the cervical level. Does not contain any brain tissue, which is clearly shown by MRI. The subcutaneous fat is normal. Treated by simple excision.
- Occipital dermoid tracts and cysts are more common. The posterior bulging mass often is inflammatory and less elastic. MRI demonstrates the lesion, which is usually extended to the cerebellum, irregular, enhanced, and sometimes infected.
- Other possible posterior masses of the upper neck include neurofibromas (NF1), hemangiomas, lymphangiomas, and lipomas.

Discussion

Background

- Chiari III malformation is extremely rare, occurring in as few as 1 per 150 of all Chiari cases, most commonly in girls.
- Carries the same genetic prognosis as other neural open dysraphisms. In experimental animals, offspring may show any of the following neural closure defects: myelomeningoceles/Chiari II, Chiari III, cranioschizis, exencephaly/anencephaly, rachischizis, and craniorachischizis.
- On the contrary, Chiari I seems not to belong to the same group of malformations and has no genetic association.

Etiology

Familial/ethnic occurrence similar to Chiari II, commonly associated with maternal dietary folate deficiency or methylene tetrahydrofolate reductase (MTHFR) mutations. Toxins such as *Tripterygium wilfordii* and arsenic also have been implicated.

Clinical Findings

- Fetal ultrasonographic or postnatal discovery of occipital mass, often associated with microcephaly. Late diagnosis has been reported to 14 years of age.
- Soft tissue mass of the upper neck with microcephaly, dystrophic skin, and abnormal hair
- Brain stem/cerebellar symptoms (cranial nerve deficits, respiratory insufficiency, spasticity, aspiration, and dysphagia)
- In the older child, symptoms of syncope and headache and signs of raised intracranial pressure may be seen as well as developmental delay.

Complications

- Mostly neurologic, due to the abnormalities of the brain stem/cranial nerves, through herniation or tethering, with ensuing respiratory infections
- In case of surgery, complications related to the amount of tissue resected and to the reduced skull capacity preventing the reintegration of the herniated tissues
- Hydrocephalus

PATHOLOGY

- Occipital meningoencephalocele containing nervous element attached to the wall of the sac, meningeal tissue, and dysplastic/necrotic nervous tissue
- No subcutaneous fat is found under the dysplastic surface epithelium.
- Cerebellar disorganization
- Brain stem distortion with cranial nerve stretching. Posterior midline diastasis of the medulla: Underneurulation of the medulla is typical of Chiari III malformation.
- Pressure necrosis of the herniated brain

HISTOLOGY

- Locally neural dysplasia, gliosis, fibrosis, and necrosis; meningeal inflammation with hypervascularity
- Brain disorganization with cortical dysplasias and gray matter heterotopia may also be associated.

Imaging Findings

Classically, low occipital–high cervical encephalomeningocele. The definition has been expanded to include any encephalomeningocele when seen in combination with the hindbrain anomalies of Chiari II malformation.

RADIOGRAPHY

- Not needed. Would show the microcephaly with sloped forehead, a posterior bony defect typically at the craniovertebral junction, and a posterior mass of soft tissues

ULTRASOUND

- Not needed, as presurgical MRI is a must.
- Might help in assessing the vascular flow

CT

- Mostly for a careful assessment of the bone defect in the cervical, occipital, and, possibly, the parietal bones
- It demonstrates the encephalomeningocele and possibly the associated hydrocephalus.
- CT angiography may demonstrate the abnormal course of the arteries and venous structures.

MRI

- MRI demonstrates the encephalomeningocele, with herniated brain, meninges, and CSF.
- No overlying subcutaneous fat
- Deformed, dysplastic brain stem; associated forebrain involvement, ventriculomegaly
- Necrosed or dysplastic tissues
- Abnormal course of the arteries, disorganization of the dural venous sinuses around the bone defect. These findings have important implications for surgical planning and prognosis.
- The associated hindbrain anomalies of Chiari II are small posterior fossa with large foramen magnum; medulla, fourth ventricle, and vermis displaced toward the cervical canal.

Treatment

- Be it with CT or MRI, a careful assessment of the viable and functional tissue, as well as of the vessels, is needed before surgery. Conventional angiography is usually not needed.
- Corrective surgery: should be applied as early as possible as the encephalomeningocele tends to expand under the pressure of the CSF (a premature cesarean delivery for early correction is advised when the malformation is diagnosed in utero). After delivery, surgical correction of the

defect is required if the child is considered as viable (resection of herniated brain preserving the venous anatomy, duroplasty, and often skin grafts). Typically most of the brain tissue herniated in the sac is nonfunctional. Some cases have been treated with secondary closure after shunting.
- Prevention: genetic counseling. In women at risk, preconceptional folate administration is indicated.

Prognosis

- Poor, dependent on the degree of cerebellar and brain stem herniation and destruction. Newborns often suffer from respiratory and feeding difficulties.
- In surviving children, spasticity and severe mental delay are common.

Embryology

Several theories exist:

- The Chiari II anomalies are thought to be linked to CSF leakage through the open lumbosacral myelomeningocele; this results in a small posterior fossa unable to accommodate the brain stem and cerebellum.
- The neural tube is known not to close in a continuous way but simultaneously at different sites. A closure defect at the craniovertebral junction would result in the Chiari III malformation. The neural tissue fails to separate from the overlying ectoderm, preventing the interposition of mesenchymal elements (especially the bone and the fat).
- A disturbance of enchondral bone formation with craniocervical defect may result from abnormality in ossification centers, but this would not explain the neural content to be tethered to the surface epithelium. This more likely explains the simple meningocele.
- Because of adjacent pressure erosion by the herniated tissues, the posterior cephalocele may involve the supraoccipital and parietal bones (membranous origin), with herniation of the occipital lobes, falx, tentorium, and dural sinuses.

Associated Conditions

- Dysplastic tentorium, midbrain deformation (**Fig. 12A4**), partial or complete agenesis of the corpus callosum/septum pellucidum, and remote dysplasias of the neural axis
- Scalloping of the petrous pyramids and clivus, aplasia of the posterior falx cerebri, and aberrant location of the venous sinuses and deep cerebellar veins
- Incomplete fusion of the posterior arches, most commonly C1, in more than 70% of cases

Pathophysiology

The initial disorder is the failed closure of the neural tube and the absence of interposition of mesenchymal covering tissues. This from the start implies a dysplasia of the corresponding neural tube. Then the pressure of the CSF tends to push more of the adjacent brain tissue through the posterior hiatus, generating new ischemic lesions of the previously normal tissue. At the same time, the calvarium does not grow sufficiently, and over time it becomes more difficult to accommodate the extruded brain substance that could be viable into the herniated pouch. Finally, the closure of the defect generates an imbalance between the secretion and resorption of CSF, with development of hydrocephalus.

PEARLS_____

- Cerebral encephalomeningocele plus Chiari II = Chiari III
- Ectasia of foramen magnum, herniation of cerebellar tissue, in girls with Klippel-Feil anomaly: subset of Chiari III malformations identified only on imaging performed for cervical spinal anomalies

PITFALL_____

- Brain stem and vascular structures may be difficult to identify.

Suggested Readings

Cakirer S. Chiari III malformation: varieties of MRI appearances in two patients. Clin Imaging 2003;27:1–4

Castillo M, Quencer RM, Dominguez R. Chiari III malformation: imaging features. AJNR Am J Neuroradiol 1992;13:107–117

Haberle J, Hulskamp G, Harms E, Krasemann T. Cervical encephalocele in a newborn: Chiari III malformation: case report and review of the literature. Childs Nerv Syst 2001;17:373–375

Lee R, Tai KS, Cheng PW, Lui WM, Chan FL. Chiari III malformation: antenatal MRI diagnosis. Clin Radiol 2002;57:759–767

McLone DG, Knepper PA. The cause of Chiari II malformation: a unified theory. Pediatr Neurosci 1989;15:1–2

Sirikci A, Bayazit YA, Bayram M. The Chiari III malformation: an unusual and asymptomatic variant in an 11-year-old child. Eur J Radiol 2001;39:147–150

CASE 13

Clinical Presentation

A 2-week-old infant presents with facial deformity.

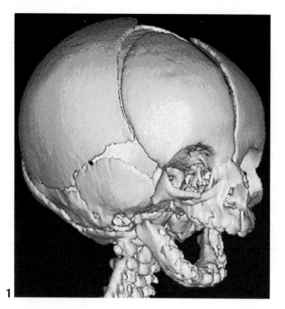 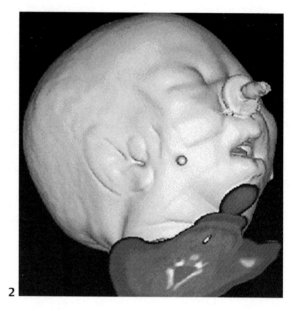

Figure 13A

Radiologic Findings

Three-dimensional CT demonstrates bilateral midfacial hypoplasia. There is hypoplasia of the malar bone, with absence of the zygomatic arch and hypoplasia of the mandibular ramus and condyle. The temporomandibular joint is absent (**Fig. 13A1**). The temporal bone is not fully developed, and the external auditory canal is abnormally located inferiorly. Soft tissue imaging demonstrates an abnormal pinna (**Fig. 13A2**). These abnormalities were essentially symmetrical.

Diagnosis

Lateral facial dysplasias: Treacher Collins syndrome (TCS), also called mandibulofacial dysostosis (MFD1) or Treacher Collins-Franceschetti syndrome (TCOF)

Differential Diagnosis

- Hemifacial microsomia (HFM) is also called oculoauriculovertebral dysplasia and Goldenhar's syndrome: coloboma of the *upper* eyelid, hemifacial microsomia (may be bilateral but asymmetrical), and vertebral defects.
- Acrofacial dysostosis 1 or Nager's syndrome: severe malar hypoplasia and micrognathia, associated with absence of radius, radio-ulnar synostosis, hypoplasia. or absence of the thumb. Gene defect located on 9q32
- Ablepharon macrostomia syndrome (AMS): absent eyelid, eyebrows, eyelashes, fusion defect of the mouth, rudimentary external ears, ambiguous genitalia, rudimentary nipples, and coarse, dry skin

Discussion

Background

TCS is a disorder of craniofacial development. An autosomal dominant syndrome, it is found in 1 per 50,000 live births. The TCOF1 mutation is found in 78% of patients. Familial in 40% of cases, it arises as new spontaneous mutation in 60%. The obligatory features of TCOF are marked hypoplasia of the malar bone, hypoplasia of the mandibular ramus and condyle, obliteration of the frontonasal angle, colobomas of the lower eyelids, and malformation of the eyelashes.

Etiology

Various explanations have been offered regarding the pathogenesis of TCS: problems of differentiation of the branchial arch mesoderm preventing normal facial bone development, abnormal ossification of the viscerocranium, even ischemia from stapedial artery hypoplasia or defect of ectomesenchymal cells within the developing trigeminal ganglia.

Genetics

TCS is a familial, autosomal dominant syndrome with penetrance near 100% but variable expression. The genetic abnormality is mapped to chromosome 5q31.3q33.3, and more than 100 mutations have been identified, mostly deletions. Prenatal diagnosis is possible from amniocentesis (at 16 to 17 weeks) or chorionic villous sampling (at 10 to 11 weeks).

Clinical Findings

- The facial abnormalities are essentially bilateral and symmetrical.
- Midfacial hypoplasia and retrognathia, with macrostomia
- Eye abnormalities: palpebral slanting, shortened palpebral fissures, colobomas (developmental cleft) of the *lower* eyelid, and absent eyelashes. Compromised extra-ocular muscle function, due to the orbital distortion. Corneal exposure due to palpebral hypoplasia.

- Ill-shaped, ill-located pinna. Moderate to major hearing loss (96% of patients)
- Abnormalities of the upper airways resulting in respiratory and speech disorders with postural adaptation, and obstructive apnea especially in sleep (25% of patients). Respiratory distress may occur when the mandible is particularly small.
- Swallowing may be impeded also because of pharyngeal narrowing, posteriorly located tongue, abnormal temporomandibular joint, and, occasionally, because of an associated cleft palate.

Imaging Findings

CT

- CT is performed before 6 months to document the extent of craniofacial skeletal dysmorphology and to assess the external auditory canal and middle ear anatomy.
- The skeletal abnormalities are bilateral and symmetrical.
- Small or absent malar bones resulting in orbital deformity (inferolateral rotation of the orbit with shortening of its floor)
- Maxillary bone abnormalities (narrow or overprojected, vertically oriented maxilla, elevated or narrow palate, cleft palate), choanal shortening
- Mandible abnormalities (hypoplasia or agenesis of the condyle and ascending ramus, retrognathia with dental malocclusion, retruded chin), hypoplastic or even absent (free-floating mandible) temporomandibular joint elements
- Nasal anomalies (broad or protruded)
- Temporal bone anomalies, atretic or stenotic external auditory canals (85%), hypoplastic and ill-shaped middle ear cavities, missing (46%) or hypoplastic/ankylosed (46%) ossicles. These external and middle ear anomalies are typically symmetrical (88%). The inner ear (cochlea, vestibule, semi-circular canals, and internal auditory canal) is normal.

FETAL ULTRASOUND

- The diagnosis of mandibular hypoplasia can be made in utero.

Treatment

- Correction of colobomas can be made early to protect the cornea.
- Pinna repair is delayed until after age 6 to allow time for adequate costal cartilage development, which is required for successful reconstruction.
- Surgical correction of the zygoma and orbit is usually not performed until the patient is 5 to 7 years of age, but earlier treatment may be required to protect the cornea. Rhinoplasty will follow.
- Maxillomandibular reconstruction should be performed in early skeletal maturity, ~15 years. Lengthening of the mandible may have to be performed earlier to prevent respiratory distress.
- Middle ear surgery is indicated in selected cases. Hearing aids are needed in all patients.

Complications

- Respiratory distress
- Psychosocial disorders

Prognosis

- Except in the event of a fatal respiratory distress, normal life expectancy and normal mentation
- The facial deformities do not change and especially do not worsen with age.

PEARLS_____

- Limb anomalies do not occur in TCS, which helps differentiate it from other syndromes that manifest with similar facial features.
- Hypoplasia or deficiency of the zygoma is considered by some investigators to be the central event of TCS.
- The findings are typically bilateral and symmetric.

PITFALL_____

- Naso- and oropharyngeal hypoplasia, and occasionally choanal atresia, can cause severe breathing problems and even death.

Suggested Readings

Arvystas M, Shprintzen RJ. Craniofacial morphology in Treacher Collins syndrome. Cleft Palate Craniofac J 1991;28:226–230

Caruso PA, Harris GJ, Padwa BL. CT imaging of craniofacial malformations. Neuroimaging Clin N Am 2003;13:541–572

Ellis PE, Dawson M, Dixon MJ. Mutation testing in Treacher Collins syndrome. J Orthod 2002; 29:293–297

Lowe LH, Booth TN, Foglar FM, Rollins NK. Midface anomalies in children. Radiographics 2000;20:907–922

Marszalek B, Wojcicki P, Kobus K, Trzeciak W. Clinical features, treatment and genetic background of Treacher Collins syndrome. J Appl Genet 2002;43:223–233

OMIM (Online Mendelian Inheritance in Man). Treacher Collins-Franceschetti syndrome TCOF; Hemifacial microsomia HFM; Acrofacial dysostosis 1, Nager type AFD1; Ablepharon-macrostomia syndrome. Baltimore: Johns Hopkins University; 2005

Posnick JC, Ruiz RL. Treacher Collins syndrome: current evaluation, treatment and future directions. Cleft Palate-Craniofacial J 2000;434:1–24

Rotten D, Levaillant JM, Martinez H, Ducou Lepointe H, Vicaut E. The fetal mandible: a 2D and 3D sonographic approach to the diagnosis of retrognathia and micrognathia. Ultrasound Obstet Gynecol 2002;19:122–130

CASE 14

Clinical Presentation

A 7-month-old male presents with triangular appearance of the forehead and flattened temporal fossae, giving a "keel-shaped" appearance to the head.

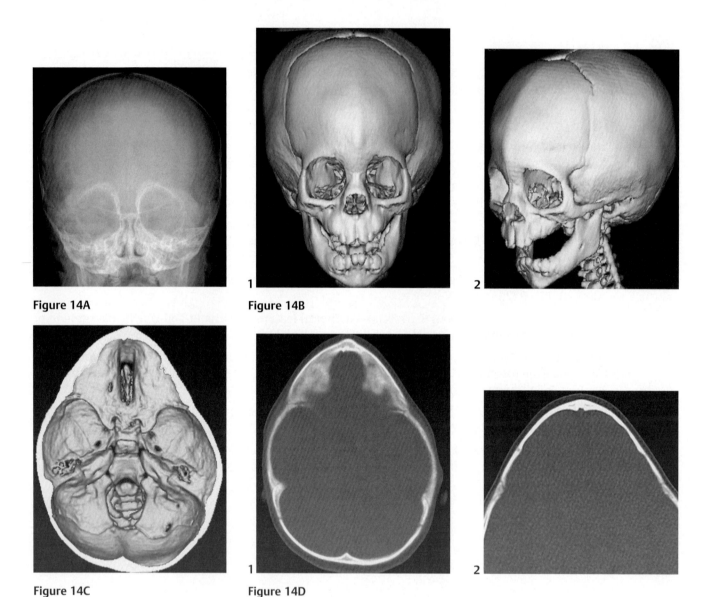

Figure 14A

Figure 14B

Figure 14C

Figure 14D

Radiologic Findings

The AP plain x-ray of the skull demonstrates hypotelorism, with medial elevation of the superior orbital rims giving the face a "quizzical" appearance (**Fig. 14A**). Selected images from 3D CT volume-rendered reconstructions: frontal (**Fig. 14B1**) and oblique (**Fig. 14B2**) show a prominent, ridged metopic suture. The frontal squama is poorly expanded, in contrast with the temporoparietal widening of the skull. The inside view of the skull (**Fig. 14C**) demonstrates its triangular shape (trigonocephaly). Note narrowing of the anterior cranial fossa, lateral shortening of the orbital roofs,

Table 14–1 The Craniosynostoses

Suture Affected	Resulting Deformity	Description
Metopic	Trigonocephaly	Triangular skull, keel-shaped, frontal median ridge, symmetrical
Coronal, bilateral	Anterior brachycephaly	Skull short anteriorly, wide parietal, symmetrical
Coronal, unilateral	Anterior plagiocephaly	Unilateral frontotemporal flattening
Sagittal	Scaphocephaly	Elongated, canoe-shaped skull, symmetrical
Lambdoid, bilateral	Posterior brachycephaly	Skull short posteriorly, anterior bulge, symmetrical
Lambdoid, unilateral	Posterior plagiocephaly	Unilateral posterior flattening
All	Oxycephaly	Small rounded skull, symmetrical; needs early surgery to allow the brain to grow
All, bone dysplastic	Acrocephaly	Syndromic, malformed face and base as well

a deep and narrow cribriform plate groove, and the bilateral bulging and widening of the middle cranial fossa. Axial imaging illustrates the trigonocephaly with the metopic beak (**Fig. 14D1**) and the endocranial metopic notch in the region of the anterior portion of the superior sagittal sinus (**Fig. 14D2**).

Diagnosis

Metopic synostosis, or trigonocephaly (the suture synostosis is the defect, trigonocephaly is its morphologic consequence)

Differential Diagnosis

- Metopic ridge due to normal fusion of the metopic suture; no significant skull deformity, endocranial ridge present
- Premature metopic fusion also may be due to failure of brain growth; imaging then demonstrates brain anomalies.
- Other craniosynostoses (**Table 14–1**)

Discussion

Background

Metopic synostosis is uncommon but is probably under-evaluated, as only the cases needing cosmetic repair are brought to medical attention. It likely represents between 5 to 7% and 14% of isolated craniosynostoses. The metopic suture is the first cranial suture to fuse. Fusion may start as early as 3 months and is normally completed by 6 to 8 months. Sutural fusion originates at the nasion and concludes at the anterior fontanelle. Patients might present early in life with a metopic ridge, which appears fused on imaging, but with a normal head shape. At the other end of the spectrum is the child with clear metopic synostosis and trigonocephaly. Male to female ratio is ~3:1.

When a suture fuses prematurely, the squamae it feeds fail to grow, leading to a focal stenosis; on the contrary, the rest of the calvarium tends to expand to accommodate the brain expansion. This double process of focal stenosis and distant expansion explains the marked deformity. In simple craniosynostosis (no bone dysplasia, skull base essentially normal), surgery is needed for cosmetic purpose only. However, when all sutures are fused prematurely (oxycephaly), surgery then is needed to allow the brain to expand.

Etiology

Metopic suture synostosis can be an isolated defect (80% of cases), or it can occur in association with other malformations including some syndromes. In most patients, craniosynostosis is a primary event and occurs sporadically. There are rare familial reports. Syndromic trigonocephaly is causally heterogeneous as metopic synostosis is found in several delineated syndromes such as *Jacobsen* (11q23 deletion: trigonocephaly, developmental delay, facial anomalies, campodactyly, and immune thrombocytopenia), *Saethre-Chotzen* (10q26, 7p21: acrocephalosyndactyly type III), *Opitz C-trigonocephaly*, *Say-Meyer* (trigonocephaly with short stature and developmental delay), and *Christian's* (Xq28: mental retardation, skeletal dysplasia, and abducens palsy) syndromes.

Other causes include head constraint in utero from either uterine deformities or from multiple births, and endocrine disorders, specifically related to thyroid metabolism, rickets, or hypercalcemia. Several metabolic conditions have been linked to metopic ridging, including mucopolysaccharidoses and mucolipidoses.

Finally, there is an increased incidence of trigonocephaly occurring after exposure to valproic acid (anti-epileptic drug) in utero that is statistically significant. Trigonocephaly is the only type of synostosis observed in this context.

Clinical Findings

Premature fusion of the metopic suture results in trigonocephaly, which is characterized by a triangular appearance of the head. Patients may present with a range of dysmorphic features, including an isolated, palpable midline ridge or a large keel-shaped prominence overlying the metopic suture; ethmoidal hypoplasia with orbital hypotelorism; a shortened anterior cranial fossa; and bitemporal narrowing with biparietal widening. In 80% of patients, the malformation is isolated. In 20% it is associated with other malformations, either syndromic (5%) or not (15%).

Visceral malformations include malformations of the heart, a wide array of genitourinary tract abnormalities, brain malformations (affecting the corpus callosum mostly). Nonvisceral anomalies affect the face (cleft palate, coloboma) and the limbs. Familial cases of isolated trigonocephaly are reported, pointing to a genetic disorder.

Imaging Findings

RADIOGRAPHY

- Hypotelorism with medial elevation of the orbital rim leads to a "quizzical" appearance on frontal plain films.
- Normal lucency of the other sutures

CT

- 3D CT should be performed in every case where surgery is contemplated.
- Demonstrates frontal beaking with bitemporal narrowing and biparietal widening
- Orbital features include a narrow interorbital distance with hypotelorism in 60%.
- Cephalic index, width of the cranial base, and ear size and shape are unaffected.
- An endocranial metopic notch is virtually diagnostic of premature suture fusion and was seen in 93% of synostotic patients in one report (Weinzweig et al, 2003).
- Metopic notch is not seen in any nonsynostotic patient.
- A complete evaluation of the cranium is needed because associated malformations of the face or the base may mean that the case is syndromic.

MRI

- MRI may be useful to evaluate the brain malformation (mostly partial or complete callosal agenesis).

Treatment

- Trigonocephaly is not self-correcting with age, and patients with otherwise normal head growth should have cranial vault reshaping surgery to correct the abnormality for cosmetic reasons but possibly also for allowing optimal mental development.
- The need for surgery is more obvious when there is marked deformity.
- Surgery is usually performed at 6 to 9 months of age.

PEARLS_____

- Abnormal head shape at birth does not necessarily mean that the child has craniosynostosis.
- Craniosynostosis generally presents a progressive deformity. However, sometimes clinical differentiation can be difficult.
- A karyotype is needed in any patient with craniosynostosis, mental retardation, and minor abnormalities.

PITFALLS_____

- In normal individuals an endocranial ridge is usually seen in the region of the metopic suture. An endocranial metopic notch occurs in nearly all cases of premature metopic fusion.
- An ectocranial ridge at the site of the suture is seen in the majority of patients with metopic synostosis; however, it is also seen in 10 to 25% of nonsynostotic patients. There is a need for CT to diagnose true craniosynostosis.

Suggested Readings

Azimi C, Kennedy SJ, Chitayat D, et al. Clinical and genetic aspects of trigonocephaly: a study of 25 cases. Am J Med Genet A 2003;117:127–135

Lajeunie E, Le Merrer M, Marchac D, Renier D. Syndromal and nonsyndromal primary trigonocephaly: analysis of a series of 237 patients. Am J Med Genet 1998;75:211–215

Weinzweig J, Kirschner R, Farley A, et al. Metopic synostosis: defining the temporal sequence of normal suture fusion and differentiating it from synostosis on the basis of computed tomography images. Plast Reconstr Surg 2003;112:1211–1218

Zumpano MP, Carson BS, Marsh JL, Vanderkolk CA, Richtsmeier JT. Three dimensional morphological analysis of isolated metopic synostosis. Anat Rec 1999;256:177–188

CASE 15

Clinical Presentation

An 8-month-old baby presents with anorectal malformation and sensori-motor deficit of the lower extremities.

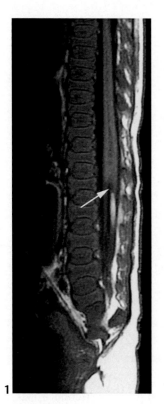 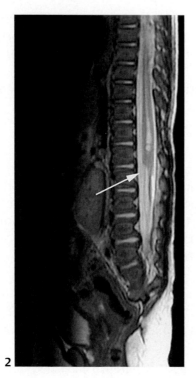 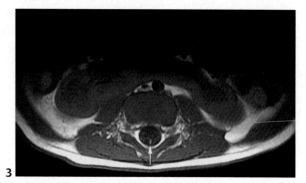

Figure 15A

Radiologic Findings

The sagittal T1-weighted (**Fig. 15A1**) and T2-weighted (**Fig. 15A2**) MRI demonstrates agenesis of the lower sacrum and coccyx. The caudal spinal cord is dysplastic and wedge-shaped (arrow). This is due to the agenesis of the conus, which is metamerically consistent with the missing spine. There also is hydrosyringomyelia, and a lipoma of the filum terminale is noted (arrow) (**Figs. 15A1** and **15A3**). The axial T1-weighted MRI (**Fig. 15A3**) demonstrates a horseshoe kidney.

Diagnosis

Partial sacral agenesis, which is part of the so-called caudal regression syndrome

Differential Diagnosis

- The terms *sacral agenesis,* or *lumbosacral agenesis,* or *thoracolumbosacral agenesis* (which are different degrees of the same defect) are purely descriptive and speak for themselves. The term *caudal regression syndrome* refers to a pathophysiology, which is only a postulate.
- The "hemisacral agenesis," or "scimitar sacrum," is a sacral defect typically related to an anterior-lateral sacral meningocele. The expansion of the meningocele generates scalloping and lateral displacement of the sacral plate, but the sacral segments are present. The association of a scimitar sacrum, a presacral mass (meningocele or lipomeningocele, or teratoma), and ano-rectal malformation makes up the Currarino syndrome.
- Sacral agenesis without spinal cord agenesis, or with tethered cord. The lower spine is lacking, whereas the cord is located below L1, its lower end being tapered instead of wedge-shaped. Although included in the group of caudal regression syndrome, this malformation may be a different entity, in which only the lower vertebral development is affected.
- Other scalloping and deformity of the caudal spine may result from malformations primarily of the cord (terminal lipoma, terminal myelocystocele).
- When the lower spine is off-midline, a false image of distal sacral agenesis is generated.

Discussion

Background

Caudal regression syndrome is a rare congenital defect, characterized by the absence of the caudal-most vertebrae and spinal cord. The defect may affect the caudal sacrum only, or it may extend upward as far as the thoracic spine, with functional defects and associated malformations in proportion with the extent of the agenesis. It may be associated with a fusion, and posterior rotation, of the lower limbs ("mermaid" appearance or sirenomelia). Other visceral malformations, especially of the pelvic organs, are common. The pathogenesis of the disorder is poorly understood. Maternal diabetes is a common factor, and insulin in excess has been shown to generate a similar malformation in the chick embryo. The role of segmentation gene defects is likely as well, as it is in other segmental spinal dysgeneses.

Embryology

Embryology holds that the cord and spine develop from two different, successive steps. The first is *primary neurulation* (week 4), in which the surface ectoderm differentiates into a neural plate that becomes a neural groove and a neural tube over which the surface ectoderm fuses again. This makes up most of the CNS, from the forebrain to the metameric level S2. Then (week 5) the totipotential caudal cell mass caudal to S2 keeps growing and differentiates to produce the terminal spine and cord, the perineum, and part of the pelvic organs (especially the structures derived from the primitive cloaca). This second step, or *secondary neurulation,* includes the development of a transient tail, which regresses secondarily to leave the coccyx and the filum terminale as residues but also the functional cord segments S3, S4, and S5, as well as the conus proper.

The caudal regression syndrome has been assumed to result from an excessive regression that could extend to the upper sacral, the lumbar, or even the thoracic levels. Yet this hypothesis does not take into account the fact that the regression is not supposed to involve the product of the primary neurulation, that is, the spine and cord above S2. It is therefore more likely that the absence of caudal spine and cord be related to a destructive/dysgenetic process, or to a defect of the segmentation genes. The former is consistent with the fact that a major etiology of the malformation is maternal diabetes; the latter would be consistent with the more general syndrome of segmental ageneses of the spine and cord.

Because the perineum and portions of the pelvic organs develop from the same caudal cell mass as the distal spine and cord, malformations of the sphincters, of the cloaca-derived structures, and of the bladder are commonly associated with sacral agenesis. Because the terminal cord is agenetic, the corresponding metameric levels are not innervated, and fatty metaplasia of the muscles occurs. The sensorimotor defect affects motor functions more extensively than the sensory function.

Pathology

In caudal regression syndrome the distal spine is lacking. The last vertebra present is usually limited to its center, with stenosis of the residual canal. If the sacral plate is entirely absent, the iliac bones rotate posteriorly and join in the midline, with everted hips; the feet face backward. Fusion of the lower limbs results in the mermaid or sirenomelia. The agenesis of the spine may extend as much as to the thoracic segment.

The spinal cord is partially absent as well, the agenesis being metamerically consistent with the agenesis of the spine (that is, the last roots present fit the level of the last complete vertebra). Its lower end is blunt and wedge-shaped, without the usual tapering of the conus. A filum may or may not be apparent.

The muscles below the metameric level of the cord agenesis are not innervated and present as fatty masses. As a consequence the vascular tree is poor, which may compromise future surgery to provide axial stability to the patient.

Histology

Besides the absence of the terminal segment of the cord, the cord tissue may be dysplastic. Fusion of the sacral roots and/or of the sensory ganglia may be present.

Clinical Findings

The clinical consequences of the disorder relate to the *cord defect* (neurological deficit), to the *spine defect* (axial stability), and to the *associated visceral malformations*. Obviously, all are proportional to the extent of the agenesis. Minor signs are clubfeet and minor distal muscle weakness. Sphincter dysfunction may be unrecognized for years and may result in neurogenic bladder. More patent perineal abnormalities usually lead to investigation of the lower spine, allowing for the diagnosis. The sensorimotor deficit may be massive, the motor defect being always more extensive than the sensory defect; this also leads to early radiologic evaluation. Extensive agenesis of the spine with instability and muscular fatty metaplasia is easily recognized clinically and makes the clinical diagnosis. Associated major malformations (sirenomelia, anal atresia, vesical extrophy, and malformed genitalia) can also be clinically identified.

Imaging Findings

RADIOGRAPHY

- Conventional radiography may demonstrate the extent of the spinal agenesis and the associated anomalies of the pelvic girdle.

ULTRASOUND

- Helpful to assess the viscera

CT

- CT of the spine, especially with 3D rendering, shows the extent of the vertebral and other skeletal abnormalities, and the fatty metaplasia of the muscles corresponding to the agenetic metameres.
- Can also show the associated visceral anomalies

MRI

- Method of choice for analysis of intraspinal findings
- In addition to other gross spinal column findings, a characteristic wedge-shaped cord terminus without a normal conus medullaris is typically seen.
- In this classic (thoraco) (lumbo) sacrococcygeal dysplasia, the end of the cord is located high in the spinal canal.
- Also depicts the atypical cases (such as the cord tethering) and allows a differential diagnosis from other spine and cord malformations.

Beyond making the diagnosis, imaging is needed to assess the extent of the defects and plan future surgery when possible.

Treatment

- If detected early, pregnancy termination can be offered. Standard prenatal care is not altered if continuation of pregnancy is opted for.
- If born alive, extensive surgery in the tertiary center is usually needed to repair the defects, mostly to ensure axial stability and compensate for sphincter anomalies.

PEARLS_____

- Wedge-shaped cord terminus is characteristic for caudal regression.
- About 10% of patients with (lumbo) sacral agenesis have OEIS (Omphalocele, cloacal Exstrophy, Imperforate anus, and Spinal deformities), and another 10% have VACTERL syndrome (Vertebral anomalies, Anorectal malformations, Cardiac malformations, TracheoEsophageal fistulae, Renal anomalies, and Limb anomalies).

PITFALLS_____

- Do not miss a subtle terminal agenesis of the cord in a patient with anomalies of the lower gastrointestinal or genitourinary system.
- On sagittal imaging, do not overread an off-plane distal spine for sacral agenesis.

Suggested Readings

Adra A, Cordero D, Mejides A, Yasin S, Salman F, O'Sullivan MJ. Caudal regression syndrome: etiopathogenesis, prenatal diagnosis and perinatal management. Obstet Gynecol Surv 1994;49:508–516

Barkovich AJ, Raghavan N, Chuang S, Peck WW. The wedge-shaped cord terminus: a radiographic sign of caudal regression. AJNR Am J Neuroradiol 1989;10:1223–1231

DeLaPaz RL. Congenital anomalies of the lumbosacral spine. Neuroimaging Clin N Am 1993;3:425–442

Julian D, Abbott UK. An avian model for comparative studies of insulin teratogenicity. Anat Histol Embryol 1998;27:313–321

Martucciello G, Torre M, Belloni E, et al. Currarino syndrome: proposal for a diagnostic and therapeutic protocol. J Pediatr Surg 2004;39:1305–1311

Nievelstein RAJ, Hartwig NG, Vermeij-Keers C, Valk J. Embryonic development of the mammalian neural tube. Teratology 1993;48:21–31

Nievelstein RAJ, Valk J, Smit LM, Vermeij-Keers C. MR of the caudal regression syndrome: embryologic implications. AJNR Am J Neuroradiol 1994;15:1021–1029

Tortori-Donati P, Fondelli MP, Rossi A, Raybaud CA, Cama A, Capra V. Segmental spinal dysgenesis: neuroradiologic findings with clinical and embryologic correlation. AJNR Am J Neuroradiol 1999;20:445–456

CASE 16

Clinical Presentation

A child presents following a motor vehicle accident (MVA). She was a backseat passenger.

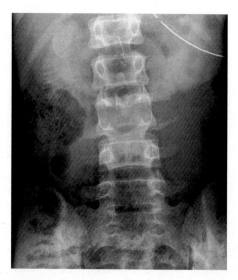

Figure 16A

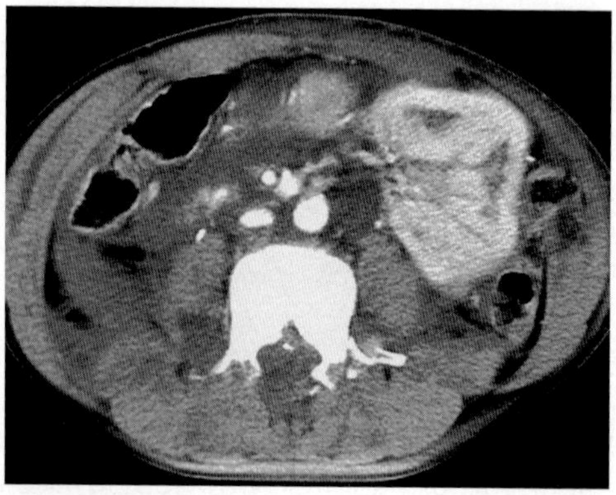

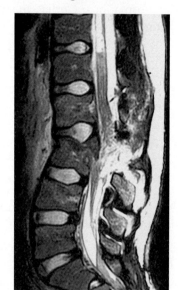

Figure 16B

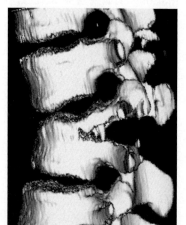

Figure 16C

Figure 16D

Radiologic Findings

The AP lumbar spine film (**Fig. 16A**) demonstrates an "empty vertebral body" due to the lack of a spinous process projecting over the vertebral body, and the diastatic fracture traversing both pedicles. The CT findings (**Fig. 16B**) show fluid in the abdomen, thickened bowel wall, and abnormal mesentery. There is blurring of the paraspinal muscle-fat planes by contusion and edema and "absent" (because dislocated) vertebral neural arch. CT surface rendering of the spine (**Fig. 16C**) shows anterior angulation of the spine centered on L3, and horizontal splitting of the vertebral body and bilateral diastasis of the pedicles. MRI sagittal T2-weighted image (**Fig. 16D**) demonstrates malformation of the cord with a low conus projecting at the L4–L5 level, laceration of the cord facing the vertebral transverse fracture, and probable laceration of the dura as well. There is rupture of the posterior elements (spinous process, interspinous ligament). There is another severe lesion of the cord (high T2 signal) located above the fracture (T12–L10), likely generated by a traction and avulsion of the cord trapped at the level of the fracture.

Diagnosis

Lap-belt or seat-belt fracture-dislocation. Also known as "fulcrum" or angular spinal fracture. Eponymous classification, for example, "Chance fracture" (see grading), relates to the type of posterior column injury.

Differential Diagnosis

- None: Clinical circumstances (traffic accident) and radiologic features are pathognomonic.

Discussion

Background

The combination of vertebral body wedge compression, facet subluxation and/or disruption, and anterior displacement of the spinal segment above the dislocation were described by G.Q. Chance, a British radiologist, in 1948. The association with lap-belt injury was noted later. Lap belts or 2-point lap restraints, are considered obsolete; however, they are still common for the middle passenger in the back seat. Similar injuries may result from a child wearing a 3-point restraint incorrectly as a 2-point restraint, or an unrestrained passenger being thrown over the front seat.

Etiology

Lap-belt restraints are associated with a variety of injuries in children, mainly bowel and upper lumbar spine, bur vascular injuries also occur. Two-point restraint seat belts tend to slip cephalad over the intended position across the anterior-superior iliac spines. The injury occurs as a result of flexion-distraction forces with the fulcrum centered in the anterior abdominal wall at the site of seat-belt contact. During deceleration MVAs, the fulcrum of flexion is moved to the anterior abdominal wall, resulting in distraction forces on the spine at the thoracolumbar junction.

The spine is divided into three columns: anterior, middle, and posterior. The anterior column includes the anterior spinal ligament, the anterior anulus fibrosus, and the intervertebral disk and anterior two-thirds of the vertebral body. The middle column includes the posterior aspect of the vertebral body, the posterior anulus fibrosus, and the posterior longitudinal ligament. The posterior column includes all structures posterior to the posterior longitudinal ligament. Injury to two or more columns is regarded as unstable. Lap-belt injures commonly cause disruption of all three columns and are, therefore, mechanically unstable. There is fracturing of the anterior spinal column, frequent anterior vertebral compression, horizontal fracture of the posterior column, and ventral shifting of the spinal column above the level of dislocation. Wedge compression, anterior displacement of the spine above the fracture, and facet subluxation are common features.

Clinical Findings

Clinically, lap-belt fractures are recognized by abdominal bruising or skin lacerations conforming to the shape of the seat belt. Clinical findings depend on the injuries presented. Abdominal and back pain are present in conscious patients. There is a variable degree of neural compromise, ranging from no neurologic findings to complete lower extremity paralysis as seen in our case, typically due to compression of the cauda equina. In the case described, the cord itself was low, and therefore more exposed to injury.

Associated Conditions

Seat-belt syndrome is present in nearly half of patients with lap-belt fractures. These include abdominal injuries (aortic rupture, hollow viscera injury, mesenteric tear) with vertebral injury and abdominal wall ecchymosis.

Pathology

Findings are of varying combinations of disrupted ligaments, vertebral disks, and fractures, with contusion and laceration of the cord or avulsion of the roots of the cauda equina.

Developmental Stages

Pure dislocations involving the intervertebral disk and ligaments in the absence of fractures are more common in the immature spine.

Grading

- **Posterior ligament disruption (pure dislocation):** This may occur as a purely ligamentous injury, or it may be associated with avulsion of the intervertebral disk, common in childhood.
- **Chance fracture:** The fracture line extends through the spinous process, pedicles, transverse processes, and up through the posterior superior corner of the vertebral body and through the intervertebral disk.
- **Horizontal fissure fracture (fulcrum fracture):** The fracture line extends horizontally through, and splits the vertebral body. Older patients with brittle bones are more likely to get this fracture type.
- **Smith fracture:** The superior articular processes and a small posterior fragment of the vertebral body are included with the posterior arch fracture. The spinous process is intact, but the interspinous and supraspinous ligaments are torn.

Imaging Findings

RADIOGRAPHY

- The AP radiograph typically shows an "empty vertebra" resulting from widening of the interspinous distance at the fracture and displacement of the spinous process.
- The lateral view may show the fracture line, splaying of the posterior elements due to disruption of the posterior interspinous ligaments and jumped or perched facet joints.
- There may be wedge compression of the anterior aspect of the vertebra.
- Signs of bowel injury, free intraperitoneal or focal bowel dilatation and thickening, may be seen on the abdominal film.

CT

- CT is modality of choice in fracture identification and depiction.

- The site of fracture on axial images is commonly marked by a paravertebral hematoma and edema.
- The actual fracture line is often in the same plane as the axial images and difficult to see; therefore, thin sections (1–3 mm) with sagittal and coronal reformats are mandatory.
- 3D reconstructions are useful.
- The fracture may pass through the disk, facet joints, and spinous ligaments without a bony fracture. Alternatively, the fracture line may pass through the posterior spinous process, articular processes, or vertebral body; the facet joints are often disrupted and may be jumped or perched.

MRI

- MRI is the best modality to demonstrate ligamentous and spinal cord injury.
- Sagittal T2-weighted fat-saturated images display edema of the fractured vertebral body, blood, high signal within injured ligaments, and edema within the cord if it is injured.
- Compression and laceration can be caused at the time of injury by displaced spinal elements, which may go back in place.
- The compression may also be associated with a herniated disk or retropulsed bone fragments. Gradient echo images are useful to demonstrate hemorrhage.
- Areas damaged by intramedullary hematoma and laceration will not recover function.
- Imaging should include the whole abdomen due to the high risk of intra-abdominal injury.
- Bowel injury is likely if there is free intraperitoneal air. Findings may be subtle, for example, focal bowel wall thickening, mesenteric hematoma, and free fluid limited to the site of injury.

Treatment

- Immobilization is required.
- Choice of closed reduction versus spinal instrumentation depends on the stability of the spinal column.
- If there is no associated neurologic injury, treatment is aimed at correcting the kyphotic deformity with traction and stabilization. However, if there is spinal cord compression, emergency decompression is required.
- Steroids may be used to treat spinal cord edema.

Prognosis

- Neurologic injury is common. Fifteen percent of survivors have permanent neural injury.
- Prognosis is dependent on the degree of neurologic compromise.

Complications

- The cord normally terminates at T12/L1; therefore, associated injury at this level results in bladder and bowel dysfunction, paralysis, and lumbosacral plexopathy.
- Belt fractures may be associated with injury to the large and small bowel, mesentery, pancreas, bladder, and aorta.
- Visceral injury may be life-threatening, and diagnosis is crucial in determining immediate management.
- Late mechanical or neurologic deterioration and kyphosis from a missed dislocation may occur.

PEARLS_____

- Seat-belt fracture, with associated intra-abdominal injury, should be considered in all patients with bruising associated with wearing a lap belt.
- Look for an "empty vertebral body" on AP abdominal and lumbar spine plain films.

PITFALLS

- Dislocations may be "relocated" prior to imaging. Always look for paraspinal soft tissue swelling and edema, even when the plain films of the spine appear normal.
- Fracture lines may be difficult to see on CT axial images. Thin-section imaging with sagittal and coronal reformats should be performed.
- Associated soft tissue injuries may be life-threatening.

Suggested Readings

Beaunoyer M, St-Vil D, Lallier M, et al. Abdominal injuries associated with thoracolumbar fractures after motor vehicle collision. J Pediatr Surg 2001;36:760–762

Brant-Zawadzki M, Jeffrey RB Jr, Minagi H, Pitts LH. High resolution CT of thoracolumbar fracture. AJR Am J Roentgenol 1982;138:699–704

Griffet J, Bastiani-Griffet F, El-Hayek T, Dageville C, Pebeyre B. Management of seat-belt syndrome in children: gravity of 2-point seat-belt. Eur J Pediatr Surg 2002;12:63–66

Neumann P, Osvalder AL, Nordwall A, Lovsund P, Hansson T. The ultimate flexural strength of the lumbar spine and vertebral bone mineral content. J Spinal Disord 1993;6:314–323

Rogers LF. The roentgenographic appearance of transverse or Chance fractures of the spine: the seat-belt fracture. Am J Roentgenol Radium Ther Nucl Med 1971;111:844–849

Rumball K, Jarvis J. Seat-belt injuries of the spine in young children. J Bone Joint Surg Br 1992;74:571–574

Sivit CJ, Taylor GA, Newman KD, et al. Safety-belt injuries in children with lapbelt ecchymosis: CT findings in 61 patients. AJR Am J Roentgenol 1991;157:111–114

SECTION II
Head and Neck

SECTION 4

Head and Neck

CASE 17

Clinical Presentation

A 4-year-old female presents with right eye swelling and is unable to open her eyelid. She has mild right proptosis.

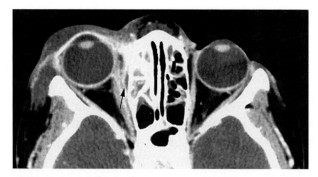

Figure 17A

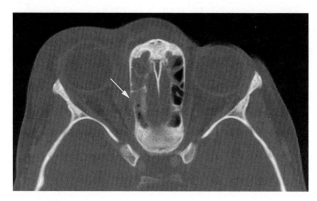

Figure 17C

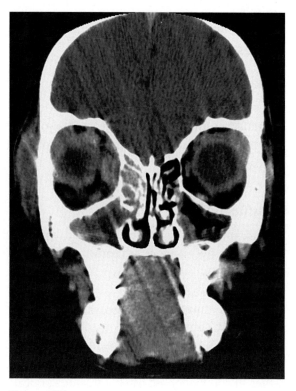

Figure 17B

Radiologic Findings

Axial contrast-enhanced CT image through the orbits at the level of the mid globes shows right preseptal soft tissue swelling with preseptal cellulitis and proptosis of the globe (**Fig. 17A**). This cellulitis also extends laterally along the superficial soft tissues of the temporal region of the face. Extensive ethmoid sinusitis (mucosal enhancement and thickening) is present. There is a small, lentiform subperiosteal fluid collection, with enhancing rim at the medial aspect of the right orbital wall (**Fig. 17A**, arrow). No intraconal fat stranding is present. On the contrast-enhanced coronal image of the orbits through the midposterior globe, the extent of the subperiosteal fluid collection, with enhancing rim, is better appreciated, as is its relationship to the lamina papyracea and the laterally deviated, slightly thickened medial rectus muscle (**Fig. 17B**). This fluid collection is adjacent to the lamina papyracea, which has undergone focal disruption (**Fig. 17C**, arrow).

Diagnosis

Subperiosteal orbital abscess

Differential Diagnosis

- Orbital pseudotumor
- Pediatric rhabdomyosarcoma of the orbit

Discussion

Background

The clinical diagnosis of orbital and periorbital infections mandates a thorough history, physical examination, and ophthalmologic evaluation. CT scanning assists in the diagnosis of orbital infections and their complications. Demonstration of orbital and/or subperiosteal abscess mandates surgical drainage.

Classification

Orbital infections have been classified with a widely accepted system proposed by Chandler et al (1970). This five-stage classification system of worsening infections and prognosis is as follows:

Stage I: Periorbital cellulitis
Stage II: Orbital cellulitis
Stage III: Subperiosteal abscess
Stage IV: Orbital abscess
Stage V: Cavernous sinus thrombosis (and other intracranial complications that are generally placed in this category)

Stages III and higher are usually treated surgically, with accompanying antimicrobial therapy, usually by empiric intravenous antibiotics, followed by oral antibiotics. Stages I and II are usually treated with antibiotics alone and are followed to ensure resolution.

Etiology

Subperiosteal orbital abscess is often due to bacterial infection that extends from adjacent paranasal sinus disease, usually the ethmoid sinus with its relatively thin lamina papyracea. Periostitis of the lateral sinus wall (medial wall of the orbit) occurs with sinus infection, and the wall can become eroded and disrupted, allowing purulent material to accumulate along the medial orbital wall. Initially, the pus is contained away from ocular muscles and intraconal space by the tough fibrous periosteum but can progress to frank intraorbital abscess.

Infection may also arise from the face, lacrimal sac, nose, or teeth and spread to the sinuses and orbits via the anterior and posterior emissary veins, which drain the face as they lack valves. Bacteremia is readily transmitted to the orbit via these emissary veins, and this can lead to cellulitis and abscess.

Pathology

Inflammatory cells, fibrous tissue, and necrotic debris along with the offending microorganism(s) are characteristics of orbital subperiosteal abscess. Mixed organisms are common, with staphylococci, streptococci, and pneumococci being most prevalent. Occasionally, anaerobes and *Haemophilus influenzae* (decreasing trend due to widespread H influenza type B vaccination) are seen. Laboratory findings show increased white blood cells with a left shift.

Imaging Findings

CT

- The CT imaging appearance depends on disease duration and course of the infection.
- Imaging early on may show an enhancing space-occupying lesion that is poorly defined and unorganized along the inner orbital wall, in keeping with a phlegmon. With time, this appearance may progress to a more organized abscess, with fluid collection centrally and periosteal elevation.
- The coronal imaging plane allows better appreciation of the extent of the intraorbital processes, in the craniocaudal dimension. The location of the abscess relative to other intraorbital structures and paranasal sinuses can be seen well in this plane.
- Other CT features include:
  - Rim-enhancing fluid density collection along orbital wall
  - Adjacent sinusitis, usually ethmoid (enhancing thickened soft tissues in sinus cavity)
  - Dehiscent sinus wall
  - Gas within fluid collection may be present
  - Proptosis of the globe, which can be deviated downward as well
  - May have swelling of the adjacent extraocular muscles

MRI

- Generally not necessary for diagnosis, but is very useful for determining the presence and extent of complications, such as cerebritis, cerebral abscess, meningitis, subdural empyema, and venous sinus thrombosis
- MRI is not particularly useful for bone changes or for assessing gas-containing areas.
- The multiplanar capability of MRI aids in diagnosis and accurate size measurement of intracranial abscesses or empyemas.
- T1-weighted contrast-enhanced images show rim-enhancing fluid collection adjacent to the sinus, within the orbit.
- T2-weighted images show increased signal intensity within fluid collection and sinus changes consistent with sinusitis.

Treatment

- Surgical drainage and debridement, usually via functional endoscopic sinus surgery
- Open sinus surgery is utilized less commonly, but may be needed in cases where the endoscopic instruments are not able to access the region of interest.
- Concomitant broad-spectrum antibiotics, usually intravenous, are then orally administered.

Prognosis

- Excellent in most cases, with the combination of antimicrobial therapy and drainage
- Poorer prognosis if it progresses to frank intraorbital abscess

Complications

- If untreated, or treatment is delayed, the infection may progress to optic nerve ischemia, with impaired visual acuity or blindness.

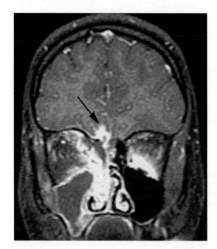

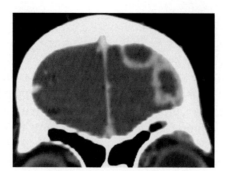

Figure   17D Coronal   T1-weighted, gadolinium-enhanced image at the level of the posterior orbit shows disruption of the bony floor of the right anterior cranial fossa, with loss of the black cortical line. There is sinusitis of the right ethmoidal and maxillary sinuses. A small, parasagittal, low-signal intensity collection, similar in signal intensity to the right maxillary and ethmoid sinuses, shows peripheral enhancement and extends through the aforementioned bone defect. This is a small, subdural abscess collection, also known as a subdural empyema (arrow).

Figure 17E Two lobulated, rim-enhancing complex subdural fluid collections along the left frontal lobe are present on the enhanced, coronal CT scan at the level of the frontal sinuses in a different patient. These are loculations of a subdural empyema. The extent of the empyema may be quite removed from the sinuses.

- Intracranial complications can occur if the infection extends via dehiscent bones or vascular or neural foramina. Sinus thrombosis, cerebritis, cerebral abscess, meningitis, and subdural empyema are the major intracranial complications (**Figs. 17D** and **17E**).
- Chronic sinusitis, chronic orbital infection, and osteomyelitis may occur in partially treated disease.

PEARLS_____

- Lentiform rim-enhancing fluid collection along orbital wall with associated bony dehiscence and adjacent sinusitis
- Most orbital abscesses are caused by adjacent ethmoid sinusitis. If sinus disease is not present, look for a foreign body and ask about a history of trauma.

PITFALLS_____

- Imaging at a stage prior to the organization of the abscess may lead to underdiagnosing subperiosteal infection. This may lead to the use of only antibiotics and not surgical drainage, which may be unsuccessful at eradicating infection, leading to chronic infection or complications.
- CT scanning may be somewhat limited in the discrimination of different soft tissue densities in acute infection.

Suggested Readings

Arjmand EM, Lusk RP, Muntz HR. Pediatric sinusitis and subperiosteal orbital abscess formation: diagnosis and treatment. Otolaryngol Head Neck Surg 1993;109:886–894

Chandler JR, Langenbrunner DJ, Stevens ER. The pathogenesis or orbital complications in acute sinusitis. Laryngoscope 1970;80:1414–1428

Younis RT, Lazar RH, Bustillo A, Anand VK. Orbital infection as a complication of sinusitis: are diagnostic and treatment trends changing? Ear Nose Throat J 2002;81:771–775

CASE 18

Clinical Presentation

A 16-year-old adolescent male presents with right-sided nasal obstruction and epistaxis.

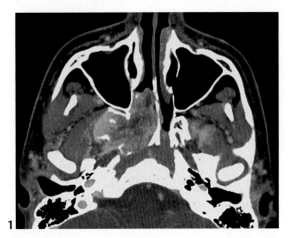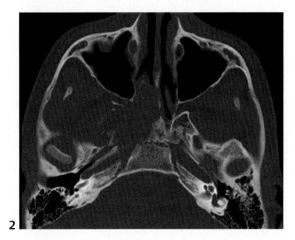

Figure 18A

Radiologic Findings

Axial CT, soft tissue (**Fig. 18A1**) and bone (**Fig. 18A2**) windows, at the level of the maxillary sinus show characteristic features of juvenile nasopharyngeal angiofibroma. There is an enhancing mass expanding and extending into the posterior nasal air space with erosion of the base of the right pterygoid plate and lateral extension to the infratemporal fossa.

Diagnosis

Juvenile nasopharyngeal angiofibroma

Differential Diagnosis

- Other causes of nasal mass lesions, for example, antrochoanal polyp, nasal polyp, encephalocele, and other rare neoplasms: inverted papilloma, squamous cell carcinoma, adenocarcinoma, esthesioblastoma, rhabdomyosarcoma
- Other causes of orbital swelling or proptosis
- Other causes of epistaxis, either local or systemic

Discussion

Background

Juvenile angiofibroma is the most common benign nasopharyngeal tumor; nevertheless, it is uncommon and accounts for only 0.05% of all head and neck neoplasms. An incidence of 1:5000 to 1:60,000 in otolaryngology patients has been reported. This tumor was described by Hippocrates, but the term *angiofibroma* was first used by Friedberg in 1940 to describe this fibrovascular tumor. It occurs almost exclusively in prepubertal and adolescent males. The age range is 7 to 20 years, median 15 years, and hence the lesion is referred to frequently as juvenile angiofibroma. The male gender predilection is so typical that some authors suggest chromosomal analysis in the rare instance it occurs in females. This is a highly vascular tumor, and severe bleeding may accompany biopsy. For this reason, surgeons are reluctant to undertake biopsy of a nasopharyngeal mass in an adolescent male patient and prefer to rely on imaging methods for deciding whether the mass is likely to be an angiofibroma or a nonvascular lesion such as an antrochoanal polyp.

Staging Systems

Different staging systems exist for nasopharyngeal angiofibroma. The two most commonly used systems for treatment planning and prognosis are those of Sessions and of Fisch.

- Classification according to Sessions:
    - Stage IA: Tumor limited to posterior nares and/or nasopharyngeal vault
    - Stage IB: Tumor involving posterior nares and/or nasopharyngeal vault with involvement of at least one paranasal sinus
    - Stage IIA: Minimal lateral extension into pterygomaxillary fossa
    - Stage IIB: Full occupation of pterygomaxillary fossa with or without superior erosion of orbital bones
    - Stage IIIA: Erosion of skull base (i.e., middle cranial fossa/pterygoid base), minimal intracranial extension
    - Stage IIIB: Extensive intracranial extension with or without extension into cavernous sinus
- Classification according to Fisch:
    - Stage I: Tumors limited to nasal cavity, nasopharynx with no bony destruction
    - Stage II: Tumors invading pterygomaxillary fossa, paranasal sinuses with bony destruction
    - Stage III: Tumors invading infratemporal fossa, orbit, and/or parasellar region remaining lateral to cavernous sinus
    - Stage IV: Tumors invading cavernous sinus, optic chiasmal region, and/or pituitary fossa

Etiology

The vast majority of angiofibromas originate from the pterygopalatine fossa in the recess behind the sphenopalatine ganglion at the anterior aperture of the pterygoid canal (Lloyd et al, 1999).

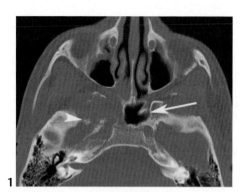
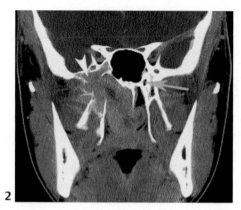

Figure 18B Axial (**1**) and coronal (**2**) CT show an enhancing mass invading and expanding the base of the right pterygoid process. There is extension along the line of the pterygoid canal (normal contralateral side indicated by arrow) with invasion of the greater wing of the sphenoid sinus (arrowhead). There is involvement of the right lateral wall of the sphenoid sinus. The mass extends into the nasal cavity, crossing the midline to involve the contralateral side.

The cause of this tumor remains unclear. Suggested theories include a hormonal theory due to the lesion's occurrence in adolescent males; a desmoplastic response of the nasopharyngeal periosteum or the embryonic fibrocartilage between the basiocciput and the basisphenoid; and origin from nonchromaffin paraganglionic cells of the terminal branches of the maxillary artery.

Clinical Findings

Symptoms of angiofibromas are numerous and nonspecific. Epistaxis (either severe or blood stained, mostly unilateral and recurrent) and nasal obstruction are the most common symptoms. There must be a high index of suspicion of this neoplasm in any prepubertal or adolescent male with a nasal mass lesion and either of these two symptoms. Other symptoms include:

- Headache, especially if paranasal sinuses are blocked
- Swelling of cheek and trismus denotes spread to the infratemporal fossa.
- Unilateral rhinorrhea, anosmia, rhinolalia (nasal speech) from the nasal mass
- Deafness or otalgia from eustachian tube blockage
- Proptosis and optic nerve atrophy from involvement of orbital fissures
- Decreasing vision due to optic nerve tenting has been reported rarely.

Pathology

Nasopharyngeal angiofibroma is a sessile, lobulated mass, and rarely the tumor is polypoid or pedunculated. The texture of the mass is rubbery and is often observed as a red-pink to tan-gray.

Histology

- Encapsulated and composed of vascular tissue and fibrous stroma with coarse or fine collagen fibers
- Vessels are thin-walled, lack elastic fibers, have absent or incomplete smooth muscle, and can vary in appearance from stellate or staghorn to barely conspicuous due to stromal compression.

Imaging Findings

RADIOGRAPHY

- A soft tissue mass in the nasopharynx that resembles an antrochoanal polyp can be seen.
- The "antral sign": anterior bowing of the posterior wall of the maxillary sinus and maxillary sinus opacification is very suggestive of juvenile nasopharyngeal angiofibroma in an adolescent male;

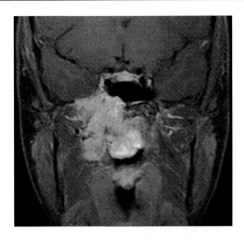

Figure 18C Coronal fat-saturated T1-weighted image postgadolinium of the same patient as **Fig. 18B**. This shows the vascular right nasopharyngeal mass protruding into the nasal cavity, involving the infratemporal fossa, and extending along the pterygoid muscles. There is involvement of the right lateral wall of the sphenoid sinus and extension to the right middle cranial fossa from involvement of the greater wing of sphenoid.

however, the sign is nonspecific and could be due to other slow-growing neoplasms such as a schwannoma.

CT

- CT has surpassed plain films in usefulness.
- Excellent for showing the osseous destruction characteristic of this locally aggressive tumor
- Characteristically shows two diagnostic features in virtually every patient:
  - Vividly enhancing mass lesion in nose and pterygopalatine fossa
  - Erosion of the bone behind the sphenopalatine foramen at the base of the medial pterygoid plate (**Figs. 18B1** and **18B2**)
- Other findings demonstrate the extent of the tumor:
  - Anterior growth occurs under the nasopharyngeal mucous membrane, displacing it anteriorly and inferiorly toward the postnasal space. Eventually, the nasal cavity is filled on one side, and the septum deviates to the other side.
  - Superior extension with erosion of the sphenoid sinus, and rarely involvement of the cavernous sinus. Of particular importance is the presence and extent of invasion of the sphenoid sinus as this is the main determinant of recurrence.
  - Lateral extension through the pterygomaxillary fissure into the infratemporal fossa
  - Orbital apex involvement via the infraorbital fissure, which can extend outside the muscle cone to involve the middle cranial fossa through the superior orbital fissure
  - Posterior growth along the line of the pterygoid canal invading and eroding the base of the pterygoid process. May progress to invasion and expansion of the diploë of the body and the greater wing of the sphenoid and, in some patients, invasion of the middle cranial fossa

MRI

- Excellent for showing the preoperative extension of angiofibroma; fat-saturated, postgadolinium sequences are especially useful (**Fig. 18C**).
- MRI characteristic features are due to the high vascularity of the tumor causing signal voids—"salt and pepper" appearance on T1 images and strong postcontrast enhancement.
- Helps define the presence and extent of invasion of the sphenoid—the main determinant of recurrence.
- Plays a vital role in postoperative surveillance: to show any residual or recurrent tumor, record tumor growth or natural involution, and monitor the effects of radiotherapy.

ANGIOGRAPHY

- Angiography shows the branches of the external carotid system to be the primary feeders.
- The main supply comes from the internal maxillary artery, but ascending pharyngeal or vidian arteries may contribute to the blood supply.
- Unnamed branches from the internal carotid artery contribute to vascularity in rare instances.

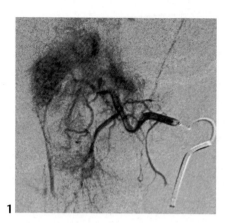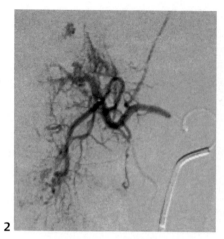

Figure 18D Preoperative embolization of right nasopharyngeal angiofibroma. Selective internal maxillary artery angiogram, lateral view, shows extensive tumor vascularity pre-embolization (**1**). Following embolization with contour particles (150–250 μm in size), there was a significant reduction in tumor vascularity (**2**).

Treatment

- Many modalities have been used for management of nasopharyngeal angiofibromas, including sclerosing agents, cryotherapy, hormonal therapy, and preoperative embolization by particulate embolic agents.
- The only techniques that appear to allow effective tumor control are external beam radiation and surgery with or without preoperative embolization.
- Surgery is the "gold standard" treatment for this tumor. The aim of surgery is complete resection with minimal morbidity and blood loss in accordance with the principles of en bloc resection for cancer surgery. The surgical approach must be tailored to tumor stage, location, and extension.
- Whether preoperative embolization predisposes to later recurrence is unclear, and conflicting opinion exists regarding the value of preoperative embolization. Embolization, perhaps paradoxically, appears to be contraindicated when there is deep invasion of the pterygoid base as tumor shrinkage may result in tumor being inaccessible to the surgeon, thus making recurrence likely. Other authors favor embolization in most cases. Intracranial extension of tumor appears to be an undisputed indication for embolization in most centers (**Figs. 18D1** and **18D2**).
- External beam radiation therapy is reserved for patients who present with unresectable intracranial disease or refuse surgery for any reason.
- Management of recurrence is controversial. Repeat surgery in association with external beam radiation therapy for uncontrolled tumors may be necessary.

Prognosis

- Recurrence is a major problem and a conspicuous feature of angiofibromas, with rates reported from 25 to 40%.
- Half of recurrences are within the first 12 months of surgery.
- Recurrence typically occurs at the initial site of origin or within the sphenoid, characteristically causing expansion of the pterygoid base and greater wing of the sphenoid sinus.
- Patients identified by CT with a high risk of tumor recurrence require early imaging surveillance 3 to 4 months after surgery.

Complications

- Excessive bleeding can occur. With improvement in diagnostic imaging techniques and preoperative embolization, the need for blood transfusion has been greatly reduced.

- Malignant transformation has been reported in six cases; five of these patients were treated with radiotherapy.
- Cranial nerve palsies have been rarely reported as a result of embolization.
- Osteoradionecrosis and/or blindness due to optic nerve damage may occur due to radiotherapy.
- Fistula of the palate at the junction of the soft and hard palate may occur with the transpalatal approach but is prevented by preservation of the greater palatine vessels during flap elevation.
- Anesthesia of the cheek is a frequent occurrence with the Weber-Ferguson incision.

PEARLS

- CT is excellent for showing the osseous destruction and characteristically shows the two primary diagnostic features in virtually every patient:
  - Vividly enhancing mass lesion in nose and pterygopalatine fossa
  - Erosion of the bone behind the sphenopalatine foramen at the base of the medial ptergoid plate
- MRI and CT are excellent for showing the preoperative extension.
- MRI plays a vital role in postoperative surveillance.

PITFALL

- Delineation of the presence and extent of invasion of the sphenoid is vital as this is the main determinant of recurrence.

Suggested Readings

Beham A, Kainz J, Stammberger H, Aubock L, Beham-Schmid C. Immunohistochemical and electron microscopical characterization of stromal cells in nasopharyngeal angiofibromas. Eur Arch Otorhinolaryngol 1997;254:196–199

Chagnaud C, Petit P, Bartoli J, et al. Postoperative follow-up of juvenile nasopharyngeal angiofibromas: assessment by CT scan and MR imaging. Eur Radiol 1998;8:756–764

Cummings BJ, Blend R, Keane T. Primary radiation therapy for juvenile nasopharyngeal angiofibroma. Laryngoscope 1984;94:1599–1605

Fagan JJ, Snyderman CH, Carrau RL, Janecka IP. Nasopharyngeal angiofibromas: selecting a surgical approach. Head Neck 1997;19:391–399

Friedberg SA. Vascular fibroma of the nasophargnx (nasopharyngeal fibroma). Arch Otolaryngol 1940;31:313–326

Howard DJ, Lloyd G, Lund V. Recurrence and its avoidance in juvenile angiofibroma. Laryngoscope 2001;111:1509–1511

Lasjaunias P. Nasopharyngeal angiofibromas: hazards of embolization. Radiology 1980;136:119–123

Lloyd G, Howard D, Lund VJ, Savy L. Imaging for juvenile angiofibroma. J Laryngol Otol 2000;114:727–730

Lloyd G, Howard D, Phelps P, Cheesman A. Juvenile angiofibroma: the lessons of 20 years of modern imaging. J Laryngol Otol 1999;113:127–134

Makek MS, Andrews JC, Fisch U. Malignant transformation of a nasopharyngeal angiofibroma. Laryngoscope 1989;99(10 Pt 1):1088–1092

Mann WJ, Jecker P, Amedee RG. Juvenile angiofibromas: changing surgical concept over the last 20 years. Laryngoscope 2004;114:291–293

Tewfik TL, Tan AK, al Noury K, et al. Juvenile nasopharyngeal angiofibroma. J Otolaryngol 1999;28:145–151

Ward PH. The evolving management of juvenile nasopharyngeal angiofibroma. J Laryngol Otol Suppl 1983;8:103–104

CASE 19

Clinical Presentation

A 4-year-old boy presents with nasal obstruction.

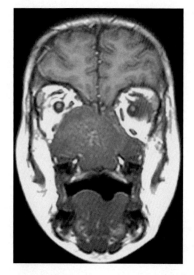

Figure 19A

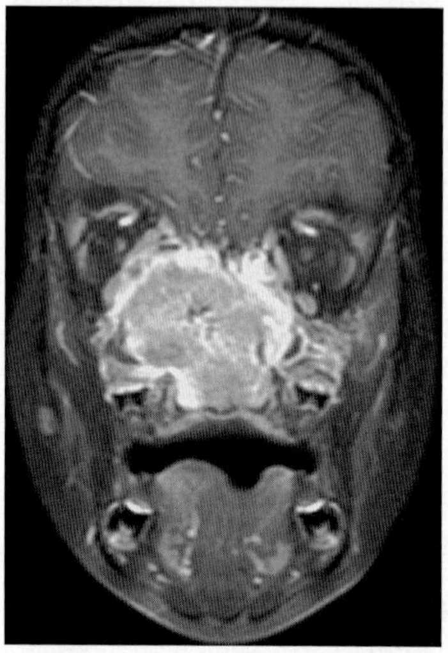

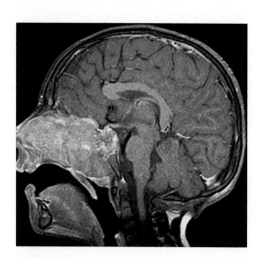

Figure 19B

Figure 19C

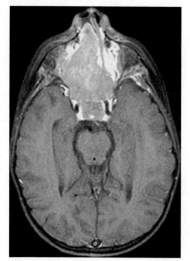

Figure 19D

Radiologic Findings

There is a huge soft tissue mass with malignant features centered in the nasopharynx. Unenhanced T1-weighted coronal image (**Fig. 19A**) shows a slightly hyperintense to muscle mass filling the nasal cavities and infiltrating the medial aspects of both orbits, greater on the right than on the left. Following contrast there is intense heterogeneous enhancement, as shown on the corresponding coronal fat-suppressed T1-weighted image (**Fig. 19B**). Sagittal and axial fat-suppressed, contrast-enhanced, T1-weighted images (**Figs. 19C** and **19D**) better show its extent. Anteriorly it involves both nasal cavities. There is destruction of part of the nasal septum, and the residual septum is displaced to the left. The tumor extends into the medial maxillary sinuses, whereas posteriorly it involves the clivus. Superiorly the cavernous sinus is infiltrated, displacing the carotid arteries laterally. It also involves the frontal bone and adjacent dura.

Diagnosis

Rhabdomyosarcoma

Differential Diagnosis

- Benign tumors, including teratoma, lymphangioma, neurofibroma, juvenile angiofibroma
- Malignant tumors, especially neuroblastoma, fibrosarcomas, malignant fibrous histiocytoma

Discussion

Background

Most masses in the pediatric head and neck are benign, consisting primarily of congenital, developmental, or inflammatory lesions. Malignant tumors are less common in children, but 35% of all pediatric sarcomas manifest in the head and neck region. The rhabdomyosarcoma family is the most common soft tissue malignancy encountered in childhood. Rhabdomyosarcoma is essentially a disease of childhood and young adults. There is a bimodal age distribution, with one peak during childhood and another peak during adolescence. Most arise before age 12 years. There is a slight male predominance.

Rhabdomyosarcomas are thought to arise from primitive mesenchymal tissue expressing myogenic (skeletal muscle) differentiation, probably satellite cells associated with skeletal muscle embryogenesis. They can develop in any part of the body, including those not containing muscle, with the exception of bone (to which it commonly metastasizes). Rhabdomyosarcomas can spread by direct extension and may erode directly through bone or extend through skull-base foramina via a perineural spread to produce epidural masses with occasional meningeal involvement. They also may extend along lymphatic vessels to lymph nodes or hematogeneously to lung, liver, bone, and bone marrow.

Classification of sarcomas according to anatomic location in the head and neck is helpful because of the influence of location on presentation and disease management. Common locations include orbital (**Figs. 19E1** and **19E2**), parameningeal, or nonparameningeal sites. Parameningeal sites are the most common locations and have a poorer prognosis. These sites include the middle ear, nasal cavity, paranasal sinuses, nasopharynx, and infratemporal fossa. Nonparameningeal regions include the parotid gland, oral cavity, oropharynx, hypopharynx, larynx, thyroid/parathyroid, and neck. Staging depends on local extension, regional and distant metastases, and amount of residual tumor remaining after surgical resection.

Etiology

The etiology of rhabdomyosarcoma is uncertain, but genetic factors may contribute to its development. Embryonal rhabdomyosarcomas show consistent loss of heterozygosity or loss of imprinting at a specific locus on the short arm of chromosome 11, whereas alveolar rhabdomyosarcomas have two distinct translocations, either *PAX3-FKHR* or *PAX7-FKHR*.

Several hereditary disorders are associated with increased risk of rhabdomyosarcoma including Li-Fraumeni (an autosomal dominant disorder involving germline mutation of p53 tumor-suppressor gene), neurofibromatosis, and Beckwith-Wiedemann syndrome.

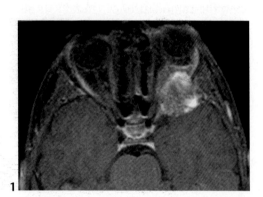
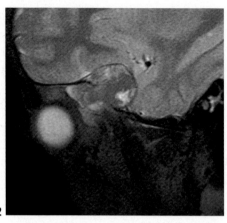

Figure 19E Five-year-old girl with proptosis of the left eye. There is a rhabdomyosarcoma involving the superolateral orbital rim on the left with a heterogeneous mass in the left lateral upper retrobulbar space extending into the middle cranial fossa (**1**). Axial contrast-enhanced T1-weighted fat-suppressed image (**2**) shows a heterogeneous mass with peripheral enhancement and extension into the left middle cranial fossa, better shown on the sagittal fast spin echo fat-suppressed image.

Clinical Findings

Most sarcomas of the head and neck present with nonspecific signs and symptoms, or often a painless mass. Symptoms generally depend on anatomic location, tumor size, and spread.

Pathology and Histology

Biopsy of the tumor is required. Histologically, rhabdomyosarcomas are generally divided into three subtypes (embryonal, alveolar, and pleomorphic) depending on differences in cellularity, spindle cell morphology, surrounding stroma, and growth pattern. The embryonal type is the most common, representing about two thirds of all head and neck cases in children. Embryonal rhabdomyosarcoma has two variants: botryoid (defined by the presence of subepithelial aggregates of tumor cells) and spindle cell (characterized by presence of spindle-shaped cells with a stroma-rich appearance). Alveolar rhabdomyosarcoma has a histologic appearance similar to pulmonary alveoli. Alveolar rhabdomyosarcomas generally have a worse prognosis.

Electron microscopy may show thin and thick filaments, myotubular intermediate filaments, and Z-band material. Rhabdomyosarcomas express several skeletal muscle markers including desmin, sarcomeric actin, and sarcomeric myosin heavy chain, which suggests myogenic cell origin or stem cell precursor.

Imaging Findings

Imaging studies augment physical examination by more accurately assessing the size and local tumor extent. Important information includes intracranial involvement, bone destruction, and regional node involvement. However, the imaging features of the various subtypes tend not to differ.

RADIOGRAPHY

- Radiography may show bone destruction but has been superseded by CT and MRI.

CT

- High-resolution CT and MRI are studies of choice.
- CT is best for assessing bone involvement (Figs. 19F1 and 19F2) and is often used in complementary fashion with MRI.

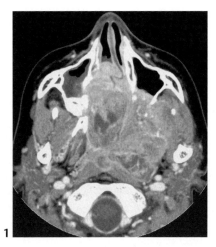
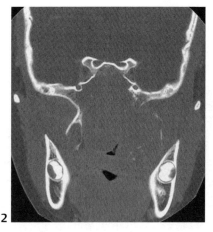

Figure 19F Twelve-year-old girl with a large nasopharyngeal rhabdomyosarcoma involving the posterior and midnasal cavity and left masticatory region. Note the intense heterogeneous enhancement of the tumor on the axial enhanced CT image with soft tissue window (**1**) and the bone destruction of the vertical plates of the maxilla on the left on the coronal CT image with bone windows (**2**).

- Unenhanced CT shows low-attenuation mass.
- Enhanced CT typically shows marked homogeneous or heterogeneous enhancement.
- May see hemorrhage, necrosis, or calcification infrequently

MRI

- Offers better soft tissue resolution, multiplanar capability
- Better able to evaluate primary lesion, perineural extension, dural involvement, bone marrow replacement, and orbital invasion
- T1-weighted imaging isointense to slightly high-signal intensity mass compared with muscle, typically homogeneous
- T2-weighted high-signal mass typically heterogeneous (**Fig. 19G**)
- May see marked heterogeneous enhancement or grape-like enhancement (botryoid sign), found typically in nasal cavity
- May see bone destruction, hemorrhage

Treatment

- Multimodality therapy common
- Surgical resection is critical; however, complete resection may not be possible because of involvement of vital structures or unacceptable functional disability.
- Chemotherapy and radiation therapy are often used as primary therapy.
- Radiation therapy may be used for incomplete tumor resection, suspicion of residual disease, or tumor recurrence.

Prognosis

- Survival now ~70%, with 5-year disease-free survival of 58 to 74%
- Generally favorable for head and neck rhabdomyosarcoma, as typically lower stage at presentation
- Poor prognostic factors include local invasiveness, presence of metastases at diagnosis, regional nodal involvement, large tumor size and high grade, alveolar histologic subtype, and CNS infiltration.

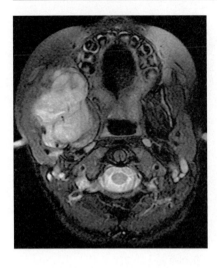

Figure 19G Four-year-old girl with rhabdomyosarcoma involving the right infratemporal fossa and right side of the mandible. Axial T2-weighted fast spin echo fat-suppressed image shows the large lobulated mass with slight heterogeneous signal intensity. Note infiltration and destruction of the right side of the mandible and adjacent regional invasion.

Complications

- Complications of therapy include facial asymmetry, visual/orbital problems, dental abnormalities, growth retardation, and cognitive deficits.
- Radiation-induced secondary malignancies, growth abnormalities, and neuroendocrine abnormalities.

PEARL_____

- Rhabdomyosarcoma is a malignant tumor that destroys bone and has a propensity for the head and neck region.

PITFALL_____

- Pay careful attention to intradural extension.

Suggested Readings

Asakura A, Rudnicki MA. Rhabdomyosarcomagenesis: novel pathway found. Cancer Cell 2003;4:421–422

Chiles MC, Parham DM, Qualman SJ, et al. Sclerosing rhabdomyosarcomas in children and adolescents: a clinicopathologic review of 13 cases from the Intergroup Rhabdomyosarcoma Study Group and Children's Oncology Group. Pediatr Dev Pathol 2004;7:583–594

Cripe TP. Rhabdomyosarcoma. (2005) Available online at http://www.emedicine.com/ped/topic2005.htm

Furze AD, Lehman DA, Roy S. Rhabdomyosarcoma presenting as an anterior neck mass and possible thyroid malignancy in a seven-month-old. Int J Pediatr Otorhinolaryngol 2005;69:267–270

Gujar S, Gandhi D, Mukherji SK. Pediatric head and neck masses. Top Magn Reson Imaging 2004;15:95–101

Hagiwara A, Inoue Y, Nakayama T, et al. The "botryoid sign": a characteristic feature of rhabdomyosarcomas in the head and neck. Neuroradiology 2001;43:331–335

Hicks J, Flaitz C. Rhabdomyosarcoma of the head and neck in children. Oral Oncol 2002;38:450–459

Kim EE, Valenzuela RF, Kumar AJ, Raney RB, Eftekari F. Imaging and clinical spectrum of rhabdomysarcoma in children. Clin Imaging 2000;24:257–262

O'Callaghan MG, House M, Ebay S, Bhadelia R. Rhabdomyoma of the head and neck demonstrated by prenatal magnetic resonance imaging. J Comput Assist Tomogr 2005;29:130–132

Paulino AC, Simon JH, Zhen W, Wen BC. Long-term effects in children treated with radiotherapy for head and neck rhabdomyosarcoma. Int J Radiat Oncol Biol Phys 2000;48:1489–1495

Sturgis EM, Potter BO. Sarcomas of the head and neck region. Curr Opin Oncol 2003;15:239–252

CASE 20

Clinical Presentation

A 5-day-old newborn was sent for imaging due to failure to pass a nasogastric tube on the right side.

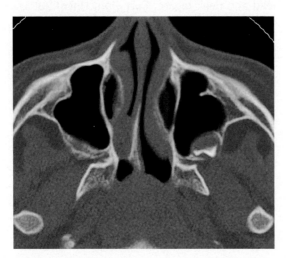

Figure 20A

Radiologic Findings

Axial CT scanning (**Fig. 20A**) shows a funnel-shaped posterior portion of the right nasal cavity. An abnormal medial deviation of the right lateral nasal wall and perpendicular palatine bone with an expanded medial pterygoid plate with a widened vomer is also seen. Soft tissue plug fills the right nasal cavity just in front of the ipsilateral closed choana.

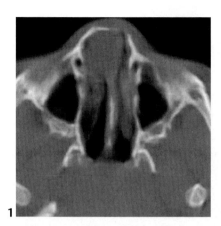

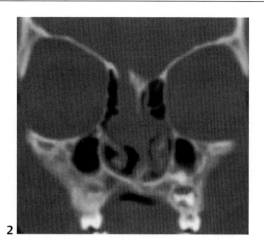

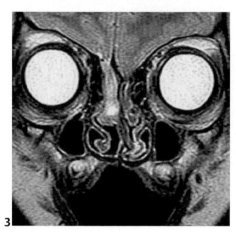

Figure 20B The following figures demonstrate right frontonasal encephalocele. Axial CT (**1**) at nasal cavity of a right frontonasal encephalocele is shown as a soft tissue mass immediately to the right of the midline in the anterior nasal cavity. The coronal CT (**2**) delineates the bone defect at the anterior portion of the right cribriform plate. The coronal MRI T2-weighted image (**3**) shows herniation of the right gyrus rectus and olfactory bulb through the defect into the nasal cavity.

Diagnosis

Choanal atresia, unilateral

Differential Diagnosis

The etiologic diagnosis of neonatal nasal obstruction includes:

- Nasopharyngeal atresia
- Encephalocele/meningoencephalocele (frontoethmoidal, sphenoethmoidal) (**Figs. 20B1** to **20B3**)
- Pyriform aperture stenosis (**Fig. 20C**)
- Binder syndrome (nasal passage stenosis with midface hypoplasia)
- Congenital cysts/tumors (dermoid cyst, hemangioma, hamartoma, nasocystocele)
- Neonatal rhinitis (viral, secondary to gastroesophageal reflux, medicamentosa)
- Foreign body

Discussion

Background

Neonates are obligate nasal breathers and nasal obstruction, especially if bilateral and complete, may cause severe respiratory distress. The posterior choanae are the orifices that connect the posterior nasal cavity with the nasopharynx. Atresia or narrowing of the posterior choanae is the most common cause of nasal obstruction in the neonate, with an incidence of 1 in 5000 to 8000 births.

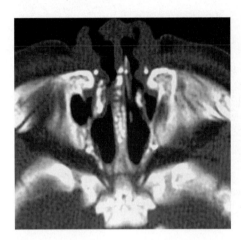

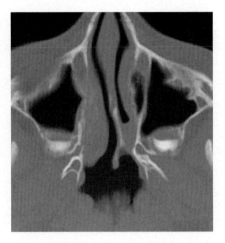

Figure 20C Nasal aperture stenosis was observed in a newborn. Axial CT of the nasal bone (angled along the hard palate) shows dysmorphic features, sacral dimple, and chondrodysplasia punctata type. There is narrowing of the piriform aperture and of the anterior nasal cavity. The maxillary spines show abnormal punctate calcification pattern.

Figure 20D Membranous type choanal atresia in a 5-year-old child. Axial CT shows slight mucosal thickening anterior to the band of left choanal atresia.

There is slight female predominance. Stenosis is more common than true atresia, and bony atresia is more common than membranous atresia. Most references state that choanal atresia is usually unilateral (**Fig. 20D**). Mixed osseous-membranous atresia is seen in ~70% of the patients versus 30% for the pure bony atresia.

Etiology

Choanal atresia results from the failure of resorption of the oronasal membrane that restricts the local growth. An alternative theory of pathogenesis is focused on the abnormal migration of neural crest cells to form the skull base/nasal cavities.

Pathology

In osseous atresia, there is incomplete canalization of the choanae. The membranous variety is secondary to incomplete resorption of epithelial plugs. Bilateral choanal atresia (**Figs. 20E1** and **20E2**) is often syndromic, and 50 to 75% of the patients have other associated congenital malformations, which may include CHARGE association (Coloboma of the eye, Heart disease, Atresia of choanae, Retarded growth, Genital abnormalities, and Ear anomalies), craniofacial syndromes (Crouzon disease, Apert's syndrome, Treacher Collins syndrome), fetal alcohol syndrome, and gastrointestinal anomalies (tracheoesophageal fistula, malrotation).

Clinical Findings

Clinical bilateral choanal atresia is life threatening, usually presenting early in life with severe respiratory distress often aggravated by feeding but relieved by crying. Unilateral choanal atresia presents classically later in life with rhinorrhea and infection, simulating a setting of nasal foreign bodies. Inability to pass a nasogastric tube (no. 5 or 6 French catheter) into the nose of a newborn with the presence of air in the lower respiratory tree is often diagnostic. It demands establishment of an oral airway and CT scanning of the nasal cavity area.

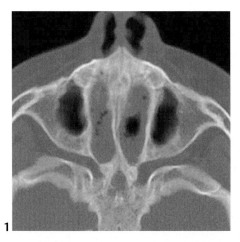
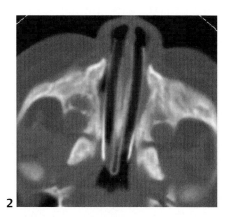

Figure 20E Bilateral choanal atresia in a newborn. Preoperative CT (**1**) of the nasal bone shows bilateral choanal atresia. Postoperative CT (**2**) at 4 weeks shows nasal tubes in place as a first stage of management to ensure nasopharynx patency.

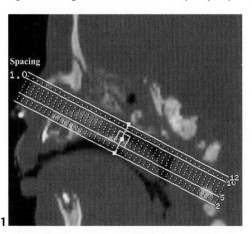
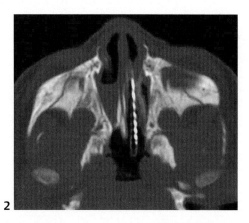

Figure 20F Unilateral choanal atresia, mixed membranous/osseous type in a newborn with CHARGE association. Scout view of CT (**1**) of the nasal cavity outlines the angulation for optimal CT scanning. CT image (**2**) demonstrates the right choanal atresia. Also, note a nasal tube going through the patent left nasal cavity and nasopharynx.

Imaging Findings

CT

- CT scan is the modality of choice for imaging patients with suspected choanal atresia.
- Axial and coronal imaging is important for complete evaluation, including views in bone window settings.
- Suctioning of nasal secretions and administration of nasal decongestants prior to imaging are recommended to better define the thickness of the obstructing membrane.
- Optimal axial CT images are obtained along a plane 10 degrees angled from the hard palate (**Fig. 20F1**).
- Characteristic features include:
  - Thick and club-shaped vomer bone (width of vomer >0.34 cm in <8 years and >0.55 cm in >8 years of age is abnormal)
  - The posteromedial maxilla and perpendicular palatine bone are medially deviated and may be fused with the lateral margins of vomer (**Fig. 20F2**).
  - Funneling of the posterior nasal cavity (width of posterior nasal cavity <0.67 cm at birth and <0.86 cm by 6 years of age is abnormal)
  - The medial pterygoid plates may be expanded and fused with the vomer.
  - In long-standing osseous atresia there can be deviation of the bony hard palate and the nasal septum to the side of the atresia.

- ○ In membranous form, there is funneling of the posterior nasal cavity with narrowing just anterior to the pterygoid plates (**Fig. 20D**). The membranous obstructions are either thin and shelflike, or they can be thick and resemble mucous plugs. Variable amounts of air, fluid, and secretions are seen in front of the obstruction, which can be differentiated by using decongestants.

Treatment

- Bilateral choanal atresia is a surgical emergency.
- Before surgery, initial treatment consists of placement of an oral airway.
- Unilateral atresia can be surgically repaired on an elective basis.
- Bony atresia requires either a transpalatal or an endoscopic approach with or without bony remodeling.
- Membranous atresias can be treated with simple perforation.
- Transnasal stenting is useful in stabilizing the airway (**Fig. 20E2**).

Complications

- Potential problems include infection from the maintained stents, postoperative stenosis in case of puncture and curettage techniques, and crossbite following transpalatal procedures.
- Transnasal interventions appear to avert many complications.

Prognosis

- Bilateral choanal atresia is a life-threatening condition in the newborn.
- Prognosis in cases associated to syndromes is rather dependent on the other congenital anomalies.

PEARLS_____

- Complete bilateral obstruction of the nasal passage in a newborn is a medical emergency.
- Nasal obstruction affects the breathing, feeding, and sleeping functions of the young infant.
- Failure to pass a nasogastric tube with air present in the lower tracheobronchial tree is a "red flag" for adequate management.
- Funneling and narrowing of the posterior nasal cavity are important CT signs.

PITFALLS_____

- Nonossification of the normal bones in the midline nasal region may pose a potential problem. This is especially true in cases with choanal atresia where the presence of retained secretions, etc., may simulate appearance of a midline encephalocele.
- Presence of retained secretions in the nasal cavity can mislead regarding the thickness of the obstructing membrane.

Suggested Readings

Black CM, Dungan D, Fram E, et al. Potential pitfalls in the work-up and diagnosis of choanal atresia. AJNR Am J Neuroradiol 1998;19:326–329

Brown OE, Pownell P, Manning SC. Choanal atresia: a new anatomic classification and clinical management applications. Laryngoscope 1996;106:97–101

Lowe LH, Booth TN, Joglar JM, Rollins NK. Midface anomalies in children. Radiographics 2000;20:907–922

Olnes SQ, Schwartz RH, Bahadori RS. Consultation with the specialist: diagnosis and management of the newborn and young infant who have nasal obstruction. Pediatr Rev 2000;21:416–420

Slovis TL, Renfro B, Watts FB, et al. Choanal atresia: precise CT evaluation. Radiology 1985;155:345–348

CASE 21

Clinical Presentation

A 3-year-old female presents with a painless palpable lump adjacent to the lateral left orbital wall and no history of trauma.

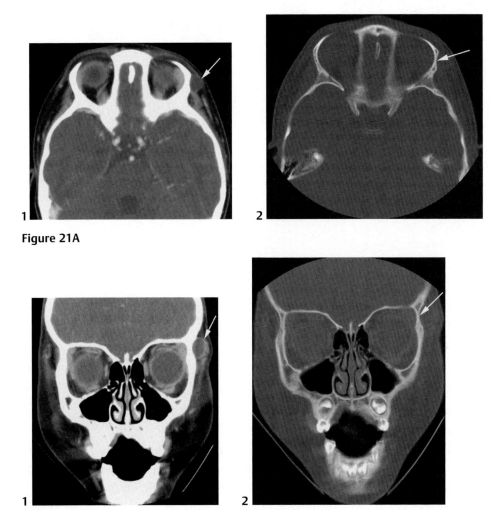

Figure 21A

Figure 21B

Radiologic Findings

Axial (**Figs. 21A1** and **21A2**) and coronal (**Figs. 21B1** and **21B2**) contrast-enhanced CT demonstrates a small hypodense subcutaneous unilocular mass (arrows) adjacent to the lateral left orbital wall. Bone algorithm (**Figs. 21A2** and **21B2**) demonstrates bone scalloping (arrows) without bone destruction. The rim of the lesion enhances, but the center does not enhance.

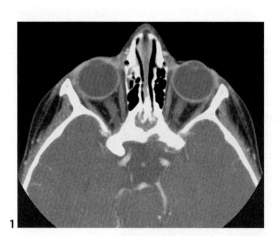
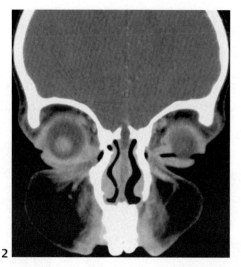

Figure 21C (1,2) Axial CT demonstrates a small midline dermoid centered on the nasal tip extending through the nasal bone and splitting the crista galli, consistent with a dermoid sinus tract.

Diagnosis

Left periorbital dermoid

Differential Diagnosis

- Epidermoid
- Sebaceous cyst

Discussion

Background

Epidermoids and dermoids are inclusion cysts derived from ectoderm. Epidermoids contain only squamous epithelium; dermoids, on the other hand, may also contain hair and sebaceous and sweat glands, along with squamous epithelium. Unlike teratomas, dermoids and epidermoids are not true neoplasms. Dermoids can be evident at birth but usually present later in life. These are slow-growing lesions that show progressive enlargement over time with bony scalloping due to pressure erosion. There is a slight male predilection.

Approximately 7% of all dermoid cysts arise in the head and neck region. They commonly occur around the orbit, in the calvarium, but can also occur in the posterior or middle cranial fossae. Extracranial dermoids are most common in the superior temporal/orbital region. Periorbital dermoids typically occur in the lateral third of the supraorbital rim and are frequently superficial and mobile. Nasal dermoids may present as a cyst, a sinus, or a fistula. Nasal dermoids may show a bifid crista galli or an enlarged foramen cecum or may have intracranial extension (**Figs. 21C1** and **21C2, 21D1** and **21D2**). Dermoids can also infrequently occur adjacent to the tongue. Intracranial dermoids are most common in the cerebellopontine angle or parasellar region.

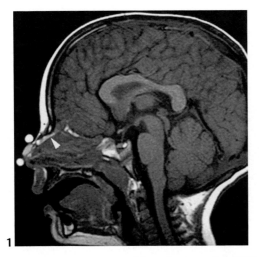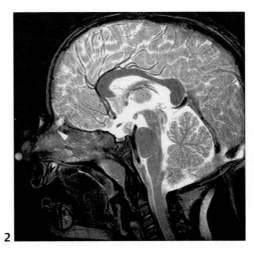

Figure 21D Sagittal T1- (**1**) and T2-weighted (**2**) images demonstrate fat-containing tract extending from a subcutaneous dermoid (arrowhead) through the foramen cecum and crista galli. Note the interruption to the normal fat-containing marrow of the crista galli. T2 hyperintense vitamin E capsule was used as a skin marker.

Etiology

Dermoids are thought to arise from failure of surface ectoderm to separate from underlying structures or possibly from sequestration or implantation of surface ectoderm. This may result in a tract or cyst as the surface ectoderm is drawn into the developing embryo. They are thought to arise early in development, most likely between 3 and 5 weeks of gestation.

Clinical Findings

Extracranial dermoids usually present in the first 4 decades of life as small, painless palpable subcutaneous masses of the head and neck, usually <1 to 2 cm. Intracranial dermoids may be associated with a dimple or sinus tract. If a dermoid is large in size, it can cause obstructive hydrocephalus and present with signs of raised intracranial pressure. Rarely, dermoids can present with chemical meningitis.

Pathology

Macroscopically, dermoids are noted as thick-walled structures that may contain dystrophic calcification; they are usually unilocular with floating lipid, cheesy material. Microscopically, dermoids are characterized as keratin-filled cysts lined by stratified squamous epithelium containing adnexal structures including sebaceous elements, sweat glands, and hair follicles within the cyst lining.

Imaging Findings

RADIOGRAPHY

- Scalloped margins with a soft tissue mass
- Rarely peripheral calcification may be evident on plain film.

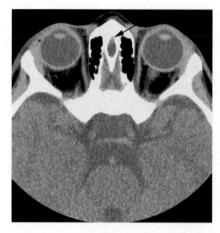

Figure 21E CT shows dilated foramen cecum (arrow).

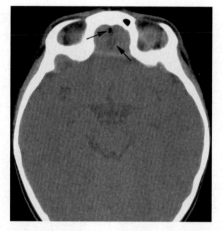

Figure 21F CT demonstrating soft tissue/fat-containing mass (arrows) in the anterior cranial fossa, which connects via the foramen cecum to a nasal tip dermoid (not shown).

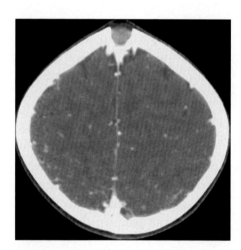

Figure 21G CT shows anterior fontanelle dermoid abutting the superior sagittal sinus with obvious implications for surgery and potential blood loss.

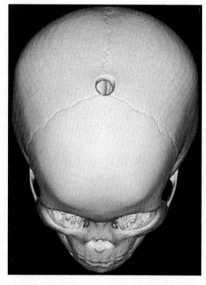

Figure 21H 3D CT demonstrates a "punched out" lesion at the anterior fontanelle.

ULTRASOUND

- Superficial dermoids can be evaluated; however, not all communication with the intracranial contents is well appreciated.

CT

- CT excellent at showing bone detail (**Figs. 21E** and **21F**)
- CT imaging characteristics depend on specific contents.
- Typically, unilocular midline cystic mass with density similar to fat and may have a fat-fluid level
- Scalloping of adjacent bone is common
- Dermoids may be intra- or extracranial (**Figs. 21G** and **21H**).

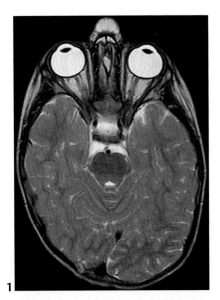 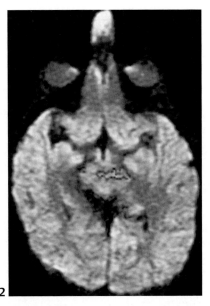

Figure 21I Axial T2-weighted (**1**) and axial diffusion sequences (**2**) demonstrate a T2 hyperintense mass at the nasal tip with diffusion restriction (apparent diffusion coefficient dark-image not shown), consistent with a nasal dermoid.

MRI

- MRI is best for visualizing intracranial extension.
- Variable appearance but typically hyperintense on T1-weighted images due to the presence of fatty components or cholesterol crystals
- On T2-weighted images, lesions are hyperintense if fat suppression is not used (**Fig. 21I1**).
- One needs to carefully assess for sinus tract, which may be present.
- Dermoids in the spine may be associated with spinal dysraphism or a fibrous band.
- Dermoid may demonstrate restricted diffusion (**Fig. 21I2**).

Treatment

- Surgical excision if large or intracranial connection/fistula
- Endoscopic excision can be used for small zygomaticofrontal lesions.

Complications

- Chemical meningitis from rupture
- Sinus tract or fistula may be associated.
- Bacterial meningitis from infected sinus tract

Prognosis

- Excellent with complete surgical excision

PEARL_____

- In a child with midline or off midline cystic mass with fat, consider dermoid/epidermoid tumor.

- Sinus tract may be difficult to visualize and may require high-resolution CT and/or MRI.

Suggested Readings

Caldarelli M, Colosimo C, Di Rocco C. Intra-axial dermoid/epidermoid tumors of the brainstem in children. Surg Neurol 2001;56:97–105

Edwards PC, Lustrin L, Valderrama E. Dermoid cysts of the tongue: report of five cases and review of the literature. Pediatr Dev Pathol 2003;6:531–535

Guerrissi JO. Endoscopic excision of frontozygomatic dermoid cysts. J Craniofac Surg 2004;15:618–622

Huisman TA, Schneider JF, Kellenberger CJ, et al. Developmental nasal midline masses in children: neuroradiological evaluation. Eur Radiol 2003;14:243–249

Rahbar R, Shah P, Mulliken JB, et al. The presentation and management of nasal dermoid. Arch Otolaryngol Head Neck Surg. 2003;129:464–471

Smirniotopoulos JG, Chiechi MV. Teratomas, dermoids and epidermoids of the head and neck. Radiographics 1995;15:1437–1455

CASE 22

Clinical Presentation

A young child presents with a midline enlarging neck lump just below the chin, above the level of the hyoid bone.

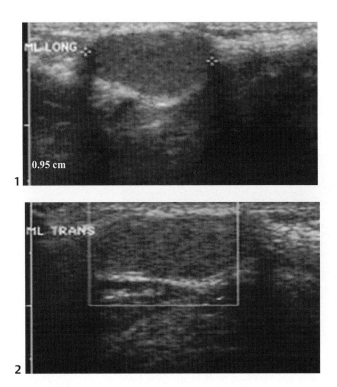

Figure 22A

Radiologic Findings

Ultrasonography of the anterior neck in the sagittal (**Fig. 22A1**) and transverse (**Fig. 22A2**) planes demonstrates a well-defined midline echogenic mass just above the hyoid bone.

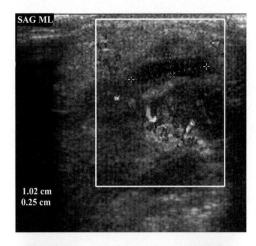

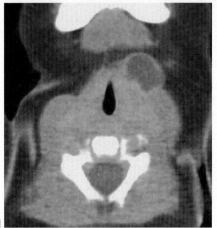

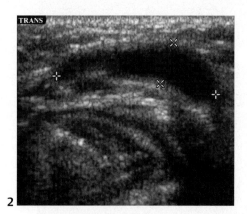

Figure 22B Midline sagittal sonogram in submental area demonstrating early abscess formation and adjacent inflamed lymph node.

Figure 22C Left anterior cystic hygroma of the neck. Axial CT (**1**) showing a well-defined hypodense cyst. Corresponding transverse sonogram (**2**) demonstrates a superficial off-midline anechoic cyst.

Diagnosis

Thyroglossal duct cyst

Differential Diagnosis

- Abscess (**Fig. 22B**)
- Lymphangioma (cystic hygroma, **Fig. 22C**)
- Hemangioma
- Enlarged lymph node (**Fig. 22B**)
- Cystic teratoma
- Lipoma
- Branchial cleft cyst
- Ectopic thyroid

Discussion

Background

The most common congenital neck anomaly, thyroglossal duct cysts, accounts for 70% of congenital neck anomalies and are frequent neck masses second only to benign lymphadenopathy. It has equal

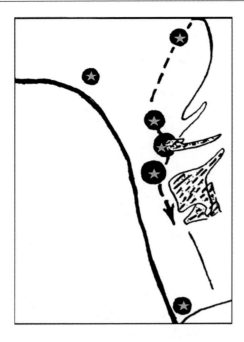

Figure 22D Diagram showing possible locations (stars) of thyroglossal duct cysts along their embryologic path. Landmarks are the foramen cecum of the tongue base, the hyoid bone, the thyroid cartilage, and the sternum.

incidence in males and females. Seven percent of the adult population may have such a remnant. Familial cases are rare but do occur, and they may be autosomal dominant or recessive.

Embryology

Thyroglossal duct cysts result from the failure of involution of the thyroglossal tract. This tract is normally patent until the eighth week of development, and it is located ventrally to the developing hyoid bone and anterior to the thyroid membrane. The thyroid anlage has formed at 4 weeks of development by invagination of the endodermal cells of the tongue. It then descends as a bilobed diverticulum toward its definitive position. These embryologic considerations explain the possible anatomic positions of the thyroglossal duct cyst (**Fig. 22D**). Four general locations are encountered: intralingual (2%), suprahyoid including submental (25%), thyrohyoid (60%), and suprasternal (13%). Entrapment of the thyroglossal tract in the midline merging of the hyoid anlage explains the involvement of the periosteum or the bone itself, and this is of therapeutic significance.

Clinical Findings

Mass and infection, single or recurrent event, are the main modes of presentation. The enlarging midline anterior neck mass has a characteristic upward movement with tongue protrusion. Other symptoms include cough and signs of otitis media. Dysphagia and airway obstruction are usually seen in the lingual form. Fistula to the skin can be seen secondary to trauma, previous surgery, or spontaneous drainage after infection.

Pathology

- Macroscopy: smooth, well-defined cyst along the route of descent of the thyroid gland, between the foramen cecum of the tongue base and the expected location of the thyroid, in the midline of the inferior neck. Ten to 24% are located just lateral to the midline, often to the left.
- Microscopy: cyst-lined by respiratory or squamous epithelium, with small deposits of thyroid tissue. Secretions likely secondary to repeated local inflammation/infection give rise to the cyst.

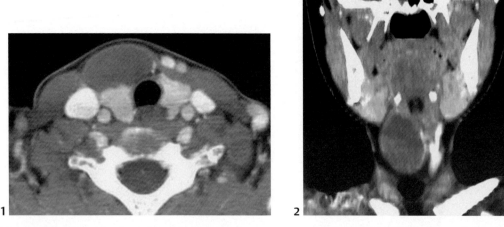

Figure 22E CT showing hypodense thyroglossal duct cyst just to the right of midline in the axial plane (**1**) with corresponding coronal reformat (**2**).

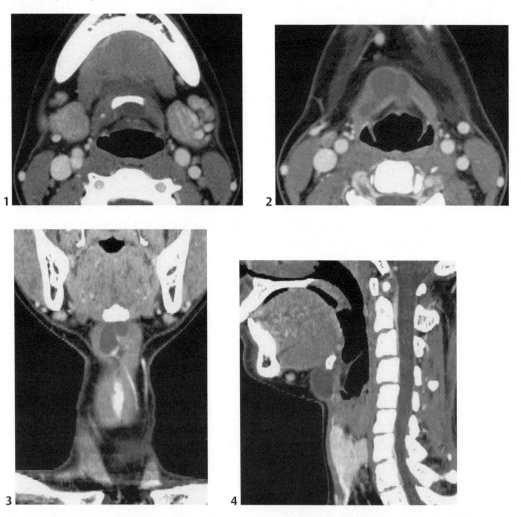

Figure 22F CT features of septated thyroglossal duct cyst closely attached to hyoid bone. Axial CT (**1**) delineating small part of the cyst posterior to hyoid bone. The adjacent axial CT (**2**) defines the multiseptated appearance of the major portion of the cyst. Coronal (**3**) and sagittal (**4**) reformats give a better overview of its anatomic relationship to the hyoid bone.

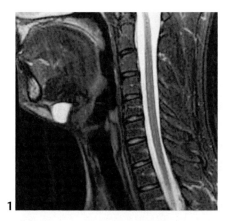
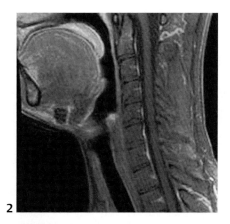
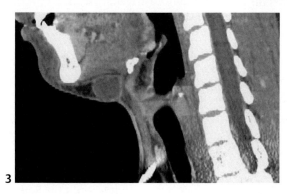

Figure 22G MRI of suprahyoid thyroglossal duct cyst. Sagittal T2-weighted (**1**) image showing increased signal intensity of fluid content. Sagittal fat-suppressed T1-weighted image (**2**) postgadolinium injection demonstrates a rim-enhancement pattern similar to sagittal contrast-enhanced CT scan (**3**).

Imaging Findings

ULTRASOUND

- Commonly as hypoechoic mass, often with increased through transmission
- May present as anechoic mass or with homogeneous (**Fig. 22A**) or heterogeneous echogenicity
- Echogenicity of content is related to proteinaceous nature of the fluid.
- Preoperative ultrasound should exclude ectopic thyroid tissue by demonstrating a normal thyroid gland.

CT

- Smooth, well-circumscribed mass with thin walls and homogeneous fluid attenuation (**Figs. 22E1** and **22E2**)
- Septations may be present (**Figs. 22F1** to **22F4**).
- Peripheral rim enhancement is classic on postintravenous contrast CT.
- Coronal and/or sagittal reformated imaging delineates the involvement of the hyoid bone (**Figs. 22F3** and **22F4**).

MRI

- Low signal on T1-weighted and high signal on T2-weighted images (**Figs. 22G1** to **22G3**)
- No peripheral enhancement after gadolinium injection, unless infected
- Thickening of rim with infection or hemorrhage

Treatment

- Sistrunk operation, with dissection of the thyroglossal tract and resection of the central portion of the hyoid bone, is the main operation of choice.
- Management of infected cyst includes antibiotics and incision or drainage when needed.

Prognosis

- Sistrunk operation bears an excellent prognosis.
- Recurrence rate approximates 2.6%.
- Recurrence rate is related to presence of recent preoperative cyst infection, incomplete resection of the tract, and presence of multiple thyroglossal duct tract.
- Carcinoma has been reported in association with thyroglossal duct cyst in <1%.

PEARLS

- Asymptomatic or infected usually midline infrahyoid neck mass in children
- Ultrasound is the modality of choice, as there is no need for radiation or sedation.
- Ultrasonographic appearance is not related to infection.
- Rapid increase in size usually represents acute infection.

PITFALLS

- Pseudosolid appearance, due to proteinaceous content, with uniform echogenicity can be seen.
- Exclude ectopic thyroid tissue by ultrasonography.

Suggested Readings

Ahuja AT, Metrevelli KC. Sonographic evaluation of thyroglossal duct cysts in children. Clin Radiol 2000;55:770–774

Brousseau VJ, Solares CA, Xu M, Krakovitz P, Koltai PJ. Thyroglossal duct cysts: presentation and management in children versus adults. Int J Pediatr Otorhinolaryngol 2003;67:1285–1290

Koeller KK, Alamo L, Adair CF, Smirniatopoulos JG. Congenital cystic masses of the neck: radiologic-pathologic correlation. Radiographics 1999;19:121–146

CASE 23

Clinical Presentation

A 4-year-old male presents with a nontender right-sided neck mass.

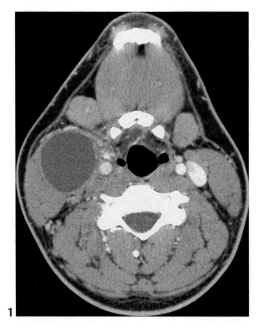 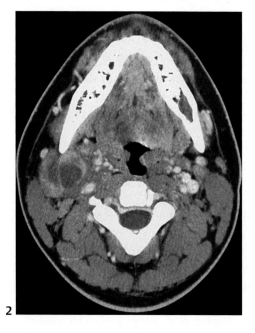

Figure 23A

Radiologic Findings

Contrast-enhanced axial CT images (**Figs. 23A1** and **23A2**) depict a well-demarcated, hypodense right-sided unilocular mass effacing the anterior margin of the right sternocleidomastoid muscle. The mass displaces the right internal carotid artery and jugular vein medially. The mass extends inferiorly from the level of the mandibular angle and displaces the right submandibular gland anteriorly. There is a thin enhancing rim, whereas centrally the lesion is nearly isointense with CSF. There is minimal associated lymphadenopathy.

Diagnosis

Second branchial cleft cyst (BCC)

Differential Diagnosis

Pertains to cystic neck masses as follows:

- Cystic hygroma
  - Typically present at birth (~60%) with 90% seen by 2 years
  - Often multilocular and may extend behind sternocleidomastoid muscle
- Dermoid cyst
  - Congenital midline mass usually present at birth
- Thyroglossal duct cyst
  - Midline in 75%
  - Approximately 65% are below hyoid bone.
  - May move upward with sticking tongue out
- Necrotic lymph node
  - Usually prominent adjacent lymphadenopathy
- Hemangioma
  - May see flow on Doppler interrogation
- Ranula
  - Usually in sublingual space
- Teratoma
  - May see soft tissue components (fat, calcium)
- Neural tumor
  - Usually primarily solid components
- External laryngocele
  - Extension from laryngeal ventricle, air or fluid filled

Discussion

Background

Embryologically, the branchial complex consists of six, paired mesodermal arches, which are separated by five clefts lined by endoderm. The fifth and sixth arches are generally rudimentary; however, the first four develop the major structures of the neck, as outlined in **Table 23–1**. There are three general types of anomalies of the branchial cleft complex. Branchial cleft sinuses are tracts, with or without a cyst, that communicate to gut or skin. Fistulae are residual tracts extending from pharynx to the skin. BCCs are isolated and have no opening to skin or pharynx.

A second BCC can arise anywhere along the embryologic path of the second branchial cleft fistula, which runs from the tonsillar fossa inferiorly along the anterior border of the sternocleidomastoid muscle to the supraclavicular location. There are four types of second BCCs based on their location along this embryologic pathway. Fistulae of second BCCs generally end around the supratonsillar fossa/pillar or directly on tonsil surface and present with recurrent attacks of inflammation.

Table 23–1   Derivatives of the Branchial Complex

Derivative	Cleft (Ectoderm)	Arch (Mesoderm)	Pouch (Endoderm)
First	External auditory canal	Mandible Muscles of mastication	Eustachian tube
Second	Sinus of His	Muscles of facial expression Malleus and incus Hyoid bone	Palantine tonsil Supratonsillar fossa
Third	Sinus of His	Hyoid bone Stylopharyngeus muscle	Inferior parathyroid glands Thymus
Fourth	Sinus of His	Epiglottis Thyroid cartilage Pharyngeal muscles Aortic arch	Superior parathyroid glands
Fifth/Sixth		Cartilage of neck	

Etiology

The most popular theory is that BCCs are remnants of the cervical sinus of His, which is formed during migration of arches between the second and seventh weeks of fetal life. Second BCCs, sinuses, and branchial fistulae can arise or extend from anywhere along the embryologic path of the second arch, which runs from the tonsillar fossa inferiorly along the anterior border of the sternocleidomastoid muscle to the supraclavicular location. There are four types of second BCCs based on location along this embryologic pathway. Fistulae of second BCCs generally end around the fauceral pillar, supratonsillar fossa, or directly on tonsil surface. Some authors support a theory of cystic cervical lymph node or salivary gland inclusion as the etiology and suggest the term *benign lymphoepithelial cysts*.

Pathology

BCCs are usually lined by stratified squamous epithelial cells and may have lymphoid tissue in their periphery. Occasionally they have a respiratory component. Fine-needle aspiration (FNA) shows straw-colored fluid with squamous and polymorphonuclear cells, lymphocytes, and cholesterol crystals.

Clinical Findings

Typically, a second BCC is a slow-growing fluctuant mass noted at the angle of the mandible, seen in patients 10 to 40 years of age, which is often moveable in all planes. There is no motion of the mass with swallowing. Up to 40% of patients relate appearance to upper respiratory tract or odontogenic infection. BCCs do not communicate with skin or pharynx. If there is drainage, then one should consider branchial fistula (both internal and external openings) or branchial sinus (one opening). Second BCCs may also present as a tonsillar mass.

First BC anomalies are usually found in middle-aged women and present as a recurrent parotid mass or abscess. Third BCCs typically occur in children and young adults and lie posterior to carotid vessels. Fourth BC anomaly is very rare and arises from the piriform sinus descending into the mediastinum.

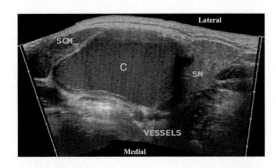

Figure 23B Axial oblique sonogram depicts second BCC (C) located anterior to sternocleidomastoid muscle (SCM) and posterior to submandibular gland (SM). Carotid vessels lie medial to cyst.

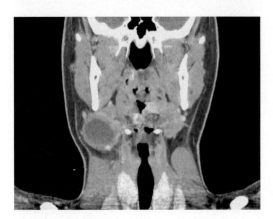

Figure 23C Coronal enhanced CT.

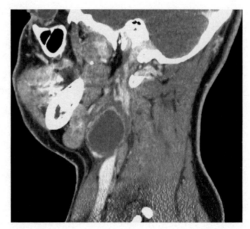

Figure 23D Sagittal reconstructed enhanced CT.

Imaging Findings

A cystic mass that demonstrates displacement of sternomastoid muscle posterolaterally, submandibular gland anteriorly, and carotid bundle medially is often considered diagnostic of a second BCC.

ULTRASOUND

- Generally a unilocular cystic mass with thin walls
- Anechoic or hypoechoic
- May become complex with thick wall if infected (**Fig. 23B**)

CT

- Well-defined mass with low attenuation and nonenhancing rim (**Fig. 23C**)
- Can become complex with thick enhancing rim if infected (**Fig. 23D**)

MRI

- Typically a hypointense lesion on T1-weighted images (**Fig. 23E1**)
- Hyperintense on T2-weighted images. Associated inflammation also has high signal areas (**Fig. 23E2**).
- Following contrast have rim enhancement (**Fig. 23E3**) or show vascular deviation, as in **Fig. 23F**, where the right carotid artery and jugular vein are displaced medially (arrow)

Complications

- BCC may become infected, resulting in a more complex cystic nature, with a thicker enhancing margin evident on US, CT, and MRI.
- Signal intensity on T1-weighted images may increase with proteinaceous/hemorrhagic components with infection.

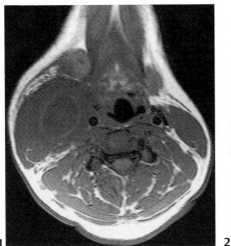
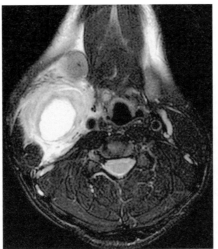
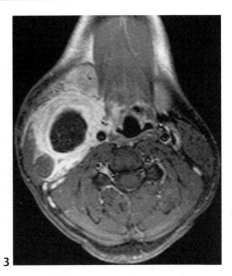

Figure 23E (**1**) Axial T1-weighted image showing irregular hypointense right-sided mass. (**2**) Axial T2-weighted image demonstrating high-signal intensity with adjacent inflammatory rim of slightly lower signal intensity. (**3**) Postcontrast axial image showing peripheral rim enhancement.

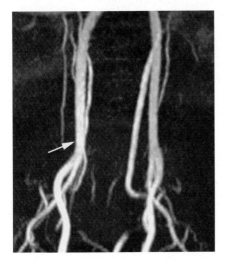

Figure 23F MR angiography showing displacement of right jugular vein and carotid artery (arrow).

Treatment

- Surgical excision required for complete cure and generally recommended
- Removal of associated sinus or fistulous tract required
- Overall recurrence rate after surgical excision is 3 to 5%, with increased incidence/risk of sinus and fistulae compared with cysts.
- Sclerotherapy has been attempted with less success.

PEARLS

- Second BCCs account for ~90% of branchial cleft anomalies.
- First BCCs account for ~8% while third BCCs account for 2%.
- PET scanning may help prove a diagnosis of neoplastic necrotic lymph node.
- Fistulae usually present in infants or young children

PITFALLS_____

- An infected cyst can be mistaken for a necrotic lymph node and vice versa.
- In adults, a search for tumors of the aerodigestive tract may be indicated.
- Cytologic appearance of an FNA of an inflamed BCC and metastatic squamous cell carcinoma can be similar.

Suggested Readings

Ahuja AT, King AD, Metreweli C. Second branchial cleft cysts: variability of sonographic appearances in adult cases. AJNR Am J Neuroradiol 2000;21:315–319

Alvarez JC, Moris C, Mendez JC, Fuente E. Imaging quiz case 2: branchial cleft cyst. Arch Otolaryngol Head Neck Surg 1998;124:603–605

Cerezal L, Morales C, Abascal F, et al. Pharyngeal branchial cyst: magnetic resonance findings. Eur J Radiol 1998;29:1–3

Coppens F, Peene P, Lemahieu SF. Diagnosis and differential diagnosis of branchial cleft cysts by CT scan. J Belge Radiol 1990;73:189–196

Donegan JO. Congenital neck masses. In: Cummings CW, Fredrickson JM, Harker LA, Krause CJ, Schuller DE, eds. Otolaryngology: Head and Neck Surgery. 2nd ed. St. Louis: CV Mosby; 1993:1554–1565.

Gadiparthi S, Lai SY, Branstetter BF IV, Ferris RL. Radiology quiz case 2: parapharyngeal second branchial cleft cyst. Arch Otolaryngol Head Neck Surg 2004;130:1121,1124–1125.

Girvigian MR, Rechdouni AK, Zeger GD, Segall H, Rice DH, Petrovich Z. Squamous cell carcinoma arising in a second branchial cleft cyst. Am J Clin Oncol 2004;27:96–100

Glosser JW, Pires CAS, Feinberg SE. Branchial cleft or cervical lymphoepithelial cysts: etiology and management. J Am Dent Assoc 2003;134:81–86

Kim KH, Sung MW, Roh JL, Han MH. Sclerotherapy for congenital lesions in the head and neck. Otolaryngol Head Neck Surg 2004;131:307–316

MacNab T, McLennan MK, Margolis M. Radiology rounds: branchial cleft cyst. Can Fam Physician 1995;41:1673,1676–1679

Ramirez-Camacho R, Garcia Berrocal JR, Borrego P. Radiology quiz case 2: second branchial cleft cyst and fistula. Arch Otolaryngol Head Neck Surg 2001;127:1395–1396

CASE 24

Clinical Presentation

A 6-month-old baby girl presents with growing right facial mass.

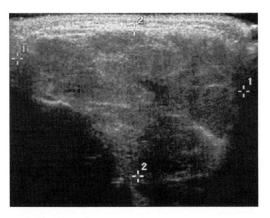

Figure 24A

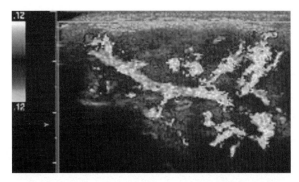

Figure 24B (See Color Plate 24B.)

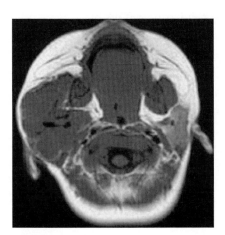

Figure 24C

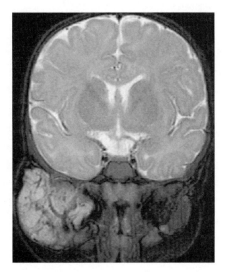

Figure 24D

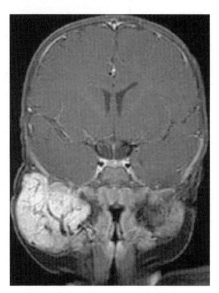

Figure 24E

Radiologic Findings

Ultrasonographic images show a large, soft tissue mass of heterogeneous echogenicity (**Figs. 24A** and **24B**). Color Doppler evaluation shows high flow and high vessel density (**Fig. 24B**). MRI including axial unenhanced T1-weighted image (**Fig. 24C**), coronal fat-suppressed T2-weighted image (**Fig. 24D**), and fat-suppressed T1-weighted image following gadolinium enhancement (**Fig. 24E**) show a large mass initially isointense to muscle within the right parotid gland extending to the right parapharyngeal region with multiple internal flow voids. The lesion shows high T2 signal intensity and intense enhancement following gadolinium administration.

Diagnosis

Hemangioma of infancy

Differential Diagnosis

Other vascular anomalies and tumors

- Kaposiform hemangioendothelioma
- Noninvoluting congenital hemangioma
- Rapidly involuting congenital hemangioma
- Vascular malformations
  - Venous malformation
  - Lymphatic malformation
  - Arteriovenous malformation
- Rhabdomyosarcoma
- Neuroblastoma
- Fibrosarcoma
- Lipoblastoma

Discussion

Background

Vascular anomalies can be classified as either tumors (most common being hemangiomas) or vascular malformations, which may be arterial, venous, lymphatic, or combined. Hemangiomas are the most common benign tumor of childhood with a predilection for the head and neck. Head and neck hemangiomas constitute 60% of all cases, followed by the trunk in 25% and the extremities in 15%. Hemangiomas are multiple in 20% of cases. Hemangiomas are seen much more commonly in girls than boys. Hemangiomas are usually not noticed at birth, most often presenting as a firm soft tissue mass a few weeks after birth. They typically have a rapid proliferation or growth phase in the first year of life, followed by spontaneous slow involution. By the age of 5 years, 50% have involuted, increasing to 70% by age 7 and 90% by age 9 years. Clinical history and physical examination make the diagnosis in 90% of the cases. Imaging is required with a large or atypical lesion for assessment of potential complications, surgical planning, and, in some cases, for evaluation of treatment.

Etiology

Usually hemangioma of infancy is sporadic; however, associations with a variety of syndromes and familial cases have also been described.

Pathology

Hemangioma of infancy is grossly characterized by lobules of capillaries with evidence of cellular proliferation. Histologically, clusters of plump endothelial cells and multilaminated endothelial basement membrane are frequently observed. Pericytes and mast cells may be seen with involution. Immunohistochemistry reveals that vascular endothelial growth factor predominates in the growth phase, and GLUT1, a glucose transporter, is normally expressed in all phases of hemangioma growth.

Clinical Findings

Clinical findings of hemangiomas in infancy depend on the site, depth, and extent of the lesion. Diagnosis is typically made on the basis of clinical history of rapid postnatal growth and clinical appearance. When superficially present, hemangiomas appear as a red or blue plaquelike firm soft tissue mass in infants. When deep in location, hemangiomas can present with airway obstruction, organomegaly, or congestive heart failure.

Imaging Findings

PLAIN RADIOGRAPHY

- Nonspecific soft tissue mass

ULTRASOUND

- Most cost-effective technique
- Well-defined lobulated variable echogenicity mass
- High flow on color and pulsed Doppler study, high vessel density with low resistance

CT

- Homogeneous, isodense to muscle mass
- Following intravascular contrast administration shows intense and diffuse enhancement

MRI

- Modality of choice due to soft tissue contrast and multiplanar capability
- Well-circumscribed lobulated mass, with flow voids at the center and periphery of the lesion, related to high flow feeding and draining vessels
- Isointense to muscle on T1-weighted imaging
- Hyperintense to muscle on T2-weighted imaging; however, less intense than CSF
- Shows homogeneous enhancement after administration of gadolinium
- Involuting hemangiomas will have areas of fibrofatty tissue that also can be seen at CT. Imaging is not usually required during involution.

ARTERIOGRAPHY

- Best reserved for patients requiring embolization

Complications

Depends on site and extent of involvement
- Ocular disturbances including visual loss, astigmatism, amblyopia, tear-duct occlusion (**Figs. 24F1 to 24F3**)
- Cosmetic scarring and disfigurement
- Ulceration and hemorrhage
- Airway compromise
- Visceral involvement
- Congestive heart failure
- Gastrointestinal hemorrhage

Treatment

- Treatment aimed at preventing life- or function-threatening complications, permanent disfigurement, and scarring

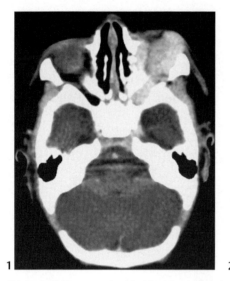 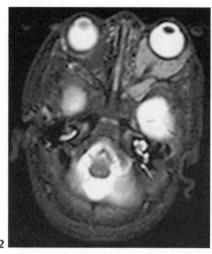 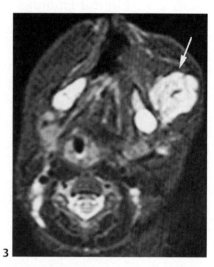

Figure 24F Two-month-old girl with multiple hemangiomas affecting head and neck region and liver. Axial CT following contrast enhancement (**1**) at the level of the orbits showing an intraorbital hemangioma on the left. Axial T2-weighted MRI (**2**) with better demonstration of the intraorbital soft tissue mass corresponding to CT shown in (**1**). Axial T2-weighted MRI (**3**) more inferiorly at the level of the left cheek showing a second separate lesion (arrow) at the mandibular level.

- When located in a non-organ/life-threatening location may have close clinical observation, so-called active nonintervention
- Complete involution does not necessarily mean complete disappearance of the lesion, with residual abnormality such as telangiectasias, scar formation, fibrous fatty tissue, or atrophic skin fairly common.
- Therapeutic intervention in children with compromised airway, deviation of the visual axis, organomegaly, or congestive heart disease may consist of systemic, topical, or intralesional steroid administration, arterial embolization, interferon a-2b, laser therapy, or surgery.

Prognosis
- Excellent prognosis in the majority of nonsyndromic head and neck cases
- Residual skin changes in up to 40 to 50% of the patients

PEARLS
- Kasabach-Merritt syndrome, the association of a vascular tumor and consumption coagulopathy, is typically not a complication of hemangioma but rather kaposiform hemangiomioendothelioma or tufted angioma.
- Acronym PHACEs: represents association of facial hemangiomas with Posterior fossa malformations including Dandy-Walker malformation, Hemangioma, Arterial anomalies, Coarctation of the aorta, Eye abnormalities, and occasional Sternal defects

PITFALL
- Other vascular lesions can occasionally be confused with hemangiomas, and biopsy may be needed.

Suggested Readings

Auriemma A, Bellan C, Poggiani C, Somaschini M, Colombo A. Imaging of neonatal hemangiomas: two cases. Eur J Ultrasound 1999;9:161–165

Bruckner AL, Frieden IJ. Hemangiomas of infancy. J Am Acad Dermatol 2003;48:477–496

Ceisler E, Blei F. Ophthalmic issues in hemangiomas of infancy. Lymphat Res Biol 2003;1:321–330

Donnelly LF, Adams DM, Bisset GS III. Vascular malformations and hemangiomas: a practical approach in a multidisciplinary clinic. AJR Am J Roentgenol 2000;174:597–608

Dubois J, Garel L. Imaging and therapeutic approach of hemangiomas and vascular malformations in the pediatric age group. Pediatr Radiol 1999;29:879–893

Werner JA, Dunne AA, Folz BJ, et al. Current concepts in the classification, diagnosis and treatment of hemangiomas and vascular malformations of the head and neck. Eur Arch Otorhinolaryngol 2001;258:141–149

CASE 25

Clinical Presentation

A 3-week-old girl presents with a newly noted neck mass.

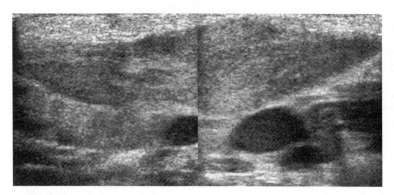

Figure 25A

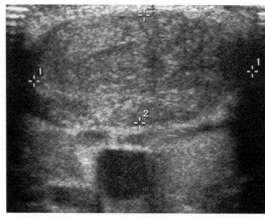

Figure 25B

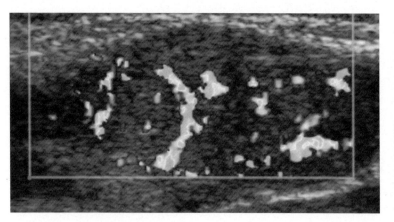

Figure 25C (See Color Plate 25C.)

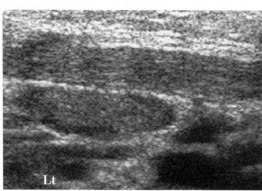

Figure 25D

Radiologic Findings

Longitudinal and transverse ultrasonographic images of the neck (**Figs. 25A, 25B, 25C, and 25D**) show diffuse fusiform enlargement of the right sternocleidomastoid muscle (SCM). There is increased slightly heterogeneous echogenicity of the right SCM, especially within its mid portion, as shown on the transverse image (**Fig. 25B**). Color Doppler longitudinal section shows increased flow within the right SCM (**Fig. 25C**). No abnormality is noted on the left (**Fig. 25D**).

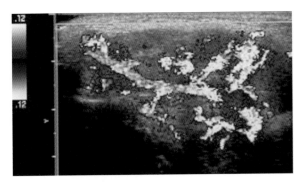

Figure 24B (See Figure 24B, p. 123.)

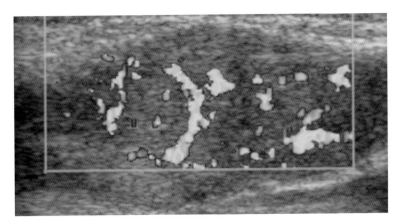

Figure 25C (See Figure 25C. p. 128.)

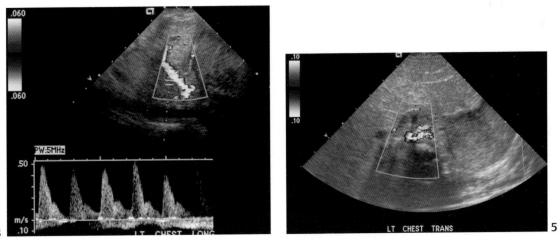

Figure 37C Frontal chest ultrasonographic images (**3** and **5**) reveal a paraesophageal echogenic mass with a prominent systemic feeding artery arising from the upper abdominal aorta in this extralobar sequestration. (See Figures 37C3 and 37C5, p. 186.)

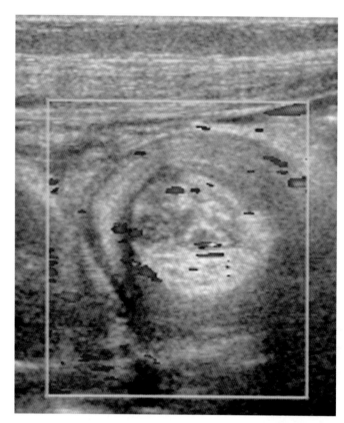

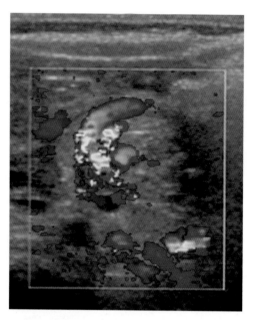

Figure 62E2 The "whirlpool sign," characterized by twisting of the superior mesenteric artery and vein, is highly specific for midgut volvulus, as seen in color Doppler (See Figure 62E2, p. 305.)

Figure 59A (See Figure 59A, p. 286.)

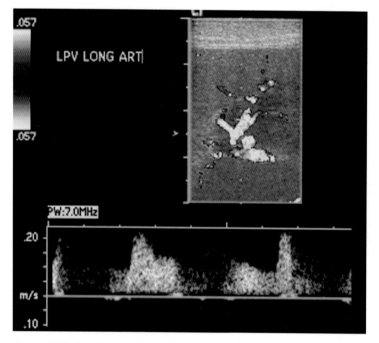

Figure 66B (See Figure 66B, p. 323.)

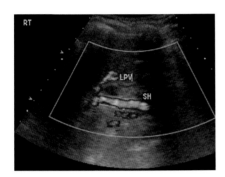

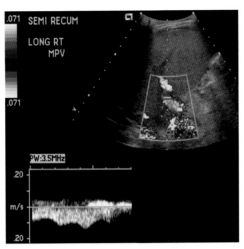

Figure 66G (Same patient as in **Fig. 66F**) Color Doppler ultrasound assessment demonstrating patency of a newly placed portomesenteric shunt (SH). LPV, left portal vein. (See Figure 66G, p. 326.)

Figure 66H Differential diagnosis: Hepatofugal portal flow demonstrated on Doppler ultrasound in a patient with veno-occlusive disease following bone marrow transplant. (See Figure 66H, p. 326.)

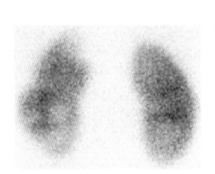

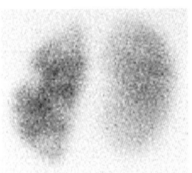

Figure 76A (See Figure 76A, p. 373.) **Figure 76B** (See Figure 76B, p. 373.)

Diagnosis

Fibromatosis colli

Differential Diagnosis

Solid and cystic soft tissue masses of the anterolateral neck in a young infant

- Rhabdomyosarcoma or other soft tissue sarcoma
- Neuroblastoma
- Inflammatory masses including infectious or metastatic adenopathy
- Rare benign soft tissue tumors including aggressive fibromatosis, cervical thoracic lipoblastomatosis, infantile myofibromatosis, and plexiform neurofibroma
- Branchial cleft cysts
- Lymphangiomas

Discussion

Background

It is important to recognize the clinical and imaging features of fibromatosis colli to avoid unnecessary biopsy or undue concern. Fibromatosis colli, often associated with birth trauma or difficult delivery, is an uncommon benign form of infantile fibromatosis with masslike enlargement of the SCM. It is seen in ~0.4% of newborns and infants, affecting male infants slightly more often than female infants. Fibromatosis colli is more commonly encountered on the right compared with the left and is rarely bilaterally. Most cases show no abnormality at birth. Frequently, the disease manifests in the late neonatal period and usually spontaneously disappears by 8 months of age. It is characterized by a firm, painless soft tissue mass in the mid to lower third of the SCM. Normal SCM has two muscular heads, which insert separately onto the sternum and clavicle. Fibromatosis colli frequently involves the distal aspect of the SCM but can also be encountered anywhere in its length and may involve either the sternal head alone or both heads. Following initial discovery, there may be a slight increase in size of the mass; however, the mass usually resolves over the next several months. Torticollis may present in 10 to 20% of cases and usually develops after the appearance of sternocleidomastoid mass.

Etiology

Although the exact cause is unclear, in some cases fibromatosis colli is likely related to birth trauma associated with a difficult or forceps delivery, as this may be noted in up to 50% of cases. The mechanism of injury to the muscle may be localized crushing and ischemia. Intrauterine torticollis or during labor has been suggested to cause pressure necrosis of the SCM and also to lead to the development of fibromatosis colli.

Associated Findings

Fibromatosis colli and congenital muscular torticollis have been associated with congenital anomalies, including foot anomalies, dislocation of the hip, and obstetrical events such as breech delivery and forceps extraction. There may be associated injury to the brachial plexus.

Clinical Findings

Most often fibromatosis colli presents with a firm, painless muscle mass, which appears within the first few weeks of life. The mass may grow slightly over the following few weeks. Lesions that present in the neonatal period usually resolve spontaneously or with physical therapy within a few months. However, lesions that present after 1 month of age may not resolve and may increase in size. Fibrous tissue within the lesion can lead to contraction and tightening of the SCM, motion restriction, and ipsilateral head tilt known as wryneck or torticollis.

Histology

Histologic analysis shows fibromatosis, which is a benign proliferation of fibrous tissue with infiltrative growth pattern. In fully developed fibromatosis colli there is dense scar tissue separating bundles of skeletal muscle. Some muscle atrophy may be present. Fine-needle biopsy can be used if there is concern regarding the diagnosis, although this is uncommonly needed.

Imaging Findings

RADIOGRAPHY

- Radiographs are usually normal.
- Rare lytic lesions have been reported within the head of the clavicle at the attachment of the fibrosed SCM from extension of fibrous proliferation into the bone.

ULTRASOUND

- Best imaging modality for diagnosis due to relative low cost and lack of radiation
- Ultrasonographic findings include focal or diffuse enlargement of the SCM, usually in a fusiform configuration and in the lower two thirds of the muscle.
- The mass moves synchronously with the SCM and can involve one or both heads of the SCM.
- The echogenicity of the mass is most frequently hyperechoic or mixed but may be isoechoic or hypoechoic relative to normal muscle. A striated pattern of alternating increased and decreased echogenicity may be noted.
- Margins of the mass are usually well defined, especially on transverse images.
- Echogenic foci with acoustic shadowing due to calcifications have been reported uncommonly.
- Ultrasonography is helpful in excluding other disorders.
- Imaging findings not characteristic of fibromatosis colli would include irregular margins, mass extending beyond the confines of the SCM, poor definition of the surrounding fascial planes, and/or mass associated with adenopathy, bone involvement, intracranial spinal extension, vascular encasement, or airway compression.

CT

- Generally not needed
- Focal or diffuse isodense enlargement of the SCM without discrete focal soft tissue mass (**Fig. 25E**)
- Mass is localized within the SCM with normal surrounding fascial planes, lack of associated adenopathy, airway compression, vascular encasement, bone involvement, or intracranial or intraspinal extension as may be seen in other neck masses.
- The mass may cause deviation of surrounding structures such as the trachea or neck but not encasement or significant compression.

MRI

- Generally not needed
- Focal or diffuse enlargement of the SCM, localized within the muscle with clear surrounding fascial planes and lack of associated adenopathy, airway compression, vascular encasement,

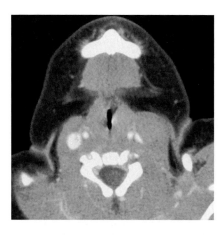

Figure 25E Axial contrast-enhanced CT image showing enlargement of the left SCM with similar density as the normal right side.

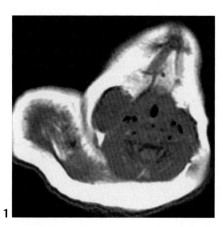

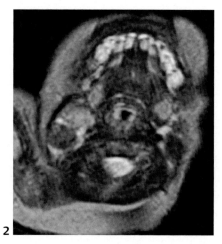

Figure 25F T1-weighted (**1**) and T2-weighted (**2**) MRI show marked enlargement of right SCM, which is isointense to surrounding muscle on T1 and hyperintense on T2-weighted images.

bone involvement, or intracranial or intraspinal extension as may be seen in other neck masses
- Isointense to muscle on T1-weighted images, higher signal than muscle or fat on T2-weighted images (**Figs. 25F1** and **25F2**)
- Low signal intensity patches and linear bands can be seen within the lesions on T2-weighted images.

ANGIOGRAPHY/CONVENTIONAL ANGIOGRAPHY OR MRA

- Not needed

Treatment

- Conservative treatment consists of passive stretching of the affected SCM and strengthening exercises of the contralateral muscle.
  In only a minority of cases ranging from 10 to 20% will surgery be required.
- Surgical lengthening is done in severe cases that fail conservative management.

Prognosis

- Most cases resolve spontaneously in a few months with conservative therapy.

Complications

- Torticollis, seen in 10 to 20% of cases

- Fusiform enlargement of the SCM in a neonate presenting clinically with an anterior neck mass is characteristic of fibromatosis colli.
- Ultrasonography may show a variety of echogenicity patterns, but all are confined solely to SCM.

- Clinical follow-up is needed to ensure appropriate resolution, as rarely other lesions can show a similar appearance early in their course.
- Imaging findings not characteristic of fibromatosis colli include irregular margins, mass extending beyond the confines of the SCM, poor definition of the surrounding fascial planes, and/or mass associated with adenopathy, bone involvement, intracranial spinal extension, vascular encasement, or airway compression.

Suggested Readings

Ablin DS, Jain K, Howell L, West DC. Ultrasound and MR imaging of fibromatosis colli (sternomastoid tumor of infancy). Pediatr Radiol 1998;28:230–233

Bedi DG, John SD, Swischuk LE. Fibromatosis colli of infancy: variability of sonographic appearance. J Clin Ultrasound 1998;26:345–348

Castellote A, Vazquez E, Vera J, et al. Cervicothoracic lesions in infants and children. Radiographics 1999;19:583–600

Chan WL, Cheng JCY. Ultrasonography of congenital muscular torticollis. Pediatric J 1992;22:256–260

Crawford SC, Harnsberger HR, Johnson L, Aoki JR, Giley J. Fibromatosis colli of infancy: CT and sonographic findings. AJR Am J Roentgenol 1988;151:1183–1184

Ekinci S, Karnak I, Tanyel FC. Infantile fibromatosis of the sternocleidomastoid muscle mimicking muscular torticollis. J Pediatr Surg 2004;39:1424–1425

Kiesewetter WB, Nelson PK, Palladino VS, Koop CE. Neonatal torticollis. JAMA 1955;157:1281–1285

Kurtycz DF, Logrono R, Hoerl HD, Heatley DG. Diagnosis of fibromatosis colli by fine-needle aspiration. Diagn Cytopathol 2000;23(5):338–342

Robbin MR, Murphy MD, Temple T, Kransdorf MJ, Choi JJ. Imaging of musculoskeletal fibromatosis. Radiographics 2001;21:585–600

Sartoris DJ, Mochzuki RM, Parker BR. Lytic clavicular lesions in fibromatosis colli. Skeletal Radiol 1983;10:34–36

Snitzer E, Fultz P, Asselint B. Magnetic resonance imaging appearance of fibromatosis colli. Magn Reson Imaging 1997;15:869–871

CASE 26

Clinical Presentation

A 23-month-old boy presents with head tilt, fever, and right-sided cervical lymphadenopathy.

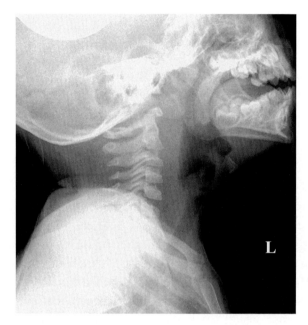

Figure 26A

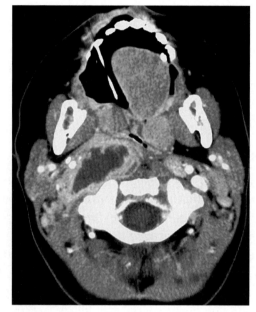

Figure 26B

Radiologic Findings

Lateral soft tissue radiograph of the neck shows increased thickness of the prevertebral soft tissues anterior to the upper cervical spine, worrisome for retropharyngeal inflammation, either abscess or cellulitis (**Fig. 26A**). CT study was performed under general anesthesia with an orotracheal tube in situ. Enhanced axial CT image shows a large, well-delineated right-sided mass with low-intensity interior and thick enhancing rim (**Fig. 26B**). There is bowing of the right internal carotid artery anterolaterally and compression of the right internal jugular vein. Mass effect is present on the right posterolateral aspect of the oropharynx, with moderate deviation of the right tonsil anteromedially. Remaining CT images show that the lesion extends from the skull base inferiorly down to the level of the mandible and into the right parapharyngeal space.

Diagnosis

Large right-sided retropharyngeal abscess (RPA)

Differential Diagnosis

- Other superficial and deep neck space infections including peritonsillar and superficial abscesses, suppurative cervical lymphadenitis
- Esophageal foreign body with perforation
- Aneurysm
- Hematoma
- Benign and malignant tumors of the retropharyngeal and surrounding region including cystic hygroma, hemangioma, rhabdomyosarcoma, cervical spine tumors, and lymphoma

Discussion

Background

The retropharyngeal area is a deep neck space extending from the skull base down into the mediastinum that normally contains lymph nodes in young children. It is bordered by buccopharyngeal fascia anteriorly, prevertebral fascia posteriorly, and carotid sheaths laterally. RPAs are potentially life-threatening deep space neck infections, which can be of medical or traumatic origin. Infrequent in occurrence, retropharyngeal infection and abscess is largely a disease of childhood, with most cases occurring in children <5 years of life. Most RPAs result from lymphatic spread of a variety of predisposing head and neck and upper respiratory tract infections, including pharyngitis and tonsillitis. Traumatic causes may follow lacerations from objects stuck in the mouth such as pencils. In early childhood, lymph nodes are located in the retropharyngeal space, generally straddling the junction of retropharyngeal and parapharyngeal spaces. Lymphadenitis in this region can subsequently lead to cellulitis, phlegmon, and abscess. With increasing age, atrophy of the retropharyngeal lymph nodes probably occurs, decreasing the disease risk in older children. Infection in older children and adults is more often due to perforation from foreign bodies and iatrogenic injury including endoscopy.

Clinical Findings

The typical presentation of retropharyngeal infection and abscess is often nonspecific, with sore throat, fever, torticollis, and neck pain commonly seen. Drooling, malaise, decreased oral intake, irritability, neck mass, and respiratory distress or stridor, decreased appetite, jaw stiffness or neck stiffness, or muffled voice can also be seen. Occasionally, upper respiratory infection can precede symptoms of RPA. Physical findings include fever, cervical adenopathy, decreased range of neck motion, neck mass, posterior pharyngeal mass, and respiratory distress.

Pathology and Laboratory Findings

Positive microbiological cultures of pus, blood, or pharyngeal space are found in roughly 50% of patients. Predominant organisms include *Streptococcus* species and *Staphylococcus aureus*. However, anaerobes and mixed flora can also be seen.

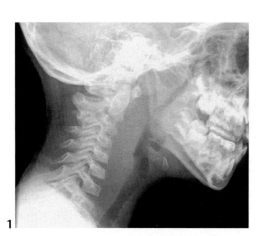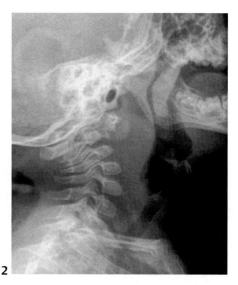

Figure 26C Two patients with RPAs and differing appearance of retropharyngeal soft tissues. The patient on the left (**1**) shows moderate diffuse soft tissue thickening and displacement of the air column anteriorly. The patient on the right (**2**) shows more marked soft tissue bulging superiorly and abnormality at the craniocervical junction.

Imaging Findings

RADIOGRAPHY

- Useful as initial screening examination but does not distinguish phlegmon from abscess
- Need appropriate technique (with neck extended and in inspiration) to decrease false-positive examination as thickening of retropharyngeal soft tissues may be simulated during expiration, during swallowing, or with the neck flexed.
- Normal prevertebral soft tissue width should be no greater than 7 mm above the glottis and 14 mm below. If anteroposterior soft tissue thickness is greater than adjacent vertebral body, this suggests inflammation and possible abscess.
- May see widening of prevertebral soft tissues often with kyphosis or loss of cervical lordosis from muscle spasm
- Can see anterior displacement of hypopharynx and tracheal air column (**Figs. 26C1** and **26C2**)
- May see gas, air-fluid level, or foreign body in retropharyngeal soft tissues
- Plain films may appear equivocal or even normal on occasion, especially with parapharyngeal collections.
- Associated complications include spinal osteomyelitis
- Chest radiography is recommended to exclude mediastinal extension or pulmonary complications.

FLUOROSCOPY

- May be helpful in differentiating false- from true-positive by monitoring the retropharyngeal thickness during breathing.

CT

- Contrast-enhanced CT is the diagnostic method of choice. Scan should be performed from skull base to T2.
- CT considered sensitive but not as specific in differentiating abscess from cellulitis/phlegmon
- Useful in initial diagnosis, determining the extent of disease, assessment of potential complications, and in monitoring treatment

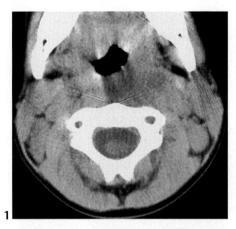 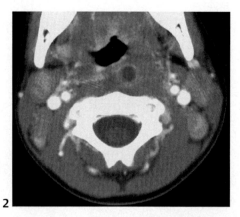

Figure 26D Axial CT showing unenhanced (**1**) and enhanced (**2**) images. Unenhanced image shows retropharyngeal hypodensity on the left with some distortion of the hypopharyngeal airway. Enhanced image shows small hypodensity with mild rim enhancement. Findings suggest early small abscess, but phlegmon may have similar appearance. Patient responded well to antibiotics without surgery needed.

- Distinguish abscess from cellulitis on CT by abscess size; the hypodensity of the abscess, which should be similar to cerebrospinal fluid; presence of complete rim enhancement; and/or gas (**Figs. 26D1** and **26D2**).
- Local tissue edema can mimic pus on occasion.
- RPAs usually appear off center due to the presence of the midline raphe formed by the superior constrictor muscle.
- Associated adenopathy is common and can be bilateral and bulky.
- Can see infrequent vascular compression, bone involvement, compression of neighboring structures
- Midline abscesses are usually in the prevertebral space.
- In patients with any degree of airway compromise, sedation of patient may lead to airway compromise. CT is not completely reliable in distinguishing phlegmon from abscess.

MRI

- MRI is usually not necessary but helpful if there is concern regarding spine or cord involvement, unusual infection, or suspicion of tumor or vascular mass (**Figs. 26E1** and **26E2**).
- Sedation is more often a concern with MRI, as young children generally require sedation; consider an anesthesia consult.
- MRI may show arterial enhancement and luminal narrowing possibly as a sign of impeding arterial damage.

ULTRASOUND

- May be of value for immediate evaluation to distinguish abscess from cellulitis or to guide aspiration
- Can show central necrosis and presence of abscess, vascular complication with color Doppler
- Drawbacks include operator dependence and limited published studies to date.
- Not considered adequate for complete surgical planning of abscess as not all loculations well seen, particularly those extending throughout the deep neck spaces
- Limited assessment posteriorly for spine and cord

ANGIOGRAPHY/CTA OR MRA

- May be needed for suspected vascular complications

Treatment

- Management depends on the maturity and size of infection.

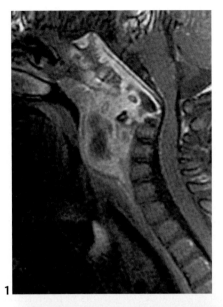

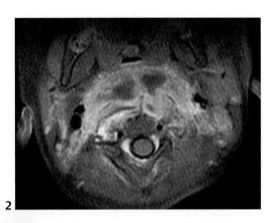

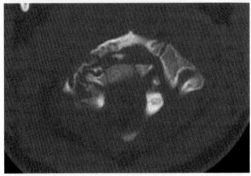

Figure 26E A 13-month-old girl presented with long-standing torticollis and initial suspicion of tumor. Midline contrast-enhanced sagittal T1-weighted fat-suppressed (**1**) and axial (**2**) images showing large prevertebral/retropharyngeal soft tissue mass with central hypointensity and involvement of the craniocervical junction, especially C2 and clivus. There is moderate spinal stenosis at the craniocervical junction. Biopsy showed abscess with granulation tissue in keeping with acute and chronic inflammation. No pathologic evidence of mycobacteria was found. Axial CT (**3**) showing bone destruction of C1 and C2 from RPA (same patient as shown in **1** and **2**), especially on the right, and associated subluxation of the C1–2 level.

- Broad-spectrum antibiotic therapy directed initially toward aerobic and anaerobic flora of nasopharynx
- Aspiration and surgical drainage of abscess as needed

Prognosis

- Generally excellent in recent reports

Complications

- Secondary to mass effect, abscess rupture, or spread of infection
- Airway compromise more likely to occur with larger pus collections
- Abscess rupture can lead to asphyxia or aspiration of pus and lead to pneumonia.
- Vascular complications include jugular vein thrombosis, carotid artery aneurysm, and rupture.
- Spread of infection either laterally, posteriorly, or inferiorly with mediastinitis, osteomyelitis, or damage to major neurovascular structures (**Fig. 26E3**)
- Can see necrotizing fasciitis and sepsis

PEARLS_____

- Proper technique for lateral radiograph (inspiratory film with neck extension) is key to minimizing false-positive examinations.
- Vascular complications of RPA are rare in postantibiotic era but should be considered if the abscess extends into the carotid space on CT.
- Air in thickened retropharyngeal soft tissues implies rupture of the abscess into pharynx or esophagus.

PITFALLS_____

- Sedation can relax airway muscles, leading to airway obstruction.
- Do not forget to look for complications, including mediastinal extension.

Suggested Readings

Brechtelsbauer PB, Garetz SL, Gebarski SS, Bradford CR. Retropharyngeal abscess: pitfalls of plain films and computed tomography. Am J Otolaryngol 1997;18:258–262

Castellote A, Vazquez E, Vera J, et al. Cervicothoracic lesions in infants and children. Radiographics 1999;19:583–600

Chao HC, Chiu CH, Lin SJ, Lin TY. Colour Doppler ultrasonography of retropharyngeal abscess. J Otolaryngol 1999;28:138–141

Cmejrek RC, Coticchia JM, Arnold JE. Presentation, diagnosis, and management of deep-neck abscesses in infants. Arch Otolaryngol Head Neck Surg 2002;128:1361–1364

Craig FW, Schunk JE. Retropharyngeal abscess in children: clinical presentation, utility of imaging and current management. Pediatrics 2003;111:1394–1398

Daya H, Lo S, Papsin BC, et al. Retropharyngeal and parapharyngeal infections in children: the Toronto experience. Int J Pediatr Otorhinolaryngol 2005;69:81–86

Glasier CM, Stark JE, Jacobs RF, Mancias P, Leithiser RE Jr, Seibert R. CT and ultrasound imaging of retropharyngeal abscess in children. AJNR Am J Neuroradiol 1992;13:1191–1195

Ide C, Bodart E, Remacle M, De Coene B, Nisolle JF, Trigauz JP. An early MR observation of carotid involvement by retropharyngeal abscess. AJNR Am J Neuroradiol 1998;19:499–501

Kuhnemann S, Keck T, Riechelmann H, Rettinger G. Rational diagnosis of pediatric pharyngeal abscess. Laryngorhinootologie 2001;80:263–268

Pontell J, Har-El G, Lucente FE. Retropharyngeal abscess: clinical review. Ear Nose Throat J 1995;74:701–704

Riccabona M, Grubbauer HM. Ultrasound diagnosis of parapharyngeal abscess in infancy. Ultraschall Med 1994;15:43–44

Roberson DW, Kirse DJ. Infectious and inflammatory disorders of the neck. In: Wetmore RF, Muntz HR, McGill TJ, eds. Pediatric Otolaryngology: Principles and Practice. New York, NY: Thieme; 2000:969–991

Singh I, Rakesh C, Gupta KB, Yadav SPS. Fatal pyothroax: a rare complication of retropharyngeal abscess. Indian J Chest Dis Allied Sci 2003;45:265–268

Stone ME, Walner DL, Koch BL, Egelhoff JC, Myer CM. Correlation between computed tomography and surgical findings in retropharyngeal inflammatory processes in children. Int J Pediatr Otorhinolaryngol 1999;49:121–125

Vural C, Gungor A, Comerci S. Accuracy of computerized tomography in deep neck infections in the pediatric population. Am J Otolaryngol 2003;24:143–148

CASE 27

Clinical Presentation

A 9-month-old male presents with a 4-week history of right esotropia (inward turning of the eye) and periorbital swelling.

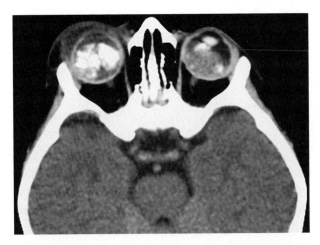

Figure 27A

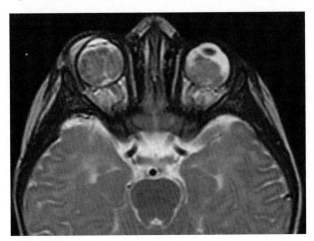

Figure 27B

Radiologic Findings

CT (**Fig. 27A**) reveals bilateral calcified mildly enhancing intraocular masses with right periorbital swelling. Axial fast spin echo T2-weighted MRI (**Fig. 27B**) demonstrates bilateral intraocular hypointense masses consistent with partly calcified retinoblastoma.

Diagnosis

Bilateral retinoblastoma

Differential Diagnosis

- Persistent hyperplastic primary vitreous
- Coats' disease
- Norrie's disease
- Retinal astrocytic hamartomas of tuberous sclerosis
- Toxocara endophthalmitis
- Retinopathy of prematurity

Discussion

Background

Retinoblastoma is the most common intraocular tumor of childhood. It occurs in 1 in 10,000 to 15,000 live births. It is nonhereditary in 60 to 80% of cases and hereditary in the remainder. The hereditary form usually presents earlier (<2 years of age) and is frequently bilateral. Trilateral retinoblastoma represents the association of a midline intracranial tumor (usually pineoblastoma) with bilateral retinoblastoma. Retinoblastoma can also be rarely tetralateral when it is associated with a suprasellar tumor.

Etiology

The etiology of retinoblastoma includes both hereditary and nonhereditary forms. The gene responsible for retinoblastoma is localized to the 13q14 locus, which is mutated or deleted in both hereditary and nonhereditary forms. The retinoblastoma gene functions as a suppressor gene. If both alleles are suppressed or deleted, then retinoblastoma can develop. The hereditary form is autosomal dominant with a penetrance of 90% and with increased risk in trisomy 21.

Embryology

Retinoblastoma arises from retinal neuroectodermal cells.

Clinical Findings

Leucocoria (white papillary reflex) or "cat's eye" is the most common presentation, often shown on photographs as loss of the red eye. Other presentations include:

- Strabismus
- Orbital inflammation
- Proptosis
- Nystagmus

Pathology

Macroscopically, retinoblastomas are noted as single or multiple white, "chalky" nodules in the retina. There are three types:

- **Endophytic:** grows into the vitreous

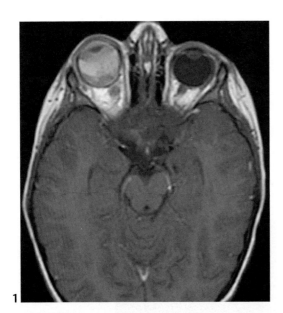 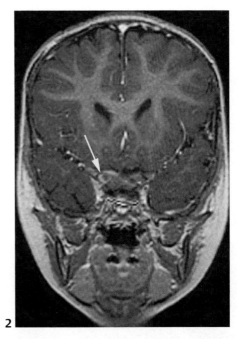

Figure 27C Axial (**1**) and coronal (**2**) contrast-enhanced T1-weighted images demonstrating a heterogeneous enhancing right intraocular mass with extension along the right optic nerve (arrow).

- **Exophytic:** grows posterior to the retina, causing retinal detachment
- **Diffuse:** plaque-like growth along the retina

Microcopically, retinoblastomas consist of a monomorphic mass of small blue cells with fleurettes, Flexner-Wintersteiner or true rosettes. Some contain Homer Wright rosettes.

Associated Conditions

Survivors of retinoblastoma are more likely to develop a nonocular malignancy, which is also more common in the hereditary form. This includes osteogenic and other soft tissue sarcomas, leukemia/lymphoma, Wilms' tumor, Hodgkin's disease, and cutaneous malignant melanoma.

Evolution

A congenital neoplasm but not normally presenting until ~2 years of age. If untreated, this disease is fatal. Retinoblastoma can spread intracranially via the optic nerve (**Figs. 27C**) and/or spread through the brain and spine via leptomeningeal dissemination.

Pathophysiology/Pathogenetic Mechanisms

The retinoblastoma gene located on the long arm of chromosome 13 produces a protein active in cell cycle suppression. Both copies of retinoblastoma gene must be affected to manifest the disease.

Imaging Findings

ULTRASOUND

- Irregular retinal-based echogenic mass with posterior shadowing (due to calcification)
- Doppler flow is detected.

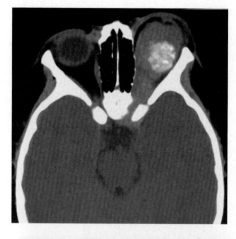

Figure 27D Axial CT image showing recurrent left retinoblastoma (note calcification) with extension through the left optic nerve canal.

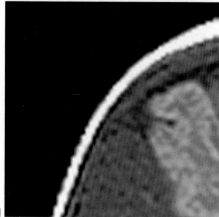

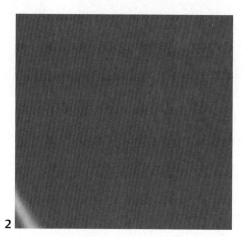

Figure 27E Coronal CT soft tissue (**1**) and bone (**2**) windows demonstrate tumor extension through an enlarged left optic nerve canal (arrows).

CT

- Fine or punctate intraocular calcification with an enhancing mass (**Figs. 27D** and **27E**)
- The mass arises from the retina, but sometimes its origin may be unclear due to border irregularity.
- May assess for extraocular extension into orbital lymphatics and optic nerve (but more sensitive on MRI)
- No microphthalmia

MRI

- T1 is variable, usually a low-signal intraocular mass that shows enhancement (**Figs. 27F, 27G**, and **27H**).
- T2 hypointense compared with normal vitreous
- Assess for extraocular extension and intracranial extension.
- Assess for pineal (trilateral) and suprasellar (tetralateral) masses.
- More sensitive to subarachnoid and intracranial spread and retinal detachment
- MRI of the spine to assess for spinal metastases

Treatment

- Treatment is dependent on staging.
- Initial treatment is tumor reduction by first-line chemotherapy. This is followed by treatment with cryotherapy, thermotherapy, plaque radiotherapy, or laser photocoagulation.

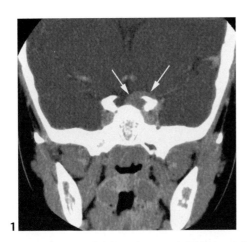
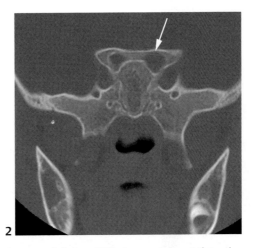

Figure 27F Axial (**1**) and coronal (**2**) T1-weighted postgadolinium MRI demonstrates trilateral retinoblastoma with a suprasellar mass (small intraocular masses may not be seen on MRI).

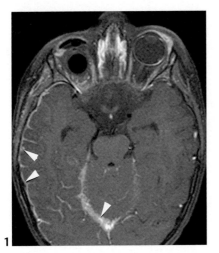
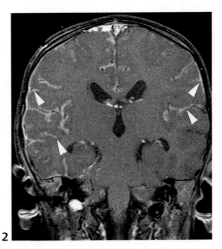

Figure 27G Right orbital prosthesis (**1**) with diffuse leptomeningeal enhancement (arrowheads) from intracranial spread of retinoblastoma shown on fat-suppressed T1-weighted images (**2**).

- Enucleation and external beam radiotherapy now not as widely used
- If bilateral, then local radiotherapy to remaining eye
- Chemotherapy and bone marrow transplant for bone marrow salvage

Complications

- Intracranial extension via the optic nerve worst prognostic factor
- Secondary nonocular malignancies such as osteosarcoma
- Radiation-induced cataracts can occur.

Prognosis

- Survival rates of 90 to 95% can be achieved with a combination of enucleation, external beam radiotherapy, laser photocoagulation, plaque radiotherapy, and cryotherapy.
- Trilateral retinoblastoma, however, is usually fatal.
- Staging based on the Reese-Ellsworth staging system.

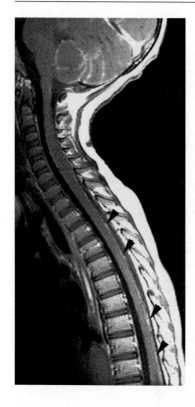

Figure 27H Sagittal T1-weighted image following gadolinium contrast shows diffuse spinal leptomeningeal enhancement (arrowheads) from retinoblastoma metastases.

PEARL

- A calcified intraocular mass in a child is retinoblastoma until proven otherwise.

PITFALL

- Calcification may not be visible on CT or MRI, but it is almost always present microscopically.

Suggested Readings

Barkovich, AJ. Pediatric Neuroimaging. 3rd ed. New York: Williams & Wilkins; 2000:324–327

Belt PJ, Smithers M, Elston T. The triad of bilateral retinoblastoma, dysplastic naevus syndrome and multiple cutaneous malignant melanomas: a case report and review of the literature. Melanoma Res 2002;12:179–182

Blaser SI, Illner A, Castillo M, Hedlund GL, Osborn A. Pocket Radiologist—Peds Neuro: Top 100 Diagnoses. Salt Lake City, UT: Amirsys; 2003

De Potter P. Current treatment of retinoblastoma. Curr Opin Ophthalmol 2002;13:331–336

Deegan W. Emerging strategies for the treatment of retinoblastoma. Curr Opin Ophthalmol 2003;14:291–295

Marcus DM, Brooks SE, Leff G, et al. Trilateral retinoblastoma: insights into histogenesis and management. Surv Ophthalmol 1998;43:59–70

Phillips C, Sexton M, Wheeler G, McKenzie J. Retinoblastoma: review of 30 years' experience with external beam radiotherapy. Australas Radiol 2003;47:226–230

Provenzale JM, Weber AL, Klintworth GK, McLendon RE. Radiologic-pathologic correlation: bilateral retinoblastoma with co-existent pineoblastoma (trilateral retinoblastoma). AJNR Am J Neuroradiol 1995;16:157–165

Skulski M, Egelhoff JC, Kollias SS, Mazewski C, Ball WS. Trilateral retinoblastoma with suprasellar involvement. Neuroradiology 1997;39:41–43

CASE 28

Clinical Presentation

A 9-year-old female presents with a "pearly white" right retrotympanic mass noted during investigation of moderate hearing loss.

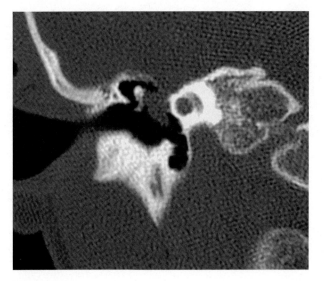

Figure 28A

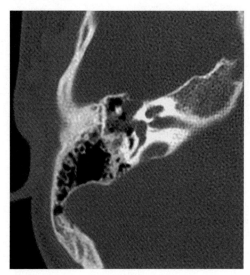

Figure 28B

Radiologic Findings

Noncontrast coronal (**Fig. 28A**) and axial (**Fig. 28B**) CT demonstrates a soft tissue mass in the right epi/mesotympanum with erosion of the medial tegmen tympani.

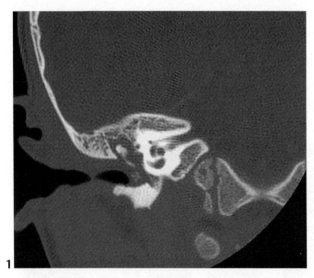 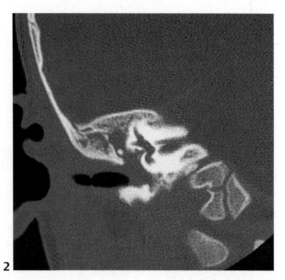

Figure 28C Coronal CT (bone algorithm) showing inflammatory soft tissue mass right middle-ear cavity (**1**). No erosion with soft tissue thickening of the superior external auditory canal (**2**).

Diagnosis

Right middle-ear cholesteatoma (**Fig. 28C**)

Differential Diagnosis

- Otomastoiditis
- Langerhans' cell histiocytosis

Discussion

Background

Congenital cholesteatoma is a keratin-filled sac in the middle ear, located medial to an intact tympanic membrane. Criteria for clinical diagnosis include a white mass medial to a normal tympanic membrane and normal pars tensa and flaccida without prior history of otorrhea, tympanic membrane perforation, or otologic surgery. There is a strong male predominance. Estimated incidence of 0.12 per 100,000. Average age at presentation is between 5 and 7 years.

Etiology

Embryonic rest cell theory proposed by Teed in 1936, who described an epithelial thickening of ectodermal origin in the upper mesotympanum medial to the malleus neck. This epithelial thickening usually involutes and becomes normal endothelium. If this does not occur, then a congenital cholesteatoma may develop.

Embryology

Embryonic epidermal inclusions fail to involute. In theory, they can form in utero, as proven when Michaels in 1986 described a structure in fetal ears at the point of transition between cuboidal and respiratory epithelium and called this "epidermoid" formation. This can be detected normally between 10 and 33 weeks' gestation; if it persists for more than 33 weeks, is abnormal

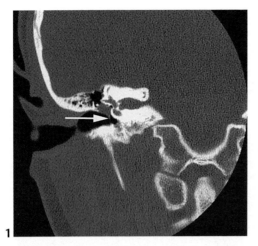 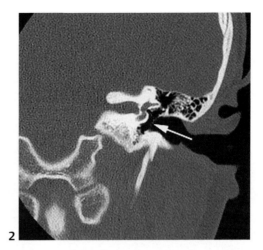

Figure 28D Coronal CT showing right middle-ear soft tissue mass (**1**) with tympanic membrane retraction (arrow). The normal side (**2**) is shown for comparison.

Clinical Findings

White pearly retrotympanic mass is usually present in the anterior-superior quadrant of the middle ear with an intact tympanic membrane. Presents most commonly with painless otorrhea and hearing loss. Rarely presents with otalgia, headache and fever, vertigo, and facial nerve palsy. Physical findings: white "pearly" retrotympanic mass with an intact tympanic membrane.

Imaging Findings

Soft tissue middle-ear mass centered on the anterosuperior quadrant and occupying to a variable extent the middle-ear cavity with or without ossicular chain erosion/destruction and mastoid air cell involvement (**Figs. 28C1** and **28C2**).

Pathology/Laboratory Findings

Macroscopically, cholesteatoma shows as white tissue mass, which are of two types: open and closed. The more common, closed type, is a closed epithelial cyst, whereas the open type diffusely "carpets" the middle-ear cleft, with matrix and keratin debris. Microscopically, cholesteatoma is characterized by a mass of squamous epithelium at the interface between pseudostratified columnar epithelium of the eustachian tube and the normal cuboidal epithelium of the middle ear.

Associated Conditions

Predisposing conditions include cleft palate and craniofacial syndromes. Blockage of the eustachian tube may cause a middle-ear effusion.

Evolution

As described by Koltai et al (2002), most cholesteatoma start as a matrix-enclosed spherical keratin pearl in the anterior-superior quadrant of the middle ear. This grows anteriorly toward the eustachian tube and may cause otitis media and a secondary middle-ear effusion. Negative pressure then causes retraction of the tympanic membrane (**Figs. 28D1** and **28D2**). Inferior growth is toward the hypotympanum, posterior growth is toward the handle of the malleus, and superior growth occurs into the anterior epitympanum. There is progressive cholesteatoma enlargement and bony erosion with final

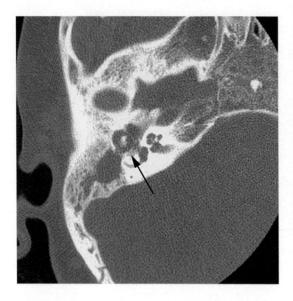

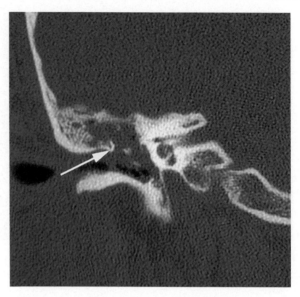

Figure 28E Axial CT (bone algorithm) showing middle-ear soft tissue mass with erosion of the right lateral semicircular canal (arrow). There is a risk of CSF fistula. There is an extension into the mastoid air cells.

Figure 28F Coronal CT (bone algorithm) demonstrates erosion of the scutum with cholesteatoma.

stages of progressive otorrhea, conductive hearing loss, tympanic membrane perforation, and cholesteatoma extension into the mastoid air cells.

Pathophysiology/Pathogenetic Mechanisms

Two main theories have been proposed: the invasion theory and the epithelial rest theory. The *invasion theory* indicates direction of migrating ectodermal cells within the developing external auditory canal is through the tympanic isthmus into the middle ear; whereas, in the *epithelial rest theory*, cholesteatoma is thought to arise from epithelial rests, which have been identified in the middle ear, most commonly in the anterosuperior quadrant in fetuses and present normally until 33 weeks' gestation.

Imaging Findings

RADIOGRAPHY

- Not useful for diagnosis

CT

- CT is the imaging modality of choice.
- Soft tissue middle-ear mass centered on the anterosuperior middle-ear cavity (**Figs. 28E, 28F,** and **28G**)
- May demonstrate erosion of the ossicular chain, tegmen tympani, mastoid air cells, and scutum. Look for dehiscence of the facial nerve canal and semicircular canal.
- CT does not differentiate between granulation tissue and cholesteatoma, so it is not precise for disease extent.

MRI

- Useful for ruling out intracranial complications including dural involvement, abscess formation, and sinus thrombosis

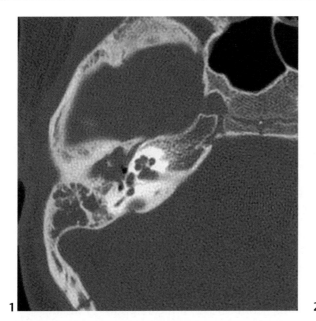
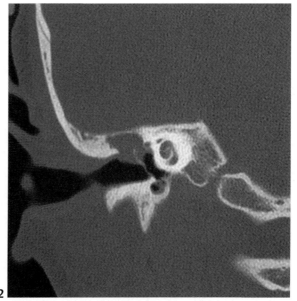

Figure 28G Axial (**1**) and coronal (**2**) CT showing eroded ossicles in a right middle-ear cholesteatoma.

Treatment

- Topical antibiotics only for superimposed infection
- Surgical management is the mainstay.
- Three main types of surgery: tympanoplasty, canal-wall-up tympanomastoidectomy, or canal-wall-down tympanomastoidectomy
- Very rarely a radical mastoidectomy is indicated.

Complications

Tympanic membrane perforation with conductive hearing loss occurs late. Erosion into the facial nerve canal causes facial nerve paralysis. Erosion into semicircular canals can cause a CSF fistula. Blockage of the eustachian tube may produce a co-existent middle-ear effusion.

Prognosis

- Staging system:
  - Stage I: single quadrant, no ossicular involvement or mastoid extension
  - Stage II: multiple quadrants, no ossicular involvement or mastoid extension
  - Stage III: ossicular involvement includes erosion of the ossicles but no mastoid involvement
  - Stage IV: mastoid extension, regardless of other findings
- There is correlation between stage of disease and probability of cholesteatoma recurrence, with ~13% recurrence rate for Stage I with linear correlation to 67% recurrence for Stage IV disease.

PEARL _____

- White "pearly" retrotympanic mass in a child is a cholesteatoma until proven otherwise.

PITFALL _____

- Early imaging may be inconclusive due to a small mass and absence of definitive erosion.

Suggested Readings

El-Bitar MA, Choi SS, Emamian SA, Vezina LG. Congenital middle ear cholesteatoma: need for early recognition: role of computed tomography scan. Int. J Pediatr Otorhinolaryngol 2003;67:231–235

Karmody CS, Byahatti SV, Blevins N, Valtonen H, Northrop C. The origin of congenital cholesteatoma. Am. J Otol 1998;19:292–297

Kazahaya K, Potsic WP. Congenital cholesteatoma. Curr Opin Otolaryngol Head Neck Surg 2004;12:398–403

Koltai PJ, Nelson M, Castellon RJ, et al. The natural history of congenital cholesteatoma. Arch Otolaryngol Head Neck Surg 2002;128:804–809

Nelson M, Rogers G, Koltai PJ, et al. Congenital cholesteatoma classification, management and outcome. Arch Otolaryngol Head Neck Surg 2002;128:810–814

Potsic WP, Samadi DS, Marsh RR, Wetmore RF. A staging system for congenital cholesteatoma. Arch Otolaryngol Head Neck Surg 2002;128:1009–1012

Shohet JA, de Jong AL. The management of pediatric cholesteatoma. Otolaryngol Clin North Am 2002;35:841–851

Soldati D, Mudry A. Knowledge about cholesteatoma, from the first description to modern histopathology. Otol Neurotol 2001;22:723–730

Teed RW. Cholesteatoma verum tympanic (its relationship to the first epibranchial placocle). Arch Otolaryngol 1936;24:455–474

SECTION III
Chest

CASE 29

Clinical Presentation

A 2-year-old presents with a sudden onset of barky cough and inspiratory stridor in the middle of the night.

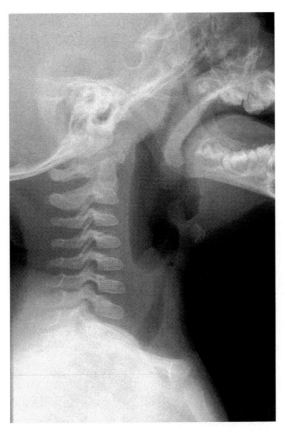

Figure 29A

Radiologic Findings

Lateral radiograph of the neck with appropriate semi-extended neck positioning and inspiration demonstrates mild subglottic narrowing and haziness (**Fig. 29A**). The glottic and supraglottic structures are well delineated and normal. There is hypopharyngeal distension from the relative subglottic narrowing.

Diagnosis

Croup

Differential Diagnosis

- Post-intubation subglottic inflammation/fibrosis
- Subglottic masses such as hemangioma
- Subglottic mucocele
- Glottic or subglottic foreign body
- Bacterial tracheitis

Discussion

Background

Croup is the most common cause of acquired upper respiratory obstruction in children. It is characterized by subglottic inflammation caused by an acute viral infection, most commonly from a parainfluenza infection. Many upper respiratory acute viral pathogens can produce a similar picture.

Clinical Findings

Croup is most commonly seen in the winter months, when parainfluenza and influenza viruses are most active. Characteristically, the child develops inspiratory stridor and intercostal retractions. The symptoms are frequently worse at night, improve with exposure to cool outside air, and commonly present in association with a nonspecific upper respiratory tract infection. Physics principles dictate that airway resistance is inversely proportional to the radius of the airway ($1/R^4$). Small decreases in the radius of the airway result in significant increases in airway resistance, an observation that is magnified by the normally smaller pediatric airway. Children, therefore, will become symptomatic earlier than adults with similar amounts of airway compromise. The age range most commonly affected is 6 months to 3 years. The diagnosis is frequently made clinically, and radiographs should only be required in clinically atypical cases.

Other causes of a croup-like syndrome include "membranous" croup and "spasmodic" croup. Membranous croup is similar to, if not the same entity as, bacterial tracheitis, and it is characterized by the presence of a mucopurulent membrane in the upper airway. It is usually caused by a bacterial infection such as *Staphylococcus aureus* alone or in combination with a viral agent. Children with membranous croup are usually older and have more toxic symptoms of severe respiratory distress and high fever. Most of these children will require intubation and intravenous antibiotics. Radiographs may demonstrate tracheal wall thickening, more severe luminal compromise, and/or intratracheal debris, which may mimic a foreign body. Spasmodic croup is due to subglottic and glottic inflammation related to an allergic reaction.

Imaging Findings

RADIOGRAPHY

- The characteristic finding in croup is found on the lateral neck radiograph, performed to optimize evaluation of the soft tissues of the neck.
- The lateral neck radiograph shows narrowing and/or poor definition to the subglottic trachea, with distention of the hypopharynx due to the relative subglottic obstruction (**Fig. 29A**).

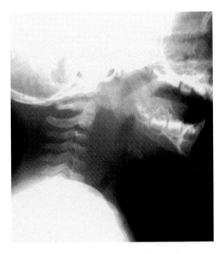

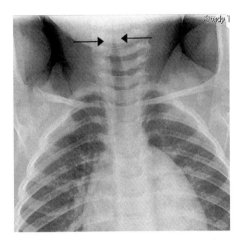

Figure 29B Expiratory lateral neck view demonstrates the subglottic narrowing to better advantage.

Figure 29C Frontal inspiratory view demonstrates tapered narrowing of the subglottic trachea (arrows), creating the "steeple" sign.

- The glottis may or may not be affected, demonstrating loss of definition of the laryngeal vestibule, although the supraglottic structures are usually spared.
- Expiratory radiographs are seldom needed but can be helpful in difficult cases (**Fig. 29B**).
- Frontal radiographs may demonstrate tapered subglottic narrowing, creating the "steeple" sign (**Fig. 29C**).
- The chest radiograph may also demonstrate bronchial wall thickening and overinflation due to the frequent inflammation of the larger airways as well (also called laryngotracheobronchitis).

Treatment

- The severity of respiratory distress in viral croup rarely requires therapeutic intervention other than ambient air humidification or aerosolized racemic epinephrine to transiently decrease the swelling.
- Endotracheal intubation is usually not needed.
- Short-term steroid administration is a controversial new mode of therapy.

Prognosis

- In the vast majority of cases, this entity is short lived and self-resolving, requiring only temporary supportive care.

PEARLS

- The radiologic diagnosis of croup depends on the appropriate clinical setting, as other causes of subglottic narrowing rarely produce such a classic clinical presentation.
- The subglottic narrowing in croup is usually symmetric. Asymmetric narrowing should raise the suspicion of focal scarring (as seen after prolonged intubation) or a focal mass (such as a hemangioma).

PITFALLS

- Beware of the poorly positioned lateral neck radiograph or one obtained in expiration as the trachea can be buckled or displaced.
- On the lateral radiograph, one must look at the epiglottis as subglottic narrowing occurs in 25% of patients.

Suggested Readings

Hedlund GL, Griscom NT, Cleveland RH, Kirks DR. Respiratory system. Chapter 7. In: Kirks DR, Griscom NT, eds. Practical Pediatric Imaging: Diagnostic Radiology of Infants and Children. 3rd ed. Philadelphia: Lippincott-Raven; 1998:651–653

Strife JL. Upper airway and tracheal obstruction in infants and children. Radiol Clin North Am 1988;26:309–322

Swischuk LE. Nasal passages, mandible and airway. Chapter 2. In: Imaging of the Newborn, Infant, and Young Child. 5th ed. Philadelphia: Lippincott, Williams & Wilkins; 2004:201–210

CASE 30

Clinical Presentation

A 3-year-old child presents to the hospital with high fever and difficulty swallowing. She has a 5-day history of preexisting upper respiratory tract infection.

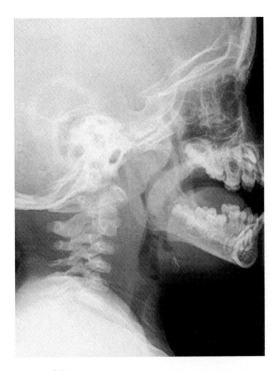

Figure 30A

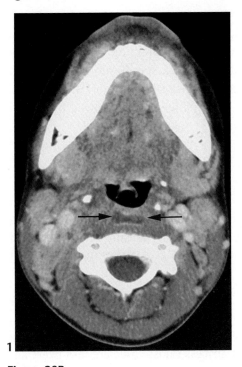
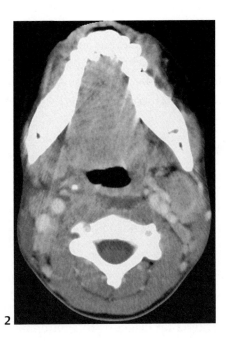

Figure 30B

Radiologic Findings

Lateral neck radiograph demonstrates prevertebral/retropharyngeal space soft tissue swelling, which bulges into the normally sharp posterior pharyngeal tissues and piriform fossae (**Fig. 30A**). Axial CT reveals low soft tissue density in retropharyngeal space between the airway and the vertebral column, with a partial ring enhancement/thickening of the regional tissues (**Figs. 30B1**, arrows, and **30B2**).

Diagnosis

Retropharyngeal cellulitis

Differential Diagnosis

- Trauma (prevertebral hematoma)
- Vertebral osteomyelitis
- Tumor (lymphoma, vertebral neoplasm)
- Inappropriate positioning of child
- Retropharyngeal vascular malformation (hemangioma, lymphatic malformation)

Discussion

Background

Retropharyngeal cellulitis and abscess usually occur in the age range of 6 months to 3 years. The retropharyngeal lymph nodes drain to the nasopharynx, middle ear, and tonsils. Bacterial superinfection of a previous viral infection in the nasopharyngeal soft tissues can result in inflammation in retropharyngeal soft tissues. Less commonly, the infection may occur from direct, foreign body penetration of the posterior pharynx.

Clinical Findings

Clinical presentation of retropharyngeal abscess is that of a febrile child who may look toxic. The presentation frequently may be similar to epiglotittis, with the child refraining from swallowing, looking toxic, complaining of a severe sore throat, and maintaining a semiflexed neck position. Whereas epiglotittis is usually clinically spontaneous, retropharyngeal abscess more frequently is predated by a typical viral upper respiratory tract infection lasting a few days, followed by sudden increase in temperature and increase in severity of symptoms.

Imaging Findings

ULTRASOUND

- Although ultrasonographic examination of the neck for cervical adenitis can be quite valuable to differentiate inflammatory adenitis from nodal abscess formation, especially with the use of Doppler interrogation, ultrasonographic evaluation of the retropharyngeal tissues may be difficult.

CT

- CT is the modality of choice to evaluate the retropharyngeal soft tissues and the cervical region for possible complications and abscess formation.
- Although total ring enhancement of a focal area of low attenuation in the retropharyngeal space defines the CT criteria for diagnosis of a retropharyngeal abscess, most cases are less overt and likely constitute retropharyngeal cellulitis rather than true abscess.

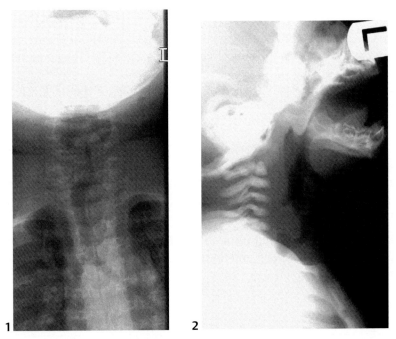

Figure 30C Frontal (**1**) and lateral plain films (**2**) of the neck reveal impressive tracheal buckling, which is commonly seen in radiographs performed in expiration or in examinations where the neck is inappropriately flexed.

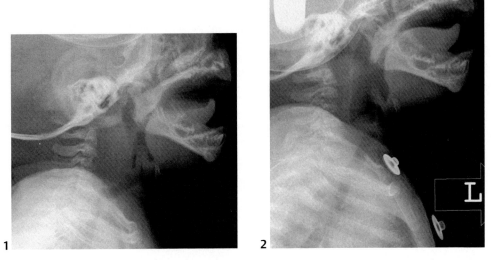

Figure 30D Initial lateral neck radiograph (**1**) demonstrates a paucity of air in the hypopharynx and excessive prevertebral tissue, likely secondary to an expiratory phase of breathing. A repeat view (**2**) in proper inspiration shows normal prevertebral soft tissue thickness.

Treatment and Prognosis

- Most cases, especially those without a true abscess but rather retropharyngeal cellulitis, respond to intravenous antibiotics and associated supportive care.
- Severe cases, especially those with significant respiratory compromise, may require intubation or surgical drainage or both.
- Intravenous antibiotics alone in milder cases, or in combination with surgical drainage in more severe cases, are usually curative.

Complications

- Possible complications include C1–2 rotary subluxation/scoliosis, abscess perforation into the airway, vascular occlusion such as jugular venous thrombosis, and, rarely, spread of infection into the mediastinum or spine.
- Whereas the diagnosis is usually made on the lateral view of the soft tissues of the neck, CT is most commonly used to identify complications.

PEARLS_____

- Expiratory tracheal buckling can create buckling of the trachea anteriorly (**Figs. 30C1** and **30C2**), causing an apparent increase in retropharyngeal soft tissues and creating a "pseudo-retropharyngeal abscess" (**Fig. 30D1**).
- Pseudo-retropharyngeal abscess can be differentiated from a true abscess when the appropriate inspiratory film demonstrates supraglottic airway and hypopharyngeal distention with air (**Fig. 30D2**).

PITFALLS_____

- Appropriate patient positioning is critical. The examination of the lateral view of the soft tissues of the neck must be performed in slight extension and during inspiration. The most common cause of a pseudo-retropharyngeal abscess is a film performed during expiration or swallowing, or an improperly positioned child.

Suggested Readings

Hedlund GL, Griscom NT, Cleveland RH, Kirks DR. Respiratory system. Chapter 7. In: Kirks DR, Griscom NT, eds. Practical Pediatric Imaging: Diagnostic Radiology of Infants and Children. 3rd ed. Philadelphia: Lippincott-Raven; 1998:246–247, 654–655

Strife J. Upper airway and tracheal obstruction in infants and children. Radiol Clin North Am 1988;26:309–322

Swischuk LE. Nasal passages, mandible and airway. Chapter 2. In: Imaging of the Newborn, Infant, and Young Child. 5th ed. Philadelphia: Lippincott, Williams & Wilkins; 2004:201–210

CASE 31

Clinical Presentation

An afebrile 18-month-old presents with acute onset of a cough, respiratory distress, and wheezing.

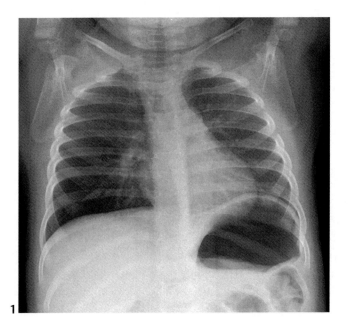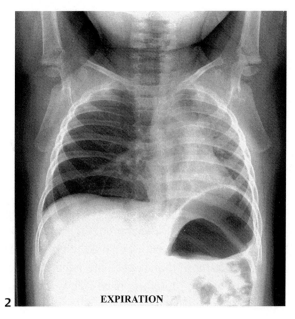

Figure 31A

Radiologic Findings

Conventional chest radiograph performed in appropriate inspiration demonstrated subtle asymmetric lucency, most obvious at the right base (**Fig. 31A1**). Mild hyperinflation of the right upper lobe also is seen with a slight shift of the mediastinal structures into the left hemithorax. Expiratory frontal view (**Fig. 31A2**) demonstrates overt mediastinal shift to the left secondary to extensive right-sided air trapping, the result of an aspirated piece of hamburger.

Diagnosis

Foreign body aspiration; aspiration of a piece of hamburger

Differential Diagnosis

- Mucous plugging
- Focal bronchostenosis or bronchomalacia
- Extrinsic bronchial compression (aberrant vessel, congenital cyst, adenopathy)
- Endobronchial lesion (rare in childhood)

Discussion

Background

Although foreign body aspiration can occur at any age, the peak age range is between 9 months and 4 years of age, when children are most likely to explore their surroundings with their mouth.

Clinical Findings

The radiographic diagnosis of foreign body aspiration requires a high index of suspicion that must be maintained when imaging children's lungs. It is noteworthy that studies have shown that up to 20% of cases present with no choking episode (Hoeve et al), and up to 30% of cases may present to medical care more than a week after the episode of aspiration (Kim et al). Both the clinician and the radiologist must, therefore, have a low threshold for considering the utility of expiratory films to demonstrate focal air trapping.

Imaging Findings

RADIOGRAPHY

- Most cases require only plain film examination, and aspirated foreign bodies are best appreciated on expiratory views.
- Conventional inspiratory radiographs may show focal lucency, focal atelectasis, or may even be normal.
- Expiratory frontal radiographs must be a standard part of the examination in any child with a choking spell or suspected foreign body aspiration. These will demonstrate focal air trapping and lack of pulmonary deflation in the affected lobe if the foreign body is causing partial obstruction.
- Complete bronchial obstruction usually causes focal atelectasis in both the inspiratory and the expiratory views.
- Foreign bodies that have been present for some time may demonstrate recurrent or persistent focal consolidation or even bronchiectasis.
- Delineation of the aspirated foreign body depends on its intrinsic radio-opacity—metal or calcific objects appear as densities, whereas most other objects are poorly appreciated due to their relative soft tissue radiographic density. In these cases, appreciation of an aspiration event depends on a high index of suspicion combined with secondary effects of partial or complete airway obstruction on the radiograph.

CT

- CT may be helpful in long-standing cases, demonstrating focal areas of atelectatic scarring or bronchiectasis.
- Multidetector CT with computerized reconstruction algorithms can provide exquisite images of intrinsic airway luminal compromise, yet are rarely needed and relatively nonspecific at determining the cause of the airway obstruction.

- Radiation dose considerations preclude widespread use of CT in the initial evaluation of an episode of foreign body aspiration.

Treatment

- Bronchoscopic removal is required to treat this condition.

Complications

- Acute complications relate to the size and position of the foreign body.
- Larger foreign bodies may lodge in the glottis and can be fatal.
- Foreign bodies that proceed distally produce a variable degree of airway compromise.
- Postobstructive pneumonitis, lobar or segmental atelectasis, or pneumothorax may complicate the acute clinical setting.
- More chronic foreign bodies can produce chronic and/or recurrent infections, resulting in focal atelectasis, scarring, and/or bronchiectasis.

PEARLS

- True expiratory films are often difficult to obtain in young children. Cross-table lateral decubitus examinations of each side in frontal projection can help in uncooperative patients; the mediastinal weight will compress the dependent lung if there is no air trapping.
- Any child with a focal area of chronic or persistent atelectasis or consolidation should be investigated for a foreign body. As most foreign bodies are radiolucent, many of these children will require bronchoscopy in the appropriate clinical setting.

PITFALLS

- At times, the normal frontal inspiratory examination may be completely normal, and abnormal air trapping may be appreciated only on the expiratory view.
- Diagnosis of foreign body aspiration requires a high index of suspicion, and a low threshold to proceed to bronchoscopic examination.
- A missed foreign body may result in delayed acute airway compromise, in an inappropriate diagnosis of recurrent airways disease such as asthma, or in subsequent recurrent pneumonias with resultant pulmonary scarring and/or bronchiectasis.

Suggested Readings

Bar-Ziv J, Koplewitz B, Agid R. Imaging of foreign body aspiration in the respiratory tract. In: Lucaya J, Strife J, eds. Pediatric Chest Imaging. Berlin: Springer-Verlag; 2002:171–186

Hedlund GL, Griscom NT, Cleveland RH, Kirks DR. Respiratory system. Chapter 7. In: Kirks DR, Griscom NT, eds. Practical Pediatric Imaging: Diagnostic Radiology of Infants and Children. 3rd ed. Philadelphia: Lippincott-Raven; 1998:802

Hoeve LJ, Rombout J, Pot DJ. Foreign body aspiration in children: the diagnostic value of signs, symptoms and pre-operative examination. Clin Otolaryngol 1993;18:55–57

Kim IG, Brummitt WM, Humphry A, Siomra SW, Wallace WB. Foreign body in the airway: a review of 202 cases. Laryngoscope 1973;83:347–354

CASE 32

Clinical Presentation

At the second day of life, a 27-week-gestational-age premature infant presents with progressive respiratory distress.

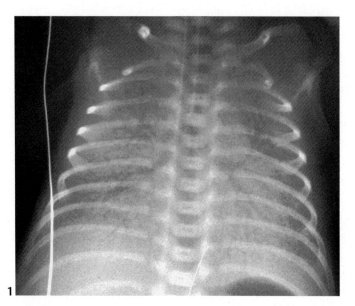 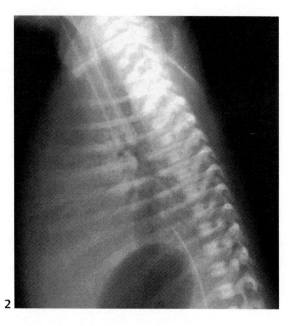

Figure 32A

Radiologic Findings

Frontal radiographic view of the intubated premature infant demonstrates diffuse, hazy "ground-glass," symmetric pulmonary opacification, and air space disease (**Fig. 32A1**). The lung volume is small due to diffuse microatelectasis from surfactant deficiency. Distended and prominent central "air bronchograms" are seen due to the relatively high-pressure ventilation and peripheral poor alveolar compliance (**Fig. 32A2**).

Diagnosis

Hyaline membrane disease (HMD)

Differential Diagnosis

- Neonatal pneumonia
- Diffuse pulmonary hemorrhage
- Diffuse pulmonary edema

Discussion

Background

HMD occurs more commonly in low-birth-weight (<2500 g) premature infants born earlier than 38 weeks of gestation.

Etiology and Pathophysiology

HMD is caused by a combination of factors. The premature lung has a paucity of type 2 pneumocytes, which form and secrete surfactant. Compared with a mature infant, the lung of a premature infant has thicker interstitium, which does not permit efficient gas exchange. This results in increased work of breathing and an increased metabolic rate. While trying to maintain a very high metabolic rate for growth, the premature infant has little respiratory capacity and poor energy reserves. These features combine to result in early respiratory failure. Furthermore, conventional treatment has used high-pressure ventilation and high oxygen concentrations, both of which cause direct lung damage. Part of this injury process involves an inflammatory reaction, including the formation of proteinaceous exudates, which fill the alveoli and constitute the "hyaline membranes."

Imaging Findings

RADIOGRAPHY

- The radiographic investigation of choice is the conventional chest radiograph.
- The lack of surfactant results in small volume, diffusely atelectatic lungs in the non-intubated state. The radiographic correlate to this is diffuse air space disease. In early or milder forms, this takes the form of diffuse ground glass density. Later or more severe cases demonstrate diffuse pulmonary dense opacification. The process is usually symmetric and worse at the lung bases.
- Intubation and pressure ventilation result in distended central bronchi and more distinct air bronchograms in the parenchyma.

ULTRASOUND

- Although ultrasound is rarely used in the diagnosis and management of this disorder, the pattern of diffuse increased pulmonary echogenicity has been described in this disorder.

Treatment

- Conventional treatment involves intubation and ventilation with high pressures. This distends the central bronchi and creates distinct air bronchograms on a pattern of diffuse air space disease.

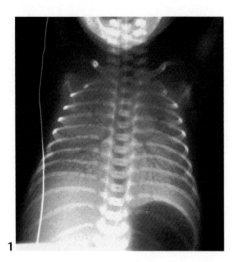 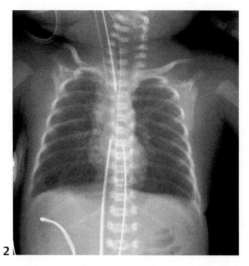

Figure 32B Frontal radiographs of a premature infant with HMD before (**1**) and after (**2**) exogenous surfactant administration. Note the marked improvements in aeration and lung volume after surfactant administration.

- Recent therapies include the administration of endotracheal exogenous surfactant. This results in immediate decreased lung compliance and alveolar distention, with rapid improvement in the radiographic pattern (**Figs. 32A** and **Fig. 32B**).
- Exogenous surfactant has been shown to decrease short-term complications.

Prognosis

- The advent of newer treatments such as exogenous surfactant administration and high-frequency ventilation have resulted in significant improvements in short-term morbidity and mortality from this process.
- Longer-term improvements in chronic lung disease and overall outcome are still controversial and will likely prove to be less impressive than the short-term improvements.
- Although the ultimate prognosis depends on a variety of confounding factors, overall prognosis is very good for uncomplicated HMD.

Complications

Complications that may be radiographically evident include:
- Pulmonary interstitial emphysema
- Asymmetric surfactant distribution causing only focal areas of improvement
- Patent ductus arteriosus (look for cardiac enlargement and pulmonary plethora/edema usually several days after birth)
- Pulmonary hemorrhage (look for sudden deterioration with diffuse alveolar opacity)
- Long-term development of fibrotic and emphysematous changes of bronchopulmonary dysplasia
- Pneumonia

PEARLS

- Radiologic differentiation of HMD from other respiratory disorders, especially neonatal pneumonia, can be impossible.

- The only radiographic finding thought to help differentiate HMD from a diffuse pneumonia, such as that due to Group B streptococcal pneumonia, is the presence of a pleural effusion, which is rarely present in uncomplicated HMD.
- The most significant utility of the plain radiograph in HMD is in the appreciation of changes due to therapeutic interventions, the identification of the positions of the various tubes and catheters used in monitoring and treating this condition, and in the appreciation of the potential complications noted previously.

PITFALL_____

- Administration of exogenous surfactant may result in nonuniform clearing, and the residual areas of opacity may resemble changes of pneumonia.

Suggested Readings

Avni EF, Braude P, Pardou A, Matos C. Hyaline membrane disease in the newborn: Diagnosis by ultrasound. Pediatr Radiol 1990;20:143–146

Donoghue V. Hyaline membrane disease and complications of its treatment. In: Donoghue V, ed. Radiological Imaging of the Neonatal Chest. Heidelberg: Springer-Verlag; 2002:33–45

Newman B. Imaging of medical diseases of the newborn lung. Radiol Clin North Am 1999;37:1049–1066

Swischuk LE. Respiratory system. Chapter 1. In: Imaging of the Newborn, Infant, and Young Child. 4th ed. Philadelphia: Lippincott, Williams & Wilkins; 1997:28–34

Twomey A. Update on clinical management of neonatal chest conditions. In: Donoghue V, ed. Radiological Imaging of the Neonatal Chest. Heidelberg: Springer-Verlag; 2002:9–33

CASE 33

Clinical Presentation

A term newborn presented with respiratory distress at birth and meconium-stained fluid.

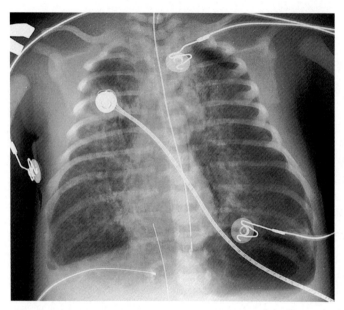

Figure 33A

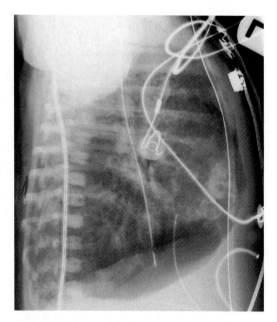

Figure 33B

Radiologic Findings

Frontal (**Fig. 33A**) and lateral (**Fig. 33B**) radiographs of a term newborn with meconium aspiration syndrome reveals bilateral combined multifocal air space, and nodular and interstitial disease in large volume lungs. The radiographs show diffuse hyperinflation and patchy areas of mixed emphysema and atelectasis, with symmetric or asymmetric bilateral nodular infiltrates. Note the moderate-sized left tension pneumothorax (manifestation of air-block phenomenon). This is commonly seen secondary to the requirement for pressure ventilation in a child with significant large and small airway obstruction by the meconium plugs (**Fig. 33A**).

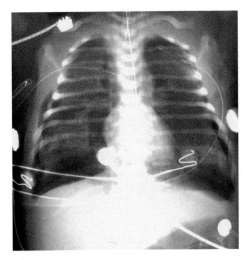

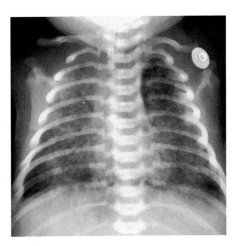

Figure 33C AP chest radiograph demonstrates bilateral pneumothoraces.

Figure 33D AP chest radiograph illustrates the common pattern of combined air space and interstitial changes in this process.

Diagnosis

Meconium aspiration syndrome

Differential Diagnosis

- Neonatal pneumonia
- Transient tachypnea of the newborn
- Amniotic fluid aspiration

Discussion

Background

Meconium aspiration occurs when the fetus passes meconium before birth, filling the amniotic fluid with meconium. Normal respiratory activity of the fetus can result in aspiration. However, a distressed fetus may be more predisposed to pass meconium and have increased respiratory activity, resulting in an increased incidence of amniotic fluid aspiration in distressed infants.

Etiology

The estimated frequency of meconium-stained amniotic fluid is 5 to 25% (median 14%) of all deliveries. Approximately 2 to 35% (median 11%) of those with meconium staining will develop respiratory difficulty and meconium aspiration syndrome. The mortality of meconium aspiration syndrome is described as between 5 and 37% (median 12%).

Pathophysiology

Respiratory problems result from a combination of factors as outlined below:
- The physical presence of meconium in airways causes partial and/or complete airway obstruction.
- Meconium itself produces a necrotizing chemical pneumonitis.

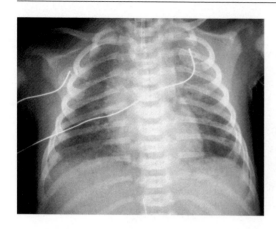

Figure 33E AP chest radiograph demonstrates the coarse interstitial changes commonly seen in this process, yet the apices demonstrate a hazy, ground-glass pattern of surfactant deficiency (ARDS). A secondary surfactant deficiency can be seen secondary to the meconium and the associated necrotizing chemical pneumonitis.

- Meconium pneumonitis causes secondary surfactant deficiency or acute respiratory distress syndrome (ARDS).
- The physical presence of meconium causes asymmetric ventilation.
- Profound initial hypoxia, hypercarbia, and respiratory acidosis predispose to persistence of fetal pulmonary arterial hypertension, resulting in "persistent fetal circulation" and right-to-left shunting, bypassing the damaged lungs through the persistently patent ductus arteriosus, resulting in hypoxia and acidosis. This is seen in up to one third of these patients.

Imaging Findings

RADIOGRAPHY

- Radiologic pattern typically demonstrates diffuse but heterogeneous lung opacity.
- Lungs are usually overinflated and of large volume.
- Mixed areas of atelectasis and emphysema secondary to small and large airways obstruction by the viscid meconium are observed.
- Pressure ventilation frequently results in air-block phenomenon, including pneumothoraces and/or pneumomediastinum, seen in up to 25% of cases (**Fig. 33C**).
- Areas of alveolar consolidation may be seen secondary to the necrotizing chemical pneumonitis incited by the presence of meconium in the airways (**Fig. 33D**).
- Bilateral symmetric or asymmetric nodular infiltrates also are frequently seen.
- As well, hazy, "ground-glass" opacity may be seen secondary to ARDS or secondary surfactant deficiency because meconium acts to degrade surfactant (**Fig. 33E**).

PEARL_____

- Meconium aspiration syndrome often occurs in infants who suffer from in utero or perinatal distress with stooling and fetal gasping.

PITFALL_____

- Most clinicians are well aware of the diagnosis, and the value of the radiograph is primarily in diagnosing complications and monitoring therapy.

Suggested Readings

Cleary GM, Wiswell TE. Meconium stained amniotic fluid and the meconium aspiration syndrome: an update. Pediatr Clin North Am 1998;45:511–529

Hedlund GL, Griscom NT, Cleveland RH, Kirks DR. Respiratory system. Chapter 7. In: Kirks DR, Griscom NT, eds. Practical Pediatric Imaging: Diagnostic Radiology of Infants and Children. 3rd ed. Philadelphia: Lippincott-Raven; 1998:712–715

Owens CM. Meconium aspiration in radiological imaging of the neonatal chest. In: Donohue V, ed. Radiological Imaging of the Newborn Chest. Heidelberg: Springer-Verlag; 2002:49–63

Swischuk LE. Respiratory system. In: Imaging of the Newborn, Infant, and Young Child. 4th ed. Philadelphia: Williams and Wilkins; 1997:41–43

CASE 34

Clinical Presentation

A term infant born by cesarean section, who develops mild tachypnea and grunting several hours after birth

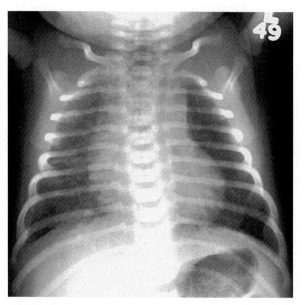

Figure 34A

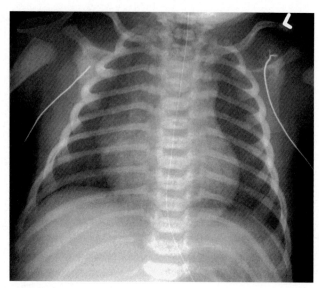

Figure 34B

Radiologic Findings

Frontal radiograph (**Fig. 34A**) of a term newborn infant demonstrates perihilar streaky opacities, mild cardiomegaly, hazy vascular markings, diffuse interstitial pulmonary edema, and prominent fissures with a small, right pleural effusion. The lung volumes are slightly increased. Frontal radiograph performed the next day (**Fig. 34B**) on the same child demonstrates rapid resolution of the previously noted abnormalities.

Diagnosis

Transient tachypnea of the newborn (TTN)

Differential Diagnosis

- Meconium aspiration
- Neonatal pneumonia
- Neonatal cardiac disease with cardiogenic pulmonary edema
- High output cardiac states such as severe neonatal anemia, hydrops, etc.

Discussion

Background

TTN, also referred to as transient respiratory distress of the newborn, neonatal retained fluid syndrome, or wet-lung disease entity, is thought to be caused by prolonged retention of fetal lung fluid due to delay in the normal clearance of resorption of fetal pulmonary fluid.

Normally, fetal pulmonary fluid is absorbed through the normal lymphatics and pulmonary venous systems. This usually occurs within the first few hours of life. In some newborns, however, the pulmonary fluid clearance is delayed. This is most commonly seen in term infants born by cesarean section or those born after a precipitous delivery. Although the proposed etiology is that these infants do not undergo the normal vaginal squeezing of the thorax during delivery, this mechanism has never been substantiated experimentally.

Imaging Findings

RADIOGRAPHY

- Mild bilateral pulmonary overinflation
- Perihilar interstitial linear opacities
- Prominent pulmonary vascularity
- Prominent fissures and/or small pleural effusions
- Mild cardiomegaly
- Rapid clearance of findings over 24 to 48 hours
- Severe cases may have air space opacities.
- Large areas of retained fluid suggest underlying congenital pathology, especially bronchial obstruction (**Fig. 34A**) or congenital lobar emphysema, especially in the polyalveolar lobe syndrome variant.

Treatment and Prognosis

- The degree of respiratory distress created by the presence of the retained fluid is usually mild, requiring only increased ambient oxygen and rarely requiring intubation and ventilation.
- By definition this condition is transient, and it rarely persists beyond 24 hours of life.

PEARLS

- It is very difficult to diagnose this entity from radiographs alone.
- The lung densities may be asymmetric and more pronounced on the right side.
- It is best to correlate radiographic findings with the clinical scenario and follow-up in the subsequent days.

- The radiograph will show at least partial clearing within the next 24 hours (**Fig. 34B**).
- However, pulmonary hyperaeration may persist longer after clear amniotic fluid aspiration, with a clearing delay up to 4 to 5 days.

PITFALL

- Some forms of cardiogenic pulmonary edema and high output cardiac states can have similar initial chest radiographic findings.

Suggested Readings

Donoghue V. Transient tachypnea of newborn. In: Donoghue V, ed. Radiological Imaging of the Neonatal Chest. Heidelberg: Springer-Verlag; 2002:45–47

Hedlund GL, Griscom NT, Cleveland RH, Kirks DR. Respiratory system. Chapter 7. In: Kirks DR, Griscom NT, eds. Practical Pediatric Imaging: Diagnostic Radiology of Infants and Children. 3rd ed. Philadelphia: Lippincott-Raven; 1998:711–712

Swischuk LE. Respiratory system. Chapter 1. In: Imaging of the Newborn, Infant, and Young Child. 5th ed. Philadelphia: Lippincott, Williams & Wilkins; 2002:38–40

CASE 35

Clinical Presentation

A newborn presents with acute onset of severe respiratory distress and hypoxia. The abdomen is scaphoid.

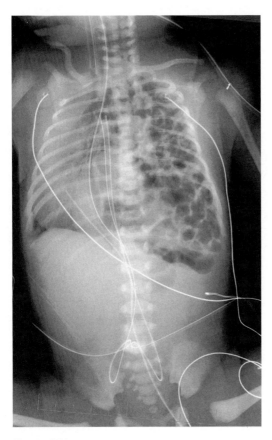

Figure 35A

Radiologic Findings

Plain film radiograph of a newborn demonstrate a lack of bowel in the abdomen and multiple air-filled bowel loops in the left hemithorax (**Fig. 35A**). The left lung is not visible, and the right lung is severely compressed by the mediastinal structures, which have been pushed into the right hemithorax.

175

Diagnosis

Congenital diaphragmatic hernia

Differential Diagnosis

- Congenital cystic adenomatoid malformation
- Pleuropulmonary blastoma
- Diaphragmatic eventration
- Focal severe pulmonary interstitial emphysema

Discussion

Background

This abnormality occurs secondary to a defect in the posterior (Bochdalek) or anterior (Morgagni) portions of the pleuroperitoneal canal at 10 to 12 weeks' gestation as the gut migrates back into the abdomen from outside the abdominal wall. The posterior, Bochdalek type is more common than the more anterior, Morgagni type by ~5:1.

Pathophysiology

The presence of the hernia causes ipsilateral and, if severe, contralateral pulmonary hypoplasia, depending on the size of the hernia and in utero timing of herniation. The clinical course is, therefore, variable, depending on the degree of pulmonary hypoplasia.

Imaging Findings

RADIOGRAPHY

- Initial plain film is usually performed after a nasogastric tube has been passed.
    - The tip of the tube may be in the chest, confirming the diagnosis, or, in the abdomen, if the stomach itself has not herniated.
- Left-sided Bochdalek hernia:
    - Some air-filled bowel loops in the chest (although the herniated bowel may be initially opaque with fluid and with air/fluid levels present over next few hours or days)
    - Areas of uniform opacity frequently represent herniated viscera or omentum, as demonstrated at ultrasonography.
    - Abdomen may demonstrate a paucity of air-filled bowel loops.

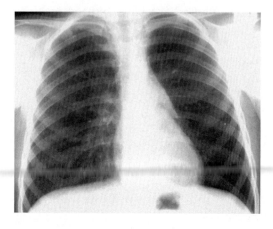

Figure 35B This film was performed 8 years after **Fig. 35A**, demonstrating a residual small left hemithorax with a relatively lucent left lung, and diminished left pulmonary vascularity, secondary to residual pulmonary hypoplasia. The child was asymptomatic.

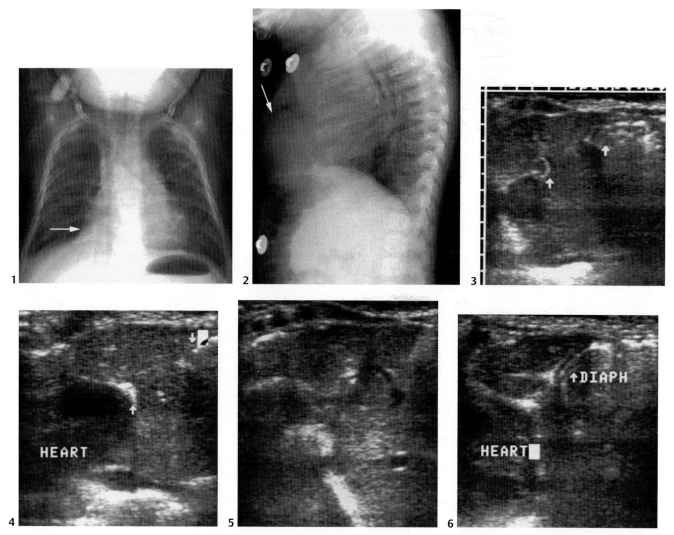

Figure 35C Plain films (**1** and **2**) of a 2-year-old demonstrate a right posteromedial cardiophrenic angle, smooth-walled soft tissue "mass" (arrows). The ultrasound examination (**3** to **6**) demonstrates a focal defect in the anterior portion of the right hemidiaphragm (arrows). Part of the liver has herniated through the defect, consistent with a Morgagni hernia.

- Radiographs performed after surgery usually demonstrate a small ipsilateral lung with some pleural fluid.
- Radiographs performed many years later show resorption of the pleural fluid with a relatively normal or slightly smaller, hyperlucent ipsilateral lung. This finding may be subtle, as lung growth continues through early childhood (**Fig. 35B**).
- Right-sided hernias:
    - Morgagni type seen more frequently on right side
    - Liver and omentum frequently seen as part of herniated structures, requiring ultrasound confirmation (**Fig. 35C**)

ULTRASOUND

- Ultrasonography is used as a confirmatory procedure when the initial radiograph is inconclusive (**Fig. 35D**).
    - Herniated structures are not air-filled (herniated viscera, omentum, or fluid-filled/collapsed loops).
    - Differentiation from cystic congenital lung lesion, for example, congenital cystic adenomatoid malformation (CCAM), is needed.
- Real-time ultrasonography demonstrates peristalsis of bowel loops.

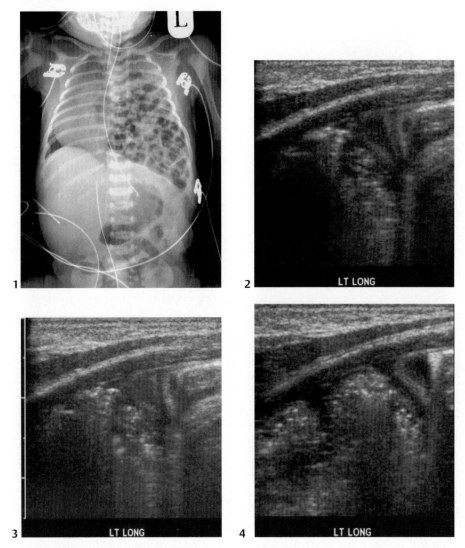

Figure 35D Frontal chest radiograph (**1**) demonstrates typical findings in a left-sided Bochdalek hernia in a newborn. Ultrasound images performed, scanning longitudinally along the left chest wall (**2** to **4**), demonstrate peristaltic bowel loops with gut signature in the left hemithorax, differentiating the lesion from a cystic lung anomaly.

Treatment

- The tracheal PLUG ("plug the lung until it grows") procedure involves in utero tracheal ligation, which enhances lung growth. The ligature is released immediately at birth, followed by transient tracheostomy tube ventilation.
- Intrauterine surgical primary repair also has been attempted. However, this is controversial and carries a varying success rate.
- Postnatal treatment consists of supportive ventilation until the infant is stable enough to undergo primary surgical repair. This will be curative of the hernia, but the outcome depends on the severity of the underlying pulmonary hypoplasia. This problem will usually be overcome with time, as postnatal lung growth results in decreasing symptoms as the child grows.

Complications

- The severity of pulmonary hypoplasia plays a role in the development and severity of persistent pulmonary hypertension (persistent fetal circulation). This results in right-to-left shunting through the persistently patent ductus arteriosus and foramen ovale, such that the infant's circulation bypasses the lungs and any potential attempts at effective ventilation.

- Therapeutic interventions for congenital diaphragmatic hernia have included inhaled nitrous oxide (pulmonary vasodilatation), newer ventilatory technologies ("jet," high-frequency oscillation), and even extracorporeal membranous oscillation (ECMO), each with varying success rates.
- Morgagni hernias are usually smaller, right-sided, rarely produce respiratory distress, and are more commonly associated with other congenital anomalies, whereas left-sided Bochdalek hernias are more frequently isolated findings.
- Prenatal ultrasonography can visualize the herniated viscera, and, as a result, several prenatal procedures have been attempted in those cases with poor prognosis (fetal hydrops, high position of liver, small right-lung-to-head ratio).

PEARLS

- Should not need to inject air/contrast, which aggravates the mass effect
- Chest ultrasound can be used in difficult cases to differentiate herniated organs and/or bowel peristalsis from alternate diagnoses such as congenital cystic adenomatoid malformation.
- Midline hernias are rare occurrences, which develop through a centrally located diaphragmatic defect. Herniated gastrointestinal tract can be encountered in the retrosternal space or inside the pericardial sac.
- Diaphragmatic hernias may be delayed in their presentation with two notable reasons having been described:
  ○ After withdrawal of positive pressure ventilation in the neonatal period for respiratory distress
  ○ After a basal pneumonia due to Group B streptococcal pneumonia

PITFALLS

- Injection of air or contrast down the nasogastric tube is to be avoided as it may aggravate the intrathoracic mass effect on the hypoplastic lungs.
- Appearance of a mass above the repaired diaphragm may signal recurrence of the diaphragmatic hernia. This mass may contain fluid or air. Similar radiographic findings are created by the presence of a residual hernia sac.
- Differentiation between Morgagni hernia and diaphragmatic eventration can be difficult. Ultrasonography may be helpful in distinguishing these entities.

Suggested Readings

Hedlund GL, Griscom NT, Cleveland RH, Kirks DR. Respiratory system. Chapter 7. In: Kirks DR, Griscom NT, eds. Practical Pediatric Imaging: Diagnostic Radiology of Infants and Children. 3rd ed. Philadelphia: Lippincott-Raven; 1998:682–683

Ryan S. Postnatal imaging of chest malformations. In: Donoghue V, ed. Radiological Imaging of the Neonatal Chest. Heidelberg: Springer-Verlag; 2002:93–111

Schwartz DS, Reyes-Mugica M, Keller MS. Imaging of surgical diseases of the newborn chest: intrapleural mass lesions. Radiol Clin North Am 1999;37:1067–1078

Swischuk LE. Respiratory system. In: Imaging of the Newborn, Infant, and Young Child. 4th ed. Philadelphia: Lippincott, Williams & Wilkins; 1997:68–73

CASE 36

Clinical Presentation

A 7-year-old was referred for suspected tuberculosis based on the provided chest radiograph.

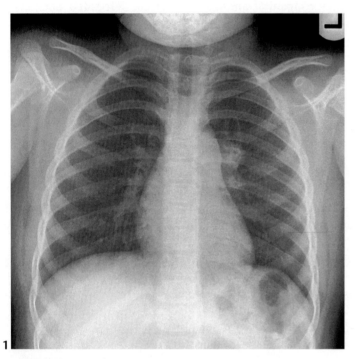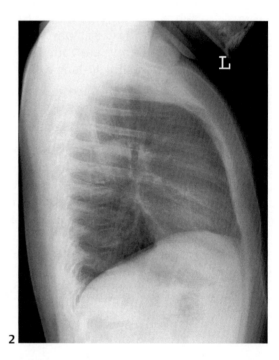

Figure 36A

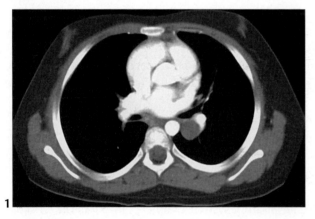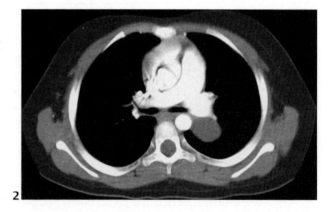

Figure 36B

Radiologic Findings

Frontal (**Fig. 36A1**) and lateral (**Fig. 36A2**) chest radiographs show left hilar enlargement, resembling adenopathy. The lateral view shows a well-defined density. Axial enhanced CT images (**Fig. 36B**) demonstrate a round, nonenhancing mass posterior to the left hilum, which is consistent with the typical appearance of a bronchogenic cyst.

180

Diagnosis

Bronchogenic cyst

Differential Diagnosis

- Other congenital cysts (e.g., esophageal duplication, bronchopulmonary foregut malformations)
- Parenchymal abscess, especially if air-filled
- Cystic adenomatoid malformation
- Hilar/mediastinal adenopathy

Discussion

Background

Bronchogenic cysts are thought to arise when a small bud of the developing tracheobronchial tree becomes amputated and isolated. These cysts may occur in the mediastinum or in the lung parenchyma. Mediastinal cysts are usually located near the carina, behind the trachea, or along the mainstem bronchi. The intrapulmonary bronchogenic cysts appear as solitary round or oval thin-walled, air-containing cysts. Bronchogenic cysts are usually isolated and, in the uncomplicated state, do not communicate with the tracheobronchial tree.

Etiology

Bronchogenic cysts usually do not present in infancy. It is estimated that over half of these cysts will present after 15 years of age. Most lesions that present in infancy do so by their mass effect on regional structures, whereas most (95%) that present after infancy do so by becoming infected.

Histology

The histology is that of a cyst lined with ciliated columnar epithelium that also contains cartilage and mucus-secreting cells. The cyst, therefore, slowly fills with fluid. Cyst fluid usually consists of mucus but can be proteinaceous or even can contain milk of calcium.

Imaging Findings

RADIOGRAPHY

- Most bronchogenic cysts are mediastinal (85–90%) in location, usually in a pericarinal distribution, with the remainder presenting anywhere throughout the lung parenchyma (**Fig. 36C**).
- These cysts can rarely be found in extrathoracic locations, including the neck and abdomen.
- Frequently, the cysts are round or oval shaped with uniform density.
- Less commonly, the cysts may have air-fluid levels when they have been filled by collateral air drift or when communication with the tracheobronchial tree has occurred through superinfection or local erosion (**Fig. 36D**).
- Rarely, a calcific rim may be seen.
- A mass effect on regional structures may produce a zone of atelectasis or obstructive emphysema. As well, regional consolidation may occur if the cyst becomes infected.

CT

- Attenuation values of bronchogenic cysts on CT are variable, although they are usually low attenuating and without demonstrable wall in the uncomplicated state.
- Internal Hounsfield unit numbers are close to water.

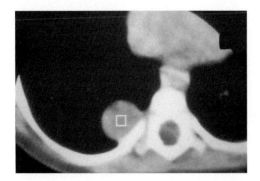

Figure 36C Axial CT image revealing a peripheral bronchogenic cyst.

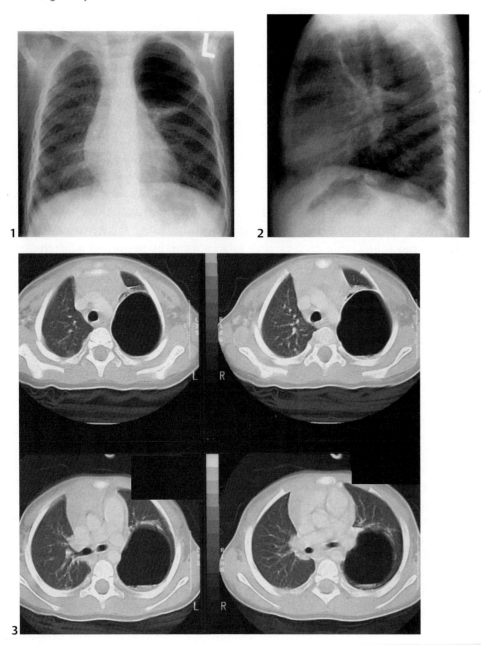

Figure 36D Erosion into a bronchus has resulted in sudden expansion of an air-filled bronchogenic cyst (**1,2**), which still has a small air-fluid level from the residual fluid still in the lesion (**3**).

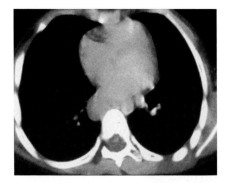

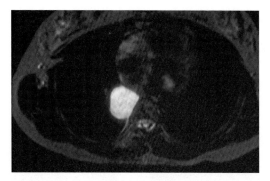

Figure 36E A right-sided mediastinal rounded mass was referred as a possible mass, with CT Hounsfield numbers suggesting that it was solid.

Figure 36F T2-weighted MRI reveals the true cystic nature of this bronchogenic cyst.

- Infrequently, these cysts have been reported to have high attenuation, mimicking a solid mass (**Fig. 36E**). This is likely due to internal milk of calcium or high internal protein concentrations. In these patients, MRI can be helpful in otherwise uncomplicated cases by the internal fluid characteristics, and the lack of surrounding tissue reaction (**Fig. 36F**). CT may also demonstrate the secondary effects of regional atelectasis or emphysema, as well as the cyst associated with focal consolidation in the case of superinfection.

MRI

- Bronchogenic cysts are primarily water signal intensity on T1- and T2-weighted sequences, but the internal characteristics can be variable depending on internal hemorrhage or infection.
- No contrast enhancement is seen following gadolinium administration.

Complications

- Bronchogenic cysts are usually isolated and, in the uncomplicated state, do not communicate with the tracheobronchial tree.
- Bronchogenic cysts may fill with air by collateral air drift, by superinfection, or by erosion into the tracheobronchial tree, which can result in sudden expansion of the lesion and at least partial filling of air.
- Infection of the cyst may result in an abscess, which may alter the underlying congenital pathologic changes.

PEARL_____

- In those cases where CT is ambiguous, MRI shows cystic nature well.

PITFALL_____

- Beware of the bronchogenic cyst with higher Hounsfield unit numbers on CT. This can occur with milk of calcium or increased protein in the fluid.

Suggested Readings

Haddon MJ, Bowen AO. Bronchopulmonary and neurenteric forms of foregut anomalies: imaging for diagnosis and management. Radiol Clin North Am 1991;29:241–254

Hedlund GL, Griscom NT, Cleveland RH, Kirks DR. Respiratory system. Chapter 7. In: Kirks DR, ed. Practical Pediatric Imaging: Diagnostic Radiology of Infants and Children. 3rd ed. Philadelphia: Lippincott-Raven; 1998:787

Mata JM, Castellate A. Pulmonary malformation and the neonatal period. In: Lucaya J, Strife J, eds. Pediatric Chest Imaging. Berlin: Springer-Verlag; 2002:94–96

Ribet ME, Copin MC, Gosselin BH. Bronchogenic cysts of the lung. Ann Thorac Surg 1996;61:1636–1640

CASE 37

Clinical Presentation

A newborn presents with mild respiratory grunting.

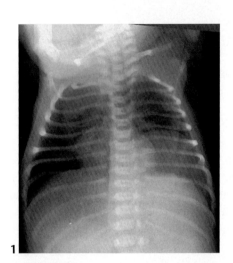
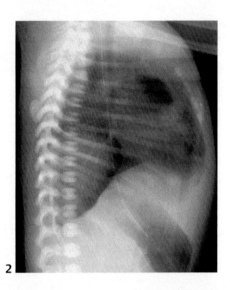

Figure 37A

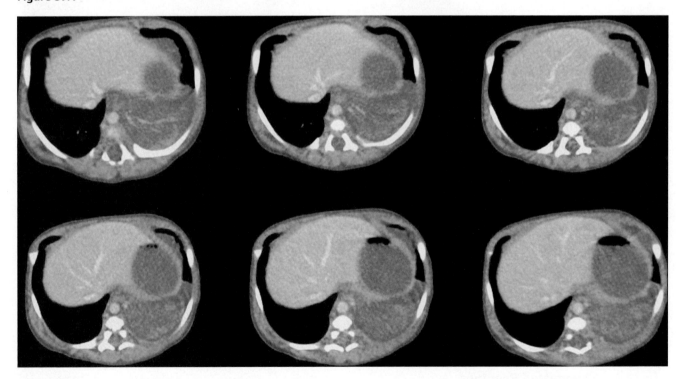

Figure 37B

Radiologic Findings

Frontal (**Fig. 37A1**) and lateral (**Fig. 37A2**) chest radiographs in a newborn with mild tachypnea reveal a uniform, well-marginated opaque mass in the posterior aspect of the base of the left hemithorax. CT examination shows a low attenuating left basal mass and an enhancing systemic artery supplying it, which arises from the descending thoracic aorta (**Fig. 37B**). This proved to be an extralobar pulmonary sequestration.

Diagnosis

Extralobar pulmonary sequestration

Differential Diagnosis

- Eventration of hemidiaphragm
- Diaphragmatic hernia
- Congenital cystic adenomatoid malformation

Discussion

Background

Pulmonary sequestration is a mass of aberrant pulmonary parenchymal tissue that has no normal connection to either the tracheobronchial tree or the pulmonary arterial system. Sequestrations receive their blood supply from the systemic arterial system and have variable pulmonary or systemic venous drainage. There are two types that are defined according to their pleural investiture: *extralobar sequestration* (~25%) is contained within its own pleural lining, whereas *intralobar sequestration* (~75%) shares the pleura with the rest of the lung. It is therefore thought that an extralobar sequestration appears after pleura is formed, whereas the intralobar variety may form earlier, that is, before pleura is formed.

Etiology

Presentation may occur through a variety of mechanisms. Traditionally, most extralobar sequestrations present earlier in life with respiratory difficulty, whereas the majority of sequestrations present in older age ranges with superinfection of the lesion. Many of these lesions, however, are now detected by prenatal ultrasound examination. Some clinical differences between intralobar and extralobar sequestrations include a male predominance when the sequestration is extralobar (80%), whereas intralobar sequestrations occur equally in males and females. As well, extralobar sequestrations in the neonatal period have an approximate 65% incidence of other congenital anomalies, which occur in only 10% of children with intralobar sequestrations.

Imaging Findings

- Demonstration of the systemic feeding artery is critical for appropriate diagnosis and surgical planning.
- Systemic artery frequently arises from the upper abdominal aorta and enters the sequestration after taking a course through the inferior pulmonary ligament. However, this can be variable, especially if the sequestration is not in the region of the lung base.
- Conventional technologies of Doppler ultrasonography, CT angiography, and dynamic enhanced MRI have made conventional angiography obsolete for this entity.

RADIOGRAPHY

- Radiographic manifestations vary depending on whether it is an intralobar or extralobar sequestration.

ULTRASOUND

- Prenatal ultrasonography demonstrates a mass of echogenic lung.
- The systemic arterial supply can be seen on prenatal Doppler study. However, differentiation from other congenital pulmonary anomalies such as cystic adenomatoid malformation of the lung can be difficult as pulmonary sequestrations may have cystic components.

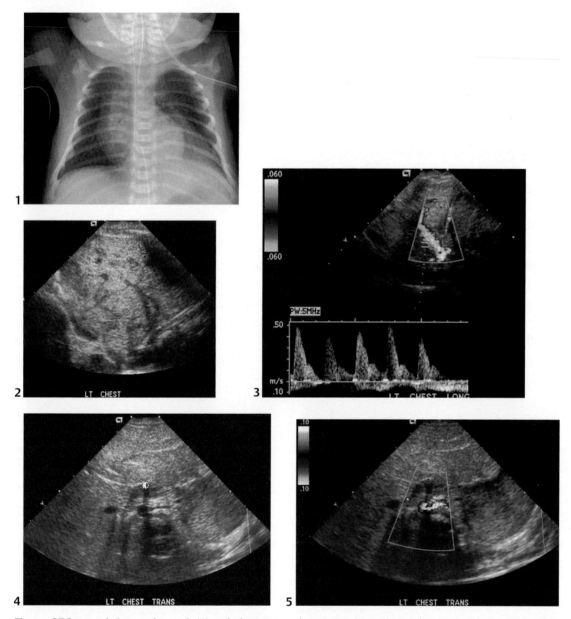

Figure 37C Frontal chest radiograph (**1**) and ultrasonographic images (**2** to **5**) reveal a paraesophageal echogenic mass with a prominent systemic feeding artery arising from the upper abdominal aorta in this extralobar sequestration. (See Color Plate 37C3 and 37C5.)

- Echogenic pulmonary lesions seen in the fetal period that are likely sequestrations may involute to some extent.
- Many of these leave behind abnormal areas of lung/pleura that are asymptomatic and whose true nature may never be known, as continued conservative management seems prudent currently.

Extralobar

- Extralobar is usually homogeneous and solid on all imaging modalities.
- Ultrasound
  - Solid mass of relatively uniform echogenicity
  - Doppler study usually demonstrates the feeding artery in the central portion of the mass.
  - The artery is sometimes traceable to the aorta if there is no interposed aerated lung (**Fig. 37C**).

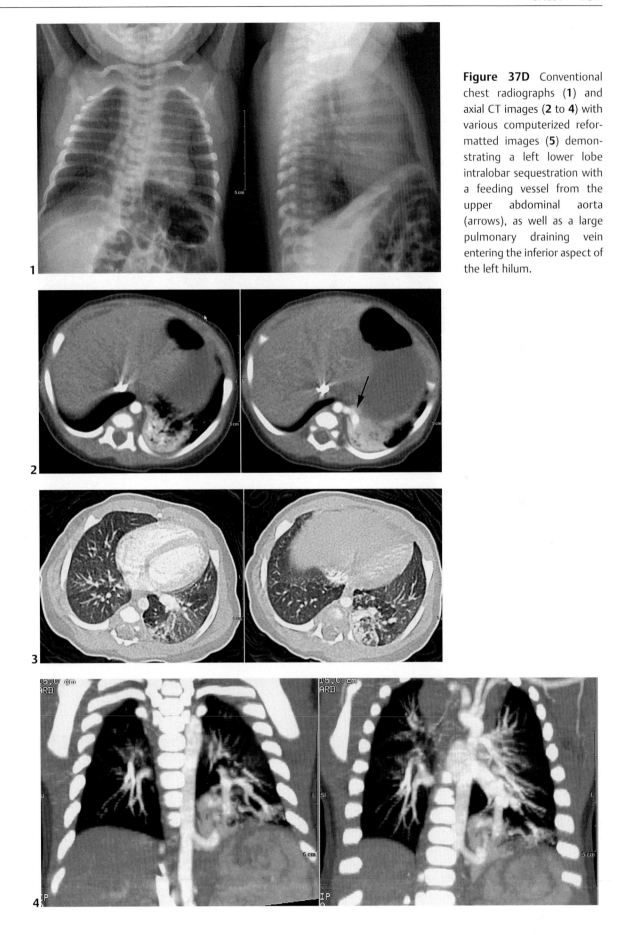

Figure 37D Conventional chest radiographs (**1**) and axial CT images (**2** to **4**) with various computerized reformatted images (**5**) demonstrating a left lower lobe intralobar sequestration with a feeding vessel from the upper abdominal aorta (arrows), as well as a large pulmonary draining vein entering the inferior aspect of the left hilum.

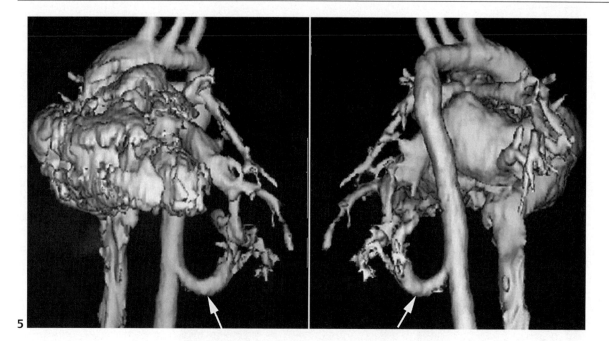

5

- CT
  - Usually a low attenuating mass of solid tissue
  - CT angiography usually demonstrates both the feeding artery and draining vein, and multiplanar reformats as well as 3D reconstruction frequently help to trace the vascularity (**Fig. 37D**).

- MRI
  - Intermediate signal on T1-weighted images, increased signal on T2-weighted sequences
  - Flow sensitive or dynamic gadolinium enhancement can be used to demonstrate the vascularity (**Fig. 37E**).

Intralobar

- Intralobar sequestrations more commonly become complicated by infection and secondary communication with the tracheobronchial tree.
- Appearances of intralobar sequestrations are quite variable on all modalities.
- Radiography
  - Intralobar sequestrations may demonstrate areas of consolidated lung, air-fluid levels, and/or pleural effusions.
- Ultrasound
  - Focal emphysema in the area around the sequestration is sometimes seen in association with intralobar sequestrations (**Fig. 37D3**).
- CT
  - The feeding and draining vessel may be more difficult to identify at ultrasonography, and CT, especially helical multislice CT angiography, is usually more successful at delineating the internal characteristics and vascularity in intralobar sequestrations (**Fig. 37D**).

Treatment

- Surgical removal is recommended, especially if recurrent infection, respiratory symptoms, or shunting are present.

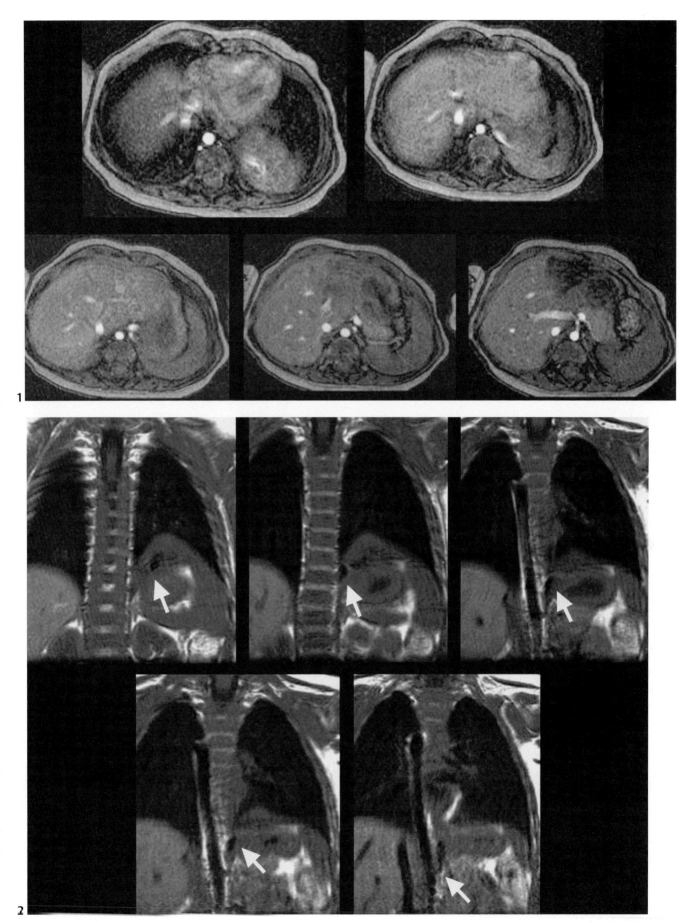

Figure 37E Axial (**1**) and coronal (**2**) MRI reveals a left lower lobe mass with a systemic arterial feeding vessel (arrows), consistent with an extralobar sequestration.

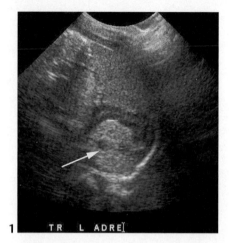 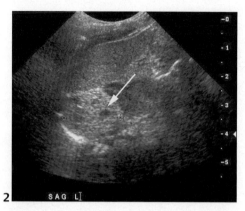

Figure 37F Transverse (**1**) and sagittal (**2**) images from an abdominal ultrasonographic examination demonstrate an echogenic mass with a few small cysts (arrows) in the region of the left adrenal gland. At surgery, this proved to be an extralobar sequestration.

PEARL

- Sequestrations may rarely be extrathoracic, especially suprarenal (**Fig. 37F**).

PITFALLS

- Other anomalies may occur that have a systemic arterial supply, and many consider these to lie within the "sequestration spectrum" or "hybrid lesions," such as bronchial supply to a cystic adenomatoid malformation of the lung, or systemic arterial supply in the case of pulmonary arterial hypoplasia.
- Be aware that not all masses with arterial flow are sequestrations as paraspinal neuroblastoma can mimic this appearance.

Suggested Readings

Hedlund GL, Griscom NT, Cleveland RH, Kirks DR. Respiratory system. Chapter 7. In: Kirks DR, ed. Practical Pediatric Imaging: Diagnostic Radiology of Infants and Children. 3rd ed. Philadelphia: Lippincott-Raven; 1998:671–679

Maya J, Castellote A. Pulmonary malformations beyond the neonatal period. In: Lucaya J, Strife J, eds. Pediatric Chest Imaging. Berlin: Springer-Verlag; 2002:99–101

CASE 38

Clinical Presentation

A 7-year-old presents with cough and fever.

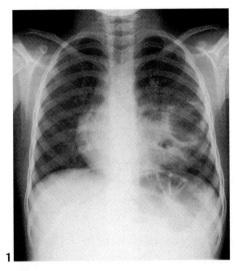 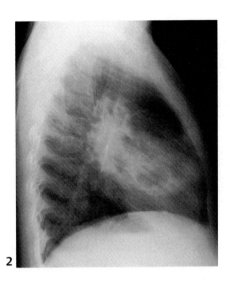

Figure 38A

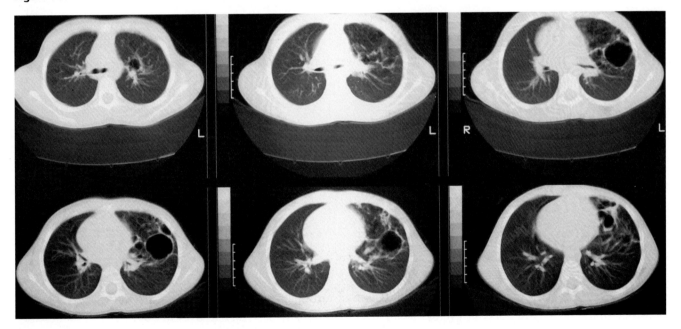

Figure 38B

Radiologic Findings

Frontal (**Fig. 38A1**) and lateral (**Fig. 38A2**) chest radiographs in a 7-year-old who presented with cough and fever demonstrate a complex cystic lesion in the region of the lingula. The radiographs show an ill-defined area of air-space opacity in the lingual, which contains several air-filled cysts with air-fluid levels. A mass effect deviating the mediastinal structures to the right is also seen. Axial CT (**Fig. 38B**) performed after a 3-week course of antibiotics reveals a mass containing multiple cysts of varying

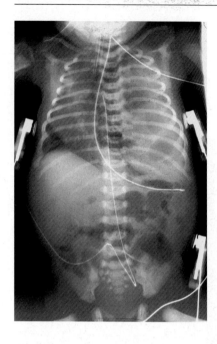

Figure 38C Frontal radiograph of a critically ill newborn, demonstrating large cysts within the left hemithorax, creating significant mass effect deviating the mediastinal structures into the left hemithorax. The child died from severe bilateral pulmonary hypoplasia.

sizes with little residual fluid within the cysts. The mass effect is persistent, and the cysts are both thick- and thin-walled, consistent with a Type II congenital cystic adenomatoid malformation of the lung.

Diagnosis

Congenital cystic adenomatoid malformation of the lung (CCAM)

Differential Diagnosis

- Pulmonary blastoma
- Diaphragmatic hernia
- Bronchogenic cyst
- Infectious pneumatoceles

Discussion

Background

CCAM is a mass consisting of disorganized overgrowth of terminal bronchiolar tissues. The etiology of formation is still a matter of controversy, having been traditionally described as a "hamartomatous" or disorganized overgrowth of terminal bronchiolar tissues. The pathologic and subsequent radiologic manifestations can be variable, depending on the presence and size of the cystic portion of the malformation. Although many appear to derive their arterial supply from the pulmonary circulation, systemic arterial supply may occur, in which case it is not easily differentiable from an intralobar pulmonary sequestration. There is, therefore, a spectrum on anomalies that fall between the various known entities. If these present after the neonatal period as a focus of infection, definitive pathologic differentiation from other congenital anomalies and/or lung abscess can be difficult.

The most widely used classification schema is based on the original system described by Stocker in the late 1970s. According to this system, Type I includes those with cysts >2 cm (50% of cases) (Figs. 38A and 38C). Type II are those with cysts that vary between subcentimeter and 2 cm (40% of

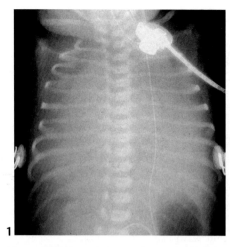
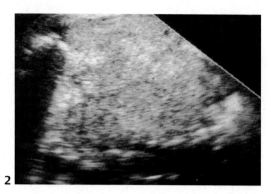

Figure 38D Frontal chest radiograph (**1**) demonstrates bilaterally opaque lungs at birth. There is, however, severe shift of the nasogastric tube and trachea into the left hemithorax. Bedside ultrasonographic examination (**2**) demonstrates a somewhat nonspecific solid mass, pathologically proven to be a Type III CCAM.

cases), and Type III are microcystic or solid (10% of cases) (**Fig. 38D**). CCAMs are usually unifocal and unilobar but can be multilobar, with no site predilection in the lung.

Clinical Findings

Approximately 70% present in the neonatal period with respiratory distress, which can be severe (**Fig. 38C**). They may be fluid-filled initially at birth and become air-filled after a few hours or even several days, depending on their extent of communication with the tracheobronchial tree. The true incidence of clinical presentation of these lesions is now uncertain, as it is thought that most are currently diagnosed by prenatal ultrasound. It is thought that those that do not present in the neonatal period will present later in life when they become superinfected. It also is thought that these lesions carry a rare malignant potential, which may result in pulmonary blastoma formation. This is thought to be a "dysontogenetic" neoplasm, which is locally aggressive and can metastasize. It is thought that this lesion may be similar to a mesenchymal sarcoma or even rhabdomyosarcoma, which has been described as originating from a CCAM in several case reports. In some of these lesions, pneumothorax has been described as the presenting clinical feature. It is well accepted that many intrathoracic cystic lesions can be appreciated at prenatal ultrasonography, although differentiation from cystic sequestration, bronchogenic cyst, and even diaphragmatic hernia can be difficult. Additionally, it is well accepted that many of these lesions involute over the length of the gestation, leaving behind asymptomatic lesions that no longer have a definitive radiologic pattern. Management of these asymptomatic lesions is controversial.

Imaging Findings

RADIOGRAPHY

- Mass with multiple cysts with or without solid or fluid-filled components
- Mass effect often observed
- With or without regional consolidation
- With or without pneumothorax as presenting feature

ULTRASOUND

- Most useful in the prenatal period—cystic mass acting as space-occupying lesion

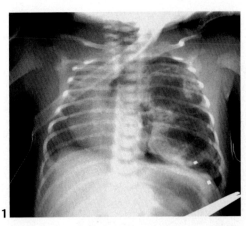 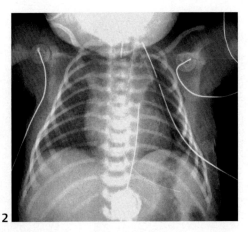

Figure 38E Frontal chest radiographs at birth (**1**) and after subsequent removal (**2**) of a Type III CCAM. At birth, initial radiograph shows at the left base the in utero drain that was placed to drain a large cyst, which was causing fetal hydrops. The postsurgical examination shows little size differential between the two lungs, and the child was sent home several days after surgery with minimal residual symptoms.

CT

- CT findings are usually similar to those on plain film.
- A mass of thick-/thin-walled cysts that may have a more solid-appearing component is seen.
- Rarely the mass may have a systemic feeding vessel.

MRI

- MRI is rarely used for CCAM because CT is usually definitive for the partially air-filled cysts.

Treatment

- Prenatal surgical shunting of cysts large enough to produce fetal hydrops (**Fig. 38E**) has been successfully performed, and those not amenable to shunting have undergone in utero resection successfully.
- Postnatal management of clearly symptomatic lesions is surgical resection due to the risk of eventual infection as well as the consideration of possible malignancy.
- Management of smaller, asymptomatic lesions that have demonstrated in utero regression is currently controversial.

PEARLS_____

- Because many prenatally diagnosed CCAMs regress over time, some of these become small enough that they are asymptomatic at birth.
- A conservative approach to these lesions is being considered as the true nature of many congenital intrathoracic cystic lesions is still unknown (**Fig. 38F**).

PITFALLS_____

- Studies have shown that a prenatally diagnosed congenital cystic lesion in the chest carries a differential diagnosis that includes CCAM, sequestration, diaphragmatic hernia, and bronchogenic cyst.

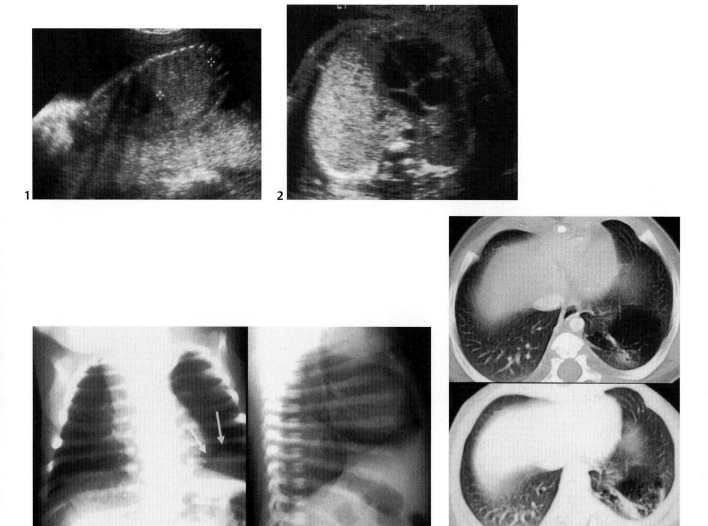

Figure 38F Ultrasonographic images in the early third trimester (**1** and **2**) reveal a large in utero intrathoracic left-sided mass with several small cysts, consistent either with a CCAM, sequestration, or a "hybrid" of both. Postnatal chest radiograph (**3**) and CT (**4**) demonstrate in utero regression, leaving a significantly smaller lesion without distinctive characteristics. As the child was asymptomatic, no surgery was performed.

- Even visualization of a systemic feeding artery does not exclude the diagnosis of a CCAM, and many "hybrid" lesions are now being identified that have pathologic characteristics of both CCAM and sequestration.

Suggested Readings

Marta JM, Costellobe A. Pulmonary malformations beyond the neonatal period. In: Lucaya J, Strife JL, eds. Pediatric Chest Imaging. Berlin: Springer-Verlag; 2002:98–100

Ryan S. Postnatal imaging of chest malformations. In: Donoghue V, ed. Radiological Imaging of the Neonatal Chest. Heidelberg: Springer-Verlag, 2002:93–111

Stocker JT, Madewell JE, Probe RM. Congenital cystic adenomatoid malformation of the lung. Hum Pathol 1977;8:155–171

CASE 39

Clinical Presentation

A 6-month-old presents with focal wheezing and mild respiratory distress.

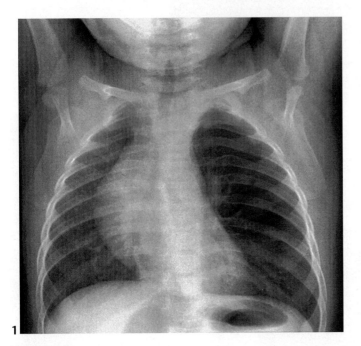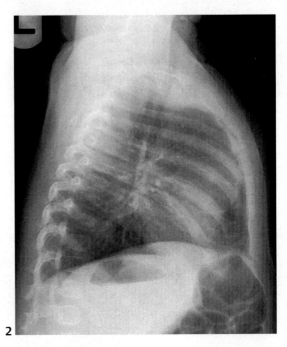

Figure 39A

Radiologic Findings

Frontal (**Fig. 39A1**) and lateral (**Fig. 39A2**) conventional chest radiographs demonstrate focal lucency and overinflation of the left upper lobe with mild shift of mediastinal structures to the right.

a bronchogenic cyst can compromise the regional bronchus and produce a similar area of hyperinflation. A small number of cases demonstrate no bronchial abnormality; yet, at pathological examination, excess numbers of alveoli are demonstrated, and this has been called the polyalveolar lobe syndrome. The most commonly involved anatomic sites are the left upper lobe and right middle lobe. Most affected children present early in life (mean age of diagnosis is 5 months) with respiratory distress and tachypnea, whereas others present later in life as incidental findings.

Imaging Findings

RADIOGRAPHY AND CT

- Lobar hyperlucency (**Fig. 39B**)
- Attenuated vascularity (**Fig. 39B**)
- Mediastinal shift (**Fig. 39B**)
- Variable compression of adjacent normal lung
- May appear mass-like in neonatal period due to delayed resorption of fetal pulmonary fluid (**Fig. 39C1**, radiographs at birth; **Fig. 39C2**, CT at 4 days of age; and, **Fig. 39C3**, radiograph at 1 week of age)

ULTRASOUND

- Prenatal ultrasonography demonstrates echogenic lung that may decrease in size during gestation.

NUCLEAR MEDICINE

- Ventilation/perfusion scans demonstrate lobar air trapping.

Treatment

- Treatment is by surgical lobectomy, depending on the severity of respiratory distress in those patients with milder symptoms who can be managed conservatively.
- Conservative management may result in a slow decrease in size of the affected lobe with respect to the remainder of the lung.

PEARL_____

- All children should probably undergo a CT scan to exclude extrinsic bronchial compression or focal extrinsic bronchial compression.

PITFALL_____

- In the appropriate age ranges, strong consideration should be given to bronchoscopy to exclude a foreign body, especially if symptoms are of acute onset. Left upper lobe foreign body aspiration is fortunately uncommon.

Suggested Readings

Hislop A, Reid L. New pathological findings in emphysema of childhood, I: Polyalveolar lobe with emphysema. Thorax 1970;25:682-690

Olutoye OO, Coleman BG, Hubbard AM, Adzick NS. Prenatal diagnosis and management of congenital lobar emphysema. J Pediatr Surg 2000;35:792–795

Ozcelik U, Gocmen A, Kiper N, Dogru D, Dilber E, Yalcin EG. Congenital lobar emphysema: evaluation and long-term follow-up of thirty cases at a single centre. Pediatr Pulmonol 2003;35:384–391

CASE 40

Clinical Presentation

A previously well 4-year-old presents with acute onset cough, leukocytosis, and fever.

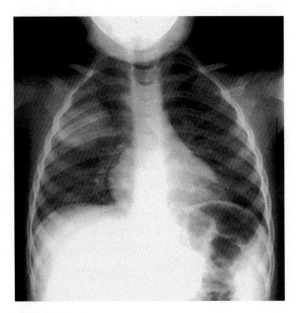

Figure 40A

Radiologic Findings

The AP chest radiograph shows spherical mass-like areas of soft tissue in the right upper lobe of the lung, which is sharply defined and with uniform opacity consistent with typical "round pneumonias" (**Fig. 40A**).

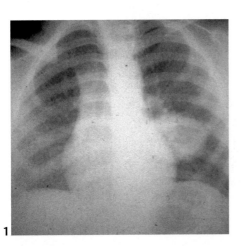 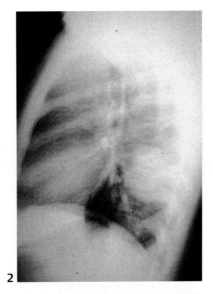

Figure 40B (1,2) Standard chest radiographs of a child with cough and fever showing well-defined and sharply marginated areas of soft tissue density within the lung, consistent with typical round pneumonias.

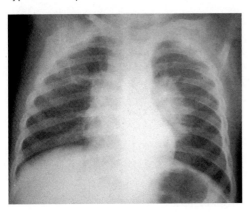

Figure 40C Large, sharply marginated left perihilar soft tissue masslike opacity in the region of the superior segment of the left lower lobe in a child with cough and fever.

Diagnosis

Round pneumonia

Differential Diagnosis

- Round atelectasis
- "Pseudo-tumor" (plasma cell granuloma)
- Neurogenic mass (if posterior)
- Solitary metastasis (rarely attain the size of a round pneumonia, especially in the absence of a known primary malignancy)

Discussion

Background

Round pneumonias are most commonly seen in children ≤8 years of age. They are a unique radiographic manifestation of a usual bacterial pneumonia in this age range.

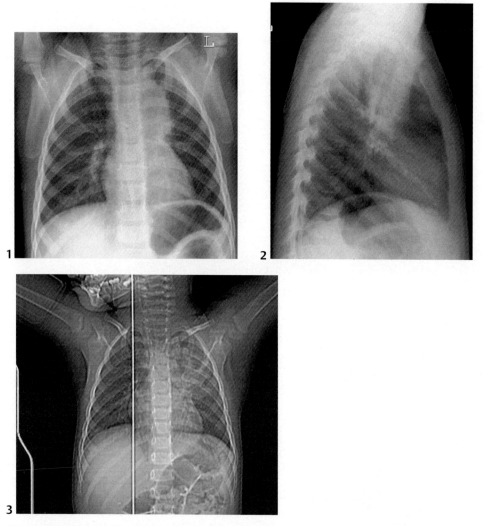

Figure 40D Frontal (**1**) and lateral (**2**) radiographs in a 2-year-old child with cough and fever revealed a well-defined soft tissue opacity in a left paramediastinal location, worrisome for an anterior mediastinal mass. The "scout" examination for the CT scan (**3**) performed 18 hours later already demonstrated air within part of the opacity, representing a rapid early response to antibiotics. (*Continued*)

Clinical Features

The child characteristically presents with typical clinical features of an uncomplicated pneumonia. These children improve with standard antibiotic care. The bacterial etiology is, therefore, thought to be primarily pneumococcal.

Pathophysiology

The pathophysiology of round pneumonias has been attributed to a combination of immature collateral pathways of ventilation, more closely apposed connective tissue septae, and smaller alveoli in children ≤8 years of age. In the older child, unusual pathogens should be considered, such as fungal disease, especially if the child is immunocompromised.

Imaging Findings

RADIOGRAPHY

- Usually seen as a large, masslike, round opacity with slightly irregular edges (**Fig. 40B**)

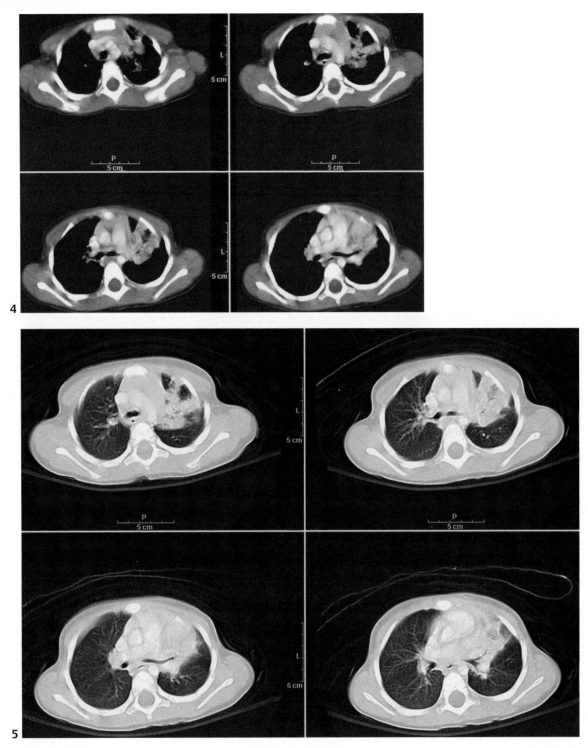

Figure 40D (*Continued*) Soft tissue (**4**) and lung (**5**) windows confirm partial lingular consolidation in this child with a paramediastinal round pneumonia.

- Round pneumonias are most often seen in the superior segments of the lower lobes (**Fig. 40C**).
- Posterior location is the most commonly affected area because gravity pools infected fluid into the most dependent bronchus.
- Round pneumonias may look indistinguishable from a solid tumor (**Fig. 40D**).
  - Round pneumonias characteristically change rapidly over 48 hours, as the infection spreads or begins to resolve, depending on whether antibiotics have been started.
  - Lateral view may look like a mass as well but sometimes demonstrates less distinct borders than the frontal view.
  - Round pneumonias may mimic primary or metastic tumor (check for rib changes to differentiate).
- Only 20% of round pneumonias contain air bronchograms.

Treatment

- For the usual case of round pneumonia, appropriate antibiotic therapy is indicated, with follow-up examination in a few days to ensure that there has been some response and there has been an appropriate change in the radiologic appearance.
- As the area of consolidation either progresses or regresses, the sharp margination is quickly lost, resulting in the more common ill-defined margination of alveolar disease.

PEARL_____

- Differentiation from a neurogenic mass can be made if there are rib or bony changes, which are never present in a typical round pneumonia.

PITFALL_____

- Although the findings are characteristic, it is critical to ensure proper clinical and radiologic follow-up to confirm this diagnosis.

Suggested Readings

Carty H, ed. Emergency pediatric radiology. Chapter 2. In: Duncan AW, ed. Emergency Chest Radiology in Children. Berlin: Springer-Verlag 2002:75

Eggli KD, Newman B. Nodules, masses and pseudomasses in the pediatric lung. Radiol Clin North Am 1993;31:651–666

Griscom NT. Pneumonia in children and some of its variants. Radiology 1988;167:297–302

Hedlund GL, Griscom NT, Cleveland RH, Kirks DR. Respiratory system. Chapter 7. In: Kirks DR, ed. Practical Pediatric Imaging: Diagnostic Radiology of Infants and Children. 3rd ed. Philadelphia: Lippincott-Raven 1998:639

Rose RW, Ward BH. Spherical pneumonias in children simulating pulmonary and mediastinal masses. Radiology 1973;106:179–182

CASE 41

Clinical Presentation

A 10-year-old recent immigrant presents with a 2-month history of intermittent fevers and cough.

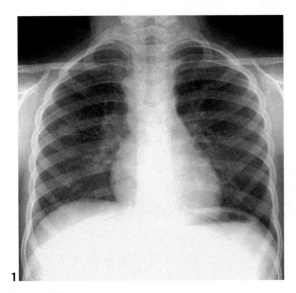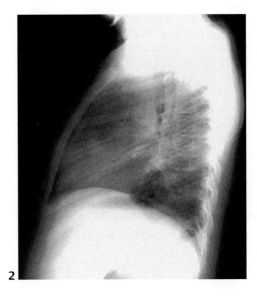

Figure 41A

Radiologic Findings

Frontal (**Fig. 41A1**) and lateral (**Fig. 41A2**) chest radiographs in a child with intermittent cough and fever reveals a small, right upper lobe peripheral focus of air-space density. Ipsilateral right superior hilar adenopathy is seen (see also **Figs. 41B, 41C**, and **41D**). A linear opacity of thickened lymphatic channel is noted between the parenchymal focus and the regional adenopathy, constituting Ranke's complex.

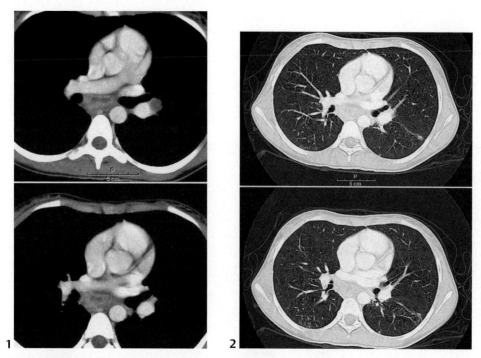

Figure 41B Soft tissue (**1**) and lung windows (**2**) from a CT scan demonstrating similar findings as in **Fig. 41A**. There is mediastinal and hilar adenopathy, which demonstrate peripheral thick enhancement and central low attenuation, consistent with caseating necrosis. The lung windows demonstrate the small peripheral parenchymal focus and the thick line of lymphatic drainage leading to the hilum.

Diagnosis

Primary tuberculosis

Differential Diagnosis

Differential diagnosis of primary tuberculous complex
- Atypical mycobacterial infection
- Histoplasmosis
- Mycoplasma pneumonia infection
- Foreign body pneumonitis

Discussion

Background

Tuberculosis is a disease undergoing an alarming, worldwide resurgence due to many factors, including the relatively recent HIV pandemic, the relative ease of worldwide travel, and the emergence of drug resistant forms. The World Health Organization estimated that 100,000 children worldwide died in 1998 from tuberculosis. Children constitute ~6% of the 22,000 new annual symptomatic cases in the United States.

Etiology

The vast majority of children become infected through inhalation of the bacillus, usually from close contact with an infected adult. Transmission from another child is extremely rare because most children do not produce sufficient sputum with coughing to spread the infection. In fact, isolation of the organism

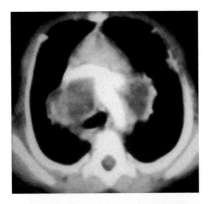

Figure 41C A more overt case of hilar adenopathy on a CT scan, with changes in the lymph nodes suggesting caseating necrosis.

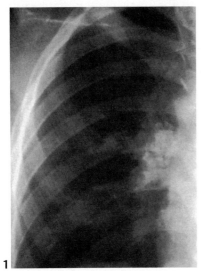

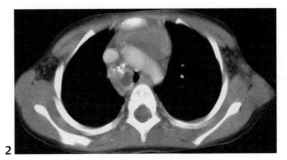

Figure 41D Coned image from a plain chest radiograph (**1**) and CT scan (**2**) demonstrating calcification in hilar and mediastinal adenopathy, frequently seen in tuberculous infection.

from children is significantly more difficult than from adults and usually requires sequential gastric aspirate as children tend to swallow their sputum. Even then, it is estimated that, depending on the study, the organism can be isolated in only approximately one third to one half of affected children.

Clinical Findings

Many children who become infected will remain asymptomatic and may never develop clinically apparent disease. Those at highest risk for clinical symptoms and/or more severe disease include those children living in closer quarters with infected adults (especially those in poverty), those exposed to more virulent forms of the organism, children <6 years of age, and children who are immune deficient (whether due to congenital, acquired, or iatrogenic causes of immunodeficiency). The most common pediatric presentation of tuberculous disease is with a primary infection complex, whereas postprimary tuberculous disease is most commonly seen in adolescents or adults. Disseminated or "miliary" disease is more common in smaller children and infants, as well as in those who are immunocompromised.

Imaging Findings

RADIOGRAPHY

Lack of ability to isolate an organism in children makes radiographic evaluation a key diagnostic modality in the evaluation of the child with suspected tuberculosis.

- Hallmark of primary infection is the presence of hilar/mediastinal lymphadenopathy, which is seen in ~90% of cases and may be the only radiologic finding, especially in younger children (~50% of cases).
- Ranke's complex includes a parenchymal focus of infection, regional lymphadenopathy, and lymphangitis between the two.
- Lymphadenopathy may be difficult to detect but the secondary signs are sometimes present, which include tracheal and/or mainstem deviation, compression, and/or narrowing.
- Complete resolution of parenchymal disease rarely occurs in <6 months, but usually occurs within 2 years.
- Both primary parenchymal and/or regional lymph nodes may demonstrate calcification, especially if present for >6 months.
- In primary disease, there is no lobar preference, in contrast to the upper lobe preference for postprimary disease.

CT

- CT is the examination of choice in unusual, complicated, or disseminated disease or when conventional radiography is equivocal.
- Lymphadenopathy demonstrated as peripheral nodal enhancement with central, low attenuating caseous necrosis
- Nodal calcification is better appreciated at CT than plain film, and heavy calcification usually infers a longer-standing infection.
- Peripheral parenchymal focus is much appreciated.
- Complications of tracheobronchial deviation/compression, endobronchial spread of "progressive primary pulmonary infection," pleural infection, and cavitation of primary foci are better seen at CT.
- Postprimary infection is demonstrated as centrilobular nodules with the tree-in-bud appearance of smaller airway involvement, cavitation, and bronchiectasis.
- Miliary disease consists of varying-sized nodules.

MRI

- Useful at delineating mediastinal complications of lymphadenopathy but high cost, need for sedation
- Poor pulmonary parenchymal visualization currently limits the use of MRI.

PEARL_____

- A positive skin test and a suggestive chest radiograph will significantly alter management, even if the organism cannot be isolated.

PITFALL_____

- Lymphadenopathy and pulmonary infection may persist or even progress (in up to one third of cases) for several months despite appropriate medical therapy.

Suggested Readings

Daltro P, Nunez-Santos E. Pediatric tuberculosis. Chapter 7. In: Lucaya J, Strife J, eds. Pediatric Chest Imaging. Berlin: Springer-Verlag, 2002:129–142

Jamieson DH, Cremin BJ. High resolution CT of the lungs in acute disseminated tuberculosis and a pediatric radiology perspective of the term "miliary." Pediatr Radiol 1993;23:380–383

Leung A, Muller NL, Rafael Pineda P, Fitzgerald JM. Primary tuberculosis in children: radiographic manifestations. Radiology 1992;182:87-91

CASE 42

Clinical Presentation

An 18-month-old girl presents with recurrent episodes of respiratory distress and suspected pneumonia.

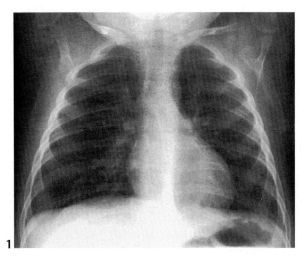 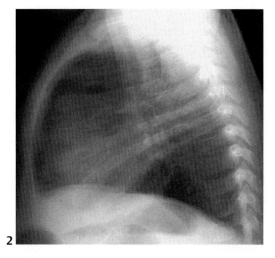

Figure 42A

Radiologic Findings

Frontal (**Fig. 42A1**) and lateral (**Fig. 42A2**) views of the chest in an 18-month-old girl reveal subtle early changes of lower airways disease, including mild diffuse overinflation and mild bilateral central bronchial wall thickening, consistent with early changes of cystic fibrosis. This was the third episode of suspected lower airway respiratory disease in the first year of life, prompting the child's physician to perform a sweat test. Note that the area of subsegmental atelectasis is greater in the right upper lobe than in the left upper lobe.

Diagnosis

Early cystic fibrosis

Differential Diagnosis

- Asthma
- Unlucky child with recurrent episodes of bronchiolitis
- Early immune deficiency, especially immunoglobulin deficiency
- Recurrent aspiration
- Primary ciliary dyskinesia

Discussion

Background

Cystic fibrosis is said to be the most common life-shortening inherited disease in the Caucasian population, affecting approximately 1 in 2500 live births in the United States and northern Europe. It is estimated that ~4% of whites are heterozygous for the most common form of the disorder.

Etiology

Current genetic technology has identified the genetic defect to be a mutation on the long arm of chromosome 7. The most common mutation is at the position dF 508 (70–80% of cases). The resultant mutation causes a physiologic disturbance in the sodium chloride ion transport system in epithelial cell membranes. This results in viscous secretions causing inspissated mucus in the tracheobronchial tree, digestive system, reproductive system, and sweat glands.

Clinical Findings

Clinically, the child has recurrent wheezing, cough, and recurrent pneumonias and/or broncholitis. In the first few years of life, any child with these symptoms should undergo a sweat test, which is a simple procedure (called the "spinal tap" of pediatric respirology; that is, if you think of it, do it). Later in childhood, the child/teenager may develop chronic obstructive pulmonary disease, emphysema, bronchiectasis, and manifestation of diffuse air trapping such as a barrel chest and kyphosis.

Respiratory manifestations include sinusitis, mastoiditis, nasal polyps (in 25%), and recurrent lower respiratory tract infections, which cause 90% of the morbidity and mortality from this disease. The gastrointestinal tract is the second most significant organ system involved, causing pancreatic insufficiency, which in turn causes malabsorption, failure to thrive, meconium ileus in the newborn, distal intestinal obstruction syndrome (DIOS) later in life, and inspissated bile-causing hepatic cirrhosis.

Imaging Findings

RADIOGRAPHY

- Demonstrates changes of small and large airways disease (**Figs. 42B1** and **42B2**) as follows:
  - Bronchial and bronchiolar wall thickening, progressing to bronchiectasis
  - Hyperinflation
  - Emphysema
  - Mucous plugging ± postobstructive pneumonitis

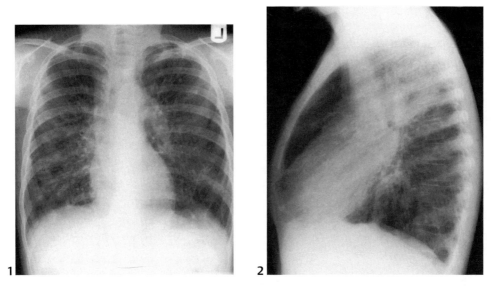

Figure 42B Frontal (**1**) and lateral (**2**) views of the chest in a young adult with cystic fibrosis, revealing more advanced changes of multifocal bronchiectasis, diffuse air trapping, hyperinflation, "barrel-shaped" thoracic cage, and enlarged hila from combined lymphadenopathy and pulmonary arterial hypertension.

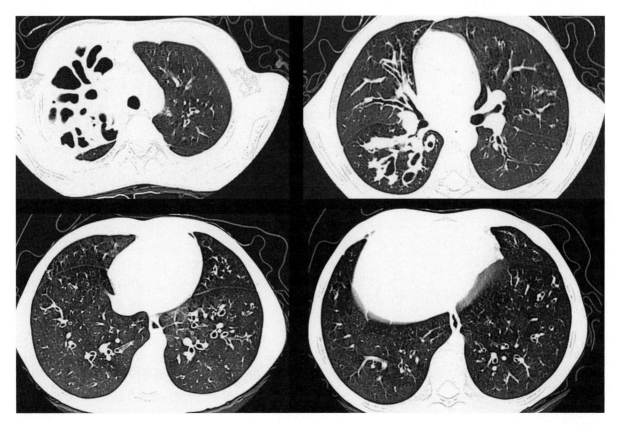

Figure 42C CT scan from a child with pronounced right upper lobe bronchiectasis as well as more diffuse multifocal bronchiectasis, bronchial wall thickening, and mosaic perfusion typical of the diffuse airways changes seen in cystic fibrosis.

- Although a diffuse process, when more focal, upper lobes tend to be more affected.
- Hilar enlargement:
  - Hilar adenopathy results from recurrent/persistent infection.
  - Appears later due to pulmonary hypertension from chronic hypoxia
- Apical blebs/air-filled cysts
- Pneumothorax common
- Barrel chest, kyphosis

CT

- Diffuse airways disease characterized by multifocal bronchiectasis (**Fig. 42C**)
- Hilar adenopathy secondary to recurrent/chronic infection
- Emphysema
- Pulmonary hypertension in later stages
- Small airways disease manifested as bronchial wall thickening, tree-in-bud appearances on high-resolution CT

Treatment

- Treatment includes multiple courses of antibiotics, aggressive respiratory therapy and physiotherapy, inhaled bronchodilators, and gastrointestinal enzyme replacement.
- Although survival rates from the disease have improved drastically (in the 1930s, almost universally fatal by school age, whereas mean survival in 1990 was 28 years), ultimate survival rates with the advent of lung transplantation have yet to be determined, as donor lungs are still difficult to find.

PEARLS_____

- A radiologist with a high index of suspicion should suggest the disease after reviewing the child's previous films.
- The failure to thrive, which may accompany the disease, can be seen as a paucity of soft tissues in the infant/young child.

PITFALLS_____

- Cystic fibrosis is included by some in the differential diagnosis of upper lobe interstitial changes; however, it would be more accurate to consider it as a diffuse process.
- Differential diagnosis of a child with chronic airways disease, nasal polyps, sinusitis, and mastoiditis includes atopy and immune deficiency.

Suggested Reading

Orenstein DM, Bowen AD. Cystic fibrosis: clinical update for radiologists. Radiol Clin North Am 1993;31:617–630

CASE 43

Clinical Presentation

A 14-year-old presents with 2 weeks of intermittent fever and swollen neck nodes on the right.

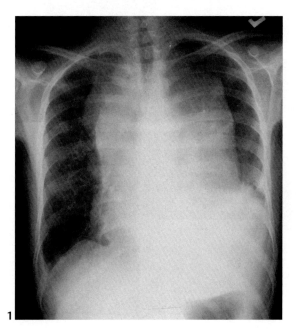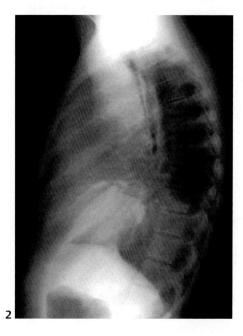

Figure 43A

Radiologic Findings

Initial frontal (**Fig. 43A1**) and lateral (**Fig. 43A2**) chest radiographs demonstrate a large anterior mediastinal mass causing posterior tracheal compression and deviation. A moderate-sized left pleural effusion is present. Multiple axial CT postintravenous contrast enhancement scans (**Figs. 43B1** to **43B4**) demonstrate a large anterior mediastinal mass. This bulky, inhomogeneous, and nodular mass causes vascular deviation and significant superior vena cava (SVC) compression. Note that the left pleural effusion is located anterior, as the child was scanned in the prone position due to respiratory compromise when in the supine position. Images using lung windows (**Fig. 43B5**) demonstrate significant tracheal narrowing.

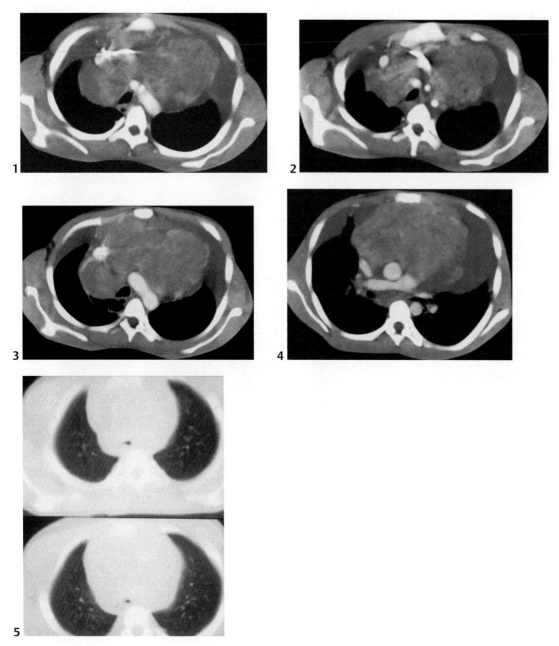

Figure 43B

Diagnosis

Hodgkin's lymphoma

Differential Diagnosis

- Mediastinal germ cell tumor
- Thymic tumor
- Leukemia, especially T cell
- Other types of lymphoma
- Langerhans' cell histiocytosis

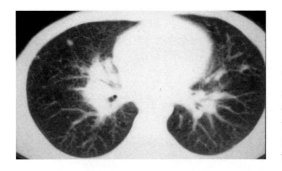

Figure 43C Axial slice at lung windows from a CT scan demonstrates a fine interstitial process of lymphatic dilatation, which could be secondary either to central lymphatic obstruction by the tumor or to interstitial spread of tumor into the lung through lymphatic channels. A nodule in the right middle lobe is in keeping with parenchymal involvement with lymphoma.

Discussion

Background

Lymphoma, the third most common malignancy in children behind leukemia (first) and CNS tumors (second), constitutes approximately one quarter of all pediatric mediastinal masses. The most common anterior mediastinal mass in children is the nodular sclerosing subtype of Hodgkin's disease. Approximately 85% of children with Hodgkin's disease have involvement of the intrathoracic lymph nodes, whereas 60% of children with non-Hodgkin's have intrathoracic/mediastinal nodal involvement.

Clinical Findings

The most clinically significant problem that occurs at presentation of a child with mediastinal lymphoma is secondary compression by the mass of regional mediastinal structures. Airway compromise of more than 25% of the tracheal lumen occurs in up to 25% of children and can be life threatening. As well, superior/inferior vena cava obstruction can be life threatening because this may cause decreased venous return to the heart, a physiologic problem that is intensified by endotracheal intubation and positive pressure ventilation, which may result in circulatory collapse if the anesthesiologist is not careful. It is imperative, therefore, that the child be interviewed carefully for *any* respiratory difficulty in the supine position before the initial staging by CT scan. Prone or decubitus scanning may be necessary.

Imaging Findings

RADIOGRAPHY

- Mediastinal widening, usually in an asymmetric fashion, often with nodular borders
- ± tracheal displacement and/or narrowing asymmetric soft tissues of the neck or axilla
- ± pleural effusions (~20% of cases—usually reactive and not malignant)
- ± hilar adenopathy
- ± pulmonary parenchymal involvement characterized by nodules or interstitial septal thickening (**Fig. 43C**)
- Concept of "bulk" disease is still used according to radiologic findings of the ratio of maximum mediastinal width of tumor to maximum thoracic wall internal diameter. The patient has bulk disease if the ratio is >0.35. However, the definition of bulk disease is variable and poorly defined in the literature.

CT

- Mediastinal widening, usually in an asymmetric fashion, often with nodular borders. CT is mainstay of staging.
- Higher speed multislice helical scanning decreases the need for sedation.

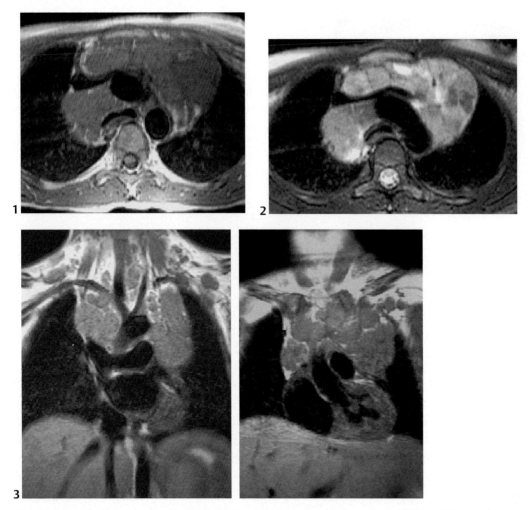

Figure 43D Axial T1- **(1)** and T2-weighted **(2)** sequences as well as coronal T1-weighted **(3)** sequence demonstrate the mediastinal mass to a better extent than on CT, yet CT remains the single staging modality of choice due to a better ability to image potential pulmonary parenchymal involvement.

- Usually consists of anterior mediastinal mass that may spread to the middle and/or posterior mediastinum; mass of lobulated lateral margins, nodular, heterogeneous
- Internal characteristics are usually solid, although internal necrosis can be seen with cystic components
- Rarely, if ever, calcifies before treatment but may show calcification or necrosis after treatment.
- CT detects degree of mediastinal compression, which is critical in the initial clinical evaluation as SVC obstruction or airway compromise may be life threatening.
- In most cases of lymphoma, the mass usually displaces and compresses mediastinal structures, rather than encasing the regional structures.
- Lung parenchymal involvement occurs in ~10% of children with Hodgkin's lymphoma. This is more likely secondary to direct spread through the lymphatics/interstitium than by hematogenous metastatic spread.
- Hilar lymphadenopathy usually occurs as contiguous spread from mediastinal nodes, especially in Hodgkin's.
- Pleural effusion, seen in ~20% of cases, can be reactive or secondary to lymphatic obstruction and is usually sterile. Pericardial effusion is seen in 5% of cases and is virtually always malignant and secondary to direct invasion of the pericardium.

MRI

- Problematic in younger children due to frequent need for sedation
- Most useful in differentiating normal thymus/thymic rebound from tumor
- Tumor demonstrates lower T1 signal, higher T2 signal than normal thymus, but inhomogeneous signal can also occur with necrosis, inflammation, and/or fibrotic scarring (**Fig. 43D**). MRI, therefore, like CT, carries a high sensitivity profile and a high negative predictive value but relatively poor specificity (75%) and positive predictive (35%) values.

PET

- Early studies suggest that PET is most beneficial at detecting active tumor even in the midst of necrotic/fibrotic residual masses, as well as at detecting subtle areas of tumor involvement in staging.

LYMPHANGIOGRAPHY

- No longer performed

PEARLS_____

- Following treatment for lymphoma, necrotic nodes are not uncommon.
- Node necrosis at presentation may be seen in nodular sclerosing Hodgkin's disease.
- Following treatment, patients may develop secondary neoplasms.
- Patients with Hodgkin's disease who are treated with chemotherapy may develop leukemia (seen in up to 5% of patients).

PITFALLS_____

- Rebound thymic hyperplasia, which may mimic recurrent tumor, frequently occurs after cessation of chemotherapy.
- No imaging modality is established as a definitive method of differentiating recurrent tumor from rebound thymic hyperplasia.
- Helpful hints include the relative homogeneity of the thymic hyperplasia in contrast to recurrent disease, and the lack of a mass effect on regional structures by thymic rebound in all imaging modalities.
- Close follow-up is always warranted.

Suggested Readings

Cohen MD. Imaging of Children with Cancer. St. Louis: Mosby-Yearbook; 1992:89–134

Kaste S. Lymphoma: Controversies in imaging the pediatric chest. Chapter 12. In: Lucaya J, Strife J, eds. Pediatric Chest Imaging. Berlin: Springer Verlag, 2002:209–224

Meza MP, Benson M, Slovis TL. Imaging of mediastinal mass in children. Radiol Clin North Am 1993;31:583–604

SECTION IV
Cardiac

CASE 44

Clinical Presentation

A newborn infant developed severe respiratory distress and cyanosis immediately after birth.

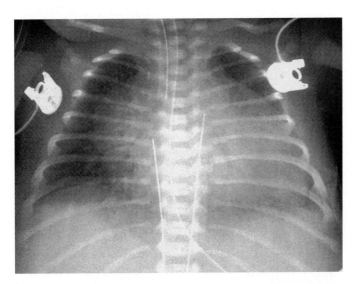

Figure 44A

Radiologic Findings

A frontal chest radiograph (**Fig. 44A**) obtained immediately after birth demonstrates a markedly enlarged heart. The right atrial border extends to the upper mediastinum and bulges far to the right. The pulmonary vascularity is slightly prominent.

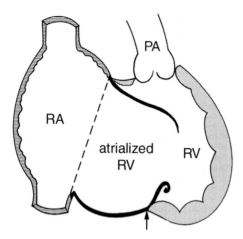

Figure 44B

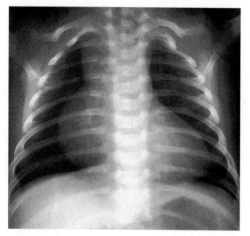

Figure 44C Frontal chest radiograph of a newborn with pulmonary atresia and intact ventricular septum shows a markedly enlarged heart with an egg-on-side appearance. The right atrial contour is prominent, and the pulmonary vascularity is reduced.

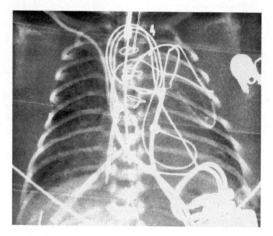

Figure 44D Frontal chest radiograph of a newborn with heart block shows severe cardiomegaly and severe pulmonary edema.

Diagnosis

Ebstein's malformation of the tricuspid valve (**Fig. 44B**) with patent ductus arteriosus

Differential Diagnosis

Severe cardiomegaly in the newborn:

- Ebstein's malformation*
- Unguarded tricuspid valve*
- Uhl's anomaly: absence of the myocardium of the right ventricle*
- Pulmonary atresia with intact ventricular septum* (**Fig. 44C**)
- Congenital heart block** (**Fig. 44D**)
- Congenital aortic insufficiency; aorto-left ventricular tunnel**
- Cardiac tumor
- Massive pericardial effusion

*Typically seen with diminished pulmonary vascularity
**Typically seen with pulmonary edema

Discussion

Clinical Findings

The clinical features vary with the severity of the lesion. The milder forms can escape detection. The most severe forms develop cyanosis in the newborn period. Cyanosis may spontaneously decrease in severity as the pulmonary vascular resistance drops, only to return after some years. Dyspnea due to severe heart failure is frequent. Dyspnea also can be due to lung hypoplasia related to long-standing cardiomegaly from the early gestational period. A systolic murmur due to tricuspid regurgitation is heard in the left sternal border. Occasionally, the patients present with supraventricular tachycardia. Cardiomegaly varies from mild to as massive as in the present case depending on the degree of tricuspid regurgitation.

Pathology

In Ebstein's malformation, all three leaflets of the tricuspid valve—the septal, anterior, and posterior leaflets—are abnormal. The most characteristic changes are seen in septal and posterior leaflets that show various degrees of hypoplasia, dysplasia, and apically displaced attachment to the septum and posterior free wall of the right ventricle. A significant part of the right ventricle is functionally incorporated into the right atrium, which is called atrialization of the right ventricle (**Fig. 44B**). Although the anterior leaflet has a normal attachment to the anterior free wall, it is usually large with an appearance of a sail. As the leaflet margins cannot oppose properly during ventricular systole, tricuspid regurgitation is the major physiologic consequence. Occasionally, the distal attachment of this sail-like anterior leaflet can be to an apical muscular shelf in the free wall of the right ventricle, separating the right ventricle into the inlet and outlet zones. This variant is called stenotic Ebstein's malformation and is not associated with significant tricuspid regurgitation. In most cases of Ebstein's malformation, an atrial septal defect is present or the foramen ovale is patent, allowing a right-to-left shunt through it.

Imaging Findings

FETAL ULTRASOUND

- Severe form of Ebstein's malformation can hardly escape detection at fetal ultrasound examination because of massive cardiomegaly.
- When there is severe cardiomegaly with predominant enlargement of the right atrium and right ventricle, the attachment of the septal leaflet of the tricuspid valve to the ventricular septum should be investigated.

RADIOGRAPHY

- Ebstein's malformation should be included in the differential diagnosis when the chest radiograph shows massive cardiomegaly and diminished pulmonary vascularity.
- The present case shows mildly increased vascularity because of persistent patency of the ductus arteriosus.

MRI

- MRI is rarely indicated.
- MRI is advantageous over echocardiography in visualizing the morphology of the anterior leaflet of the tricuspid valve and right ventricular free wall.

ECHOCARDIOGRAPHY

- Postnatal follow-up is usually by echocardiography.

Treatment and Prognosis

- Asymptomatic patients with minor forms of Ebstein's malformation do not need any treatment.
- Most symptomatic patients require surgical treatment to ameliorate the hemodynamic problems.
- The surgical treatment includes plication of the atrialized portion of the right ventricle and tricuspid annulopasty.
- Tricuspid valve replacement can be considered in larger patients.
- The outcome of the surgical treatment in neonates with severe cardiomegaly and congestive heart failure is poor.
- It is unlikely that these neonates would be candidates for cardiac transplantation because of impaired development of the lungs and pulmonary arteries.

PEARLS_____

- The most common cause of massive cardiomegaly in the newborn is Ebstein's malformation.
- Although the pulmonary vascularity is usually diminished, it may be increased with patent ductus arteriosus.
- The outcome depends on both the severity of tricuspid regurgitation and the severity of lung hypoplasia.

Suggested Readings

Anderson KR, Zuberbuhler JR, Anderson RH, Becker AE, Lie JT. Morphologic spectrum of Ebstein's anomaly of the heart: a review. Mayo Clin Proc 1979;54:174–180

Chaoui R, Bollmann R, Goldner B, Heling KS, Tennstedt C. Fetal cardiomegaly: echocardiographic findings and outcome in 19 cases. Fetal Diagn Ther 1994;9:92–104

Freedom RM, Benson LN. Ebstein's malformation of tricuspid valve. In: Freedom RM, Benson LN, Smallhorn JF, eds. Neonatal Heart Disease. London: Springer-Verlag; 1992:471–483

Hornberger LK, Sahn DJ, Kleinman CS, Copel JA, Reed KL. Tricuspid valve disease with significant tricuspid insufficiency in the fetus: diagnosis and outcome. J Am Coll Cardiol 1991;17:167–173

CASE 45

Clinical Presentation

A term newborn developed severe hypoxemia, cyanosis, and tachypnea immediately after birth. The obstetric history was unremarkable.

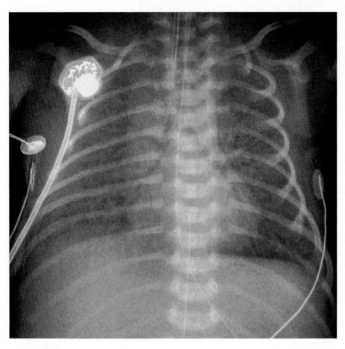

Figure 45A

Radiologic Findings

A frontal chest radiograph (**Fig. 45A**) shows moderately hyperinflated lungs with generalized increase in interstitial lung markings. The heart is normal in size and configuration.

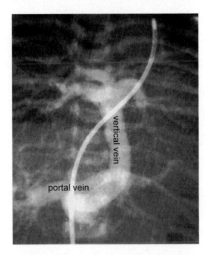

Figure 45B Injection into the main pulmonary artery at cardiac catheterization shows that all pulmonary veins make a confluence at a vertical vein that connects to the portal vein in the liver.

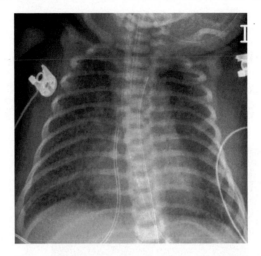

Figure 45C Plain chest radiograph, of a patient with hypoplastic left heart syndrome and restrictive atrial communication, shows generalized increase in interstitial lung markings and air trapping as in **Fig. 45A**.

Diagnosis

Total anomalous pulmonary venous connection (TAVPC) to the portal vein (**Fig. 45B**)

Differential Diagnosis

- Obstructive type of TAVPC; most commonly seen with anomalous connection to the portal vein
- Stenosis of the individual pulmonary veins
- Hypoplastic left heart syndrome with restrictive atrial communication (**Fig. 45C**)
- Congenital lymphangiectasia
- Transient respiratory distress of the newborn
- Interstitial viral pneumonia
- Hyaline membrane disease in the term infant with surfactant deficiency

Discussion

Clinical Findings

The clinical manifestation of TAPVC to the portal vein is significantly different from those of anomalous connection to the other sites. In the typical form of TAPVC, the venous drainage is directly or indirectly into the right atrium via a vascular channel, whereas in this form, the pulmonary venous drainage is into the hepatic parenchyma that has high vascular resistance. In fetal life, the high vascular resistance within the liver is not transmitted to the pulmonary veins because the pulmonary venous blood drains freely into the right atrium through the ductus venosus. However, pulmonary venous obstruction suddenly develops immediately after birth with closure of the ductus venosus. Therefore, the patients become cyanotic and very sick soon after birth with clinical features similar to those of severe hyaline membrane disease. Hepatomegaly is occasionally considerable. On auscultation there usually is no murmur. Rarely, the symptoms develop later in life with delayed closure of the ductus venosus.

Pathology

TAPVC is a condition in which all pulmonary veins of both lungs are abnormally connected to a structure or structures other than the left atrium. The most common location of an abnormal connection is to the left innominate vein, followed by the coronary sinus, portal vein, right superior vena cava, right atrium, and multiple sites. When the connection is to the portal vein, the pulmonary veins form a confluence into a vertical channel that courses to the abdomen through the esophageal hiatus to connect to the portal vein (**Fig. 45B**).

Imaging Findings

FETAL ULTRASOUND

- Anomalous pulmonary venous connection can easily escape detection at fetal ultrasound if connection of the individual pulmonary veins is not carefully investigated.

RADIOGRAPHY

- Chest radiographs in the newborn typically show no abnormality in heart size and contour (**Fig. 45A**). The heart size can even be small because moderate to severe air trapping is common.
- The lungs show a generalized increase in interstitial markings. This pattern of pulmonary venous hypertension is somewhat different from that seen in older children. Vascular redistribution and Kerley's B lines are rarely seen in newborns with pulmonary venous obstruction.
- The diagnosis in newborns can be delayed because the radiographic features are primarily interstitial lung pattern, whereas there is neither audible murmur nor cardiomegaly.
- Similar radiographic and clinical features are also seen in TAPVC to other sites when there is severe stenosis of the pulmonary venous confluence or pathway to the abnormal draining site.
- Hypoplastic left heart syndrome can also show similar radiographic features when the atrial septum is intact or an atrial communication is restrictive (**Fig. 45C**).
- The radiographic findings resemble those of transient respiratory distress of the newborn and congenital lymphangiectasia.
- The patients are often diagnosed with interstitial pneumonia of viral etiology based on the radiographic features. The abnormal densities in interstitial pneumonia, however, show uneven distribution and are associated with patchy distribution of consolidation, atelectasis, and hyperinflation.

ECHOCARDIOGRAPHY

- The diagnosis of TAPVC is usually made by echocardiography.
- The initial abnormality detected is usually the presence of right-to-left shunting at the atrial level.
- Although the overall heart size is normal, the right atrium, right ventricle, and main pulmonary artery are enlarged, whereas the left atrium, left ventricle, and aorta are small.
- The pulmonary veins are not connected to the left atrium but form a confluence into a vertical vascular channel behind the small left atrium. The vertical vein descends in the posterior mediastinum adjacent to the descending aorta and connects to the portal venous system.
- The abdominal ultrasonography shows the unusually dilated portal veins and vascular channel.

MRI

- When echocardiographic visualization of the pulmonary venous drainage is incomplete, MRI with contrast-enhanced angiography can be performed, and cardiac catheterization with angiography can be avoided.

Treatment and Prognosis

- The patient's condition can temporarily be improved with administration of E-type prostaglandin, keeping the patency of the ductus venosus.
- Urgent surgical correction is mandatory.
- Surgical mortality is reported up to 40%, which is significantly higher than in other forms of TAPVC.
- Although the late result of repair is generally excellent, pulmonary venous obstruction is not uncommon.

PEARLS_____

- Although the diagnosis of obstructive type of TAPVC should be made by echocardiography, MRI, or angiography, this rare entity can be considered as a strong possibility based on plain radiographic findings.
- The cardinal plain radiographic feature is a generalized increase in interstitial markings in a cyanotic newborn.
- Air bronchograms are usually absent with obstructed TAPVC, but they will commonly be seen with hyaline membrane disease. The lungs are often hyperaerated with TAPVC and underaerated with hyaline membrane disease.

PITFALL_____

- Because of the severe venous obstruction and frequently present patent ductus, it may be angiographically difficult or impossible to demonstrate the draining vessel on the levophase of a pulmonary arteriogram.

Suggested Readings

Anderson RH, Marcartney FJ, Shineborne EA, Tynan M. Pulmonary venous abnormalities. In: Anderson RH, Marcartney FJ, Shineborne EA, Tynan M, eds. Paediatric Cardiology. Edinburgh: Churchill Livingstone; 1987:509–539

Lucas RV Jr, Lock JE, Tandon R, Edwards JE. Gross and histological anatomy of total anomalous pulmonary venous connection. Am J Cardiol 1988;62:292–300

Musewe NN, Smallhorn JF, Freedom RM. Anomalies of pulmonary venous connections including cor triatriatum and stenosis of individual pulmonary veins. In: Freedom RM, Benson LN, Smallhorn JF, eds. Neonatal Heart Disease. London: Springer-Verlag; 1992:309–331

CASE 46

Clinical Presentation

A newborn presents with mild cyanosis and failure to thrive.

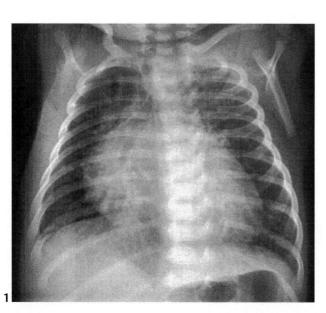 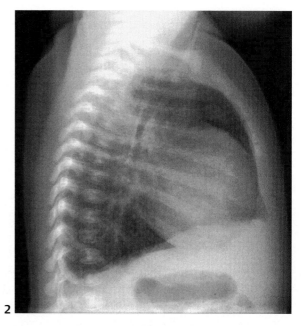

Figure 46A

Radiologic Findings

The frontal chest radiograph (**Fig. 46A1**) shows a moderately enlarged heart with an egg-on-side configuration and increased pulmonary vascularity. The superior mediastinum is narrow because of thymic hypoplasia. Note that the anterior upper mediastinum is empty in lateral view (**Fig. 46A2**).

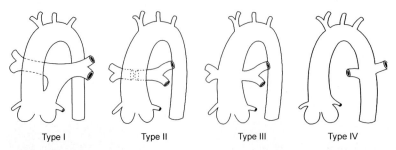

Type I   Type II   Type III   Type IV

Figure 46B Schematic diagram of four types of truncus arteriosus as described by Collet and Edwards.

Diagnosis

Truncus arteriosus with DiGeorge syndrome

Differential Diagnosis

- Egg-on-side appearance:
  - Complete transposition of the great arteries: pulmonary vascularity, variable
  - Pulmonary atresia with intact ventricular septum: diminished pulmonary vascularity
  - Truncus arteriosus: increased pulmonary vascularity
- Boot-shaped heart: In truncus arteriosis the heart may also be boot shaped, but this is less common.
  - Tetralogy of Fallot: normal heart size and diminished pulmonary vascularity
  - Pulmonary atresia with ventricular septal defect: normal heart size with diminished pulmonary vascularity or enlarged heart with increased pulmonary vascularity
  - Truncus arteriosus: moderate cardiomegaly with increased pulmonary vascularity
- Narrow superior mediastinum:
  - Complete transposition of the great arteries with postnatal regression of the thymus
  - Truncus arteriosus with thymic hypoplasia in association with DiGeorge syndrome or postnatal regression of the thymus

Discussion

Clinical Findings

Most patients with truncus are recognized as having congenital heart disease during the neonatal period. During the first few weeks of life, persistence of increased pulmonary vascular resistance results in mild cyanosis with little evidence of heart failure. As the pulmonary vascular resistance decreases, cyanosis may disappear and be replaced by signs of congestive heart failure. When the truncal valve is severely regurgitant, the signs of congestive heart failure may manifest immediately after birth. Generally, the heart is overactive, and a pansystolic murmur is heard at the left precordium. Microdeletion of chromosome 22q11 is seen in ~40% of patients with truncus, and patients with this deletion include DiGeorge and velocardiofacial syndrome cases.

Pathology

Truncus arteriosus is characterized by a single arterial vessel arising from the heart through a single arterial valve giving origin to the systemic, pulmonary, and coronary arteries. According to the origin of the pulmonary arteries from the single arterial trunk, four types of truncus have been described (**Fig. 46B**) (Collett and Edwards). In type I, a short pulmonary trunk originates from the truncus and then bifurcates into the branch pulmonary arteries. In type II, the branch pulmonary arteries arise directly from the truncus with the orifices close together. In type III, the branch pulmonary arteries arise from the truncus with the orifices wide apart. In type IV, the branch pulmonary arteries arise from the descending aorta. This form is now considered to represent a form of pulmonary atresia with ventricular septal defect rather than truncus arteriosus, the branches being considered as major aortopulmonary collateral arteries. With rare exceptions, a large ventricular septal defect is present immediately underneath the truncal valve. The truncal valve has three leaflets in approximately two thirds of patients. In the remaining patients, the truncal valve has two or four to six leaflets. Truncal valve leaflets are often dysplastic, causing valvar regurgitation or, uncommonly, stenosis.

The most common associated cardiovascular anomalies include right aortic arch with a mirror-image branching pattern, interrupted aortic arch, stenosis of the pulmonary arterial ostia or branches, and unilateral absence of a pulmonary artery.

Imaging Findings

FETAL ULTRASOUND

- Truncus arteriosus rarely escapes detection at fetal ultrasound screening.
- When the diagnosis of truncus is made at fetal ultrasound, chromosomal study including FISH (fluorescent in situ hybridization) for microdeletion of chromosome 22 is performed. The baby should be delivered in a tertiary care center.

RADIOGRAPHY

- The initial chest radiographs obtained after birth show mild to moderate cardiomegaly and mildly increased pulmonary vascularity (**Fig. 46A**). In a few weeks the heart shows progressive enlargement with increasing pulmonary vascularity as the pulmonary vascular resistance decreases with age.
- The overall cardiac configuration often resembles a side view of an egg or a boot, or it can be nonspecific. An egg-on-side appearance is related to absence of subpulmonary right ventricular outflow tract. In a normal heart, the slight bulge of the left upper heart border below the pulmonary arterial segment is partly due to the presence of underlying right ventricular outflow tract, although it may not be a border-forming structure. In truncus, this part is absent, and the left heart border is flatter than normal.
- A similar configuration is also seen in pulmonary atresia with intact ventricular septum and complete transposition of the great arteries. In pulmonary atresia with intact ventricular septum, the left upper heart border is flat due to hypoplasia of the right ventricular outflow tract. In complete transposition, a different mechanism is responsible for flatness of the left upper heart border. As the right ventricular outflow tract is displaced to the right to support the ascending aorta in complete transposition, the left upper heart border is less convex.
- A boot-shaped heart is due to elevation and rounding of the cardiac apex and concavity of the pulmonary arterial segment. It is classically seen in tetralogy of Fallot and pulmonary atresia with ventricular septal defect. It is also seen in some truncus cases in which the main pulmonary arterial segment is short or absent, or the left pulmonary artery arises directly from the posterior wall of the truncal root.
- Occasionally, an abnormally high origin of the left pulmonary artery can be seen.
- The superior mediastinum is narrow in patients with DiGeorge syndrome because of thymic hypoplasia. The superior mediastinum can also be narrow in the absence of DiGeorge syndrome when the chest radiographs are obtained a few days or weeks after birth. This is due to postnatal atrophy of the thymus in response to stress.
- The vascular pedicle itself may be narrower than normal in truncus, as only one arterial trunk is present.

ECHOCARDIOGRAPHY

- Postnatal diagnosis depends mostly on echocardiography with Doppler interrogation.
- Intracardiac anatomy of truncus can be somewhat similar to that of tetralogy of Fallot and pulmonary atresia with ventricular septal defect.
- Direct visualization of the origins of the pulmonary arteries in high parasternal short-axis views will usually differentiate truncus from other two defects.
- Aortopulmonary window may mimic truncus both clinically and echocardiographcially. In aortopulmonary window, a ventricular septal defect is not a part of the anomaly and separate semilunar valves are present.
- Cardiac catheterization is not required in young infants. However, when the patient is older, catheterization should be performed to assess severity of pulmonary vascular disease.

Treatment and Prognosis

- The patients need operative repair in early infancy before the significant pulmonary vascular disease develops.
- Operative mortality is higher after the age of 6 months.
- The operative repair procedure includes closure of the ventricular septal defect so that the left ventricular outflow tract is directed to the truncal valve, detachment of the pulmonary arterial confluence from the truncus, and placement of a right ventricle-to-pulmonary artery conduit.
- With successful neonatal surgery, ~70 to 80% of patients survive.
- When the fixed pulmonary vascular disease is diagnosed, only a palliative treatment is an option. More than 80% patients with untreated or palliated truncus die by the age of 1 year.

PEARLS_____

- Truncus arteriosus can be suspected when a newborn with signs of congestive heart failure shows enlarged heart with either egg-on-side appearance or boot shape and increased pulmonary vascularity.
- Absent or small thymic shadow suggests association with DiGeorge syndrome.

Suggested Readings

Ceballos R, Soto B, Kirklin JW, Bargeron LM Jr. Truncus arteriosus: an anatomical-angiographic study. Br Heart J 1983;49:589–599

Collet RW, Edwards JE. Persistent truncus arteriosus: a classification according to anatomic types. Surg Clin North Am 1949;25:1245–1270

Yoo SJ, Kim YM, Bae EJ, et al. Cardiac imaging in common arterial trunk. Prog Pediatr Cardiol 2002;15:41–51

CASE 47

Clinical Presentation

A newborn presents with cyanosis and tachypnea.

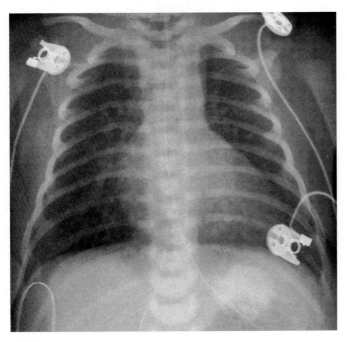

Figure 47A

Radiologic Findings

A frontal chest radiograph (**Fig. 47A**) shows a mildly enlarged heart with an egg-on-side configuration and mildly increased interstitial markings.

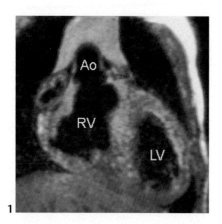

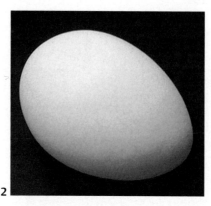

Figure 47B T1-weighted coronal MRI (**1**) of a patient with complete transposition of the great arteries shows an egg-on-side appearance, as shown in **2**. Ao, aorta; LV, left ventricle; RV, right ventricle.

Figure 47C Diagram showing complete transposition of the great arteries. Ao, aorta; LA, left atrium; LV, left ventricle; PA, pulmonary artery; RA, right atrium; RV, right ventricle.

Diagnosis

Complete transposition of the great arteries. A T1-weighted MRI in coronal plane (**Fig. 47B1**) shows that the aorta arises from the morphologically right ventricle. Note that the cardiac configuration in both plain radiograph and MRI is egg-shaped (**Fig. 47B2**).

Differential Diagnosis

Egg-on-side appearance:

- Complete transposition of the great arteries: pulmonary vascularity, variable
- Pulmonary atresia with intact ventricular septum: diminished pulmonary vascularity
- Truncus arteriosus: increased pulmonary vascularity

Discussion

Clinical Findings

The circulatory arrangement of complete transposition is such that all patients have significant desaturation from birth. Cyanosis is usually evident from the first day of life when the ventricular septum is intact or within a week or month when there is a large ventricular septal defect.

Pathology

Transposition of the great arteries is defined as discordant connection between the ventricles and great arteries; that is, the morphologic right ventricle connects to the aorta and the left ventricle to the pulmonary artery. Complete transposition of the great arteries is defined as the combination of normal concordant atrioventricular connection and discordant ventriculoarterial connection (**Fig. 47C**). Thus the systemic venous return is recirculated to the body via the right atrium, right ventricle, and aorta, whereas the pulmonary venous return is recirculated to the lungs via the left atrium, left ventricle, and pulmonary artery. Therefore, the systemic and pulmonary circulations are in parallel and separate, resulting in severe systemic desaturation. A prerequisite of life is intercirculatory mixing. The

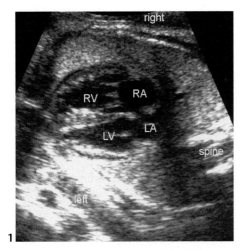 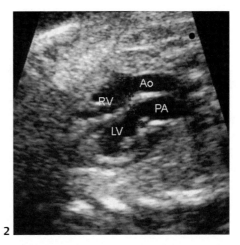

Figure 47D (1) Four-chamber fetal echocardiogram shows a normal anatomy. LA, left atrium; LV, left ventricle; RA, right atrium; RV, right ventricle. **(2)** Ventricular outflow tract view shows that the aorta (Ao) arises from the right ventricle and the pulmonary artery (PA) from the left ventricle.

sites of intercirculatory mixing include normally occurring foramen ovale and, in the newborn, a patent ductus arteriosus. Usually, there is bidirectional flow between the two atria, and left-to-right shunt through the patent ductus arteriosus. There may be additional defects such as an atrial septal defect or a ventricular septal defect. Complete transposition is commonly associated with a ventricular septal defect and/or left ventricular outflow tract obstruction, both of which also change the level of systemic desaturation. Right ventricular outflow tract obstruction is less common.

Imaging Findings

FETAL ULTRASOUND

- Although many cases of complete transposition are detected with fetal ultrasound, a significant number of cases may escape detection if only a four-chamber view (a basic screening view) is obtained. This is because uncomplicated complete transposition shows normal anatomy in the four-chamber view (**Fig. 47D1**).
- It is important to obtain a ventricular outflow tract view in which both right and left ventricular outflow tracts are parallel (**Fig. 47D2**).

RADIOGRAPHY

- At birth, the heart is of normal size but often shows an egg-on-side appearance. This appearance is due to the right ventricular outflow tract being displaced to the right to support the aorta on the right side in complete transposition. As the right ventricular outflow tract normally contributes to the bulk that forms the left upper heart border below the pulmonary arterial segment, its rightward displacement results in flattening of the left upper heart border (**Fig. 47B**).
- The pulmonary vascularity is usually normal. Not infrequently, the pulmonary vascularity can be asymmetric with preferential flow to the right lung. With time, there is progressive cardiac enlargement and gradual increase in pulmonary vascularity when the left ventricular outflow tract is unobstructed. The pulmonary vascularity can be diminished and the heart size can be normal with significant left ventricular outflow tract obstruction.
- At birth, the superior mediastinum is unremarkable. Within a week, the thymus may shrink with stress, uncovering the narrow vascular pedicle in typical cases. The narrow vascular pedicle is due to anteroposteriorly related great arteries with a parallel course that is the most common great arterial relationship encountered in transposition.

ECHOCARDIOGRAPHY

- Postnatal diagnosis depends mostly on echocardiography with Doppler interrogation.
- The atria have normal connection to the underlying ventricles.
- The right ventricle gives rise to the aorta on the right side, whereas the left ventricle gives rise to the pulmonary artery on the left posterior aspect of the aorta.
- Typically the ventricular outflow tracts leading to the great arteries are parallel and can be imaged in a long axial oblique view.
- Although the aorta is typically to the right of and anterior to the pulmonary artery in most cases, the left-sided or posterior aorta does not exclude complete transposition.
- An associated ventricular septal defect and/or left ventricular outflow tract obstruction can also be demonstrated in long axial oblique view.
- As the most desirable surgical procedure is an arterial switch operation with coronary arterial transfer, coronary arterial origins from the aortic sinuses should be defined before the surgery.

Treatment and Prognosis

- When the diagnosis of complete transposition is made at fetal ultrasound, the baby should be delivered in a tertiary center where a surgical repair can be performed immediately after birth.
- Infusion of prostaglandin E_1 should be started as soon as possible to keep the ductus arteriosus open for adequate mixing between pulmonary and systemic circulations.
- For critically ill neonates, balloon atrial septostomy is performed for adequate mixing at the atrial level.
- Neonates with complete transposition with or without ventricular septal defect that is not complicated by significant left ventricular outflow tract obstruction are treated with an arterial switch operation, ideally within the first week of life.
- When the surgery is postponed or delayed beyond the "safe" period for an arterial switch operation, pulmonary arterial banding and a modified Blalock-Taussig shunt can be required to train the left ventricle before the definitive surgery.
- When there is a ventricular septal defect and the left ventricular outflow tract obstruction cannot be repaired by resection, a Rastelli operation or its modified procedure is performed. In a Rastelli operation, the left ventricle is tunneled to the aorta by closing the ventricular septal defect with a baffle, and a conduit is interposed between the right ventricle and distal main pulmonary artery.
- Mustard and Senning operations, in which the systemic and pulmonary venous returns are rerouted into the left and right ventricles, respectively, are now rarely performed.
- The overall mortality rate for the arterial switch operation in large centers is typically <5%. The mortality rate for the Rastelli operation is ~10% with its higher rate of late surgical complications.
- The long-term outcome after an uncomplicated surgery is excellent.

PEARL_____

- Complete transposition of the great arteries should be suspected when a baby develops severe cyanosis immediately after birth and the frontal chest radiograph shows mild cardiomegaly with an egg-on-side appearance and mildly increased pulmonary vascularity.

Suggested Readings

Freedom RM, Mawson J, Yoo S-J, Benson LN. Complete transposition of the great arteries (atrioventricular concordance and ventriculoarterial discordance). In: Congenital Heart Disease. Textbook of Angiocardiography. Armonk NY: Futura Publishing Co.; 1997:987–1070

Muster AJ, Paul MH, Van Grondelle A, Conway JJ. Asymmetric distribution of the pulmonary blood flow between the right and left lungs in d-transposition of the great arteries. Am J Cardiol 1976;38:352–361

CASE 48

Clinical Presentation

A newborn presents with cyanosis and tachypnea.

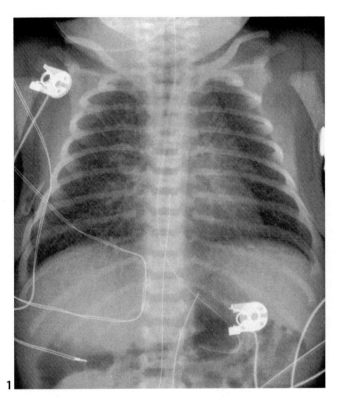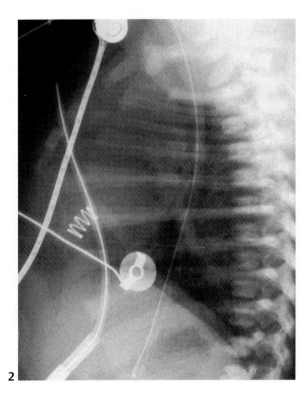

Figure 48A

Radiologic Findings

A frontal chest radiograph (**Fig. 48A1**) shows the stomach bubble in a left paramedian location and the transverse liver. There is a levocardia. In the lateral chest radiograph (**Fig. 48A2**), the upper lobar bronchi are located in similar horizontal levels. The pulmonary arterial shadow is seen mostly in front of the airway. Both lungs show increased interstitial markings due to pulmonary venous hypertension secondary to obstructive type of total anomalous pulmonary venous connection.

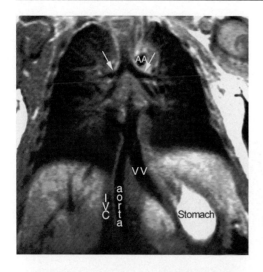

Figure 48B T1-weighted coronal MRI shows right-isomeric branching pattern of the bronchi (arrows), juxtaposition of the aorta and inferior vena cava (IVC) on the right side, and a left-sided stomach. All pulmonary veins make a confluence at a vertical vein (VV) that drains into the portal vein. AA, aortic arch.

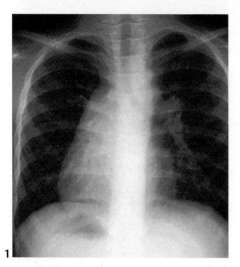

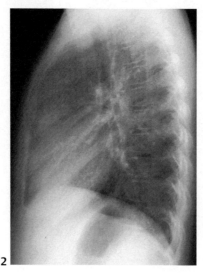

Figure 48C Chest radiographs in a patient with left isomerism. The frontal view (**1**) shows symmetrically long bronchi, right-sided stomach, and levocardia. The lateral view (**2**) shows end-on shadows of both upper lobar bronchi in similar horizontal levels. The pulmonary arteries are seen above and behind the upper lobar bronchi.

Diagnosis

Right isomerism with transverse liver and asplenia. A T1-weighted MRI (**Fig. 48B**) shows symmetrically short bronchi. Neither right nor left pulmonary artery is above the main bronchus. The abdominal aorta and inferior vena cava are juxtaposed on the right side of the spine. The pulmonary veins make a confluent channel to connect to the portal vein via a vertical vein.

Differential Diagnosis

- Left isomerism: Transverse liver and abnormally positioned stomach may also be seen in left isomerism. However, left isomerism tends to have one side of the liver larger than the other (**Fig. 48C**).

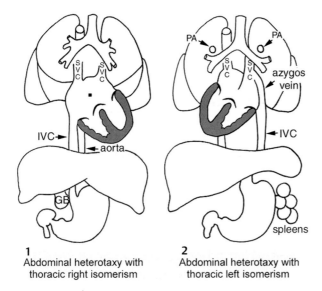

1
Abdominal heterotaxy with
thoracic right isomerism

2
Abdominal heterotaxy with
thoracic left isomerism

Figure 48D Diagrams show visceral heterotaxy with thoracic right isomerism and asplenia (**1**) and visceral heterotaxy with thoracic left isomerism and polysplenia (**2**) gastric bubble; IVC, inferior vena cava; PA, pulmonary artery; SVC, superior vena cava

Discussion

Clinical Findings

Patients with right isomerism frequently come to medical attention early in life because of associated complex congenital heart disease. The most common cardiac defects include atrioventricular septal defect, transposition of the great arteries or double outlet right ventricle, and pulmonary stenosis or atresia. Neonates with this common association develop severe cyanosis early in life. The extracardiac type of total anomalous pulmonary venous connection is present in >50% of cases. In nearly 50% of these, the anomalous connection is an obstructive type, which causes intractable hypoxemia and tachypnea.

Pathology

The term *situs* refers to the arrangement of the internal organs of the body. The normal arrangement is called situs solitus, whereas the mirror-image arrangement is called situs inversus. Rarely, the abdominal visceral arrangement is neither normal nor inverted, which is called visceral heterotaxy (**Fig. 48D**). Although visceral heterotaxy is characterized by a disorganized arrangement of the abdominal organs, the lungs and bronchi show abnormally symmetric arrangement, both sides resembling either the normal right or the left. Thus, visceral heterotaxy can be further divided into those with thoracic right isomerism or those with thoracic left isomerism. The right or left isomeric characteristics are also seen in the morphology of the atria. In right isomerism, both atria show the characteristics of the morphologically right atrium. In left isomerism, both atria show the characteristics of the morphologically left atrium. With few exceptions, right isomerism is associated with asplenia, and left isomerism with polysplenia. Right isomerism with asplenia is always associated with complex cyanotic congenital heart disease. Association with congenital heart disease is common but not a rule in left isomerism with polysplenia.

Imaging Findings

FETAL ULTRASOUND

- Cardiac defects in right isomerism should be detected with fetal ultrasound, although the diagnosis of right isomerism can often be missed.

- The fetal diagnosis of right isomerism can be made if one investigates the arrangement of the abdominal organs.

RADIOGRAPHY

- After birth, the diagnosis can be strongly suspected when the severely cyanotic newborn shows abnormal location of the stomach and unusually symmetric transverse liver in chest radiographs or on physical examination (**Fig. 48A**).
- The heart position is variable. Frequently, the cardiac apex is on the same side of the stomach.
- Presence of a minor fissure or fissures could provide a convincing clue. For instance, bilateral minor fissures suggest right isomerism. Even if a minor fissure is seen unilaterally, its presence on the same side of the stomach is almost always a definitive sign of right isomerism.
- In lateral chest radiograph (**Fig. 48C2**), because both main bronchi are symmetrically short, the upper lobar bronchi cast round lucent shadows at similar horizontal levels.
- Pulmonary arteries are seen only in front of the upper lobar bronchi because neither pulmonary artery passes over the mainstem bronchus to descend behind it. This is in contrast to left isomerism where both pulmonary arteries pass over the upper lobar bronchi and the pulmonary arteries cast shadows above and behind the end-on lucent shadows of the upper lobar bronchi (**Fig. 48D**).
- As pulmonary stenosis or atresia is associated in most cases, the heart is usually normal in size, and the pulmonary vascularity diminished.

ECHOCARDIOGRAPHY

- Diagnosis is usually made by echocardiography.
- As in fetal ultrasound, investigation of the arrangement of the abdominal organs is important.
- A very helpful clue to the diagnosis is juxtaposition of the abdominal aorta and inferior vena cava on either side of the spine, which is visualized in 90% of right isomerism.
- Absence of a spleen should be investigated by scrutinizing the upper abdomen along the greater curvature side of the stomach.
- Right isomerism is associated with multiple complex congenital cardiac defects, therefore the cardiac anatomy should be evaluated segment by segment.
- In >70% of cases, there is a univentricular–atrioventricular connection, necessitating a Fontan-type of surgery.
- Systemic and pulmonary veins show complex anatomy in all patients.
- Proper atrial septation at cardiac surgery requires clear depiction of the venous anatomy. Although the venous anatomy can be defined by echocardiography, MRI or CT angiography is perhaps the most accurate.

Treatment and Prognosis

- Most neonates with right isomerism have inadequate pulmonary blood flow, and they usually require infusion of prostaglandin.
- In some patients, prostaglandin infusion unmasks obstructed pulmonary venous connection and may precipitate pulmonary edema.
- Complex cardiac defects preclude a biventricular repair in the majority of patients, hence requiring multiple-staged operations to the Fontan circuit.
- Prognosis depends on the associated cardiac defects and is usually poor.
- The mortality of surgery is especially high in neonates with obstructive pulmonary venous connection, severe regurgitation of the common atrioventricular valve, and diminutive pulmonary arteries.
- The clinical course of patients with right isomerism and asplenia can be further complicated by two problems: bacterial sepsis related to the absence of a spleen and intestinal volvulus secondary to intestinal malrotation.

PEARL_____

- Right isomerism is suspected when a plain chest or abdominal radiograph in a cyanotic newborn shows a transverse liver and an abnormally positioned gastric bubble.

PITFALLS_____

- A right-sided stomach does not necessarily mean that there is situs inversus. A right-sided stomach can also be seen in both right and left isomerisms.
- Be persistent in trying to distinguish polysplenia from asplenia as it makes a big difference in prognosis.

Suggested Readings

Anderson RH, Becker AE. Hearts with isomeric atrial appendages. In: Controversies in the Description of Congenitally Malformed Hearts. London: Imperial College Press; 1997:67–112

Van Praagh R. Terminology of congenital heart disease: glossary and commentary. Circulation 1977;56:139–143

CASE 49

Clinical Presentation

A 15-year-old girl presents with exertional dyspnea and exercise intolerance.

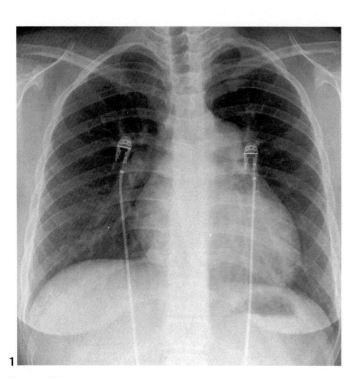
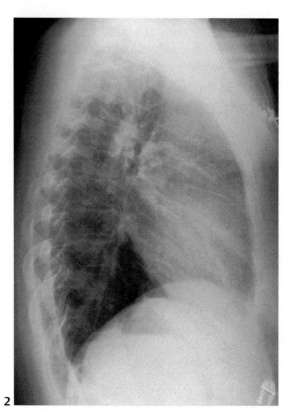

Figure 49A

Radiologic Findings

A frontal chest radiograph (**Fig. 49A1**) at presentation shows mild cardiomegaly, convex bulging of pulmonary arterial segment of the left heart border. The central pulmonary arteries are dilated, whereas peripheral pulmonary vessels are attenuated. The lateral chest radiograph (**Fig. 49A2**) also shows central-peripheral discrepancy in pulmonary artery size. The retrosternal space is obliterated because of right ventricular hypertrophy.

Diagnosis

Primary pulmonary hypertension

Differential Diagnosis

- Congenital heart disease with left-to-right shunt
- Chronic thromboembolism
- Pulmonary venous obstructive lesions including veno-occlusive disease
- Chronic lung disease
- Miscellaneous conditions (Chatterjee et al, 2002)

Discussion

Clinical Findings

The clinical features of primary pulmonary hypertension vary with the severity of the lesion. Patients frequently complain of unusual fatigue, shortness of breath, and chest pain on minor exertion. The chest pain is attributable to increased myocardial oxygen demand from increased right ventricular workload. Some patients present with episodes of fainting or loss of consciousness. On physical examination, the most consistent finding is an increased pulmonic component of the second heart sound. Elevation of jugular venous pulsation and ankle swelling are secondary findings of right heart failure.

Pathophysiology

Pulmonary hypertension is diagnosed when mean and systolic pulmonary arterial pressures exceed 20 and 30 mm Hg, respectively. Pulmonary hypertension is usually classified as primary or secondary. Secondary pulmonary hypertension is diagnosed when pulmonary hypertension is presumed to result from a coexisting disease, such as chronic pulmonary thromboembolism. In primary pulmonary hypertension, no obvious causes are recognized. Primary pulmonary hypertension is a relatively rare disease, with an annual incidence of 1 to 3 per million population. Most cases of primary pulmonary hypertension are sporadic, but there is a 6 to 12% familial incidence. The pulmonary vasculature is the exclusive target of disease, although the precise pathogenetic mechanisms are not known. Pulmonary arteriopathy as seen in primary pulmonary hypertension is characterized by obliteration of small vessels with vasoconstriction and thrombosis in situ. The increased pulmonary blood pressure leads to remodeling of the pulmonary arteries and also to right heart insufficiency.

Imaging Findings

RADIOGRAPHY

- Chest radiograph shows mild enlargement of the heart with rounded cardiac apex.
- Pulmonary arterial segment of the left heart border shows a round bulge, which may be similar to what is seen with poststenotic dilatation of the main and left pulmonary artery in pulmonary valvar stenosis.
- Central pulmonary arteries around the hilar regions are dilated, whereas the peripheral vessels are abnormally small. This causes so-called central-peripheral discrepancy of pulmonary vascularity.

MRI

- Although right heart catheterization is the "gold standard" diagnostic tool, both echocardiography and MRI are useful adjuncts or alternatives.

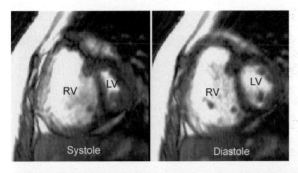

Figure 49B Cine MRI in systole and diastole shows right ventricular (RV) hypertrophy. The ventricular septum bulges into the left ventricle (LV) on systole, suggesting suprasystemic right ventricular pressure.

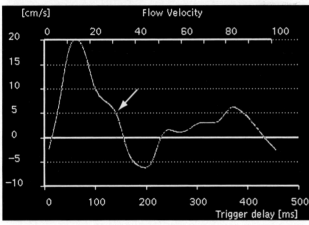

Figure 49C Time-velocity curve derived from phase-contrast velocity mapping of the main pulmonary artery at MRI shows early systolic peak, an additional peak (arrow) during deceleration phase of the systolic flow, and increased retrograde flow in late systole. The systolic forward flow declines earlier than normal.

- MRI is increasingly used for evaluation of patients with pulmonary hypertension because both pulmonary blood flow and right ventricular changes can be more accurately evaluated.
- A simple measurement of the pulmonary arterial size is a good screening tool for pulmonary hypertension. In adults, a right pulmonary artery diameter >28 mm is highly suggestive of chronic pulmonary hypertension.
- Right ventricular hypertrophy can be accurately assessed by cine imaging (**Fig. 49B**).
- Phase-contrast velocity mapping at MRI shows abnormal pulmonary hemodynamics with a blood flow pattern that includes an early systolic peak, additional second or third peaks in mid-systole, and early decline of the systolic velocity. There is greater retrograde flow after middle or late systole (**Fig. 49C**).

Treatment and Prognosis

- Prognosis is guarded, as no curative method exists for primary pulmonary hypertension.
- Patients are treated with medication to reduce pulmonary arterial pressure and to prevent blood clotting.
- To reverse the effect of endothelin, endothelin receptor antagonists have also been used with variable results.
- Patients with intractable pulmonary hypertension with medical treatment are candidates for a lung or heart and lung transplantation.

PEARLS

- Plain chest radiographic findings of pulmonary hypertension include mild cardiomegaly with right ventricular hypertrophy pattern, convex bulging of pulmonary arterial segment of the left heart border, and central-peripheral discrepancy of the pulmonary vascularity.

- The severity of pulmonary hypertension can be evaluated with MRI by performing cine imaging for a right ventricular functional evaluation and phase-contrast velocity mapping for evaluation of pulmonary arterial blood flow pattern.
- Careful examination of the pulmonary arteries is needed to exclude chronic thromboembolism.

Suggested Readings

Chatterjee K, Marco T, Alpert JS. Pulmonary hypertension: hemodynamic diagnosis and management. Arch Intern Med 2002;162:1925–1933

McGoon MD. The assessment of pulmonary hypertension. Clin Chest Med 2001;22:493–508

Mousseaux E, Tasu JP, Jolivet O, et al. Pulmonary arterial hypertension: non-invasive measurement with indexes of pulmonary flow estimated at velocity-encoded MR imaging—preliminary experience. Radiology 1999;212:896–902

CASE 50

Clinical Presentation

A 2-month-old infant presents with cyanosis.

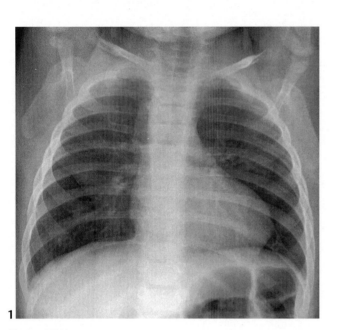
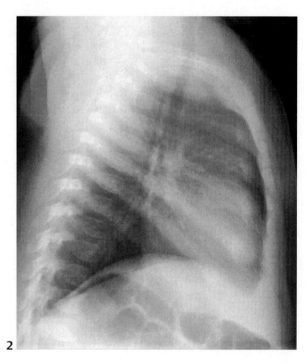

Figure 50A

Radiologic Findings

A frontal chest radiograph (**Fig. 50A1**) shows situs solitus and levocardia. The heart is normal in size, but its apex is uplifted, and the pulmonary arterial segment is flat. The overall cardiac configuration is boot shaped. The aortic arch is right sided. The pulmonary vascularity is decreased, which is more evident in the lateral view (**Fig. 50A2**). The perception in the lateral view can be facilitated by one's level of familiarity with normal vascularity.

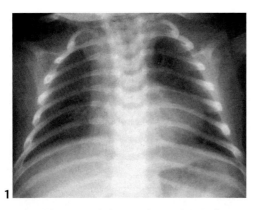
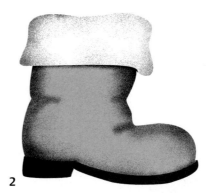

Figure 50B Frontal chest radiograph (**1**) of a patient with pulmonary atresia with ventricular septal defect and small patent ductus arteriosus. The cardiac configuration is very similar to a boot (**2**).

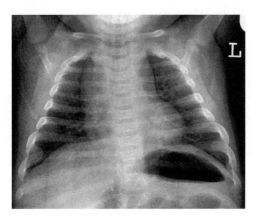

Figure 50C Frontal chest radiograph obtained in a lordotic projection from a normal infant shows a cardiac configuration similar to those of **Figs. 50A1** and **50B1**.

Diagnosis

Tetralogy of Fallot with a right aortic arch. A chest frontal view of another patient with tetralogy and pulmonary atresia shows more typical appearance of a boot (**Fig. 50B**).

Differential Diagnosis

Boot-shaped heart:

- Tetralogy of Fallot
- Pulmonary atresia with ventricular septal defect (**Fig. 50B**)
- Truncus arteriosus
- Lordotic radiographic positioning (**Fig. 50C**)

Discussion

Clinical Findings

The severity of the pulmonary outflow tract obstruction is the key as to when children with tetralogy begin to manifest significant symptoms and signs. Infants with a moderate degree of pulmonary outflow tract obstruction do well for the first few months of life with minimal or no evidence of cyanosis. With milder degree of obstruction, the patients can develop congestive heart failure due to left-to-right shunt. These patients develop cyanosis or cyanotic spells later in life as the pulmonary outflow tract

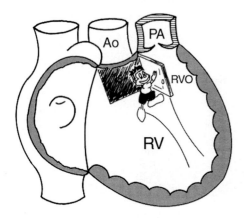

Figure 50D Cartoon showing pathogenetic mechanism of tetralogy of Fallot. The trap door is the outlet or infundibular septum. Ao, aorta; PA, pulmonary artery; RV, right ventricle; RVO, right ventricular outflow.

becomes narrower, allowing right-to-left shunt. Severe cyanosis and hypoxemia in the newborn period means that the obstruction is severe or there is pulmonary atresia.

Pathology

The four components of tetralogy of Fallot are a ventricular septal defect, pulmonary stenosis, overriding aorta, and right ventricular hypertrophy. The first three components are in fact the consequences of a single pathogenetic mechanism: the anterior, superior, and leftward deviation of the outlet septum in relation to the rest of the ventricular septum (**Fig. 50D**). Deviation of the outlet septum in such a direction causes an anterior malalignment type of ventricular septal defect and stenosis of the subpulmonary outflow tract. In addition, the aortic valve is displaced rightward and anteriorly through the ventricular septal defect to override the ventricular septum. The degrees of subpulmonary stenosis and aortic overriding are quite variable. The last component of tetralogy, the right ventricular hypertrophy, is a result of elevated right ventricular pressure.

Imaging Findings

FETAL ULTRASOUND

- Fetal sonographic diagnosis of tetralogy of Fallot can be made by using ventricular outflow tract views.
- Tetralogy not uncommonly escapes fetal detection as only a subtle abnormality is seen in four-chamber view.

RADIOGRAPHY

- Postnatal imaging evaluation includes plain chest radiography and echocardiography.
- Typically, the heart is normal in size, and the pulmonary vascularity is reduced.
- When the pulmonary outflow tract obstruction is not severe, the heart can be enlarged and the pulmonary vascularity can be mildly plethoric. With progression of pulmonary outflow tract obstruction, the shunt flow through the ventricular septal defect becomes less conspicuous, and eventually a right-to-left shunt ensues.
- The temporal changes can be appreciated in sequential plain chest radiographs.
- Boot-shaped heart is known as a typical cardiac configuration of tetralogy of Fallot. This configuration comprises uplifted cardiac apex, concave pulmonary arterial segment, and prominent aortic knob.
- It is important to note that typical boot-shaped heart is not always present.
- The cardiac apex in tetralogy is often normal in configuration.
- It is usually impossible to appreciate the concavity of the pulmonary arterial segment because the thymic shadow overlies this segment of the left heart border.
- The aortic arch is right-sided in ~30% of cases (**Fig. 50A1**).

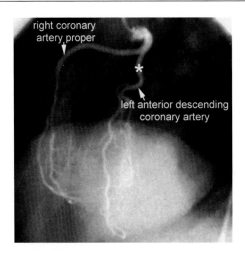

Figure 50E Selective injection into the right coronary artery. It bifurcates into the right coronary artery proper and left anterior descending coronary artery. The segment marked by an asterisk is the segment that crosses the subpulmonary outflow tract where a surgical incision is usually made.

ECHOCARDIOGRAPHY

- Diagnosis of tetralogy of Fallot is usually made by echocardiography.
- The ventricular septal defect is seen below the overriding aortic valve in parasternal long-axis view.
- The pulmonary outflow tract narrowing due to deviated outlet septum is best seen in short-axis or right anterior oblique view.
- The pulmonary valve is commonly bicuspid or unicuspid, and stenotic.
- The main pulmonary artery is small and may show supravalvar narrowing.
- The origins of the left and, less commonly, the right pulmonary artery can be stenotic.
- The sizes of the pulmonary arteries are measured in the mediastinum for evaluation of eligibility for total one-stage repair.
- Uncommonly, there is an additional source of pulmonary blood supply, which can be either a patent ductus arteriosus or major aortopulmonary collateral arteries (MAPCAs).
- When the ductus is patent and there is a left aortic arch, it connects the undersurface of the aortic arch and the proximal left pulmonary artery.
- The MAPCAs usually arise from the thoracic descending aorta or the bracheocephalic branches of the aortic arch. When there are MAPCAs, the anatomy should be evaluated by using either contrast-enhanced MR, CT angiography, or conventional x-ray angiography.
- As the surgical incision will be made in the pulmonary outflow tract, it is important to check whether there is any major coronary arterial branch crossing the free wall of the subpulmonary right ventricular outflow tract. The dangerous coronary anatomy includes the left anterior descending coronary artery arising from the right coronary artery, the single left coronary artery, and the prominent conal branch of the right coronary artery (**Fig. 50E**). When the coronary anatomy is difficult to evaluate, catheterization with aortic root injection should be performed.

Treatment and Prognosis

- When the diagnosis of tetralogy of Fallot is made at fetal ultrasound, delivery in a tertiary center can be considered when there is severe pulmonary outflow tract obstruction and the pulmonary arteries are very diminutive, and thus the patient is dependent on the patency of the ductus arteriosus.
- The definitive surgical treatment of tetralogy of Fallot is performed usually in infancy or early childhood and rarely in the neonatal period.
- When the risk of the one-stage complete repair is high while the patient is too young, an interim palliative procedure with a modified Blalock-Taussig anastomosis between the innominate artery and the branch pulmonary artery on the same side can be performed.
- The overall mortality of surgical repair of tetralogy of Fallot is <5% in most institutions.

- Although the long-term outcome is also excellent, postoperative morbidity is not uncommon.
- Chronic pulmonary regurgitation, an inevitable consequence of a transannular patch repair and/or pulmonary valvotomy, has become a significant determinant of late symptoms and long-term outcome including exercise intolerance, ventricular dysfunction, arrhythmia, and the risk of sudden death.

PEARLS

- The plain radiographic features of tetralogy of Fallot vary according to the severity of obstruction of the pulmonary outflow tract.
- Typically, the heart is normal in size and shows a boot shape.
- The pulmonary vascularity is typically reduced, which is often better appreciated in a lateral radiograph.
- The patient with a milder degree of stenosis may show mildly enlarged heart and increased pulmonary vascularity, the uplifted cardiac apex being a clue to the right diagnosis.
- Up to 30% of patients with tetralogy of Fallot have a right arch. Right arch occurs most frequently in the patients with severe pulmonary stenosis or pulmonary atresia.
- The right arch present with cyanotic heart disease is usually the mirror-image branching type that does not have a retroesophageal component by esophagogram.
- Up to 9% of patients with tetralogy will have coronary artery anomalies. The most common variation in tetralogy patients is an anomalous anterior descending coronary artery that courses over the right ventricular outflow tract. Occasionally it can be mistakenly incised at surgery.

PITFALLS

- Infundibular stenosis frequently progresses with advancing age.
- In infants, the heart size and contour are most often normal. The classic boot-shaped heart may not be present until later childhood, adolescence, or even adulthood.
- Tetralogy with very mild pulmonary stenosis, sometimes referred to as pink tetralogy, may appear radiographically similar to a simple ventricular septal defect with increased pulmonary arterial vascularity and cardiomegaly.

Suggested Readings

Anderson RH, Allwork SP, Ho SY, Lenox CC, Zuberbuhler JR. Surgical anatomy of tetralogy of Fallot. J Thorac Cardiovasc Surg 1981;81:887–896

Soto B, Pacifico AD, Ceballos R, Bargeron LM Jr. Tetralogy of Fallot: an angiographic-pathologic correlative study. Circulation 1981;64:558–566

CASE 51

Clinical Presentation

A newborn presents with respiratory distress and cyanosis.

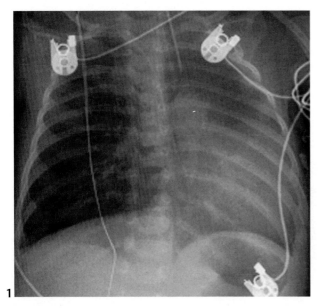
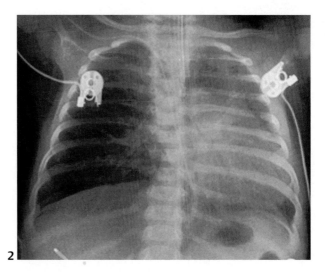

Figure 51A

Radiologic Findings

A frontal chest radiograph (**Fig. 51A1**) shows situs solitus and levocardia. The heart is displaced to the left side in association with collapse of the left lower lobe and lingular segment of the left upper lobe. The right lung is hyperinflated. On follow-up examination (**Fig. 51A2**), the left lower lobe is expanded, but there is a new area of segmental collapse in the left upper lung.

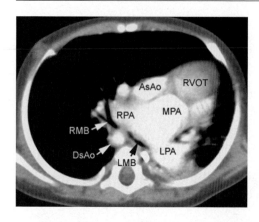

Figure 51B Contrast-enhanced CT angiogram. AsAo, ascending aorta; DsAo, descending aorta; LMB, left main bronchus; LPA, left pulmonary artery; MPA, main pulmonary artery; RMB, right main bronchus; RPA, right pulmonary artery; RVOT, right ventricular outflow tract.

Diagnosis

Tetralogy of Fallot with absent pulmonary valve syndrome. A contrast-enhanced CT image (**Fig. 51B**) shows markedly dilated main, right, and left pulmonary arteries in the mediastinum. The left main bronchus is compressed between the dilated pulmonary artery and the spine. The right main bronchus also shows a lesser degree of compression. The hyperinflated right lung is herniated into the left thorax, whereas the left lower lobe shows collapse.

Differential Diagnosis

Cyanotic newborn with hyperinflated lungs or mixture of lobar or segmental emphysema and collapse.
- Tetralogy of Fallot with absent pulmonary valve syndrome
- Pulmonary artery sling

Discussion

Clinical Findings

Patients are usually symptomatic from the newborn period, with varying degrees of heart failure, cyanosis, and respiratory distress. A loud systolic and diastolic to-and-fro murmur is audible in the left sternal border. Patients develop variable degrees of wheezing. The liver can be palpable below the costal margins because of depression of the diaphragm secondary to air trapping in the lungs.

Pathology

Absent pulmonary valve syndrome is a rare but distinct pathologic entity. In this condition, the pulmonary valve is guarded by very rudimentary leaflet(s) or is absent. It is commonly associated with tetralogy of Fallot and less commonly with a ventricular septal defect. When it is associated with tetralogy, the pulmonary valve is not only regurgitant but also stenotic because of a small pulmonary valve anulus and infundibular narrowing. Characteristically, the main and branch pulmonary arteries are aneurysmally dilated. The airway compression due to dilated pulmonary artery is the major problem in most patients. In the majority of the patients with tetralogy and absent pulmonary valve syndrome, the ductus arteriosus is congenitally absent. It is postulated that the fetus with absent ductus arteriosus develops severe pulmonary regurgitation as the fluid-filled lungs cannot accommodate the whole right ventricular output. As a consequence, the pulmonary valve leaflets are severely damaged, and the central pulmonary arteries become aneurysmally dilated.

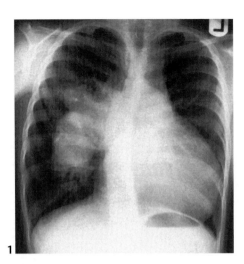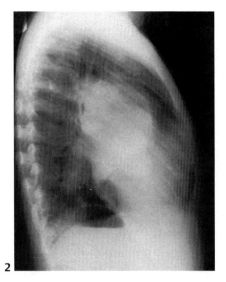

Figure 51C Frontal (**1**) and lateral (**2**) chest radiographs in a patient with tetralogy of Fallot and absent pulmonary valve syndrome show markedly dilated central pulmonary arteries that taper abruptly.

Imaging Findings

FETAL ULTRASOUND

- Fetal ultrasonographic diagnosis of tetralogy of Fallot with absent pulmonary valve syndrome can be made by recognizing the aneurysmally dilated central pulmonary arteries and small pulmonary valve anulus.
- The ductus arteriosus cannot be identified because it is usually absent.

RADIOGRAPHY

- Postnatal imaging evaluation includes plain chest radiography and echocardiography.
- Typically, the heart is normal in size, but it may show variable degrees of enlargement due to volume overload.
- Both hila can be exceptionally prominent with dilated branch pulmonary arteries (**Fig. 51C**). The dilated branch pulmonary arteries taper down abruptly as they branch in the lungs.
- Depending on the severity and distribution of airway compression by dilated pulmonary arteries, the lungs show variable patterns of abnormal aeration. The lungs may show generalized air trapping or mixture of lobar or segmental emphysema and collapse, which show rapid interval changes on follow-up (**Fig. 51A**).

ECHOCARDIOGRAPHY

- The final diagnosis is made by echocardiography.
- The intracardiac anatomy is the same as for a simple tetralogy, although subpulmonary outflow tract obstruction is usually mild.
- In contrast to classic tetralogy, the pulmonary arteries are markedly dilated.
- The small pulmonary valve anulus is seen as a ringlike constriction between the right ventricular outflow tract and aneurysmally dilated main pulmonary artery.
- Although it is named as absent pulmonary valve syndrome, vestigial leaflet tissue is usually identified.

Treatment and Prognosis

- Medical management with bronchodilators has been disappointing
- Usually complete repair can be attempted in the neonatal period, which consists of closure of the

ventricular septal defect, insertion of a valve in the pulmonary valve position, and plication of the dilated pulmonary arteries.

- For desperately ill babies, palliative pulmonary artery banding can be performed first, with complete repair later in life.
- Surgical mortality is high, and persistent airway obstruction with reduced pulmonary function is common after the surgery.

PEARLS_____

- Absent pulmonary valve syndrome should be suspected when a tachypneic baby's chest radiographs show unusual air trapping with or without segmental or lobar collapse.
- The radiographic findings may change very rapidly even without any change in symptoms and signs.

Suggested Readings

Fischer DR, Neches WH, Beerman LB, et al. Tetralogy of Fallot with absent pulmonic valve: analysis of 17 patients. Am J Cardiol 1984;53:1433–1437

Milanesi O, Talenti E, Pellegrino PA, Thiene G. Abnormal pulmonary artery branching in tetralogy of Fallot with "absent" pulmonary valve. Int J Cardiol 1984;6:375–380

Owens CM, Rees P, Elliot M, Shaw D. Plain chest radiographic changes of the absent pulmonary valve syndrome. Br J Radiol 1994;67:248–251

CASE 52

Clinical Presentation

An 11-year-old boy presents with systolic murmur and dyspnea on exertion.

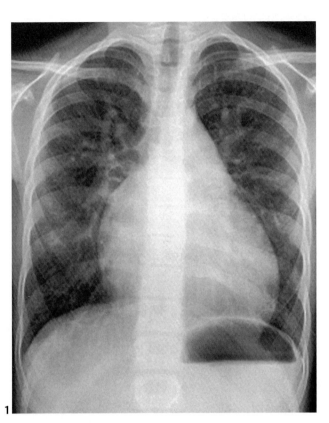
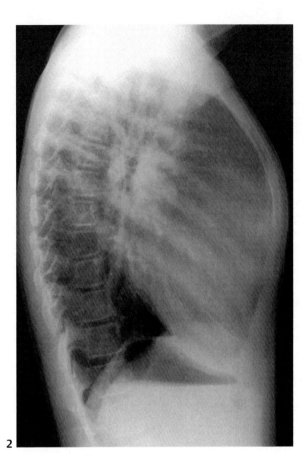

Figure 52A

Radiologic Findings

A frontal chest radiograph (**Fig. 52A1**) shows situs solitus and levocardia. The heart is moderately enlarged, and pulmonary vascularity is markedly increased. Increased vascularity is more evident in lateral view (**Fig. 52A2**) The degree of cardiomegaly reflects the amount of left-to-right shunting. The sternum shows anterior bowing due to cardiomegaly. There is left atrial enlargement. The aortic knob, however, is not prominent.

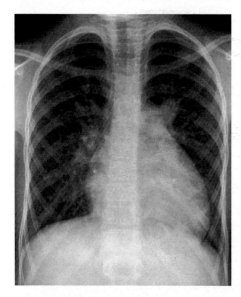

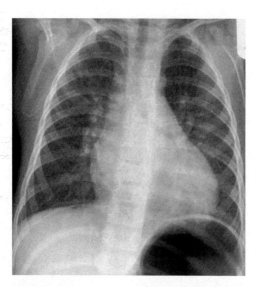

Figure 52B Frontal chest radiograph of a patient with an atrial septal defect shows enlarged heart and increased pulmonary vascularity. There is no evidence of left atrial enlargement. The aortic knob is small.

Figure 52C Frontal chest radiograph of a patient with a patent ductus arteriosus shows enlarged heart and increased pulmonary vascularity. The aortic knob is prominent. The enlarged left atrium forms a double contour on the right side.

Diagnosis

Ventricular septal defect (VSD)

Differential Diagnosis

Other causes of left-to-right shunt should be considered.

- Atrial septal defect, not associated with left atrial enlargement (**Fig. 52B**)
- Patent ductus arteriosus, usually shows a prominent aortic knob (**Fig. 52C**)
- Atrioventricular septal defect, variable features

Discussion

Clinical Findings

The symptoms and signs of isolated ventricular septal defect depend on two variables, the size of the defect and the pulmonary vascular resistance. A small defect causes little functional disturbance, with a systolic murmur being the only clinical finding. Patients having a moderate-sized defect with low pulmonary vascular resistance develop symptoms and signs of pulmonary overcirculation, left heart failure, and airway compression by dilated pulmonary vessels. Progressive pulmonary vascular disease is not common. Both small- and moderate-sized defects tend to decrease in size with time. Large, nonrestrictive defect with elevated but variable vascular resistance is associated with progressive pulmonary vascular disease, ultimately causing right-to-left shunting.

Pathology

VSD is the most ubiquitous congenital cardiac defect. It occurs either in isolation or as an associated lesion with more complex cardiac defects. VSD is classified (**Fig. 52D**) into:

- Perimembranous defect: involves the membranous septum and adjacent muscular septum

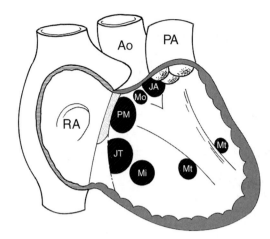

Figure 52D Illustration showing various types of ventricular septal defects. Ao, aorta; JA, juxta-arterial defect; JT, juxtatricuspid and nonperimembranous defect; Mi, Mt, Mo, muscular inlet, trabecular, and outlet defect; PA, pulmonary artery; PM, perimembranous defect; RA, right atrium.

- Muscular defect: is surrounded by a muscular rim in its entire circumference when it is seen from the right ventricle
- Doubly committed juxta-arterial defect: involves the outlet component of the septum and thus is roofed by the aortic and pulmonary valves
- Juxtatricuspid and non-perimembranous defect: involves the inlet septum along the tricuspid valve but does not extend to the membranous septum

The most common is the perimembranous type. If it is not large, it often closes spontaneously by adhesion of the adjacent tricuspid valve leaflet tissue. Small muscular defects can also close spontaneously by development of fibrous tissue plugs. The perimembranous and doubly committed juxta-arterial defects, and muscular defects involving the outlet component of the septum, are all below the aortic valve. These defects can be complicated by prolapse of the aortic valve. Although the defect can become smaller with aortic valve prolapse, aortic regurgitation is an inevitable consequence.

Imaging Findings

FETAL ULTRASOUND

- Although large ventricular septal defects may readily be detected at fetal ultrasound examination, smaller defects are often not diagnosed.

RADIOGRAPHY

- Postnatal chest radiographic features vary according to the size of the defect and pulmonary vascular resistance. When the defect is small or moderate sized, the heart is not large, and pulmonary vascularity is only mildly increased or normal in the first few days of life. As the pulmonary vascular resistance decreases with time, the heart becomes enlarged, and the pulmonary vascularity increases.
- Severe cardiomegaly and marked plethora are uncommon in the newborn period even if the defect is large and unrestrictive.
- With increasing pulmonary vascular resistance, the heart becomes smaller and vascularity less prominent.
- Significant pulmonary hypertension is characterized by normal or slightly enlarged cardiac silhouette, dilated central pulmonary vessels, and small peripheral branches.

Treatment and Prognosis

- As spontaneous closure of VSD can be expected for small- or moderate-sized defects, serial follow up with medical treatment for congestive heart failure and respiratory infection is recommended.

- When the defect is large and spontaneous closure is unlikely, a surgical closure should be considered.
- Recently, more patients are treated with device closure of the defect by an interventional procedure.

PEARLS

- A classic plain radiograph of VSD shows cardiomegaly with prominent main pulmonary artery, left atrial and biventricular enlargement, and increased pulmonary vascularity.
- If the descending branch of the right pulmonary artery is larger in diameter than the trachea, shunt vascularity is present.
- Left atrial enlargement excludes the possibility of atrial septal defect, whereas a small aortic knob is unusual in patients with a patent ductus arteriosus.

PITFALLS

- Small VSDs with less than a 2:1 shunt cannot be identified by chest radiograph.
- In the early newborn period, the presence of high pulmonary vascular resistance prevents shunt vascularity. Therefore, radiographs performed at this time usually appear normal.

Suggested Readings

Freedom RM, Bawson J, Yoo SJ, Benson LN. Ventricular septal defect. In: Bawson JB, Yoo SJ, Benson LN, Freedom RB, eds. Congenital Heart Disease: Textbook of Angiocardiography. Armonk, NY: Futura; 1997:189–218

Soto B, Becker AE, Moulaert AJ, Lie JT, Anderson RH. Classification of ventricular septal defects. Br Heart J 1980;43:332–343

Yoo SJ, Seo JW. Ventricular septum: anatomy, pathology and imaging. In: Freedom RM, ed. Atlas of Heart Diseases, Congenital Heart Disease. Philadelphia: Current Medicine; 1997:11.1–11.7

CASE 53

Clinical Presentation

A 5-month-old infant presents with Down syndrome.

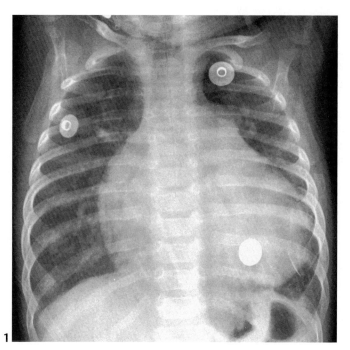
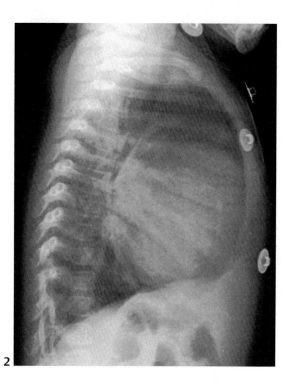

Figure 53A

Radiologic Findings

A frontal chest radiograph (**Fig. 53A1**) shows situs solitus and levocardia. The heart is moderately enlarged with a globular appearance. The pulmonary vascularity is moderately increased, and pulmonary arterial segment is convex. Both lungs are hyperinflated, with flattening of diaphragms in lateral view (**Fig. 53A2**).

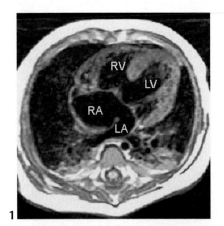 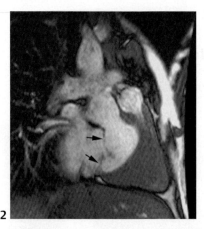

Figure 53B (1) T1-weighted axial MRI shows a large atrioventricular septal defect with a free-floating common atrioventricular valve. LA, left atrium; LV, left ventricle; RA, right atrium; RV, right ventricle. A frame of cine MRI through the ventricular septum (2) called en face image of the ventricular septum, shows a large atrioventricular septal defect and free-floating atrioventricular valve leaflets (arrows).

Diagnosis

Atrioventricular septal defect. A black-blood MRI in axial plane (**Fig. 53B1**) shows a large confluent defect involving the atrioventricular junction. A free-floating atrioventricular valve divides the defect into interatrial and interventricular components. A bright-blood MRI through the ventricular septum (**Fig. 53B2**) shows the scooped-out defect and free-floating atrioventricular valve leaflets (arrows).

Differential Diagnosis

Babies with Down syndrome should be examined with a high suspicion for congenital heart disease. The overall incidence of congenital heart disease in Down syndrome is ~40%. The common cardiac defects include:

- Atrioventricular septal defect (50–60%)
- Ventricular septal defect
- Atrial septal defect
- Tetralogy of Fallot
- Patent ductus arteriosus

Discussion

Clinical Findings

The clinical manifestation depends on the size of the defect, the presence of an interventricular component of the defect, the severity of atrioventricular valve regurgitation, and the severity of pulmonary vascular disease. Ostium primum defect with minor atrioventricular valve regurgitation is associated with mild symptoms and signs that are similar to those of a simple atrial septal defect. Complete form with severe atrioventricular valve regurgitation develops symptoms and signs of congestive heart failure in early life. Complete form is commonly associated with Down syndrome or, less commonly, other forms of aneuploidy.

Pathology

Atrioventricular septal defect is characterized by a large confluent septal defect in the atrioventricular junction (**Fig. 53B**). The normal atrioventricular septum is absent, and the defect extends in variable degrees to the adjacent atrial septum (primum septum) and inlet component of the ventricular septum. The atrioventricular junction is then demarcated by a common junction. As this common junction does not allow the so-called wedged positioning of the aortic valve between the tricuspid and mitral valves, the aortic valve is displaced anterosuperiorly. The common junction is guarded by an abnormal valve that has either a common orifice or partitioned orifices. When there is a common orifice, the valve leaflets tend to have floating positions across the defect, dividing the defect into interatrial and interventricular components. This condition with a common atrioventricular orifice and both interatrial and interventricular communications is commonly called the complete form of atrioventricular septal defect. When the common atrioventricular junction is partitioned, the valve leaflets tend to adhere to the underlying ventricular septal crest, leaving the defect completely inter-atrial. This latter condition is often designated the partial form of atrioventricular septal defect or ostium primum defect. Variable degree of atrioventricular valve regurgitation is almost always seen in both variants.

Imaging Findings

FETAL ECHOCARDIOGRAPHY

- Complete form of atrioventricular septal defect rarely escapes fetal detection, whereas partial form or ostium primum defect often does.
- A large sepal defect in the atrioventricular junction can easily be recognized at four-chamber view of the heart.
- Once atrioventricular septal defect is diagnosed, fetal karyotyping should be undertaken.
- Pelvic findings associated with Down syndrome have also been described on prenatal ultrasound.

RADIOGRAPHY

- Postnatal chest radiographic features vary according to the size of the defect, degree of atrio-ventricular valve regurgitation, and pulmonary vascular resistance.
- When there is only an interatrial shunt and the atrioventricular valve regurgitation is mild or absent, cardiomegaly is mild, and pulmonary vascularity is minimally increased.
- A complete form of atrioventricular septal defect often produces significant cardiomegaly, increased pulmonary vascularity, and vascular congestion from the newborn period. This is attributed to the atrioventricular regurgitation, which is, in effect, a large obligatory shunt from the high-pressured left ventricle into the low-pressured right atrium. It is in contrast to the atrial and ventricular septal defects in which the left-to-right shunt is relatively small in the newborn period because of a relatively small pressure gradient across the septal defect.
- With a large amount of left-to-right shunt, the lungs may show generalized air trapping, or mixture of lobar or segmental emphysema and collapse.

ECHOCARDIOGRAPHY

- The final diagnosis is made by echocardiography.
- The basic pathology is best seen in a four-chamber view.
- The defect involves the whole atrioventricular septum and adjacent atrial and ventricular septum.
- A common atrioventricular valve extends from one chamber to the other.
- In complete forms, the defect is divided into the interatrial and interventricular components by the atrioventricular valves that may either be free-floating or have chordal insertion to the septal crest.

- In partial forms, the atrioventricular valve leaflets are adherent to the septum, and only an interatrial communication is present.
- The defect can also be shown en face (**Fig. 53B2**). The degree of atrioventricular regurgitation also should be assessed by using color and spectral Doppler interrogation.

Treatment and Prognosis

- As there is no chance of spontaneous closure, the defect should be surgically closed and the incompetent atrioventricular valve repaired.
- One-stage surgical correction is usually performed before 6 months of age.
- Because Down syndrome is associated with early development of pulmonary vascular obstructive disease, surgical correction at an early stage is recommended.
- Surgical mortality is <9% for repair of patients with the complete form of atrioventricular septal defect and <3% for repair of those with the partial form.
- The postoperative course is often complicated by regurgitation or stenosis of the left atrioventricular valve, left ventricular outflow tract obstruction, residual shunt, or arrhythmia.

PEARLS_____

- There are two forms of atrioventricular septal defect: complete and partial.
- The complete form is more often associated with Down syndrome than the partial form.
- A bell-shaped chest can be seen in as many as 80% of infants with Down syndrome, likely secondary to hypotonia, which is common in trisomy 21 patients.
- Prominent conoid processes of the clavicles have been recently described as a roentgenologic finding seen on chest x-ray in patients with Down syndrome.
- The complete form is associated with large amount of left-to-right shunt from the newborn period and, therefore, shows significant cardiomegaly and increased pulmonary vascularity.
- Differentiation from other lesions with left-to-right shunt is difficult.

PITFALLS_____

- Shunt vascularity in atrioventricular septal or ventricular septal defect may not be radiographically evident in the early neonatal period secondary to the high pulmonary artery pressures seen in the first few days of life.
- Decreased acetabular angles can also be seen in normal infants and in achondroplasia and Ellis-van Creveld syndrome.

Suggested Readings

Becker AE, Anderson RH. Atrioventricular septal defect: what's in a name? J Thorac Cardiovasc Surg 1982;83:461–469

Freedom RM, Benson LN, Olley PM, Rowe RD. The natural history of the complete atrioventricular canal defect: an analysis of selected genetic, hemodynamic, and morphological variables. In: Gallucci V, Bini RM, Thiene G, eds. Selected Topics in Cardiac Surgery. Bologna: Patron Editore Bologna; 1890:45–72

Marino B, Vairo U, Corno A, et al. Atrioventricular canal in Down syndrome: prevalence of associated cardiac malformations compared with patients without Down syndrome. Am J Dis Child 1990;144:1120–1122

Clinical Presentation

An infant presents with stridor.

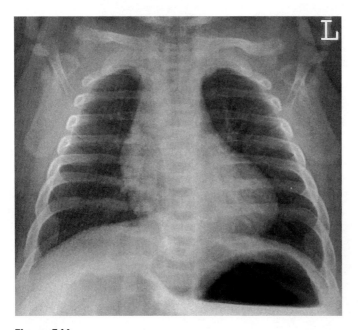

Figure 54A

Radiologic Findings

A frontal chest radiograph (**Fig. 54A**) shows situs solitus and levocardia. The heart is normal in size and configuration. The pulmonary vascularity is normal. The trachea is not bent to either side and shows concentric narrowing above the carina. The descending parts of aortic knobs are seen in both sides of the distal trachea and spinal column.

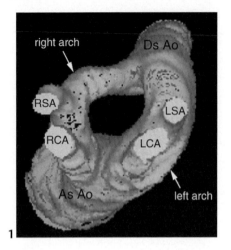
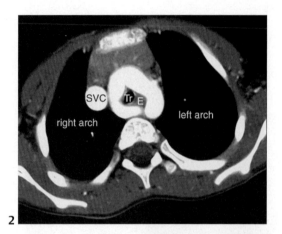
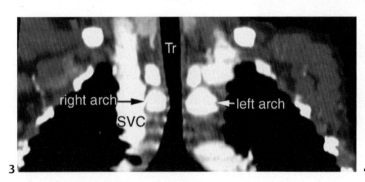
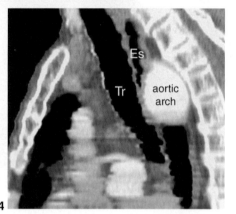

Figure 54B Three-dimensional CT angiogram (**1**) shows double aortic arch. AsAo, ascending aorta; DsAo, descending aorta; LCA, left common carotid artery; LSA, left subclavian artery; RCA, right common carotid artery; RSA, right subclavian artery. An axial CT angiogram (**2**) shows double aortic arch encircling the trachea (Tr) and esophagus (E). SVC, superior vena cava. CT angiogram reconstructed in coronal plane (**3**) shows concentric narrowing of the trachea (Tr) by compression from the aortic arches. SVC, superior vena cava. CT angiogram reconstructed in sagittal plane (**4**) shows the large aortic arch compressing the esophagus (Es) from behind. Tr, trachea. (*Courtesy of Dr. Yang Min Kim, Seoul, Korea*)

Diagnosis

Double aortic arch. CT angiograms from a different patient (**Fig. 54B**) show that the vascular ring surrounds the trachea and esophagus. The tracheal compression is well shown in the coronal image, and the esophageal compression in the sagittal image.

Differential Diagnosis

- A right aortic arch with an aberrant left subclavian or innominate artery and a left-sided ductus arteriosus also forms a complete vascular ring around the trachea and esophagus and can show similar plain radiographic features (**Fig. 54C**).
- A circumflex retroesophageal aortic arch, which is a very rare form of aortic arch anomaly, also shows similar features (**Fig. 54D**).

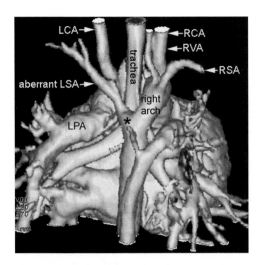

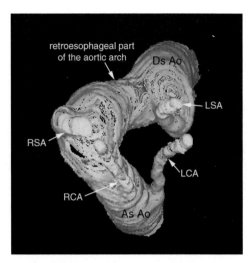

Figure 54C Three-dimensional CT angiogram viewed from behind shows that the left subclavian artery (LSA) has an aberrant arising from the diverticulum (asterisk) of the descending aorta. LCA, left common carotid artery; LPA, left pulmonary artery; RCA, right common carotid artery; RSA, right subclavian artery; RVA, right vertebral artery.

Figure 54D Three-dimensional CT angiogram seen from above shows a circumflex retroesophageal aortic arch. AsAo, ascending aorta; DsAo, descending aorta; LCA, left common carotid artery; LSA, left subclavian artery; RCA, right common carotid artery; RSA, right subclavian artery.

Discussion

Clinical Findings

The clinical manifestations vary according to the severity of tracheal and esophageal compression. Noisy breathing and stridor (with or without cough) are the most common manifestations. As the airway compression is within the thorax, the stridor is heard typically with inspiration, but it can be both inspiratory and expiratory. In contrast to other forms of vascular ring, double aortic arch manifests early in the neonatal period or infancy. As wheezing can be a predominant symptom, the problem can be mistaken for an allergy or asthma. There can be recurrent episodes of respiratory infection. Dysphagia is not common in the early pediatric age group, although the child does not favor a large lump of food.

Pathology

Double aortic arch is the most primitive form of aortic arch anomaly (**Fig. 54B1**). The ascending aorta bifurcates into the right and left arches that course backward around the trachea and esophagus, making a confluence at the descending aorta. As the trachea and esophagus are encircled by a complete vascular ring, both structures show mechanical compression (**Figs. 54B2 to 54B4**). Each arch gives rise to its own common carotid and subclavian arteries. The arches are asymmetric in most cases. Usually the right arch is larger and higher than the left arch. The descending aorta is usually on the same side of the larger arch, and the ductus arteriosus is on the opposite side. Occasionally, a segment of either the left or the right arch can be atretic. Approximately one fifth of the cases of double aortic arch are associated with congenital heart disease, such as tetralogy of Fallot, ventricular septal defect, and complete transposition of the great arteries.

Imaging Findings

RADIOGRAPHY

- Vascular ring can be suspected by plain radiographic features.
- Midline trachea with a concentric narrowing is a classic feature of double aortic arch (**Fig. 54A**).

ESOPHAGOGRAMS

- Barium esophagogram shows rather large posterior indentation in lateral view. However, this finding is also seen in other forms of vascular rings or slings.
- In frontal esophagograms, the esophagus shows bilateral indentations.

CT

- Contrast-enhanced CT is the choice of imaging modality because it shows not only the vascular anomaly but also the airway and lungs (**Fig. 54B**).
- As the aortic arches are asymmetric in size and position in most cases, the arches are rarely visualized in a single axial view.
- The whole anatomy can easily be understood by 3D CT reconstruction.

Treatment and Prognosis

- A surgical intervention is usually undertaken in early infancy because unnecessary delay may cause irreversible damage to the tracheobronchial tree.
- The smaller of the two arches is divided, and the ligamentum or patent ductus arteriosus should also be divided.
- Severe tracheomalacia may require a direct surgical repair of the trachea.
- The postoperative course can be variable. Although symptomatic relief can occur shortly after surgery, persistent symptoms and signs of airway obstruction are not unusual.
- Generally, the long-term prognosis is good.

PEARL

- Always look for the side of the arch on the frontal radiograph. If the trachea is deviated to the left, the arch is on the right. If there is tracheal narrowing on the lateral radiograph, perform a barium swallow to evaluate for a vascular ring.

PITFALL

- Double aortic arch malformations with left arch atresia may be indistinguishable at angiography or CT/MRI from right arch anomalies with aberrant left subclavian and ligamentum arteriosum because of inability to image the atretic segment.

Suggested Readings

Edwards JE. Vascular rings and slings. In: Moller JH, Neal WA, eds. Fetal, Neonatal, and Infant Cardiac Disease. Norwalk, CT: Appleton & Lange; 1990:745–754

Moes CAF. Vascular rings and related conditions. In: Freedom RM, Mawson JB, Yoo SJ, Benson LN, eds. Congenital Heart Disease: Textbook of Angiocardiography. Armonk, NY: Futura; 1997:947–983

CASE 55

Clinical Presentation

A 12-year-old girl presents with hypertension.

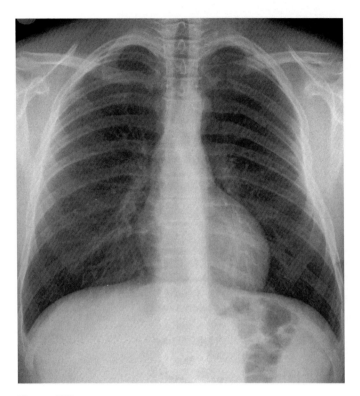

Figure 55A

Radiologic Findings

A frontal chest radiograph (**Fig. 55A**) shows situs solitus and levocardia. The heart is mildly enlarged with elongation of the left ventricular border. The prominent ascending aorta forms the right upper heart border. The aortic knob is large for the patient's age. The proximal descending aorta shows mild indentation, producing a so-called 3 sign. A few ribs show small sclerotic changes along the inferior margins.

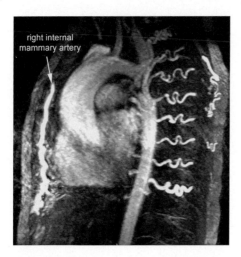

Figure 55B1 Contrast-enhanced MR angiogram shows discrete coarctation of aorta. Note the collaterals.

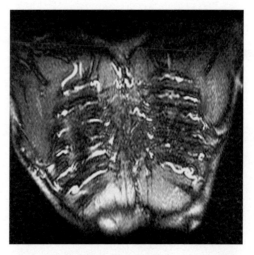

Figure 55B2 Bright-blood MRI of the posterior wall of the chest of the same patient shows dilated intercostal arteries coursing along the inferior margins of the ribs.

Diagnosis

Coarctation of the aorta. A contrast-enhanced MR angiogram (**Fig. 55B1**) in left anterior oblique view from the same patient shows tight discrete stenosis of the aorta at the junction between the isthmic segment of the aortic arch and descending aorta. Notice the dilated intercostal and internal mammary arteries functioning as collateral channels. A bright-blood MRI of the posterior chest wall in coronal plane (**Fig. 55B2**) shows that the tortuous dilated intercostal arteries course along the inferior borders of the ribs.

Differential Diagnosis

- Similar cardiac configuration can also be seen with systemic hypertension, aortic valve stenosis, and aortic root dilatation related to Marfan syndrome.
- Indentation in the prominent proximal descending aorta and sclerotic changes are the definitive clues to the diagnosis.
- Takayasu's arteritis can also involve the descending aorta and show indentation(s) in the descending aortic contour, but the changes are usually more irregular.
- One should also be aware that there are numerous other conditions that may cause rib changes such as neurofibromatosis.

Discussion

Clinical Findings

The clinical manifestations of coarctation vary according to the severity of obstruction and development of collateral circulation. Severe coarctation is associated with development of left ventricular failure immediately after birth. The lower body is underperfused, and the patient may develop metabolic acidosis, bowel ischemia, and oliguria. Once past infancy, patients are usually asymptomatic or complain of nonspecific symptoms, such as headache, frequent episodes of epistaxis, and easy fatigue on walking. With advancing age, the symptoms and signs of systemic hypertension develop. On physical examination, abnormal differences in arterial pulses and blood pressures of the upper

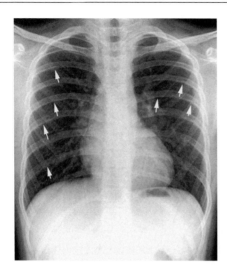

Figure 55C Frontal chest radiograph of another patient shows rib notches (arrows).

and lower extremities are the hallmarks of this disease. The femoral pulses are either absent or reduced. Major complications include congestive heart failure, rupture or dissection of the aorta, infective endocarditis or endarteritis, and cerebral hemorrhage. The physical appearance of Turner's syndrome increases clinical suspicion.

Pathology

Coarctation of the aorta is typically located near the aortic attachment of the ductus arteriosus. The convex wall of the aorta exhibits a sharp indentation. Isolated coarctation usually develops with closure of the ductus arteriosus after birth, although the obstruction may become more pronounced with time. On histologic examination, the coarctation segment contains an abnormal circumferential distribution of ductal tissue that is considered to cause constriction with closure of the ductus arteriosus after birth. In contrast to this localized form of aortic narrowing, more uniform narrowing of a part or whole aortic arch is called tubular hypoplasia. Coarctation and tubular hypoplasia may coexist or occur independently. Isolated coarctation is often associated with bicuspid aortic valve.

Imaging Findings

FETAL ULTRASOUND

- On fetal ultrasound, so-called right-side dominance is a warning sign of coarctation.
- Right-side dominance refers to a situation in which the right atrium and right ventricle are larger than the left atrium and left ventricle. However, its positive predictive value is not high.
- When severe coarctation develops in early infancy, cardiomegaly is associated with pulmonary congestion. In late childhood or adulthood, the heart is normally sized or slightly enlarged with left ventricular hypertrophy pattern. The pulmonary vascularity is normal. The aortic knob is prominent, and the indentation of the descending aorta can be seen. Dilated intercostal arteries may cause typical notches along the inferior margins of the posterior parts of the third to eighth ribs in late childhood or adulthood (arrows in **Fig. 55C**). More often, only sclerotic margins can be identified (**Fig. 55A**).

CT/MRI

- CT or MR angiography is the most useful diagnostic test. It visualizes not only the coarctation but also the extent of collateral channels (**Fig. 55B**).

Treatment and Prognosis

- When coarctation of aorta is suspected at fetal ultrasound, the baby should be delivered in a tertiary hospital.
- When coaractation is diagnosed in infancy or childhood, surgical augmentation is performed.
- For adolescents or adults with coarctation, dilatation with balloon or by placement of a stent is preferred.
- Restenosis is not uncommon after either surgical or interventional dilatation of the coarctation.
- Usually, long-term prognosis is excellent.

PEARLS_____

- Rib notching is rarely seen above the third or below the ninth ribs.
- A low-appearing aortic knob on frontal chest radiograph is another described finding with coarctation. It is caused by nonvisualization of the superior aspect of aortic 3 sign with prominent poststenotic dilation in the lower half of the 3.
- Wavy retrosternal soft tissue on lateral chest radiograph caused by enlarged mammary arteries can be seen in up to 30% of patients.
- A balloon angioplasty may be performed rather than surgical correction in some cardiovascular centers.

PITFALLS_____

- Rib notching is uncommon in children <2 years of age and is seen in only ~32% of children between 2 and 6 years of age.
- Prominent thymic tissue may obscure aortic contour abnormalities in the newborn and neonate.

Suggested Readings

Elzenga NJ, Gittenberger-de Groot AC, Oppenheimer-Dekker A. Coarctation and other obstructive aortic arch anomalies: their relationship to the ductus arteriosus. Int J Cardiol 1986;13:289–308

Ho SY, Anderson RH. Coarctation, tubular hypoplasia, and the ductus arteriosus: histological study of 35 specimens. Br Heart J 1979;41:268–274

Strife JL, Bisset GS III. Cardiovascular system. In: Kirks DR, Griscom NT, eds. Practical Pediatric Imaging: Diagnostic Radiology of Infants and Children. 3rd ed. Philadelphia: Lippincott-Raven; 1998:511–618

CASE 56

Clinical Presentation

A 5-year-old child presents with recurrent pneumonia.

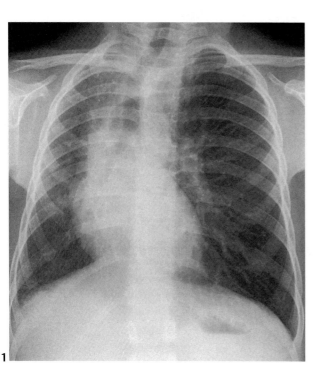 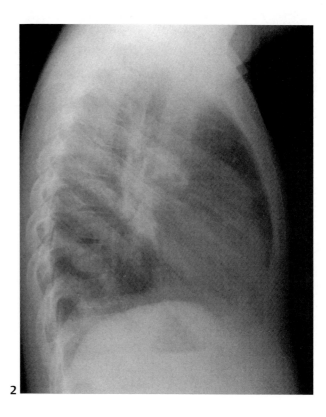

Figure 56A

Radiologic Findings

A frontal chest radiograph (**Fig. 56A1**) shows situs solitus and levocardia. The heart is positioned on the right side with small right lung volume. The pulmonary vascularity is asymmetric with prominent vessels in the left lung. The right lung shows reticular pattern. The lateral view (**Fig. 56A2**) is not remarkable.

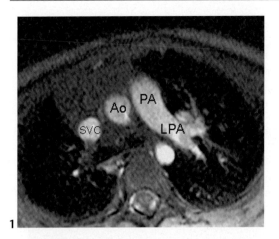 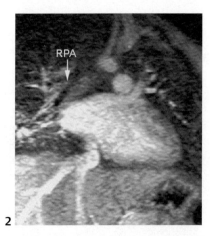

Figure 56B Bright-blood MRI in axial plane (**1**) shows that right pulmonary artery is missing. Ao, aorta; LPA, left pulmonary artery; PA, main pulmonary artery; SVC, superior vena cava. MR angiogram in an oblique coronal view (**2**) of the same patient shows tiny right pulmonary artery (RPA) in the right lung hilum.

Diagnosis

Unilateral absence of the right pulmonary artery. An axial bright-blood MRI (**Fig. 56B1**) shows absence of the mediastinal segment of the right pulmonary artery. A contrast-enhanced MR angiogram (**Fig. 56B2**) shows the tiny right pulmonary artery and its branches in the right lung.

Differential Diagnosis

Hypoplastic right lung

- Unilateral agenesis of right pulmonary artery
- Scimitar syndrome (**Fig. 57A**)
- Primary hypoplasia of right lung
- Swyer-James syndrome

Discussion

Clinical Findings

The clinical presentation of congenital unilateral absence of a pulmonary artery may be subtle. Patients often have a history of recurrent pulmonary infections. Hemoptysis from dilated bronchial arteries may develop in older children and adults. Once one is familiar with the diagnosis, it may be suspected from a chest radiograph.

Pathology

Unilateral absence of a pulmonary artery is a rare entity in which the mediastinal segment of a branch pulmonary artery is absent. It almost always involves the pulmonary artery opposite to the aortic arch. The involved pulmonary artery, although small, is invariably present in the lung and is termed *isolated*. At the lung hilum, it is connected to the ipsilateral innominate or subclavian artery through the obliterated or ligamentous ductus arteriosus. The ductal remnant can be identified as a

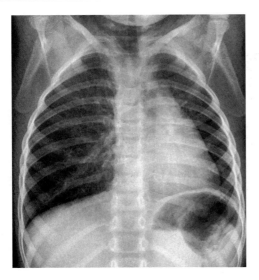

Figure 56C Frontal chest radiograph of a patient with absent left pulmonary artery and right aortic arch. The left lung volume is reduced.

small pouch arising from the undersurface of the innominate or subclavian artery. Progressive diminution in the size of the isolated pulmonary artery, lung, and hemithorax is an inevitable consequence of this condition. The distal isolateral aspect of the pulmonary artery acquires collateral blood flow from the bronchial and chest wall arteries and rarely from the coronary arteries. Absent right pulmonary artery is more commonly an isolated lesion, whereas absent left pulmonary artery often is associated with tetralogy of Fallot (**Fig. 56C**).

Imaging Findings

FETAL ULTRASOUND

- The initial step to the correct fetal diagnosis, which is often a challenge, is the appreciation of unilateral lung hypoplasia on transverse scan of the fetal thorax.
- The differential diagnoses for unilateral lung hypoplasia include absence of a branch pulmonary artery, scimitar syndrome, and primary unilateral lung hypoplasia.
- Color or power Doppler interrogation facilitates the diagnosis of the unilateral absence of a branch pulmonary artery.

RADIOGRAPHY

- The plain radiographic finding is characteristic.
- With right pulmonary arterial involvement, the right lung is small and contains small vessels that are often reticular in appearance because of collateral channels. As the left lung receives the whole right ventricular output, the left lung is plethoric.
- The heart and mediastinal structures are displaced to the right.
- In contrast to scimitar syndrome, in which the right heart border is blurred, the heart contour is usually preserved.
- The diagnosis can often be made with high index of suspicion.
- Chest radiographs of patients with pulmonary infection may show reduced lung volume due to associated atelectasis. On follow-up after antibiotic treatment, one should suspect the diagnosis of absent pulmonary artery when reduced lung volume persists with the consolidation having improved.

ANGIOGRAPHY

- The diagnosis can be made by pulmonary vein wedge angiography.

CT/MRI

- Pulmonary arterial anatomy can clearly be depicted by either CT or MR angiography (**Fig. 56B**). The missing pulmonary artery can easily be recognized in transverse axial view.
- Pulmonary artery anatomy within the lung can better be appreciated in reconstructed images in coronal planes.

Treatment and Prognosis

- Ideally, the isolated pulmonary artery should be connected to the main pulmonary artery. This procedure often initially requires some form of systemic-to-pulmonary artery anastomosis.
- When the reconstruction of the pulmonary arterial confluence is difficult and hemoptysis or pulmonary infection is intractable, pneumonectomy should be performed.

PEARLS_____

- Diagnosis of absent right pulmonary artery can be suspected when the right lung shows diminished volume with shift of the heart and mediastinal structures to the right side and diminished pulmonary vascularity with reticular pattern.
- In contrast to scimitar syndrome, in which the right heart border is blurred, the heart contour is usually preserved.

Suggested Readings

Apostolopoulou SC, Kelekis NL, Brountzos EN, Rammos S, Kelekis DA. "Absent" pulmonary artery in one adult and five pediatric patients: imaging, embryology, and therapeutic implications. AJR Am J Roentgenol 2002;179:1253–1260

Pfefferkorn JR, Loser H, Pech G, Toussaint R, Hilgenberg F. Absent pulmonary artery: a hint to its embryogenesis. Pediatr Cardiol 1982;3:283–286

Pool PE, Vogel JHK, Blount SG. Congenital unilateral absence of a pulmonary artery. Am J Cardiol 1962;10:706–732

CASE 57

Clinical Presentation

A 5-year-old child presents with recurrent pneumonia.

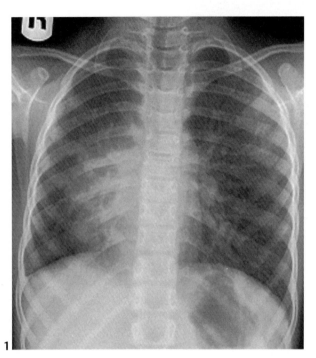
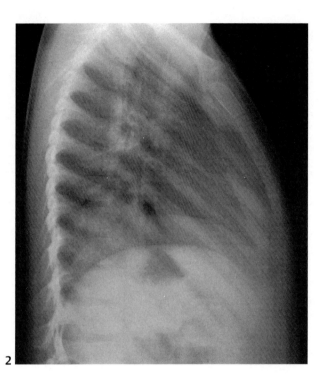

Figure 57A

Radiologic Findings

A frontal chest radiograph (**Fig. 57A1**) shows situs solitus. The heart is positioned on the right with small right lung volume. The right mediastinal border is indistinct. In lateral view (**Fig. 57A2**), there is a band of increased density behind the sternum. The pulmonary vascularity is asymmetric with prominent vessels noted on the left.

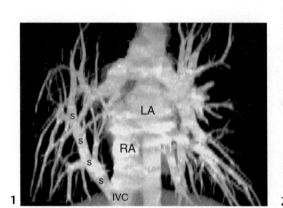
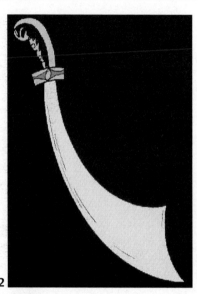

Figure 57B CT angiogram reformatted in coronal plane (**1**) shows a vertical vein (ss) that drains all pulmonary veins from the right lung into the right atrium (RA)–inferior vena cava (IVC) junction. The vertical vein is similar to a scimitar (**2**), a Turkish sword. The left pulmonary veins connect to the left atrium (LA).

Diagnosis

Scimitar syndrome. A CT angiogram (**Fig. 57B1**) shows a scimitar-shaped vein draining the entire right lung to the inferior vena cava at its junction with the right atrium.

Differential Diagnosis

Hypoplastic right lung

- Scimitar syndrome
- Unilateral agenesis of right pulmonary artery (**Fig. 56A**)
- Primary hypoplasia of right lung
- Swyer-James syndrome

Discussion

Clinical Findings

The clinical expression of this syndrome is diverse. Some patients present with severe congestive heart failure, whereas others show pulmonary artery hypertension in infancy or early childhood. Not infrequently, scimitar syndrome is recognized in a child with recurrent pulmonary infections. It is often an incidental finding at a routine chest radiographic check in an otherwise asymptomatic adult. Factors contributing to early presentation include severely obstructed pulmonary venous connections, association with other complex cardiac malformations, and/or the presence of a large aberrant systemic arterial supply.

Pathology

A scimitar is a short, curved Turkish sword (**Fig. 57B2**). Scimitar syndrome has come to designate a curved vascular channel in the right lower lung that drains a part or all of the pulmonary venous return from the right lung to the inferior vena cava at its junction with the right atrium or directly to the latter structure. The scimitar vein is often stenotic as it approaches its connection to the inferior vena cava or right atrium. Although this interesting malformation is named after the anomalous pulmonary vein, this anomalous pulmonary venous return is only a part of a more complex lung malformation involving the airway, lung tissue, arterial supply, and venous drainage. Almost invariably the right lung is hypoplastic, and the heart and mediastinal structures are displaced to the right side. A part of the right lower lung often extends to the left thorax through the defects in the parietal pleural layers; this condition is called horseshoe lung. Occasionally the extension of the right lower lung is a simple "crossover" to the left side with all pleural layers intact. Regardless of whether it is a true horseshoe lung or a simple crossover, this part of the lung is supplied by a pulmonary arterial branch that has an early takeoff from the right pulmonary artery. The right pulmonary artery and its branches are usually hypoplastic and look bizarre. Also, the bronchial branching pattern is not normal in most cases. Almost always, the basal area of the right lower lobe is supplied by an aberrant arterial branch or branches that arise from the abdominal aorta or its major branch. Usually this area has patent connections to the normal bronchial system. Occasionally the segment is also sequestered from the bronchial connection, completing the features of pulmonary sequestration. The venous drainage of the lung tissue supplied by a systemic arterial branch or branches is either to the left atrium or to the scimitar vein. Occasionally the right diaphragm is abnormally formed or defective with fusion of the lung and liver tissue.

Imaging Findings

FETAL ULTRASOUND

- Fetal diagnosis of scimitar syndrome starts with high suspicion of this rare condition when the right lung is small and the heart is positioned on the right side.
- The differential diagnoses for right lung hypoplasia include absent right pulmonary artery, scimitar syndrome, and primary hypoplasia of the right lung.
- A correct diagnosis can be made by identification of the scimitar vein and aberrant systemic arterial supply of the right lower lung.

RADIOGRAPHY

- The plain radiographic findings are very characteristic, with small right lung and the heart and mediastinal structures displaced to the right.
- The right mediastinal and heart borders on frontal radiographs are indistinct in most cases. This is because the mediastinal soft tissue extends laterally in front of the right lung and the interface between the two structures is not tangential to the radiographic beam.
- The mediastinal soft tissue is seen as a vertical curvilinear band of haziness behind the anterior chest wall.
- The scimitar vein can often be clearly seen in the frontal radiograph. However, one should not exclude the diagnosis of scimitar syndrome solely because it is not seen on a plain radiograph.
- Occasionally, an aberrant systemic arterial channel can be seen.

CT

- Although the diagnosis can be made by echocardiography, contrast-enhanced CT is most useful in defining not only the vascular anatomy but also the abnormalities of the lungs and airways (**Fig. 57B**).

Treatment and Prognosis

- Not all patients with scimitar syndrome require surgical intervention.
- Asymptomatic patients with a small left-to-right shunt and normal pulmonary artery pressures can be followed conservatively.

- Some patients with intractable recurrent infection may benefit from lobectomy.
- Other patients may benefit solely from interruption of the collateral supply, either by catheter-based occlusion or surgical ligation, assuming that there is dual vascular supply to the involved lung segment.
- Anomalously connected right pulmonary veins can be directly reimplanted into the left atrium or tunneled to the left atrium through the right atrium and atrial septal defect. However, both procedures are frequently complicated by postoperative stenosis.

PEARLS

- The diagnosis of absent right pulmonary artery can also be suspected when the right lung shows diminished volume with shift of the heart and mediastinal structures to the right side. In most cases of absent right pulmonary artery, the right heart border is clear, whereas most scimitar cases show indistinct right mediastinal or cardiac border.
- The presence of abnormal vertical vascular channel in the medial aspect of the right lower lung leads to the diagnosis.
- Absence of a visible scimitar vein on plain radiographs does not exclude the diagnosis of scimitar syndrome.

Suggested Readings

Najm HK, Williams WG, Coles JG, Rebeyka IM, Freedom RM. Scimitar syndrome: twenty years' experience and results of repair. J Thorac Cardiovasc Surg 1996;112:1161–1168

Schramel FM, Westermann CJ, Knaepen PJ, van den Bosch JM. The scimitar syndrome: clinical spectrum and surgical treatment. Eur Respir J 1995;8:196–201

Valsangiacomo ER, Hornberger LK, Barrea C, Smallhorn JF, Yoo SJ. Partial and total anomalous pulmonary venous connection in the fetus: two-dimensional and Doppler echocardiographic findings. Ultrasound Obstet Gynecol 2003;22:257–263

SECTION V
Abdominal

CASE 58

Clinical Presentation

A 6-day-old baby born at 27 weeks of gestation presents with a distended abdomen and hemodynamic instability.

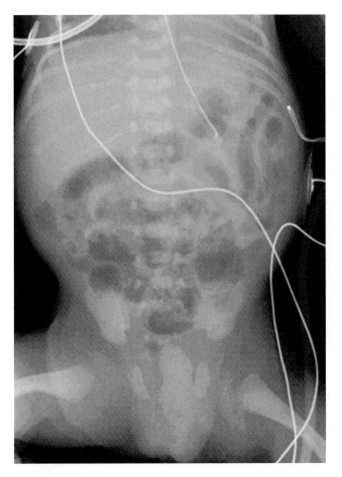

Figure 58A

Radiologic Findings

Supine radiograph (**Fig. 58A**) demonstrates a bubbly appearance in the lower abdomen consistent with pneumatosis in association with increased interloop distance in the left upper quadrant secondary to bowel wall thickening.

Diagnosis

Necrotizing enterocolitis (NEC)

Differential Diagnosis

- Intraluminal fecal residue may resemble mottled appearance of pneumatosis but rarely present in the first 2 weeks of life.
- Focal intestinal perforation without NEC and idiopathic gastric perforation present with pneumoperitoneum but without evidence of pneumatosis
- Mesenteric thromboembolism (catheter-related)
- Hirschsprung's enterocolitis (term infant)
- Malrotation and volvulus
- Other causes of neonatal sepsis may mimic clinical features of NEC and cause generalized bowel dilatation.

Discussion

Background

NEC is a severe inflammatory enteritis occurring in up to 35% of premature infants, the majority <2000 g. Any part of the bowel may be affected from the esophagus to the rectum, although the distal ileum and ascending colon are most frequently involved.

Etiology

- Multiple etiologic factors have been implicated, including hypoxia, sepsis, hypotension, intrauterine growth retardation, exchange transfusion, and umbilical arterial catheterization. Case clusters suggest an infectious agent is involved, but this may be a secondary event following compromise of the intestinal mucosal barrier. Early introduction of enteral nutrition (particularly formula feeds) and rapid increases in feed volume are associated with a higher incidence. Bowel ischemia appears to be the common pathway, with proliferation of the intestinal flora leading to bowel necrosis and perforation.
- Experimental evidence suggests that the balance of inflammatory mediators, including tumor necrosis factor, platelet activating factor, nitric oxide, and free radicals, influences intestinal perfusion and the integrity of the mucosal barrier. Disturbance of this balance increases vulnerability to NEC.
- NEC may also occur in term infants. Predisposing factors include congenital heart disease (decreased systemic perfusion) or recent abdominal surgery (particularly gastroschisis or intestinal atresia repair), polycythemia, and maternal cocaine abuse.

Clinical Findings

Symptoms usually occur in the first week of life, with very low birth weight infants (<1000 g) often presenting slightly later, after 2 weeks. Clinical signs are varied and may be nonspecific. Abdominal distension, vomiting, diarrhea, or blood per rectum occurs in association with systemic signs including fever, apnea, metabolic acidosis, and, in advanced cases, circulatory collapse. On examination there may be erythema of the abdominal wall and palpable distended bowel loops.

Complications

- Acute complications include bowel necrosis, abscesses, septicemia, disseminated intravascular coagulation (DIC), and multisystem failure in addition to iatrogenic complications associated with central venous access, total parenteral nutrition (TPN), and mechanical ventilation.

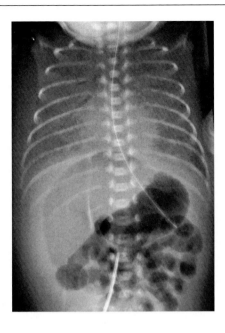

Figure 58B Thoracoabdominal radiograph demonstrating pneumoperitoneum the "football sign" with the falciform ligament outlined by air. The lungs demonstrate bilateral diffuse granular shadowing consistent with respiratory distress syndrome.

- Strictures develop in 10 to 20% of cases and can manifest as early as 1 to 2 months, even in patients in whom the initial episode was apparently mild. Most strictures (80%) occur in the colon, commonly in the region of the splenic flexure. Balloon catheter dilatation is successful in many cases.
- Adhesions may result in intestinal obstruction months or years later. Fistulae and enterocysts are rare late complications.
- The most significant long-term sequela is short gut syndrome in patients with extensive or multiple small bowel resections, with <40 cm remaining small bowel. Malabsorption, failure to thrive, and the complications of long-term TPN carry a significant morbidity and mortality.

Pathology

- Ischemic necrosis of the mucosa with microemboli results in edema, ulceration, and hemorrhage into the bowel wall. Involvement may be diffuse and contiguous or may include skip lesions. Perforation may result in localized abscess formation or generalized peritonitis.

Imaging Findings

ABDOMINAL RADIOGRAPHS

- Diffuse gaseous distension is the earliest radiographic sign of NEC, but this is very nonspecific. Loss of the normal symmetric bowel gas pattern may then occur with relative paucity of gas in one region and dilation in another. Bowel wall thickening is manifest as increased interloop distance.
- Intramural air (pneumatosis intestinalis) allows the diagnosis of NEC. It may be localized or diffuse, most frequently affecting the distal small bowel and ascending colon. Bubbly, round lucencies are believed to represent submucosal air, and curvilinear lucencies subserosal pneumatosis.
- Branching lucencies extending from the region of the porta hepatis in the right upper quadrant represent portal venous air.
- A persistent, dilated loop of bowel unaltered over serial examinations may indicate impending perforation, but this persistent loop sign is not specific nor of high sensitivity.
- A large amount of free air secondary to perforation will result in the "football sign" (round lucency over the upper abdomen and outlining the hemidiaphragms), Rigler's sign (air outlining both sides of the bowel wall), and visualization of the falciform ligament on supine radiograph (**Fig. 58B**).

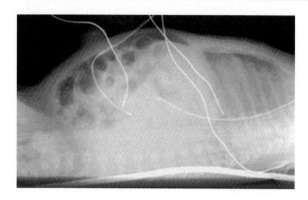

Figure 58C Cross-table lateral abdominal x-ray demonstrating free intraperitoneal air immediately beneath the anterior abdominal wall. Pneumatosis is seen in the lower abdomen.

Lesser amounts require a horizontal beam view to detect small triangles of free air immediately beneath the anterior abdominal wall on cross-table lateral view (**Fig. 58C**) or anterior to the liver on left-side-down decubitus view. However, perforation does not always result in radiographically detectable free air.

ULTRASOUND

- Bowel wall thickening, pneumatosis, portal venous air (moving high echogenicity foci), free fluid, and localized abscesses can be seen. Recent work suggests reduction in bowel wall Doppler flow may be helpful in identifying segments of impending necrosis.

CONTRAST STUDIES

- Not indicated acutely due to the risk of colonic perforation
- Post-NEC strictures may be demonstrated, commonly in the splenic flexure.
- Following bowel resection, both upper gastrointestinal (GI) follow-through and enema examinations are necessary to exclude further stricture formation in the remaining bowel prior to final reanastomosis.

Treatment

- Conservative measures are the mainstay of treatment with cessation of enteral feeding, TPN, broad-spectrum antibiotics, and inotropic support.
- Serial abdominal radiographs (12–24 hourly) monitor disease progression, development of portal venous air, or perforation resulting in free air.
- Close cooperation among neonatologist, surgeon, and radiologist is essential for optimal management. Indications for surgery include perforation, obstruction, and clinical deterioration despite aggressive medical therapy. Nonviable bowel is resected, attempting to preserve as much bowel as possible. Primary peritoneal drainage is an alternative therapeutic approach, particularly in very low birth weight infants (<1000 g). Some infants recover without subsequent GI symptoms, others require definitive operation after clinical stabilization.

Prognosis

- Mortality rates are 20 to 40%, usually associated with DIC and septicemia. Increased mortality is seen in low birth weight and gestational age infants. Advances in neonatology leading to improved survival in infants <1000 g mean that there has been an increase in the mortality from NEC in the past decade despite the overall decrease in neonatal mortality.
- Prognosis among survivors depends on GI complications, particularly short gut syndrome, and any neurodevelopmental complications of prematurity.

PEARLS_____

- The bubbly appearance of submucosal pneumatosis may be misinterpreted as stool or meconium within a normal colon. However, this pattern is rarely seen in the first 2 weeks of life, and in the clinical context of a recently delivered premature infant, a bubbly appearance should always suggest the diagnosis of NEC.
- Although the presence of portal venous air is associated with more severe disease, it does not, in contrast to the adult population, necessarily indicate a fatal outcome.

PITFALL_____

- A small amount of free air may be undetectable on supine radiographs. In the initial stages of disease, when most perforations occur, horizontal beam radiographs should also be performed. Either a supine cross-table lateral or a left-side-down decubitus view may be obtained, the cross-table lateral having the advantage of not requiring an unstable baby to be moved.

Suggested Readings

Buonomo C. The radiology of necrotising enterocolitis. Radiol Clin North Am 1999;37:1187–1198

Daneman A, Woodward S, de Silva M. The radiology of neonatal necrotising enterocolitis: a review of 47 cases and the literature. Pediatr Radiol 1978;7:70–77

Morrison SC, Jacobson JM. The radiology of necrotising enterocolitis. Clin Perinatol 1994;21:347–363

CASE 59

Clinical Presentation

A 10-month-old child presents to the emergency department with intermittent episodes of drawing his legs up to his chest and inconsolable crying.

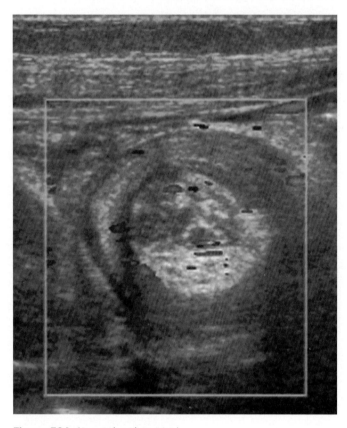

Figure 59A (See Color Plate 59A.)

Radiologic Findings

Abdominal ultrasound (**Fig. 59A**) demonstrates a soft tissue mass in the right flank with multiple hypoechoic concentric rings, central echogenic mesentery, and a few small, trapped lymph nodes. Color Doppler flow is demonstrated within the mass.

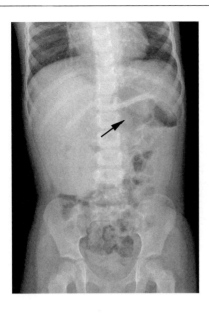

Figure 59B Supine abdominal x-ray shows a large soft tissue mass in the right flank with air in the transverse colon outlining the leading edge of the intussusception, the "crescent sign" (arrow).

Diagnosis

Intussusception

Differential Diagnosis

- Bowel wall thickening due to inflammation, infection, or hematoma

Discussion

Background

Intussusception is the invagination of a segment of bowel (the intussusceptum) into the contiguous segment (the intussuscipiens). The vast majority of symptomatic cases (90%) involve the ileocolic segment, but ileo-ileal, ileo-ileocolic, and colocolic intussusception may also occur. Peak age incidence is between 4 months and 2 years of age, but patients outside of this range are not infrequently encountered. Boys are more frequently affected than girls.

Etiology

The majority of cases are associated with inflammation and enlargement of the lymphoid tissue of Peyer's patches following a viral gastroenteritis. In a small number (5%) there is a pathologic lead point, such as a Meckel's diverticulum, duplication cyst, polyp, or, uncommonly, non-Hodgkin's lymphoma.

Clinical Findings

The classic clinical triad is of episodic abdominal pain associated with the passage of blood and mucus per rectum ("red currant jelly") and a palpable abdominal mass. However, this is present in <50% of children. Vomiting is relatively frequent, as is lethargy, which can be the major presenting feature. Considerable fluid shifts can result in hemodynamic instability. Advanced disease with established bowel ischemia or perforation presents with peritonism and shock.

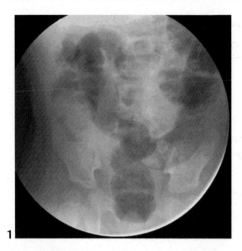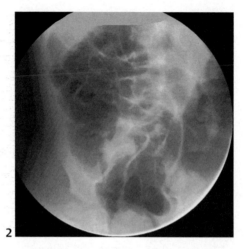

Figure 59C Fluoroscopy images prior to air insufflation (**1**) demonstrating the soft tissue mass of the intussusception in the right lower quadrant and (**2**) following successful reduction with resolution of the mass and flooding of the small bowel with air.

Complications

- Small bowel obstruction
- Bowel wall ischemia and perforation
- Hemodynamic shock

Pathology

- Venous obstruction leads to edema and hemorrhage into the bowel wall, which may progress to small bowel obstruction, bowel wall necrosis, and perforation.

Imaging Findings

RADIOGRAPHY

- Absence of bowel gas in the right iliac fossa, lateralization of air within the distal small bowel, a rounded soft tissue mass, a crescent of air at the apex of the intussusception, or small bowel obstruction may be seen (**Fig. 59B**). However, in most cases, radiographs are unremarkable and cannot exclude the diagnosis. Free air in the absence of clinical signs of peritonitis is rare.

ULTRASOUND

- Diagnostic modality of choice, with 100% sensitivity using a high-frequency linear array transducer and following appropriate training
- Soft tissue mass, 3 to 5 cm in diameter, most frequently anterior to the right kidney, just below the abdominal wall. Transverse images demonstrate multiple concentric hypoechoic rings, with a characteristic central but eccentric hyperechoic crescent of mesenteric fat drawn into the intussusception with vessels and small mesenteric lymph nodes.
- Other solid or cystic masses within the intussusception suggest a pathologic lead point.
- Small to moderate amounts of free fluid are common. Large amounts may reflect necrosis or perforation, but not invariably.

DIAGNOSTIC ENEMA

- Some institutions still perform a diagnostic enema, with air or barium, to demonstrate the soft tissue mass, and then proceed directly to a therapeutic procedure.

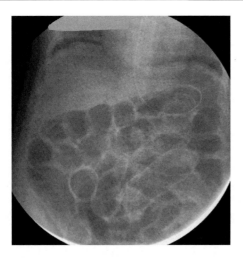

Figure 59D Radiologic pneumatic reduction under fluoroscopic control carries a small risk of inducing or uncovering a preexisting perforation. The presence of free air should be promptly recognized.

SMALL BOWEL FOLLOW-THROUGH/CT/MR

- May be useful in selected patients, particularly to delineate a suspected pathologic lead point.

Treatment

- Hemodynamic assessment and fluid resuscitation are essential prior to imaging and reduction.
- Radiologic reduction by air under fluoroscopic guidance is now the treatment of choice. The only absolute contraindications are peritonitis and perforation. Air has replaced barium in most pediatric centers as it is easier to use, has a higher success rate (70–90%), and avoids the risks of barium peritonitis.
- Precise protocols vary between institutions. A large (16 to 20 French) catheter is inserted into the rectum and securely taped. Various devices, both commercially available and locally constructed, are used to insufflate air at pressures increasing from 80 mm Hg to 110–120 mm Hg. A pressure release valve is necessary to prevent excess pressure being delivered. Pneumatic pressure is maintained for 1 to 3 minutes per attempt. The soft tissue mass of the intussusception is followed as it moves to the ileocecal junction, where there is often a transitory holdup. Disappearance of the mass and flooding of air into the small bowel indicate successful reduction (**Figs. 59C1** and **59C2**).
- Air reduction carries a 0.5 to 1% risk of inducing or uncovering a preexisting perforation (**Fig. 59D**). Tension pneumoperitoneum can result in cardiorespiratory compromise and require relief by needle puncture of the abdomen. Pediatric surgical and anesthetic support must be available on-site. Informed consent is obtained from the child's parents or guardian, with explanation of the procedure, including risks of perforation and recurrence.
- Indications for surgical reduction and/or resection are an unstable child with clinical signs of peritonitism, or following failed radiologic reduction or perforation. If radiologic reduction is unsuccessful and the patient is stable, some institutions may undertake a repeat attempt after 2 to 8 hours, with careful surgical liaison and clinical monitoring.
- Ultrasonographic guidance of air enema reduction has been described but is not in widespread use.

Prognosis

- Excellent in uncomplicated, promptly treated cases
- Morbidity and, uncommonly, mortality are associated with delay in diagnosis and inadequate resuscitation.

PEARLS_____

- Presentation outside the peak age incidence should raise the suspicion of an underlying lead point.
- Various factors are associated with lower success rates and prompt a more cautious reduction attempt but do not preclude it. Clinical factors include a long history (several days), age <6 months or >2 years, and the presence of small bowel obstruction. Ultrasound features that may be associated with a more difficult reduction of the intussusception include poor color Doppler flow, trapped peritoneal fluid, or a visible lead point.
- There is increasing recognition of small bowel intussusceptions, which are generally asymptomatic and transient. These should be regarded as a separate entity from those discussed above. They are often an incidental finding, but may also occur in Henoch-Schönlein purpura, in the setting of trauma, and in postoperative patients. Although most are not pathologically significant, they should not be dismissed unless they are transient and disappear by the end of the ultrasound study. Gastrojejunal feeding tubes may also act as a lead point for intussusception, when symptoms are more likely, and may require tube replacement.

PITFALLS_____

- A residual soft tissue mass can sometimes be seen along the medial wall of the cecum following filling of small bowel with air and apparent successful reduction. This is usually due to edema of the ileocecal valve, and can be confirmed on ultrasound if there is diagnostic uncertainty.
- Following successful radiologic reduction, there is a 5 to 10% recurrence rate, which can be multiple. These usually occur within the following 12 to 24 hours, and therefore continued clinical observation is mandatory. Recurrence can be successfully managed by repeat air enema reduction. Ultrasound search for a pathologic lead point should be made.

Suggested Readings

Daneman A, Navarro O. Intussusception, I: A review of diagnostic approaches. Pediatr Radiol 2003;33:79–85

Del-Pozo G, Albillos JC, Tejedor D. Intussusception: US findings with pathological correlation—the crescent-in-doughnut sign. Radiology 1996;199:688–692

Del-Pozo G, Albillos JC, Tejador D, et al. Intussusception in children: current concepts in diagnosis and enema reduction. Radiographics 1999;19:299–319

Gu L, Zhu H, Wang S, Han Y, Wu X, Miao H. Sonographic guidance of air enema for intussusception reduction in children. Pediatr Radiol 2000;30:339–342

Verschelden P, Filiatrault D, Garel L, et al. Intussusception in children: reliability of ultrasound diagnosis—a prospective study. Radiology 1992;184:741–744

CASE 60

Clinical Presentation

Term neonate presents with a distended abdomen and failure to pass meconium after 48 hours.

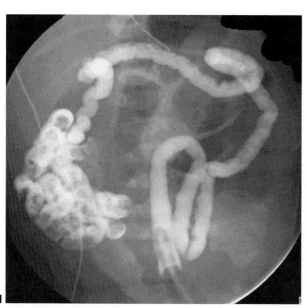
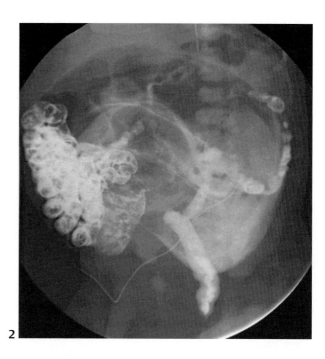

Figure 60A

Radiologic Findings

Non-ionic contrast enema (**Fig. 60A1**) in a 2-day-old girl demonstrates a microcolon. Reflux of contrast has occurred into mildly dilated loops of distal ileum, containing meconium plugs, but does not reach the more proximal dilated air-filled loops. Further reflux was achieved during a repeat examination the following day (**Fig. 60A2**), with opacification of significantly more dilated loops in the mid-ileum, containing further inspissated meconium.

Diagnosis

Meconium ileus

Differential Diagnosis

- Low gastrointestinal (GI) obstruction on abdominal radiograph–wide differential
  - ○ Ileal atresia
  - ○ Hirschsprung's disease
  - ○ Functional immaturity/left colon syndrome
  - ○ Anorectal anomaly
  - ○ Colonic atresia
  - ○ Sepsis/electrolyte disturbance
  - ○ Megacystis-microcolon-hypoperistalsis syndrome (rare)
- Microcolon on enema
  - ○ Ileal atresia—microcolon with reflux of contrast into nondilated distal ileum. If contrast reaches the atretic segment, an abrupt convex termination is seen, with residual unopacified dilated proximal small bowel loops.
  - ○ Megacystis-microcolon-hypoperistalsis syndrome (rare)—transient neonatal microcolon in association with a large-volume bladder and a variable degree of upper renal tract dilatation. Malrotation is common.
  - ○ Total colonic Hirschsprung's disease (may present as a small-caliber colon, although not usually as small as a "microcolon")

Discussion

Background

Meconium ileus is a neonatal obstruction of the ileum by abnormally viscid, inspissated pellets of meconium.

Etiology

- Almost all cases are associated with an underlying diagnosis of cystic fibrosis (CF). Conversely, meconium ileus is the initial presentation of 10 to 15% of CF cases.
- Rare cases have been described in association with partial pancreatic aplasia or stenosis of the pancreatic ducts.

Clinical Findings

Low GI obstruction—abdominal distension, failure to pass meconium, and sometimes vomiting—within the first 48 hours of life

Associated Conditions

Respiratory and other GI symptoms of CF develop later in childhood.

Complications

- Prenatal complications occur in ~50% and include perforation, which may result in meconium peritonitis and/or pseudocyst formation (walled-off local perforation), intestinal atresia, and closed-loop segmental volvulus. Migration of intraperitoneal meconium through the patent

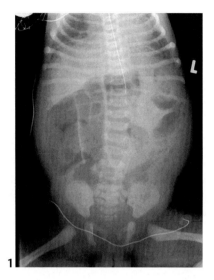
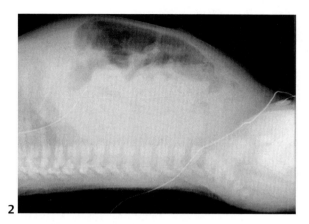

Figure 60B Supine (1) and cross-table lateral (2) abdominal x-ray of a 2-day-old girl showing generalized bowel dilatation with a mottled appearance of air mixed with meconium, in this case more prominent in the left flank. Enema confirmed meconium ileus with an underlying diagnosis of CF.

processus vaginalis testis can result in multiple small calcified scrotal masses. Rare labial meconium masses are described in girls.
- Postnatal perforation resulting in pneumoperitoneum
- Iatrogenic perforation during diagnostic or therapeutic contrast enema

Pathology

- CF is an autosomal recessive disease due to various mutations on chromosome 7 (e.g., d F508) coding for the CF transmembrane regulator (CFTR), a cyclic AMP-activated chloride channel blocker. Abnormalities in ion transport result in increased sodium influx into cells and higher viscosity of secretions, in addition to exocrine abnormalities.
- Meconium in CF contains 85% protein with a high albumin content compared with 7% protein in normal individuals.
- Macroscopically, the distal ileum is filled with dense gray meconium with the consistency of putty, with greater dilatation of the mid-ileum filled with dark gelatinous, tar-like meconium. Pseudo-cysts are collections of soft meconium walled off by peritoneal fibrosis. Meconium leakage causes an aseptic chemical peritonitis, resulting in peritoneal fibrosis, calcification, and sometimes adhesions.
- Microscopically, the intestinal villi are distorted and the mucosal glands dilated and plugged with inspissated secretions continuous with the focally calcified intraluminal meconium.

Imaging Findings

RADIOGRAPHY

- Low GI obstruction—multiple loops of dilated bowel. Distinguishing dilated small from large bowel radiographically is unreliable in neonates.
- The following radiographic features may suggest the diagnosis of meconium ileus, but none are of high specificity or sensitivity:
  - A bubbly appearance, often in the right iliac fossa, due to mixing of meconium with air, and a relative paucity of fluid levels on horizontal beam radiographs are classically described (**Fig. 60B**). Mass effect may be observed from a large pseudocyst.
  - Greater dilatation of one bowel loop—in this case the terminal ileum—may be seen, but a similar appearance can occur in ileal and colonic atresias.

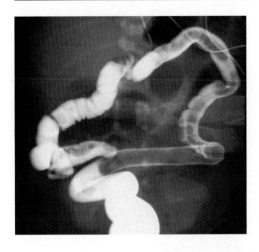

Figure 60C Non-ionic contrast enema demonstrating a microcolon with reflux into a nondilated blind-ending terminal ileal segment, with persistent air-filled dilated loops proximally. Laparotomy confirmed ileal atresia.

- ○ Scattered peritoneal calcification (meconium peritonitis) or intramural calcification of a pseudocyst may be seen, but both are also encountered in ileal atresia.

CONTRAST ENEMA

- The entire colon is of very small caliber—a microcolon. This "unused" colon implies that insufficient succus entericus reached the colon in utero as a result of a high-grade distal ileal obstruction. Its presence essentially limits the differential diagnosis to meconium ileus and ileal atresia. Differentiation depends on the appearance of the mid-to-distal ileum.
- The diagnosis of meconium ileus requires identification of dilated small bowel loops filled with meconium plugs. In some cases, the terminal ileum is clearly dilated and packed with inspissated meconium, allowing easy diagnosis. However, the degree of terminal ileal dilatation may not be marked, and the more significant dilatation is often found in the mid-ileum, requiring the opacification of more proximal small bowel loops for identification.
- In comparison, the distal ileum of ileal atresia is not dilated, and contrast should outline the convex, blind-ending segment distal to the atresia, with residual dilated air-filled, nonopacified loops seen proximally (**Fig. 60C**).

ULTRASOUND

- Prenatal signs. Dilated, echogenic bowel after 20 weeks of gestation raises the possibility of meconium ileus but is not of high specificity or sensitivity.
- Postnatally, ultrasound may demonstrate complications. Inspissated echogenic meconium within a calcified cyst is typical of a pseudocyst. Meconium peritonitis is demonstrated as scattered dense echogenic foci along peritoneal surfaces and within the scrotum.

Treatment

- Conservative management involves the use of serial contrast enemas, often in association with oral N-acetyl cysteine to soften the impacted meconium and induce its passage. Practice varies with institution; there is no clear consensus as to the optimal composition and dilution of contrast agent or the frequency of enemas.
- Low osmolar (near iso-osmolar) non-ionic contrast media are most frequently used, sometimes containing additional N-acetyl cysteine.
- Meglumine diatrizoate is less frequently used than in the past. Its high osmolarity carries a risk of precipitating circulatory collapse, and therefore a dilute solution should always be used with adequate hydration of the baby prior to and during the procedure.
- Serial enemas can be performed daily provided there is evidence of continuing clinical improvement. Reflux of contrast further into the small bowel is often possible with successive examinations.

- Surgical intervention with direct irrigation of the small bowel is indicated in complicated cases or if there is no significant clinical improvement after several enema attempts.

Prognosis

- Radiologic treatment is successful in ~60% of uncomplicated cases. The remainder will require surgical intervention.
- Complicated cases requiring surgical intervention are associated with a greater morbidity, including subsequent adhesive small bowel obstruction and blind loop syndrome.
- However, in general, the long-term nutritional and hepatobiliary status of patients with CF presenting with meconium ileus appears similar to those patients with CF with other presentations.
- It has been clearly shown that the management of patients with CF in specialized centers improves survival.

PEARL_____

- Neonatal enema technique: Water-soluble contrast is used—the consequences of perforation are less severe than barium peritonitis, and it carries a therapeutic benefit in meconium ileus and functional immaturity. An 8 French feeding tube or small Foley catheter is inserted into the rectum and taped securely. A lateral view of the rectum and rectosigmoid junction is obtained on initial filling (important in the diagnosis of Hirschsprung's disease), with further views in the prone or supine position, as the colon is opacified. Contrast may be injected manually by syringe or using gravity from a suspended source. Attempts should be made to reflux contrast into the distal ileum for both diagnostic and therapeutic reasons. However, hand injection should be cautious, as perforation of a microcolon is a well-documented risk.

PITFALLS_____

- If reflux into the most dilated loops of ileum is not achieved, then differentiation from ileal atresia is difficult. If a clearly blind-ending, nondilated segment of distal ileum is opacified, the diagnosis of ileal atresia can be made. However, if there is opacification of normal or mildly prominent distal ileum containing some meconium plugs, but contrast does not reach more significantly dilated proximal loops, then both diagnoses remain possible, as in **Fig. 60A1**. A repeat study after 24 hours is often successful in achieving further reflux into markedly dilated loops filled with meconium, and the diagnosis of meconium ileus can then be confirmed.
- There remain a small number of cases where small bowel reflux is not achieved or findings are equivocal and an atresia proximal to the opacified loops cannot be excluded. Explorative laparotomy may then be necessary.

Suggested Readings

Abramson SJ, Baker DH, Amodio JB, Berdon WE. Gastrointestinal manifestations of cystic fibrosis. Semin Roentgenol 1987;22:97–113

Berdon WE, Baker DH, Santulli TV, Amoury TV, Blanc WA. Microcolon in newborn infants with intestinal obstruction: its correlation with the level and time of onset of obstruction. Radiology 1968;90:878–885

Fuchs JR, Langer JC. Long-term outcome after neonatal meconium obstruction. Pediatrics 1998;101:E7

Jamieson D, Stringer DA. The small bowel. In: Stringer DA, Babyn PS, eds. Pediatric Gastrointestinal Imaging and Intervention. 2nd ed. Hamilton, ON: BC Decker; 2000:475–534

Leonidas JC, Berdon WE, Baker DH, Santulli TV. Meconium ileus and its complications: a reappraisal of plain film roentgen diagnostic criteria. Am J Roentgenol Radium Ther Nucl Med 1970;108:598–609

CASE 61

Clinical Presentation

Contrast enema was performed on a 2-day-old term baby who had failed to pass meconium.

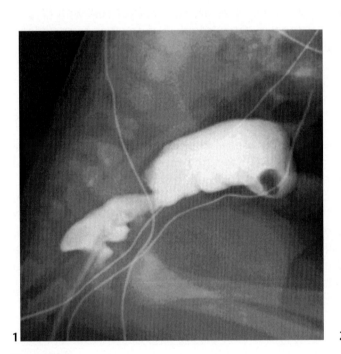 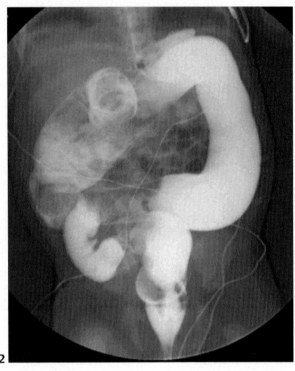

Figure 61A

Radiologic Findings

An abrupt transition zone is seen at the rectosigmoid junction (**Fig. 61A1**), with mild dilatation of the remainder of the colon (**Fig. 61A2**).

Diagnosis

Hirschsprung's disease

Differential Diagnosis

- Neonatal low obstruction:
  - Functional immaturity/left colon syndrome
  - Meconium ileus
  - Ileal atresia
  - Colonic atresia
  - Megacystis-microcolon-intestinal hypoperistalsis syndrome (rare)
- Constipation in the older child:
  - Functional megarectum
  - Motility disorders (primary and secondary visceral myopathies and neuropathies)
  - Metabolic disorders (e.g., hypothyroidism)
- Histologic findings:
  - Rare—Chagas' disease (destruction of ganglion cells)

Discussion

Background

Hirschsprung's disease, named eponymously following a report of two cases of megacolon in 1887, is due to aganglionosis of the distal bowel. It occurs with an incidence of ~1:4500 live births and demonstrates an overall 4:1 male-to-female ratio.

Etiology

- The primary abnormality is failure of the normal craniocaudal migration of vagal neural crest cells between weeks 5 and 12 of gestation. This results in distal absence of ganglion cells in the myenteric (Auerbach) plexus and submucosal (Meissner) plexus of the bowel wall. The aganglionic segment begins at the anal sphincter and extends proximally for a varying length of the colon. It is continuous, the presence of "skip" lesions being extremely rare.
- The physiology of the disease is more complex than pure aganglionosis. Abnormalities of both adrenergic and cholinergic fibers can be demonstrated, and function of the internal anal sphincter is also abnormal.

Classification

- Short segment disease (70% cases): The aganglionic segment involves the rectum and distal sigmoid colon.
- Long segment disease (25%): The aganglionic segment extends to the splenic flexure or transverse colon.
- Total colonic aganglionosis (Zuelzer-Wilson syndrome) (5%): The entire colon is involved with occasional extension into the small bowel. Total colonic disease demonstrates a strong familial tendency.
- Ultrashort segment disease: This remains a controversial entity in which the abnormality is limited to the anal sphincter. A manometric and clinical diagnosis, there are no abnormal radiologic or histologic findings.

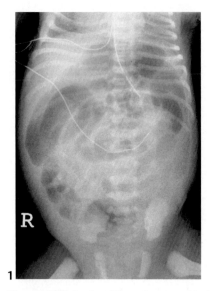
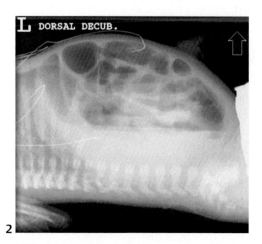

Figure 61B Supine (**1**) and cross-table lateral (**2**) abdominal x-ray demonstrating multiple dilated loops of bowel with air-fluid levels.

Clinical Findings

Most patients present with abdominal distension and failure to pass meconium within the first 48 hours of life. Explosive, foul-smelling stool on rectal examination is classic. Older infants and children develop chronic, severe constipation. Occasionally presentation may be delayed until adulthood. Diagnosis may often be suggested by contrast enema findings, but rectal biopsy is required for definitive diagnosis. In older children rectal manometry is a useful diagnostic adjunct.

Associated Conditions

- Trisomy 21 (5% of patients with Hirschsprung's disease)
- Congenital heart disease (2.5%)
- Genitourinary abnormalities (2%), for example, megaureter
- Congenital neuroblastoma (also due to neural crest maldevelopment)
- Ondine's curse (congenital central hypoventilation syndrome)
- Rare reports: Waardenburg's syndrome, congenital deafness, cartilage hair dysplasia

Complications

- Enterocolitis
  - Patients may develop enterocolitis prior to or following surgery. In a few children it is the initial presentation. Severe diarrhea may progress to dehydration and septic shock.
- Perforation
  - Usually in long segment or total colonic disease

Pathology

- Histologic diagnosis is made by the absence of ganglion cells in the submucosal plexus on a rectal mucosal suction biopsy. Full-thickness rectal biopsies are less frequently performed today but will demonstrate aganglionosis within the myenteric plexus. The biopsy must be obtained at least 2 cm

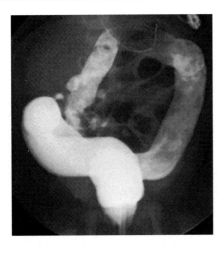

Figure 61C A rather featureless, shortened colon can be a feature of total colonic Hirschsprung's disease.

above the mucocutaneous junction, as normal rectal tissue close to the internal anal sphincter contains few or no ganglion cells.
- Macroscopically, the affected segment is narrow and contracted, with dilated bowel proximally.

Imaging Findings

RADIOGRAPHY

- Neonates: findings of low obstruction with multiple dilated loops of bowel and air-fluid levels (**Figs. 61B1** and **61B2**). In total colonic disease, calcification within the small bowel lumen and perforation resulting in pneumoperitoneum, have been described.
- Infants/older children: distended colon with marked fecal impaction

ENEMA

- In neonates, non-ionic contrast should be used to avoid the risks associated with barium and bowel perforation, and it has an equal diagnostic accuracy. In older children barium may be used.
- The most specific sign is the presence of a transition zone between narrow or normal caliber affected distal bowel and normally innervated dilated proximal bowel. This may lie at any point along the colon but is most frequent in the sigmoid region.
- In neonates, the classic transition zone may be absent and the rectosigmoid ratio is a useful indicator of abnormality. The normal neonatal and infant rectum is of greater caliber than the sigmoid colon. In Hirschsprung's disease this ratio is reversed.
- Irregular contractions within the aganglionic segment causing a sawtooth appearance may be seen, although they are not a frequent finding.
- The presence of irregular mucosa or thumb printing may indicate the presence of enterocolitis. Enemas should be avoided if clinical symptomatology suggests enterocolitis, due to the risk of perforation.
- Delayed evacuation of contrast on a 24-hour film is an unreliable sign.
- A normal examination does not exclude the diagnosis.

Treatment

- Initial treatment is usually a staged repair by defunctioning colostomy or ileostomy, followed by a definitive pull-through procedure anastomosing normal bowel to the distal rectum or anal canal by a modified Duhamel, Soave, or Swenson approach.
- Primary one-stage pull-through is now performed in some cases.
- Limited surgery—posterior rectal myotomy—may be appropriate for some older children.

Prognosis

- Bowel habit improves with time. On long-term follow-up the majority of patients have a normal bowel habit, some require stool softeners or enemas to facilitate stooling, and a few have chronic severe constipation or soiling.
- Total colonic disease has a poorer prognosis with a high mortality and morbidity rate.
- Enterocolitis is also associated with increased morbidity and mortality.

PEARLS_____

- Enema technique: A small 8 to 10 French catheter should be used in neonates and placed just inside the anus. If a Foley catheter is used, the balloon should not be inflated (at least, not until rectosigmoid views have been obtained), as it may distort the rectal appearances and obscure a transition zone. It is important to obtain a lateral rectal view in early filling to document the rectosigmoid ratio and any irregular contractions.
- Presentation in preterm infants is almost unknown.

PITFALLS_____

- The classic transition zone is more commonly demonstrated in older children than in neonates and infants.
- Although a good screening examination, a normal enema does not exclude the diagnosis, and definitive diagnosis relies on histology.
- Total colonic disease is particularly difficult to diagnose. Enema findings may be nonspecific and subtle (**Fig. 61C**). These include a short colon with hepatic and splenic flexures lying more medial than usual, a small caliber colon, a transition zone in the ileum, or a normal examination.

Suggested Readings

Berlin S, Sivit CJ, Stringer DA. The large bowel. In: Stringer DA, Babyn PS, eds. Pediatric Gastrointestinal Imaging and Intervention. 2nd ed. Hamilton, ON: BC Decker; 2000:475–534

Blane CE, Elhalaby E, Coran AG. Enterocolitis following endorectal pullthrough procedure in children with Hirschsprung's disease. Pediatr Radiol 1994;24:164–166

DeCampo JF, Mayne V, Boldt DW, et al. Radiological findings in total aganglionosis coli. Pediatr Radiol 1984;14:205–209

Pocharzevsky R, Leonidas JC. The rectosigmoid index: a measurement for the early diagnosis of Hirschsprung's disease. AJR Am J Roentgenol 1977;123:770–777

Rescorla FJ, Morrison AM, Eagles D, West KW, Grosfeld JL. Hirschsprung's disease: evaluation of mortality and long-term function in 260 cases. Arch Surg 1992;127:934–941

Rosenfield NS, Ablow RC, Marcowitz RI, et al. Hirschsprung's disease: accuracy of the barium enema examination. Radiology 1984;150:393–400

CASE 62

Clinical Presentation

A 3-week-old boy presents with sudden-onset bilious vomiting.

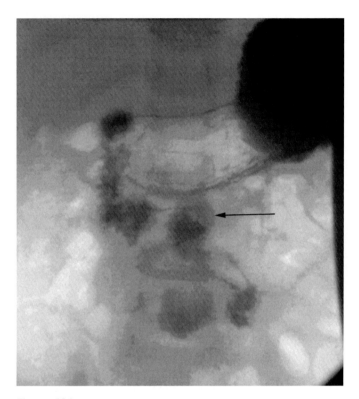

Figure 62A

Radiologic Findings

Upper gastrointestinal (GI) study (**Fig. 62A**) demonstrates an abnormally low position of the duodenojejunal junction (DJJ) (arrow), below the level of the duodenal bulb.

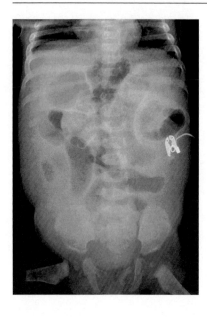

Figure 62B Abdominal x-ray of a 5-month-old girl presenting in hypovolemic shock. Thickened bowel loops secondary to ischemia are seen in the left upper quadrant.

Diagnosis

Malrotation

Differential Diagnosis

- Displacement of the DJJ by distended bowel loops or intra-abdominal masses
- Nonrotation (duodenal loop and small bowel to the right of the midline with the entire colon on the left. May be considered a subset of malrotation, but only rarely associated with volvulus)

Discussion

Background

Malrotation and midgut volvulus is potentially one of the most serious pediatric surgical emergencies, and the role of radiology in its diagnosis is critical. Delay in diagnosis carries the risk of infarctive necrosis of the entire small bowel and is potentially fatal.

Etiology/Embryology

- Around the sixth week of gestation, the duodenojejunal and ileocolic segments of the primitive gut herniate into the extraembryonic coelom in the umbilical cord. Both loops elongate and rotate 270 degrees anticlockwise around the axis of the superior mesenteric artery. The bowel loops return to their final positions within the abdominal cavity by the 11th week, and their mesenteries become fixed to the parietal peritoneum.
- The duodenal loop is fixed with the DJJ in the left upper quadrant at the ligament of Treitz. The ileocecal junction is fixed in the right lower quadrant. The normal small bowel mesentery therefore has a broad diagonal base across the abdomen.
- Any arrest in this 270-degree anticlockwise rotation during physiologic umbilical herniation results in malrotation and malfixation of the small bowel. The DJJ is displaced medially and inferiorly and/or the cecum medially and superiorly. The small bowel mesentery is therefore shortened and the risk of the entire small bowel twisting on its narrow pedicle increased (volvulus).

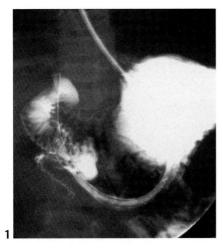 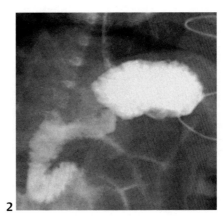

Figure 62C Signs of volvulus on upper GI study include the classic "corkscrew" appearance (**1**) and almost complete obstruction of the third part of the duodenum (**2**).

- Midgut volvulus leads to small bowel obstruction, occlusion of the superior mesenteric vessels, ischemia, and, if there is delay in diagnosis and treatment, complete small bowel infarction.
- Abnormal peritoneal bands—Ladd's bands—are often found in association with malrotation, passing from the cecum to the right lateral abdominal wall, crossing the duodenum. They may contribute to duodenal obstruction but are rarely the sole cause.

Clinical Findings

Eighty to 90% of children present with bilious vomiting at <1 year of age, 65 to 75% within the first month of life. However, volvulus can occur at any age, including adulthood, and the diagnosis should always be considered. Late presentation can result in a hypovolemic, shocked patient.

In older children, intermittent obstruction can cause chronic or recurrent abdominal pain, vomiting, and failure to thrive. Rarely, a malabsorption syndrome results from chronic venous and lymphatic obstruction. Melena due to bleeding from mesenteric and intramural varices secondary to chronic venous obstruction has been described.

Associated Conditions

- Congenital abnormalities of the abdominal wall (omphalocele, gastroschisis, and diaphragmatic hernia) are all associated with some degree of malrotation, but clinical symptoms are rare.
- Malrotation associated with visceral heterotaxy syndromes is more controversial and may require surgical intervention.
- Duodenal atresia, stenosis, and webs are associated with malrotation in ~10% of cases.
- Malrotation presenting in a child without these known clinical diagnoses is usually an isolated anomaly.

Complications

- Volvulus leading to midgut necrosis, peritonism, electrolyte abnormalities, sepsis, and shock
- Short gut syndrome following small bowel resection
- Internal hernia (rare)
- Prenatal volvulus can be a cause of small bowel atresias, which are often extensive and/or multiple.
- Malabsorption and superior mesenteric vein thrombosis secondary to chronic volvulus

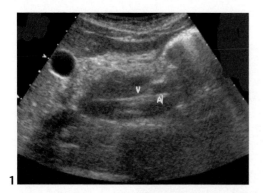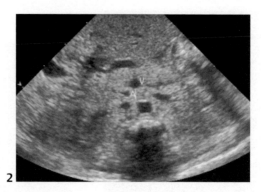

Figure 62D Transverse ultrasound demonstrating (**1**) the normal superior mesenteric artery/ superior mesenteric vein relationship and (**2**) reversed relationship, with the superior mesenteric artery lying abnormally to the right of the superior mesenteric vein.

Pathology

- Ischemic necrosis of the entire small bowel if volvulus is not promptly reduced

Imaging Findings

RADIOGRAPHY

- Unremarkable in many cases and cannot exclude the diagnosis
- Partial, and occasionally complete, duodenal obstruction
- Generalized small bowel dilatation or bowel wall thickening is a late finding, suspicious for small bowel ischemia (**Fig. 62B**).

UPPER GI STUDY

- In the neonate or sick child, non-ionic contrast is administered via a nasogastric tube. In the older or clinically well child, barium is ingested orally.
- On a well-aligned frontal image with the patient in a supine position, the normal DJJ lies to the left of the midline (at least over the left lumbar vertebral pedicle) at the level of the duodenal bulb.
- In malrotation, the DJJ is displaced medially, inferiorly, or both. The proximal jejunum may lie abnormally to the right.
- Signs of volvulus include partial or complete duodenal obstruction (second or third part) with a dilated proximal portion, or the classic "corkscrew" appearance of the duodenum and proximal jejunum twisting around its mesenteric axis (**Figs. 62C1** and **62C2**).
- The presence of volvulus is not always detectable on contrast study, and malposition of the DJJ may be the only radiologic abnormality.

CONTRAST ENEMA

- No longer performed routinely
- The cecum is quite mobile, especially in neonates (15%), and its position on fluoroscopy may not accurately reflect the true site of fixation.
- Malrotation and volvulus can occur with a normal cecal position but abnormal DJJ (16%). A normal enema cannot therefore exclude the diagnosis.
- Contrast enema is occasionally useful in defining the cecal position if upper GI study findings are equivocal. The length of the small bowel mesentery between the cecum and DJJ is the critical factor determining the risk of volvulus. A high cecum, particularly if directed medially, supports the diagnosis.

ULTRASOUND

- Seventy percent of malrotated patients show inversion of the normal relationship of the superior mesenteric artery and vein, with the vein abnormally to the left and/or anterior to the artery

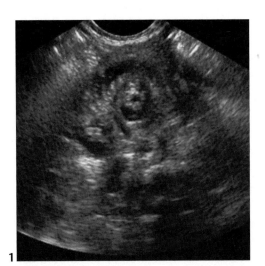
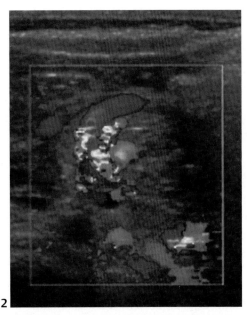

Figure 62E The "whirlpool sign," characterized by twisting of the superior mesenteric artery and vein, is highly specific for midgut volvulus, as seen in (**1**) ultrasound and (**2**) color Doppler. (See Color Plate **62E2**.)

(**Figs. 62D1** and **62D2**). However, sensitivity and specificity are not sufficient for use as a screening examination.

- The "whirlpool" sign—twisting of the superior mesenteric vein and mesentery around the artery—is a very specific sign of volvulus but of low sensitivity (**Fig. 62E**).
- The role of ultrasound remains ancillary to the upper GI study.

CT/MRI

- Malrotation can be demonstrated on cross-sectional imaging as malposition of the superior mesenteric vessels, usually as a fortuitous finding.

Treatment

- Ladd's procedure: Peritoneal bands are divided and any volvulus reduced or resected if nonviable. The small bowel is returned to the right side of the abdomen and the large bowel to the left. Adhesions subsequently develop making recurrent volvulus rare. The procedure may be performed endoscopically in uncomplicated cases.
- The management of older children with radiologic evidence of malrotation found incidentally is more controversial. Most surgeons will perform a Ladd's procedure in view of the small but potentially disastrous risk of volvulus later in life. In cases with subtle radiologic signs on contrast examinations and ultrasound, direct laparoscopic visualization of the duodenal and cecal fixation sites and/or Ladd's bands is helpful in determining the need for operative fixation.
- An upper GI study performed on a child having previously undergone Ladd's procedure will show an appearance similar to nonrotation.

Prognosis

- Excellent if promptly diagnosed and managed
- If extensive resection of ischemic or necrotic small bowel is required, short gut syndrome and the sequela of long-term total parenteral nutrition carry considerable morbidity and mortality.
- There is still a small but significant mortality rate from delayed presentation or diagnosis.

PEARL

- Upper GI study technique: It is essential to obtain a "first-pass" image of the duodenal loop for confident evaluation of the DJJ. With the patient in a prone right anterior oblique position contrast is observed entering the duodenal loop, and as it passes into the third and fourth parts, the infant is promptly turned supine for documentation of the location of the DJJ. It is critical that the patient is completely straight in the supine position without any element of rotation. Observing the position of the heart, the alignment of the vertebral pedicles, and rib symmetry is helpful in achieving this.

PITFALLS

- A normal DJJ can be mildly displaced inferiorly in the presence of generalized bowel dilatation from another cause, by masses or by an enlarged spleen, resulting in a false-positive diagnosis.
- Failure to obtain a true supine image can result in both false-positive and false-negative results as rotation alters the relationship of the DJJ to the vertebral pedicle landmarks.
- A redundant duodenum with excessive loops makes confident identification of the DJJ difficult.
- Displacement of the DJJ can be subtle. Surgical liaison and clinical correlation are particularly important in these cases.

Suggested Readings

Jamieson D, Stringer DA. The small bowel. In: Stringer DA, Babyn PS, eds. Pediatric Gastrointestinal Imaging and Intervention. 2nd ed. Hamilton, ON: BC Decker; 2000:475–534

Long FR, Kramer SS, Markowitz RI, Taylor GE. Radiographic patterns of intestinal malrotation in children. Radiographics 1996;16:547–556

Long FR, Kramer SS, Markowitz RI, Taylor GE, Liacouras CA. Intestinal malrotation in children: tutorial on radiographic diagnosis in difficult cases. Radiology 1996;198(3):775–780

Pracros JP, Sann L, Genin G, et al. Ultrasound diagnosis of midgut volvulus: the "whirlpool" sign. Pediatr Radiol 1992;22:18–20

Zerin JM, DiPietro MA. Superior mesenteric vascular anatomy at US in patients with surgically proved malrotation of the midgut. Radiology 1992;183:693–694

CASE 63

Clinical Presentation

This 3-day-old neonate with a known prenatal ultrasound diagnosis was intubated and ventilated following delivery. Extracorporeal membranous oxygenation (ECMO) was then instigated.

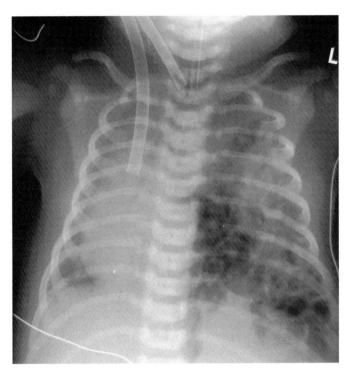

Figure 63A

Radiologic Findings

Chest radiograph (**Fig. 63A**) demonstrates multiple rounded lucencies within the left hemithorax with mediastinal shift to the right. The tips of the arteriovenous ECMO catheters are positioned in the right atrium (radiodense dot distal to the opaque linear portion of the venous catheter) and in the origin of the right common carotid artery or aortic arch (there is a small radiolucent portion beyond the apparent radiodense tip).

Diagnosis

Left congenital diaphragmatic hernia (CDH)

Differential Diagnosis

- Congenital cystic adenomatoid malformation (CCAM)
- Bronchopulmonary sequestration
- Pleuroparenchymal disease ± abscess or pneumatocele formation
- Intrathoracic solid masses
- Diaphragmatic eventration (attenuated or absent striated muscle within the peripheral muscular diaphragm)

Discussion

Background

CDH occurs with an incidence of 1 to 2 in 3000 live births. The vast majority occur posterolaterally, through the foramen of Bochdalek, with 75% of cases on the left. Herniation of abdominal contents into the thoracic cavity through a defect in the diaphragm results in varying degrees of pulmonary hypoplasia.

Clinical Findings

Most Bochdalek hernias are detected on prenatal ultrasound or present with respiratory distress and difficulty in resuscitation at birth. The abdomen is scaphoid with absent breath sounds in the affected hemithorax and displacement of the apex beat. Smaller lesions may present in later childhood with recurrent respiratory infections, constipation, or symptoms of GI obstruction. Strangulation or volvulus is an unusual but potentially fatal presentation. There is an increased incidence of delayed right-sided Bochdalek hernia following neonatal streptococcal pneumonia, the etiology of which is not fully understood. Further cases are associated with trauma, either acutely or with a delayed presentation. Small lesions may be asymptomatic, an increasing number of which are now being recognized on CT as an incidental finding.

Morgagni hernias generally present later in childhood or in adult life, often as an asymptomatic finding but sometimes associated with abdominal pain, vomiting, or chest pain. Rare neonatal cases present with respiratory distress.

Pathology/Embryology

- CDH results from a failure of normal diaphragmatic division of the thoracic and abdominal cavities between weeks 8 and 10 of gestation.
- The septum transversum forms the ventral part of the diaphragm. Defects anteriorly may occur on either side of the sternum, resulting in Morgagni hernias, which are more frequent on the right. Defects further posteriorly result in peritoneopericardial hernias. The dorsal part of the diaphragm is formed by the pleuroperitoneal membrane, which grows in to close off the pleuroperitoneal canals on either side of the mesoesophagus. Defects within this membrane are called Bochdalek's hernias.
- Traditionally, lung hypoplasia has been viewed as a secondary consequence to in utero compression. However, experimental evidence is now increasing for a primary defect in lung development.

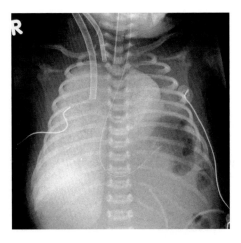

Figure 63B Chest x-ray of a 4-day-old neonate receiving liquid ventilation and ECMO support. The volume of the hypoplastic left lung and well-developed right lung can be directly visualized due to perfluorocarbon opacification. Intrathoracic location of the stomach is noted.

Associated Conditions

- CDH may be an isolated finding or occur in association with other anomalies including congenital heart disease, tracheobronchial and chromosomal anomalies.
- Bochdalek hernias are invariably associated with malrotation/malfixation of the midgut.

Complications

- Neonatal period:
  ◦ Persistent fetal circulation/pulmonary hypertension with right-to-left shunting
  ◦ Iatrogenic complications of ventilation, central venous access, total parenteral nutrition, ECMO
  ◦ GI obstruction and ischemia (rare)
- Long term:
  ◦ GI: hiatus hernia and gastroesophageal reflux (can be severe leading to growth failure)
  ◦ Respiratory: Although abnormalities in lung perfusion and reduced alveolization can be demonstrated years later, overall function is generally good. A small number of survivors will require supplemental oxygen.
  ◦ Neurologic: neurodevelopmental delay, cerebral palsy, seizures, hearing impairment as sequelae to hypoxia and ECMO complications (intracranial hemorrhage and ischemia)

Imaging Findings

PRENATAL IMAGING

- Ultrasound may demonstrate a solid or cystic thoracic mass, mediastinal shift, small abdominal circumference, and absent intra-abdominal stomach.
- MRI may be a useful adjunct in cases of diagnostic uncertainty. Future role may include fetal lung volume calculation.

RADIOGRAPHY

- Multiple radiolucencies due to bowel gas are projected over the thorax, with mediastinal shift to the contralateral side and a relative absence of bowel gas in the abdomen. Lateral films confirm the posterior or anterior location of a Bochdalek or Morgagni hernia, respectively. The position of the nasogastric tube indicates the site of the stomach; an intrathoracic location is an adverse prognostic factor.
- In patients where liquid ventilation is used, the lungs are opacified in a gravity-dependent distribution (**Fig. 63B**). Neonatal lung growth may be observed as increasing volume of opacified parenchyma.
- Further imaging is not usually required in neonatal cases. However, various modalities may be useful in cases of diagnostic uncertainty, late presentations, and posttrauma cases, and in the investigation of possible postsurgical recurrence.

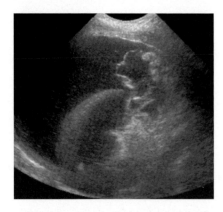

Figure 63C Thoracic ultrasound demonstrating intrathoracic bowel, pleural fluid, and herniation of the spleen in a late-presenting left-sided diaphragmatic hernia.

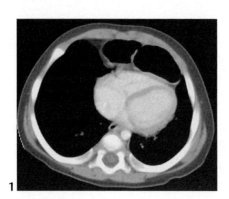

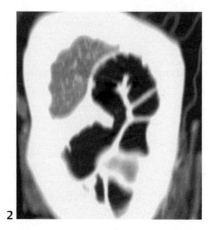

Figure 63D Axial CT (**1**) and coronal reconstruction (**2**) demonstrating a large anterior hernia of Morgagni containing transverse colon and the splenic flexure.

ULTRASOUND

- Fluid-filled loops of bowel with gut wall signature and a variable degree of peristalsis are seen within the thoracic cavity (**Fig. 63C**). Herniated liver, spleen, kidney, or other intra-abdominal organs can also be confirmed.

FLUOROSCOPY

- Contrast follow-through examination is a well-proven and reliable method of demonstrating the segments of the GI tract involved in a hernia.

MRI

- Multiplanar images, especially coronal sequences, provide excellent visualization of the defect and nature of the herniating abdominal contents without the use of ionizing radiation.

CT

- The axial imaging plane of CT is not well suited to optimal demonstration of diaphragmatic hernia. Signs include discontinuity of the diaphragm, superior positioning of abdominal viscera, and narrowing of the bowel with an hourglass configuration. Multiplanar reconstructions aid diagnosis (**Figs. 63D1** and **63D2**).

Treatment

- At birth, resuscitation with bag and mask ventilation should be avoided as this will cause gastric distension and further respiratory compromise. Neonates are intubated and ventilated, preferably before the first spontaneous respiratory effort, and a nasogastric tube passed to decompress the stomach

- A period of stablization follows, which may include correction of metabolic acidosis, pharmacologic treatment of pulmonary hypertension, high-frequency oscillatory ventilation, and ECMO support. In some centers, liquid ventilation (perfluorocarbon) is used, which may accelerate neonatal lung growth and improve gas exchange in infants with severe lung hypoplasia.
- Delayed surgical repair has now generally replaced emergent surgery. The bowel and other organs are reduced and the diaphragmatic defect repaired, often with a prosthetic patch.

Prognosis

- Mortality rates remain high (30–70%), with a 1-year survival rate of live births of ~50%.
- Major prognostic factors are the degree of ipsilateral and contralateral pulmonary hypoplasia, the severity of pulmonary hypertension, and the presence of associated malformations, especially congenital heart disease.
- However, if the infant survives the neonatal period, pulmonary prognosis is generally good.
- Late presentations are associated with a good prognosis.

PEARL_____

- During ECMO, the lungs are "rested" using low-pressure ventilation and therefore appear as a white-out. The role of chest radiographs in management is limited to the detection of large pneumothoraces or effusions that may require intervention, and monitoring catheter placement. The venous catheter tip should lie within the right atrium (placement within the superior or inferior vena cava may cause venous obstruction), and the arterial tip within the origin of the right common carotid artery or aortic arch, directed down the descending aorta (cranial direction) will result in volume overload to the heart.

PITFALLS_____

- Initial neonatal chest radiographs may demonstrate an opaque hemithorax or apparent soft tissue mass associated with mediastinal shift. The air-filled nature of the intrathoracic bowel loops may only manifest several hours later, as air is swallowed.
- The most common herniating tissue in a Morgagni hernia is omentum. The cardiophrenic mass may therefore appear solid rather than cystic on radiographs.
- Late presentations, particularly right-sided lesions, are often associated with delay in diagnosis and radiologic misinterpretation as pleuroparenchymal disease, pulmonary abscesses, or pneumatoceles. Subtle signs on the right can include a rounded superior margin of the liver with a small pleural effusion blunting the costophrenic angle.

Suggested Readings

Bohn D. Congenital diaphragmatic hernia. Am J Respir Crit Care Med 2002;166:911–915

Dillon E, Renwick M, Wright C. Congenital diaphragmatic hernia: antenatal detection and outcome. Br J Radiol 2000;73:360–365

Fauza DO, Hirschl RB, Wilson JM. Continuous intrapulmonary distension with perfluorocarbon accelerates lung growth in infants with congenital diaphragmatic hernia: initial experience. J Pediatr Surg 2001;36:1237–1240

Liu X, Ashtari M, Leonidas JC, Chan Y. Magnetic resonance imaging of the fetus in congenital intrathoracic disorders: preliminary observations. Pediatr Radiol 2001;31:435–439

Smith NP, Jesudason EC, Losty PD. Congenital diaphragmatic hernia. Paediatr Respir Rev 2002;3:339–348

CASE 64

Clinical Presentation

A 6-year-old boy presents to the emergency department with a 24-hour history of lower abdominal pain and fever.

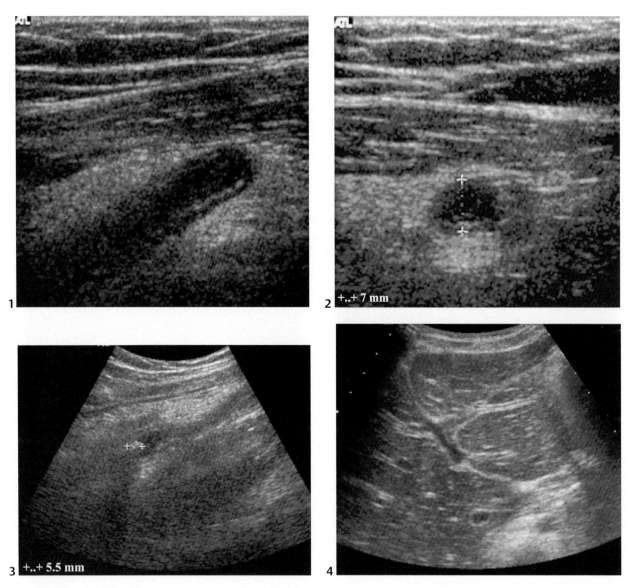

Figure 64A

Radiologic Findings

Longitudinal (**Fig. 64A1**) and transverse (**Fig. 64A2**) ultrasound images demonstrating a fluid-filled tubular structure in the right iliac fossa (7 mm diameter), which was noncompressible and could be traced to the cecum. A 5.5 mm high echogenicity focus with acoustic shadowing is seen at the base (**Fig. 64A3**); the surrounding mesenteric fat is markedly echogenic, and increased periportal echoes are noted in the liver (**Fig. 64A4**).

Diagnosis

Acute appendicitis with appendicolith

Differential Diagnosis

- Normal appendix: blind-ending and in continuity with the cecum, but ≤6 mm in diameter and without hyperemia or surrounding inflammatory changes
- Normal terminal ileum: not in continuity with the cecum, not blind-ended, and shows frequent peristalsis
- Terminal ileitis: thickened, hypoperistaltic terminal ileum of inflammatory or infectious etiology
- Mesenteric adenitis: multiple small mesenteric lymph nodes and small amounts of free fluid, but the appendix appears normal
- Colitis (e.g., Crohn's disease, typhlitis, pseudomembranous colitis): may involve the appendix, but more extensive colonic thickening and pericolic inflammatory changes should allow differentiation

Discussion

Background

Acute appendicitis is the most common acute surgical condition in childhood, with a lifetime risk of 7 to 9%. The optimal imaging and diagnostic strategy is one of the most currently controversial topics in pediatric radiology.

Etiology

- The presence of an appendicolith (inspissated fecal material and inorganic salts) in ~50% of cases suggests that luminal obstruction is a central etiologic factor. Luminal distension, ischemia, and secondary bacterial infection follow. Inflammatory changes spread from the mucosa through the appendiceal wall to the serosa. Necrosis of the appendiceal wall results in perforation, abscess formation, and peritonitis.
- In a small number of cases, appendiceal obstruction is secondary to foreign bodies, parasites, or neoplasms (e.g., carcinoid, adenocarcinoma, lymphoma).

Clinical Findings

Peak age of presentation is between 10 and 15 years of age. However, appendicitis may occur at any age, including in children as young as 1 year of age. Classic presentation is with ill-defined abdominal pain moving to the right iliac fossa, accompanied by fever, vomiting, and a raised white cell count. However, the diagnosis is often more complex in adolescent girls, in whom gynecologic conditions may show similar presentation. In young children, an atypical presentation with malaise, anorexia, vomiting, and diarrhea is more common. Delay in diagnosis is relatively common in children <10 years of age, especially in infants/toddlers, many of whom present following a 1- to 2-week history of pain with established pelvic abscesses secondary to perforation.

Complications

- Perforation most frequently leads to localized pelvic abscess or phlegmon (inflammatory mass without significant liquification) formation. Less commonly, generalized peritonitis results in multiple intra-abdominal abscesses that may involve the pelvis, paracolic gutters, and subhepatic, subphrenic, or hepatorenal spaces.

- Acute small bowel obstruction secondary to entrapment of the distal ileum is less common than paralytic ileus secondary to generalized peritonitis.
- Dilatation of the right renal collecting system is usually due to a "ureteral ileus" with atony secondary to adjacent inflammation. Less often, it may reflect true obstruction related to extrinsic compression or an inflammatory distal ureteric stricture from a pelvic abscess or phlegmon.
- Contiguous inflammatory spread may involve the bladder, with rare appendiceal fistulae and perforation into the bladder.
- Pylephlebitis (inflammation of the portal vein) with consequent portal vein thrombosis and intrahepatic abscesses, although frequent in the past, is now a rare complication.
- Adhesive small bowel obstruction is the most frequent late complication.

Pathology

- Macroscopically, the appendix is congested, the lumen commonly distended with pus and containing an obstructing fecolith. The serosa may be covered with exudate.
- Microscopically, mucosal ulceration and neutrophilic infiltration are required for diagnosis. Transmural inflammation with necrosis and perforation and/or serosal inflammation with periappendicitis are also frequently present.

Imaging Findings

ABDOMINAL RADIOGRAPHY

- Of low sensitivity and specificity and therefore not recommended as routine
- Often normal or shows nonspecific findings of right iliac fossa inflammation such as localized dilated loops, an indistinct right psoas margin, loss of the right-sided properitoneal or obturator internus fat planes, and scoliosis convex to the left
- A radiodense appendicolith is highly specific in the symptomatic patient but only seen in 5 to 10% cases.
- Generalized small bowel dilatation may indicate partial obstruction from a localized phlegmon/abscess or paralytic ileus secondary to generalized peritonitis.
- Free air is very uncommon.

ULTRASOUND

- The "graded compression" technique was described by Puylaert in 1986. A linear array transducer (5–10 MHz) is used, gradually compressing over the right iliac fossa and point of maximum clinical tenderness. The cecum, iliac vessels, and psoas muscle are identified as landmarks, and bowel is slowly displaced to visualize the appendix.
- The normal appendix is a tubular structure traceable to the cecum at its proximal end and blind-ending distally. It is <6 mm in diameter, compressible, and with minimal demonstrable color Doppler flow within its wall. Identification can be difficult, especially in younger children; published rates vary between 5 and 50%.
- The inflamed appendix is non- or only mildly compressible, fluid-filled, and >6 mm in diameter. It may contain an obstructing calcified appendicolith, identified as a high echogencity focus with acoustic shadowing. The mucosal/submucosal layer is echogenic, which, when surrounding intraluminal fluid, produces a "target" appearance.
- Supporting signs include increased echogenicity of the surrounding mesenteric fat (**Fig. 64A**) and hyperemia of the appendix. Increased periportal echoes within the liver, a small amount of free fluid, and small mesenteric nodes are often present but are nonspecific.
- Following perforation, an inflammatory phlegmon is visualized as a mixed echogenicity mass in the right iliac fossa, with surrounding echogenic inflammatory changes and often containing an appendicolith (**Figs. 64B1** and **64B2**). Hypoechoic, liquified pelvic abscesses can be identified,

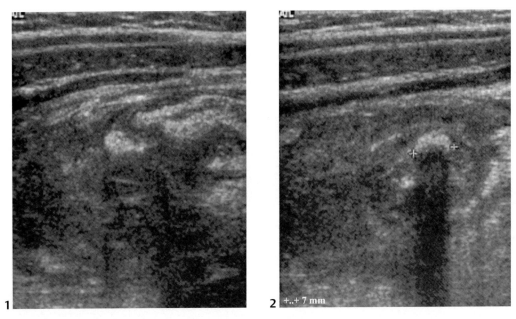

Figure 64B Ultrasound demonstrating appendiceal perforation with phlegmon formation. A mixed echogenicity mass is seen below the abdominal wall in the right iliac fossa (**1**) and containing a 7 mm appendicolith with acoustic shadowing (**2**).

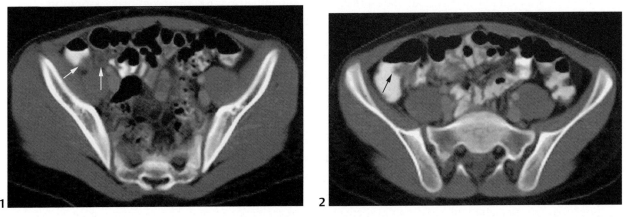

Figure 64C CT of pelvis with intravenous and oral contrast in a 13-year-old boy, demonstrating an acutely inflamed enlarged tubular appendix seen in transverse section (**1**, arrows) with adjacent cecal thickening (**2**, arrow).

although their full extent deep in the pelvis may be difficult to appreciate on ultrasound. The appendix itself is visible in only 40 to 60% of patients with appendiceal perforation.

CT

- CT protocol varies considerably with local practice. Some practitioners limit coverage to the pelvis, whereas others include the upper abdomen. The use of oral contrast, rectal contrast, and intravenous contrast is also variable, and at present there is no consensus as to the optimal protocol.
- The normal appendix is ≤6 mm (as on ultrasound), tubular, and without significant wall enhancement. It may be collapsed or partially filled with fluid, contrast media, or air. The relative lack of intra-abdominal fat makes identification of the normal appendix more difficult in children than in adults, but nevertheless it can be identified in ~75% of patients.
- The inflamed appendix is ≥7 mm in size with a thickened, enhancing wall and frequently contains a calcified appendicolith. Adjacent inflammatory soft tissue stranding and cecal apical thickening (arrowhead sign) are supporting signs (**Figs. 64C1** and **64C2**). A small amount of free fluid and small mesenteric nodes are frequent but nonspecific findings.

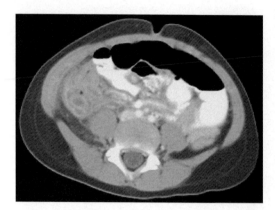

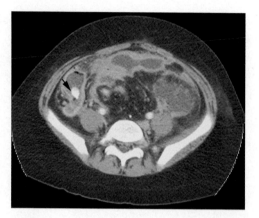

Figure 64D CT of pelvis of the same patient illustrated in **Fig. 64B**, confirming the presence of a complex mixed attenuation inflammatory phlegmon in the right iliac fossa, containing a few air bubbles but no large liquified abscess amenable to drainage. The calcified appendicolith was visualized just inferior to this level (not shown).

Figure 64E CT of pelvis in an 11-year-old girl following intravenous and oral contrast demonstrating a large 15 mm appendicolith (arrow) in the right iliac fossa with multiple low-attenuation, rim-enhancing abscesses throughout the pelvis, some of which contain a few bubbles of air. Percutaneous drainage was performed successfully.

- CT has a well-established role in "late-presenting" appendicitis with symptoms suggesting an established pelvic abscess or phlegmon. It optimally demonstrates the full extent of pelvic abscesses, determining the relative size of liquified and nonliquified components, and is used to guide percutaneous or transrectal drainage procedures (**Figs. 64D** and **64E**).
- Pneumoperitoneum with subdiaphragmatic free air is rare. However, localized small extraluminal air pockets or bubbles trapped by inflamed mesentery or from gas-forming bacterial infection may be seen.

Treatment

- Children presenting with acute uncomplicated appendicitis undergo appendectomy, which may be performed laparoscopically.
- Conservative management with comprehensive antibiotic cover is now the preferred management if perforation has resulted in a significant inflammatory phlegmon or pelvic abscess(es). Established abscesses are drained by the interventional radiologist via a percutaneous or rectal route.
- Following conservative management, ~10 to 15% of patients will experience recurrent symptoms, those patients with a residual appendicolith being at greatest risk. Depending on local practice and patient preference, interval appendectomy may therefore be performed after 6 to 8 weeks.

Prognosis

- Postoperative recovery is usually prompt. Complications include wound infections and postoperative abscess formation, both of increased incidence if the appendix is necrotic and perforated at surgery.
- Speed of recovery following percutaneous drainage is variable, with some patients requiring several drainage procedures.
- The clinical impact of the increasing use of imaging in the management of acute appendicitis remains under debate. However, there is now growing evidence for a favorable effect on false-negative laparotomy rates, perforation rates, and length of hospital stay.
- Appendicitis is associated with an ~5% lifetime risk of adhesive small bowel obstruction.

PEARLS_____

- The principle advantages of ultrasound are its lack of ionizing radiation, lower cost, ability to assess compressibility and vascularity, and value in depicting alternative genitourinary diagnoses. The principle advantages of CT are its lower operator dependency and higher sensitivity in many series, easier visualization in obese patients, and superior delineation of disease extent in perforated appendicitis, where it has a well-established role in planning interventional procedures.

- Both ultrasound and CT have high reported specificities for the diagnosis of acute appendicitis in children—both in the range of 90 to 98%. CT sensitivity is consistently between 85 and 95%. Reported ultrasound sensitivities are more variable, largely in the range of 75 to 90%, but with some centers reporting results as low as 44%. Operator dependence appears a more significant factor in ultrasound than in CT.

- There are undoubtedly multiple factors that may influence the choice of imaging modality. These include local ultrasound expertise, availability of skilled ultrasonographic personnel out of routine hours, diagnostic confidence of radiology residents and surgeons, financial considerations, and the radiation burden associated with CT. All will influence whether ultrasound is employed as the major diagnostic tool, with CT reserved for cases of persistent diagnostic uncertainty, or whether CT is utilized as the primary imaging modality.

- CT involves a relatively high radiation dose. If used as a screening method for the large number of children presenting with undiagnosed abdominal pain, the population radiation burden is considerable. The non-ionizing nature of ultrasound makes it the initial investigation of choice to many pediatric radiologists.

- Although imaging is undoubtedly useful in the management of children with suspected appendicitis, it should not be utilized in the absence of careful clinical assessment. Surgical liaison remains essential, and findings must be interpreted in conjunction with the patient's clinical status.

- Both ultrasound and CT are useful in providing supportive evidence for alternative differential diagnoses in children with lower abdominal pain, although CT may be less useful in genitourinary disease. Diagnoses to be considered include gastrointestinal pathologies (mesenteric adenitis, terminal ileitis, omental infarction, Henoch-Schönlein purpura), urinary tract pathology (pyelonephritis, cystitis, calculi), and gynecologic conditions (ovarian cyst torsion/rupture/hemorrhage, pelvic inflammatory disease, mittelschmerz).

PITFALLS_____

- Both ultrasound and CT are associated with false-negative and false-positive results.

- False-negative ultrasound may occur in retrocecal appendicitis, if inflammation is localized to the tip of the appendix or if perforation has recently occurred with decompression of the distended appendix but no organized collection. Severe pain preventing adequate compression or unfavorable body habitus is also a contributing factor. False-negative CT is less frequent but may occur if the inflamed appendix is not identified among small bowel loops or is mistaken for unopacified bowel, or if inflammatory change confined to the appendiceal tip is not appreciated.

- Both ultrasound and CT may be associated with false-positive results in ileocolitis with secondary inflammatory changes of the appendix, if normal terminal ileum is misinterpreted as the appendix, or from "overcalling" of a normal appendix. Most ultrasound and CT practitioners use a 6 mm diameter as the upper limit of a normal appendix, independent of patient age. However, there are undoubtedly a small number of patients in whom appendices several millimeters larger than this are identified in the absence of clinical symptoms, and therefore these must lie within the "normal" range.

- Both modalities are subject to the same limitations in symptomatic but "borderline" imaging cases—such as a 6 to 8 mm appendix but no or relatively minimal inflammatory signs—and clinical liaison is essential in these children. There is evidence that some cases of mild acute appendicitis may resolve spontaneously with or without antibiotic treatment, perhaps due to expulsion of a soft appendicolith from the lumen. Some of these patients suffer recurrent symptoms. However, for the purposes of diagnostic efficacy studies, they are classified as false-positive imaging results.

Suggested Readings

Birnbaum BA, Wilson SR. Appendicitis at the millenium. Radiology 2000;215:337–348

Hopkins KL, Patrick LE, Ball TI. Imaging findings of perforative appendicitis: a pictorial review. Pediatr Radiol 2001;31:173–179

Jamieson DH, Chait PG, Filler R. Interventional drainage of appendiceal abscesses in children. AJR Am J Roentgenol 1997;169:1619–1622

Kaiser S, Frenckner B, Jorulf HK. Suspected appendicitis in children: US and CT: a prospective randomised study. Radiology 2002;223:633–638

Puylaert JB. Acute appendicitis: US evaluation using graded compression. Radiology 1986;158: 355–360

Rao PM, Rhea JT, Novelline RA, Mostafan AA, McCabe CJ. Effect of computed tomography of the appendix on treatment of patients and use of hospital resources. N Engl J Med 1998;338:141–146

Sivit CJ, Siegel MJ, Applegate KE, Newman KD. When appendicitis is suspected in children. Radiographics 2001;21:247–262

CASE 65

Clinical Presentation

A 5-week-old boy presents to the emergency department with a 4-day history of nonbilious projectile vomiting.

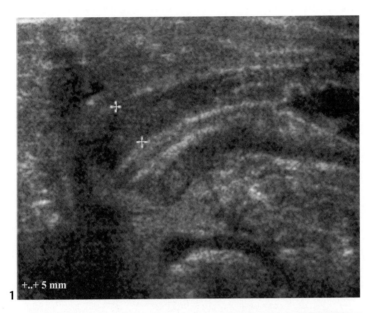

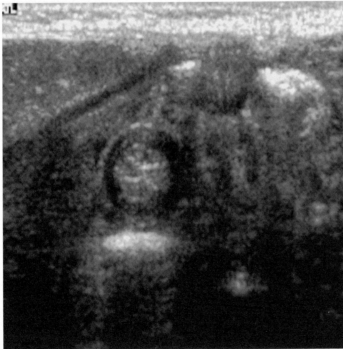

Figure 65A

Radiologic Findings

Longitudinal and transverse images of the pylorus (**Figs. 65A1** and **65A2**) demonstrate an elongated, thickened pylorus, with a muscle wall thickness of 5 mm. Fluid was seen within the gastric antrum, with no transit of gastric contents into the duodenum.

Diagnosis

Hypertrophic pyloric stenosis (HPS)

Differential Diagnosis

- Pylorospasm
- Other mechanical causes of gastric outlet obstruction (e.g., atresias/webs, prostaglandin-induced foveolar hyperplasia, eosinophilic gastroenteritis, extrinsic mass lesions, annular pancreas)
- Gastroesophageal reflux
- Metabolic and infectious causes of vomiting (clinical findings)

Discussion

Background

HPS is an acquired hypertrophy of the circular muscle of the pylorus, causing progressive gastric outlet obstruction, It occurs with an incidence of ~3 per 1000 live births. There is an increased incidence in boys (male:female 4:1), first-born children, and Caucasian race. Some cases show a strong familial tendency.

Etiology

The etiology remains largely unknown, although abnormal innervation to the circular muscle has been implicated.

Clinical Findings

Classically, infants present between 2 and 6 weeks of life with projectile nonbilious vomiting occurring 10 to 20 minutes after feeding. Occasional cases as early as the first week of life and as late as 5 months have been described. Infants fail to thrive and may become dehydrated. The classic metabolic abnormality of hypokalemic hypochloremic alkalosis is now rare. On clinical examination, gastric peristaltic activity may be seen and a palpable small mass, the "olive," may be felt in the right upper quadrant, although earlier diagnosis has reduced the incidence of this finding over the past 2 decades.

Pathology

- A pale fusiform muscle mass is seen macroscopically with a clear transition to normal gut wall distally.
- The muscle mass comprises mainly circular muscle fibers, but all layers are involved.
- Secondary mucosal changes of edema or ulceration can occur in long-standing cases.

Imaging Findings

ULTRASOUND

- Ultrasound has replaced the upper gastrointestinal (GI) study as the first-line investigation for infants with nonbilious vomiting. It is a quick, non-ionizing investigation that is both highly specific and sensitive.
- The infant is positioned in the left anterior oblique position and scanned over the epigastrium with both linear high-frequency and curvilinear transducers.

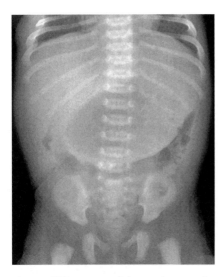

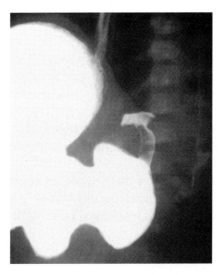

Figure 65B Supine abdominal x-ray of a 16-day-old infant demonstrating a distended air-filled stomach with relative paucity of gas distally.

Figure 65C Upper GI study demonstrating an elongated pyloric canal, concave superiorly, with a double-track appearance and shouldering at the duodenal bulb.

- A fluid-filled gastric antrum (unless a nasogastric tube has been placed) and hyperperistaltic waves are seen.
- The hypertrophied pylorus is generally hypoechoic to the adjacent liver, with a double line of hyperechoic mucosa seen centrally. Measurements of muscle width and canal length are obtained. Overreliance on absolute measurements should be avoided (especially in infants born prematurely). but a muscle width >3 to 3.5 mm and length >16 mm are usually taken as diagnostic of HPS. Measurements of muscle width <2 mm and length <14 mm are taken as normal.
- Observation of gastric outlet function is equally important. A hyperperistaltic antrum with diminished passage of gastric contents into the duodenum is strong supportive evidence in cases with intermediate measurements.

RADIOGRAPHY

- Rarely required, but will demonstrate a distended air-filled stomach with a relative paucity of gas distally (**Fig. 65B**)

UPPER GI STUDY

- Delayed gastric emptying with eventual passage of barium into an elongated, curved pyloric canal, concave superiorly (**Fig. 65C**)
- The soft tissue mass of hypertrophied muscle indents the antrum and duodenal bulb (shouldering), antral hyperdynamic peristalsis results in the "pyloric tit," and a "double-track" appearance of the pyloric canal is seen.
- Gastroesophageal reflux, with or without a hiatal hernia, is commonly demonstrated, likely secondary to gastric outlet obstruction.

Treatment

- Nasogastric drainage, intravenous rehydration, and correction of any acid–base imbalance
- Ramstedt's pyloromyotomy with incision of the hypertrophied muscle almost to the level of the mucosa. This may now be performed endoscopically.

Prognosis

- Most babies make a quick, uneventful recovery.
- Vomiting in the first 24 hours postoperatively may occur, perhaps due to preoperative gastritis.
- If vomiting is persistent, then incomplete pyloromyotomy should be considered. Evidence of ongoing gastric outlet obstruction such as hyperperistalsis and failure of passage of gastric contents into the duodenum may be demonstrated on ultrasound or upper GI study. The morphologic appearance of the pylorus is less useful, as it remains thickened even after successful pyloromyotomy for several weeks. Return to normal morphology occurs over 6 weeks to 6 months.
- Rare postoperative complications include duodenal perforation.
- Long-term follow-up shows normal overall gastric emptying in subjects having undergone pyloromyotomy as infants, although pyloric tone is higher and the amplitude of pyloric pressure waves reduced.

PEARL

- Premature infants present at an appropriate interval after birth. Pyloric measurements need to be adjusted for the patient's weight and are smaller than those given above. Correlation should be made with supportive signs of gastric outlet obstruction on ultrasound and clinical findings.

PITFALLS

- Overdistension of the stomach can result in posterior displacement of the pylorus and difficulties in visualization. Placement of a nasogastric tube and evacuation of the gastric contents will remedy this.
- Intermediate measurements of 2 to 3 mm pyloric muscle width can be seen in pyloric spasm. However, continued dynamic observation of the pylorus on ultrasound or fluoroscopy will reveal relaxation and opening with passage of gastric contents into the duodenum. The differential diagnosis is early HPS, and if there is persistent clinical suspicion, repeat ultrasound should be performed.

Suggested Readings

Haider N, Spicer R, Grier D. Ultrasound diagnosis of infantile hypertrophic pyloric stenosis: determinants of pyloric length and the effect of prematurity. Clin Radiol 2002;57:136–139

O'Keeffe FN, Stansberry SD, Swischuk LE, Hayden CK Jr. Antropyloric muscle thickness at US in infants: what is normal? Radiology 1991;178:827–830

Papadakis K, Chen EA, Luks FI, et al. The changing presentation of pyloric stenosis. Am J Emerg Med 1999;17:67–69

Sauerbrei EE, Paloshi GGB. The ultrasonic features of hypertrophic pyloric stenosis, with emphasis on the post-operative appearance. Radiology 1983;147:503–506

Stunden RJ, LeQuesne GW, Little KET. The improved ultrasound diagnosis of hypertrophic pyloric stenosis. Pediatr Radiol 1986;16:200–205

Sun WM, Doran SM, Jones KL, et al. Long-term effects of pyloromyotomy on pyloric motility and gastric emptying in humans. Am J Gastroenterol 2000;95:92–100

CASE 66

Clinical Presentation

A neonate born to a diabetic mother presents with hypoglycemia and hypertension.

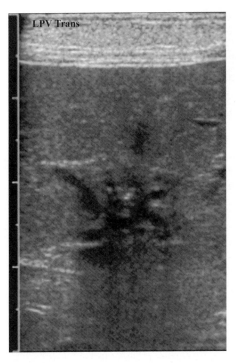

Figure 66A

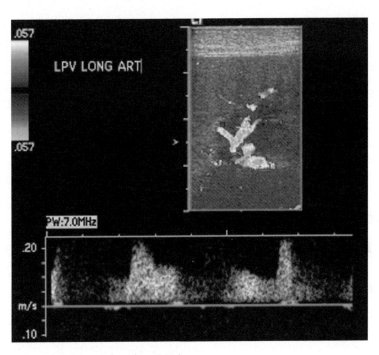

Figure 66B (See Color Plate 66B.)

Radiologic Findings

Ultrasonography shows an echogenic thrombus within the left portal vein (**Fig. 66A**), which is occluded. Patency of the left hepatic artery (**Fig. 66B**) is noted. The left hepatic artery flow was prominent compared with the right hepatic artery.

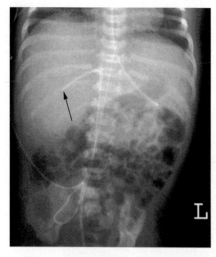

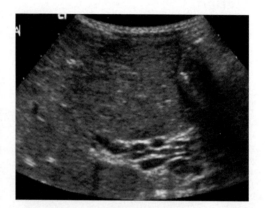

Figure 66C Abdominal radiograph of a newborn showing the tip of the umbilical vein catheter projecting in the region of the right portal vein (arrow).

Figure 66D Axial image at the level of the porta hepatis demonstrates multiple anechoic areas of vascular origin on ultrasound representing cavernous transformation of the portal vein.

Diagnosis

Thrombosis of the left portal vein

Differential Diagnosis

- Acute portal vein thrombosis:
  - Umbilical vein catheterization
  - Underlying clotting anomalies including antithrombin III deficiency and protein C or S deficiency, antiphospholipid antibody syndrome
  - Pylephlebitis complicating an intra-abdominal inflammation (appendicitis, pancreatitis)
- Chronic portal vein thrombosis:
  - Idiopathic
  - Sequelae of omphalitis or umbilical vein catheterization in newborns
  - Portal hypertension (prehepatic)
- Different conditions:
  - Veno-occlusive disease (hepatic block)
  - Congenital absence of portal vein

Discussion

Background

Portal venous thrombosis is the major cause of extrahepatic portal hypertension and gastrointestinal bleeding in children. Umbilical vein catheterization, commonly used in neonatal intensive care units, is a major cause of portal venous thrombosis (**Fig. 66C**). Thrombosis may only be detected later in life when established collateral venous circulation, including gastroesophageal varices and cavernous transformation of the portal vein, have already occurred.

Etiology

Portal vein thrombosis is frequently associated with prolonged placement of an umbilical vein catheter. Risk factors include low birth weight, reduced blood flow, hypoxia, and hypercoagulability

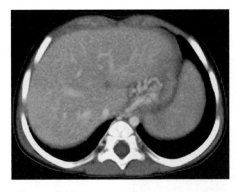

Figure 66E CT demonstrating varices along the lesser curvature of the stomach in a child with splenomegaly.

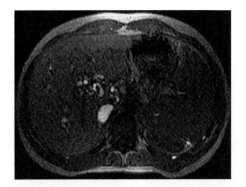

Figure 66F Preoperative MR venography (2D time-of-flight) of cavernous transformation of portal vein in a patient with splenomegaly, under consideration for placement of a portomesenteric shunt.

disorder. Malposition of the catheter in the left portal vein is most problematic, with the umbilico-portal confluence (space of Rex) being the main site of thrombosis. Spontaneous resolution is the usual outcome.

Clinical Findings

The signs and symptoms are insidious and include abdominal pain, abdominal distension, ascites, and splenomegaly. Chronic thrombosis will be evident with hematemesis due to esophageal varices as well as hemorrhoids, ascites, and signs of hypersplenism.

Complications

- Development of collateral circulation of portal hypertension:
  - Cavernous transformation of portal vein (**Fig. 66D**)
  - Varices: esophageal fundal (**Fig. 66E**), mesenterohepatic collaterals
  - Upper gastrointestinal bleeding
- Splenomegaly

Pathology

- Nonocclusive thrombosis attached to catheter
- With main portal vein obstruction, development of cavernous transformation of the portal vein, dilatation of patent paraumbilical vein, portosystemic, splenohepatic, and mesenterohepatic collaterals
- Increase of hepatic arterial flow may be seen in the area of reduced portal flow.
- Chronic perfusion deficit can lead to regional fatty infiltration.

Imaging Findings

RADIOGRAPHY

- Malposition of umbilical vein catheter projecting over one branch of portal vein (**Fig. 66C**)
- Location of catheter tip at liver level
- Rarely, calcific thrombus can be seen.

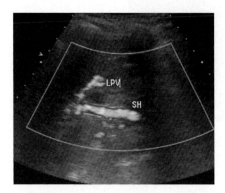

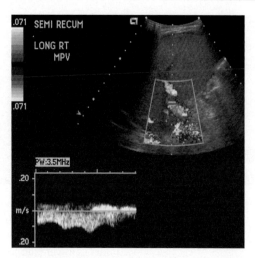

Figure 66G (Same patient as in **Fig. 66F**) Color Doppler ultrasound assessment demonstrating patency of a newly placed portomesenteric shunt (SH). LPV, left portal vein. (See Color Plate 66G.)

Figure 66H Differential diagnosis: Hepatofugal portal flow demonstrated on Doppler ultrasound in a patient with veno-occlusive disease following bone marrow transplant. (See Color Plate 66H.)

ULTRASOUND

- Ultrasound monitoring allows early detection of thrombi.
- Echogenic thrombus may be seen in the lumen of the umbilical vein extending into a branch of portal vein or ductus venosus.
- Dilatation of the involved intrahepatic portal vein branch may be seen.
- Characteristic appearance of cavernous transformation of portal vein (**Fig. 66D**).

DOPPLER ULTRASOUND

- Color/duplex Doppler can assess whether the occlusion is complete or partial.
- Loss of respiratory variation of hepatopetal flow, then flow reversal
- Portal vein pulsatility with arterial systole seen in severe cases
- Prominence of hepatic artery flow (**Fig. 66B**)
- Focal hepatic lesions (anechoic or heterogeneous suspicious for focal liver abscess)

CT

- Calcified thrombus (chronic)
- Focal hepatic infarction as hypodense area
- Signs of portal hypertension (esophageal, paravertebral varices) (**Fig. 66E**)
- Cavernous transformation of portal vein, at porta hepatis, with network of serpiginous vessels
- Focal hyperattenuation in the liver related to arterial hyperperfusion
- Varices in gallbladder wall, atrophy of the affected liver area (usually left lobe) with compensatory hypertrophy of caudate lobe
- Hepatic abscess with peripheral enhancement
- Ascites, splenomegaly

MRI

- Used less often than ultrasound or CT (**Fig. 66F**)
- Gradient echo sequences identify vascular patency.
- Spatial presaturation helps to characterize the direction of blood flow.
- MR angiography can be helpful in pre- and postoperative assessment of surgical portosystemic shunting.

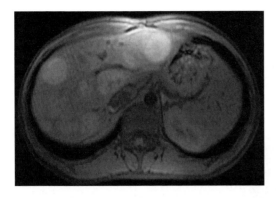

Figure 66I Differential diagnosis: Congenital absence of the portal vein. Axial MRI (spoiled gradient recall echo [SPGR] in phase) of the liver delineating multiple foci of focal nodular hyperplasia and abnormal hepatic venous anatomy with absence of the portal vein.

Treatment

- Acute thrombosis:
  - ○ Prophylactic use of heparin, thrombolytic therapy such as regional streptokinase infusion for extensive portal vein thrombus
  - ○ Medical supportive therapy
  - ○ Removal of catheter as soon as possible after detection of thrombus is the best strategy.
- Chronic thrombosis:
  - ○ Management of portal hypertension: sclerotherapy of esophageal varices, venous shunting (portocaval, mesocaval, splenorenal, mesenteric) (**Fig. 66G**)

PEARLS_____

- Catheterization of the umbilical vein is a major cause of portal vein thrombosis.
- Portal vein thrombosis is a major cause of extrahepatic portal hypertension and gastrointestinal bleeding in children.
- Controlling catheter location so it does not terminate in liver or using a smaller catheter lowers the incidence of thrombosis.

PITFALLS_____

- Hepatofugal portal vein flow can be seen in hepatic veno-occlusive disease in an acute setting (bone marrow transplant) (**Fig. 66H**).
- Congenital absence of portal vein is rare but can mimic portal vein thrombosis (**Fig. 66I**).
- Portal vein pulsatility with arterial systole on Doppler ultrasound can also be seen in congestive heart failure and tricuspid regurgitation.

Suggested Readings

Gallego C, Velasco M, Marcuello P, et al. Congenital and acquired anomalies of the portal venous system. Radiographics 2002;22:141–159

Kaushik S, Federle MP, Schur PH, et al. Abdominal thrombotic and ischemic manifestations of the antiphospholipid antibody syndrome: CT findings in 42 patients. Radiology 2001;218:768–771

Kim JH, Lee YS, Kim SH, et al. Does umbilical vein catheterization lead to portal venous thrombosis? Prospective US evaluation in 100 neonates. Radiology 2001;219:645–650

Wachsberg RH, Bahramipour P, Sofocleous CT, Barone A. Hepatofugal flow in the portal venous system: pathophysiology, imaging findings, and diagnostic pitfalls. Radiographics 2002;22:123–140

CASE 67

Clinical Presentation

A 2½-year-old boy was followed since prenatal ultrasonographic diagnosis of abdominal abnormalities.

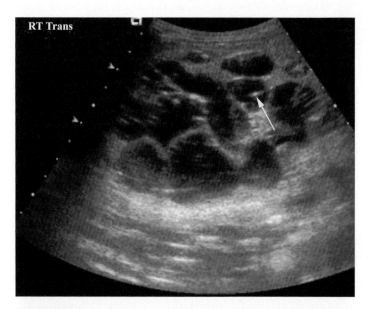

Figure 67A

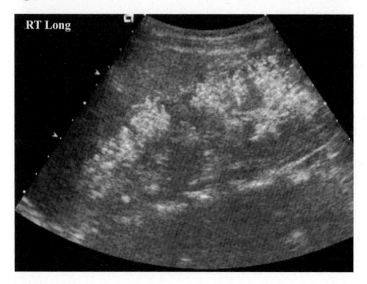

Figure 67B

Radiologic Findings

Ultrasonographic examination (transverse scan of the liver) shows extensive saccular dilatation of intrahepatic biliary tree with the "dot sign" (**Fig. 67A**, arrow). Renal enlargement (14.7 cm long) with hyperechoic parenchyma is noted (**Fig. 67B**).

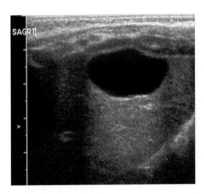

Figure 67C Differential diagnosis: simple liver cyst on routine ultrasound of an infant.

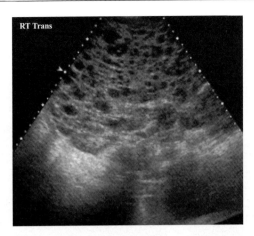

Figure 67D Differential diagnosis: extensive hepatic involvement on ultrasound of a 16-year-old girl with abdominal lymphangioma.

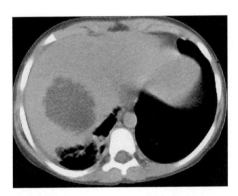

Figure 67E Differential diagnosis: CT of amebic abscess of liver dome in a child with cough and febrile illness.

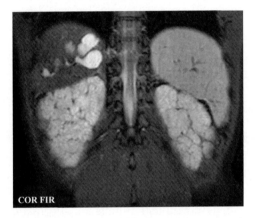

Figure 67F Coronal MRI (inversion recovery) demonstrating saccular dilatation with high signal intensity within the liver from Caroli's disease. There also is bilateral renal enlargement of autosomal recessive polycystic kidney disease.

Diagnosis

Caroli's disease

Differential Diagnosis

- Recurrent pyogenic cholangitis
- Primary sclerosing cholangitis
- Biliary tract obstruction
- Mesenchymal hamartoma of the liver
- Developmental hepatic cyst (**Fig. 67C**)
- Dysontogenetic cyst
- Lymphangioma of liver (**Fig. 67D**)
- Liver abscess (amebic) (**Fig. 67E**)
- Hydatid cyst (*Echinococcus granulosus*)

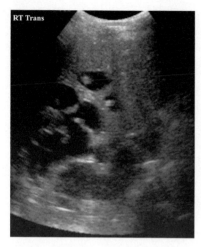

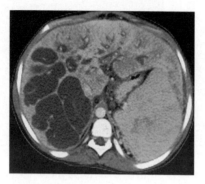

Figure 67G Sonogram of a 12-year-old patient with gastrointestinal bleeding, splenomegaly, and congenital cystic renal disease. The dot sign is pathognomonic of Caroli's disease.

Figure 67H (Same patient as in **Fig. 67G**) CT target sign, a constant feature. The right liver lobe is more severely involved.

Discussion

Background

Caroli's disease, also referred to as communicating cavernous ectasia of the intrahepatic bile ducts, is a congenital disease of an autosomal recessive type. This saccular dilatation of the intrahepatic biliary tree results from a complete or partial arrest of remodeling of the ductal plate, the hepatic precursor cells, which surround the portal venous network. There are two forms of Caroli's disease. The rare *simple form*, described by Caroli, is a malformation involving the ductal plate of central bile ducts. The *second form* is the periportal fibrosis type with ductal plate maldevelopment extending from the central to the smaller peripheral bile ducts. This is usually associated with renal cystic disease, most often, renal tubular ectasia, and also recessive polycystic renal disease (**Fig. 67F**).

Clinical Findings

The simple form typically presents with pain without jaundice and frequent episodes of infection. The periportal fibrosis type is characterized by hepatosplenomegaly and episodes of gastrointestinal bleeding related to variceal hemorrhage, due to portal hypertension. Infection is also part of its clinical features.

Complications

- The simple form is subject to bile stasis, intraductal calculi formation, cholangitis, and hepatic abscesses.
- The periportal fibrosis form manifests by cirrhosis, upper gastrointestinal bleeding, and portal hypertension.
- Chronic renal failure

Pathology

- Saccular dilatation of segmental bile ducts is the main finding.
- Normal liver parenchyma is observed in the simple form.
- The second form has additional features of proliferation of the bile ductules and fibrosis.

Imaging Findings

ULTRASOUND

- Dilatation of segmental intrahepatic bile ducts
- Echogenic septa (intraductal bridging) traverse the lumen of dilated ducts.
- Small portal vein branches are surrounded by the dilated ducts giving rise to the dot sign (**Figs. 67A** and **67G**).
- There may be:
  ○ Characteristic renal enlargement (**Fig. 67B**)
  ○ Hyperechogenicity of renal parenchyma (**Fig. 67B**)
  ○ Renal tubular ectasia with calculi (also seen on nonenhanced CT)
  ○ Renal medulla with cysts

CT

- Dilatation of bile ducts along portal vessels, directed toward the porta hepatis (**Fig. 67H**)
- Saccular appearance of the ducts that communicate with the biliary system
- The central dot sign refers to the portal vein branches, surrounded by the dilated duct.
- Sludge or calculi can be identified in the ducts.

CHOLANGIOGRAPHY

- This examination is via percutaneous transhepatic approach or via endoscopic retrograde cholangiopancreatography.
- Demonstration of the intrahepatic biliary dilatation
- In 50% of cases, there is also a fusiform distention of the extrahepatic bile tree.
- Segmental involvement, more frequently in right lobe of liver
- A beading cholangiographic pattern can be visualized.

MAGNETIC RESONANCE CHOLANGIOPANCREATOGRAPHY

- Noninvasive method to delineate the appearance and location of the saccular biliary dilatation (**Fig. 67F**)

Treatment

- External biliary drainage or biliary enteric anastomosis. These methods do not prevent cholangitis or persistent biliary dilatation.
- Hepatic lobectomy or segmentectomy in case of focal disease
- Extracorporeal shock wave lithotripsy
- Hepatic transplantation

Prognosis

- Poor long-term prognosis due to occurrence of cholangitis, cirrhosis, and portal hypertension
- Higher incidence of cholangiocarcinoma

PEARLS_____

- Although Caroli's disease is often classified as a type of choledochal cyst, it represents a different underlying etiology.
- The large intrahepatic bile ducts involvement determines Caroli's disease.
- Small interlobular duct involvement leads to congenital hepatic fibrosis.
- Caroli's syndrome is the combination of the two entities (Caroli's disease and congenital hepatic fibrosis).

PITFALL

- Recurrent pyogenic cholangitis is the most difficult differential diagnosis.

Suggested Readings

Fulcher AS, Turner MA, Sanyal AJ. Case 38: Caroli disease and renal tubular ectasia. Radiology 2001;220:720–723

Levy AD, Rohrmann CA Jr, Murakata LA, Lonergan GJ. Caroli's disease: radiologic spectrum with pathologic correlation. AJR Am J Roentgenol 2002;179:1053–1057

Mortele KJ, Ros PR. Cystic focal liver lesions in the adult: differential CT and MR imaging features. Radiographics 2001;21:895–910

Sherlock S. Cystic diseases of the liver. In: Schiff ER, Sorrell MF, Maddrey WC, eds. Schiff's Diseases of the Liver. 8th ed. Philadelphia: Lippincott; 1999:1083–1090

CASE 68

Clinical Presentation

A 1-month-old infant presents with tachypnea associated with decreased oxygen saturation.

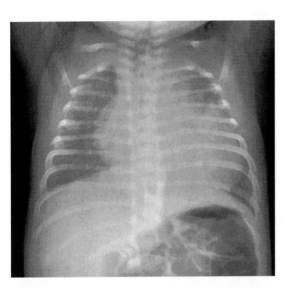

Figure 68A

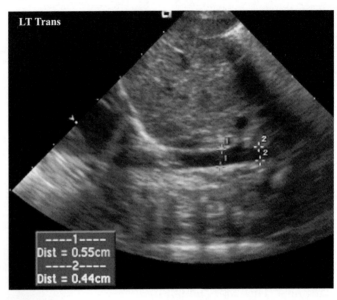

Figure 68B

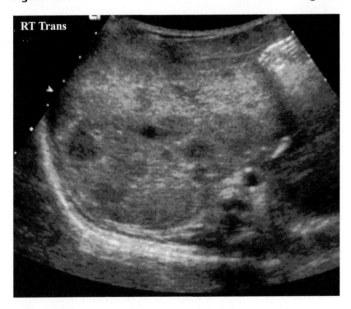

Figure 68C

Radiologic Findings

An AP chest radiograph demonstrates cardiac enlargement (**Fig. 68A**). A longitudinal ultrasonogram shows a smaller caliber of the aorta below the celiac level (**Fig. 68B**). On transverse view, the liver is occupied by multiple round hypoechoic areas (**Fig. 68C**).

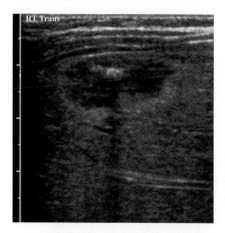

Figure 68D Differential diagnosis: hemangioma with a focal right lobe mass with central calcification.

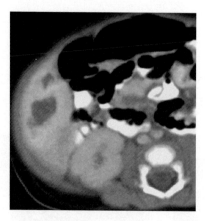

Figure 68E Differential diagnosis: The CT image shows a typical enhancement pattern of hemangioma at early scanning.

Diagnosis

Infantile hemangioendothelioma of the liver

Differential Diagnosis

- Hemangioma (**Figs. 68D** and **68E**)
- Arteriovenous malformation of the liver (**Fig. 68F**)
- Rhabdomyosarcoma of the biliary tree
- Metastatic disease, especially neuroblastoma

Discussion

Background

A rare entity, hemangioendothelioma is the most common benign hepatic tumor and is seen primarily in young infants (95% of cases <1 year of age). This vascular lesion acts as an arteriovenous fistula. It is twice as common in girls. Fifty percent of patients have associated skin hemangiomas.

Clinical Findings

Most affected infants present with congestive heart failure due to high cardiac output during the first 6 months of life. Asymptomatic hepatomegaly, jaundice, anemia, and hemoperitoneum (due to rupture) occur less commonly. A loud systolic bruit may be heard over the liver. Severe arteriovenous shunting may induce fetal hydrops. Serum a-fetoprotein level is typically mildly elevated. Spontaneous involution is observed in small lesions.

Complications

- Congestive heart failure from severe arteriovenous shunting has a 75% mortality rate if untreated.
- Kasabach-Merritt syndrome is an ominous bleeding diathesis due to platelet sequestration with thrombocytopenia and disseminated intravascular coagulopathy.

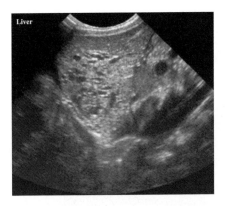

Figure 68F Differential diagnosis: hepatic arteriovenous malformation on ultrasound in a patient with cutaneous hemangiomas and congestive heart failure.

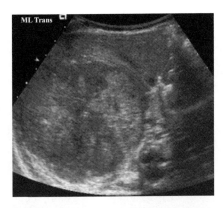

Figure 68G Two-month-old infant with hepatomegaly. Ultrasound shows large heterogeneous mass of hemangioendothelioma in the right lobe.

Gross Pathology

- Single or multiple nodules from a few millimeters to 20 cm in diameter
- Variable appearance, cystic/solid with foci of hemorrhage, hypervascular areas, and fibrosis
- Pseudocapsule made by compressed normal hepatic tissue

Histology

- Type 1: dilated vascular channels lined by plump epithelial benign cells
- Type 2: irregularly branched vascular channels lined by tufted pleomorphic endothelial cells with papillary structures building into the vessels. These type 2 lesions may resemble angiosarcoma.

Imaging Findings

RADIOGRAPHY

- Calcifications

ULTRASOUND

- Typical features of a well-circumscribed solid mass of heterogeneous echo texture. Internal calcifications are occasional (**Fig. 68G**).
- Anechoic zones representing vascular channels, identifiable on color Doppler, which demonstrates increased intratumoral vascularity.
- Enlarged hepatic artery and proximal abdominal aorta
- Multiple lesions scattered in liver parenchyma

CT

- Well-circumscribed mass (**Fig. 68H**), with early peripheral enhancement (**Fig. 68I**)
- Central enhancement can be homogeneous or patchy (hemorrhage/infarct).
- Multifocal hyperattenuation of liver on enhanced CT in case of multiple lesions

MRI

- Typically, high signal intensity on T2-weighted images; however, fibrosis may give decreased signal intensity on T2-weighted images.
- Decreased signal intensity on T1-weighted images, except at sites of calcification or hemorrhage.
- Flow void zones of high blood flow

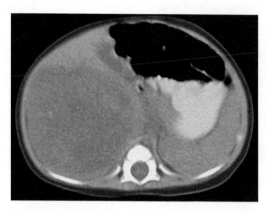

Figure 68H (Same patient as in **Fig. 68G**) Nonenhanced CT image shows the extent of the mass in the right lobe.

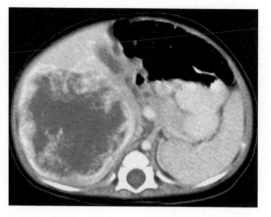

Figure 68I (Same patient as **Fig. 68G**) Early peripheral enhancement demonstrated on CT.

ANGIOGRAPHY

- Indicated when intervention is needed based on CT findings and/or lack of response to medical therapy
- Tortuous dilated hepatic artery
- Early hepatic vein filling
- Extrahepatic collateral arterial supply from superior mesenteric artery, intercostal arteries, and phrenic artery
- Nodule enhancement at parenchymal phase

Treatment

- Observation in small lesions for spontaneous involution
- Medical therapy of congestive heart failure (diuretics and digitalis)
- High-dose steroids to stimulate regression of hemangioendothelioma
- Interferon a2a, an antiangiogenesis factor, used to inhibit endothelial cell migration and proliferation
- Radiotherapy/chemotherapy (cyclophosphamide/adriamycin)
- Embolization of feeding arteries (hepatic necrosis risk related to portal venous supply to the lesion)
- Hepatectomy/orthotopic liver transplantation

Prognosis

- Spontaneous involution over a period of 8 to 12 months following initial phase of proliferation of 6 months
- In asymptomatic forms, no therapy is needed.
- In those untreated, congestive heart failure has a high mortality rate.

PEARL_____

- Ninety-five percent of liver hemangioendotheliomas present in the first year of life.

- Hypervascular hepatoblastoma can mimic hemangioendothelioma, which may lead to medical mismanagement.

Suggested Readings

Daller JA, Bueno J, Gutierrez J, et al. Hepatic hemangioendothelioma: clinical experience and management strategy. J Pediatr Surg 1999;34:98–106

Fellows KE, Hoffer FA, Markowitz RI, O'Neille JA Jr. Multiple collaterals to hepatic infantile hemangioendotheliomas and arteriovenous malformations: effect on embolization. Radiology 1991;181: 813–818

Keslar PJ, Buck JL, Selby DM. From the archives of the AFIP: infantile hemangioendothelioma of the liver revisited. Radiographics 1993;13:657–670

CASE 69

Clinical Presentation

An 8-year-old boy presents with abdominal pain.

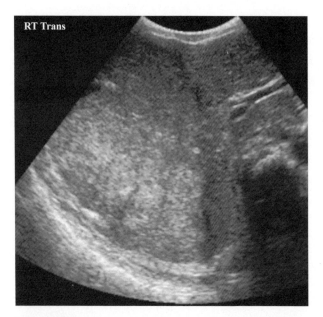

Figure 69A

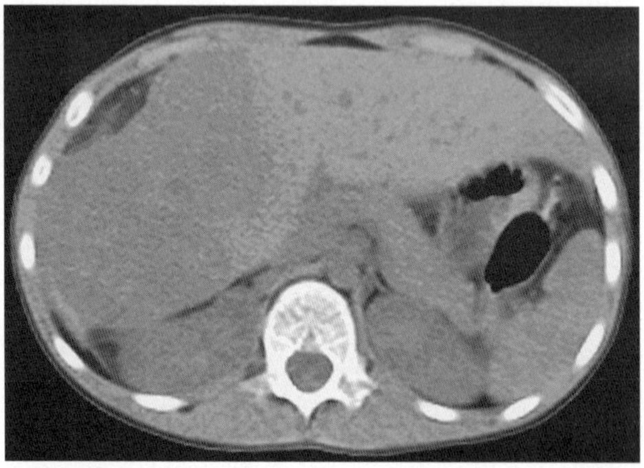

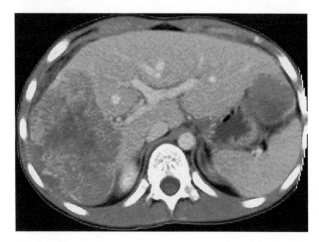

Figure 69B

Figure 69C

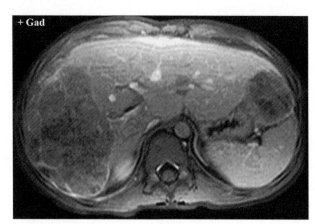

Figure 69D

Radiologic Findings

A large echogenic mass, poorly marginated, is noted in the right lobe of the liver on ultrasonography (**Fig. 69A**). A heterogeneous mass without calcification is shown on nonenhanced CT (**Fig. 69B**). Following contrast administration, peripheral enhancement of two lesions, one in the right lobe and one in the left lobe (**Fig. 69C**), is noted. The corresponding delayed T1-weighted fat suppressed MRI postgadolinium reveals heterogeneous signal of the masses, which are not hypervascular (**Fig. 69D**).

Diagnosis

Hepatoblastoma

Differential Diagnosis

- Hepatocellular carcinoma
- Infantile hemangioendothelioma
- Fibrolamellar hepatocellular carcinoma (age >5 years)
- Mesenchymal hamartoma
- Rhabdomyosarcoma of the biliary tract
- Metastatic disease, especially from neuroblastoma

Discussion

Background

Hepatoblastoma is the most common pediatric hepatic malignancy (>50%) and is most prevalent in children <3 years of age.

Etiology

Male to female ratio is 1.2–3.3:1. An increased incidence has been reported in Beckwith-Wiedemann syndrome, hemihypertrophy, familial adenomatous polypi, glycogen storage disease, Wilms' tumor, Gardner's syndrome, and fetal alcohol syndrome. Low birth weight is associated with a higher risk for hepatoblastoma.

Molecular Biology

Cytogenetic abnormalities have been noted with mainly abnormalities of chromosome 20, and a recurring aberration der (4) t (1q;4q). Alteration in the adenomatous polyposis coli (APC) gene and the b-catenin pathway are implicated in the pathogenesis of hepatoblastoma. Changes in the expression of *H19* and *IGF2* genes have also been found.

Clinical Findings

An asymptomatic mass is the most common mode of presentation. Anorexia, weight loss, jaundice, and abdominal pain can also be observed. Precocious puberty (related to chorionic gonadotropin secretion) has been described. Osteopenia is frequent. Serum a-fetoprotein levels (AFP) are increased in up to 90% of patients. Thrombocytosis is commonly reported. The right liver lobe is more frequently involved than the left (3:1 ratio). Bilobar location is seen in 20 to 30% of cases, and the disease can be multicentric. Persistence or recurrence of elevated AFP is a sensitive marker of the disease.

Complications

- Metastases at diagnosis in up to 20% of cases
- Porta hepatis, lung metastases
- Distant spread to brain and skeleton
- Intra-operative complications include hemorrhage and damage to hepatic vessels and ducts.
- Postoperative complications include subphrenic abscess, bile leak, and small bowel obstruction.

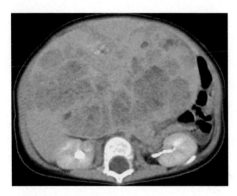

Figure 69E Hepatoblastoma stage IV. Enhanced CT showing heterogeneous density and calcifications.

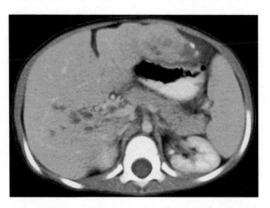

Figure 69F CT of bilobar hepatoblastoma with portal vein thrombosis, cavernous transformation of portal vein. Patient underwent liver transplantation.

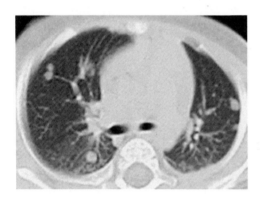

Figure 69G (Same patient as in **Fig. 69E**) CT showing multiple lung metastases.

Pathology/Histology

- Epithelial form: with the following subtypes:
  - Fetal, embryonal
  - Macrotrabecular
  - Small cell undifferentiated
- Mixed epithelial/mesenchymal form:
  - The most common mesenchymal elements are cartilage and osteoid.
- Pure fetal histology confers a better prognosis, whereas undifferentiated histology is related to poor outcome.

Imaging Findings

ULTRASOUND

- Should include color Doppler evaluation
- Helps locate the mass, defines its relationships with the portal and hepatic veins, and guides percutaneous biopsy
- The mass is solid (**Fig. 69A**), often with calcifications.
- Hemorrhagic necrosis in the center of the mass after chemotherapy

CT

- Used for initial staging of the tumor and to assess resectability (**Figs. 69B** and **69E**), also used to monitor response to preoperative chemotherapy and to assess tumor recurrence (**Fig. 69F**)
- Enhanced CT (spiral) at late arterial (**Fig. 69F**)/early portal phases is most optimal because the mass is not very hypervascular.
- CT should include evaluation of the lungs for metastases (**Fig. 69G**).

MRI

- Variable appearance showing solitary or multifocal or infiltrating mass (**Fig. 69D**)
- Vascular anatomy can be delineated on MR or CT.
- Portal venous invasion/compression may result in thrombosis with cavernous transformation.
- Typically, hypointense liver signal on T1-weighted images and hyperintense on T2-weighted images.
- Heterogeneity of the mass due to hemorrhage, fat necrosis

Staging

- Staging (four stages) relies on surgical exploration to assess spread of tumor and to ensure completeness of resection.
- Resectability of primary tumor does not influence staging when metastases (stage IV) are present.

Treatment

- Complete surgical excision is curative.
- Chemotherapy:
  - Shrinkage postchemotherapy allows easier resection.
  - Reason for nonresectability includes:
    - Large tumor (excessive bleeding)
    - Involvement of major hepatic veins, portal vein, inferior vena cava (**Fig. 69F**)
    - Bilobar, or multifocal disease (**Fig. 69D**)
- Failure of AFP to return to normal level dictates reevaluation for recurrence and metastases.
- Liver transplantation: an option for unresectable tumor or after local recurrence
- Aggressive approach at excision of lung metastases can lead to long-term survival.

Prognosis

- Fetal histology, preoperative chemotherapy, aggressive therapy of metastases—all improve prognosis.
- Nonresectable and recurrent disease carry a poor prognosis.
- Overall 2-year survival is 65%.

PEARLS_____

- Hepatoblastoma predominates in children <3 years of age, whereas hepatocellular carcinoma occurs in children >4 years of age.
- Ultrasound is good at assessing the vascular involvement, whereas CT/MRI define the extent of disease.
- Primary therapy is surgical resection, but chemotherapy increases the number of resectable tumors.

PITFALLS_____

- Presentation with congestive heart failure may lead to an unsuccessful therapy aimed at hemangioendothelioma, whereas diagnosis of hepatoblastoma is made on pathology specimen.
- AFP can be elevated, although usually not to such high levels as seen in hepatoblastoma, in the absence of demonstrable tumor, and in tyrosinemia as well as ataxia-telangiectasia.

Suggested Readings

Arcement CM, Towbin RB, Meza MP, et al. Intrahepatic chemoembolization in unresectable pediatric liver malignancies. Pediatr Radiol 2000;30:779–785

Boechat MI, Kangarloo H, Gilsanz V. Hepatic masses in children. Semin Roentgenol 1988;23:185–193

Finegold MJ. Liver tumors. Chapter 58. In: Walker WA, Durie PR, Hamilton JR, Walker-Smith JA, Watkins JB, eds. Pediatric Gastrointestinal Disease, Pathophysiology, Diagnosis and Management. 3rd ed. Hamilton, ON: BC Decker; 2000:1033–1047

Ingram JD, Yerushalmi B, Connell J, et al. Hepatoblastoma in a neonate: a hypervascular presentation mimicking hemangioendothelioma. Pediatr Radiol 2000;30:794–797

Powers C, Ros PR, Stoupis C, Johnson WK, Segel KH. Primary liver neoplasms: MR imaging with pathologic correlation. Radiographics 1994;14:459–482

CASE 70

Clinical Presentation

A 2-week-old neonate presents with jaundice (conjugated hyperbilirubinemia).

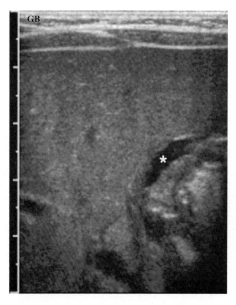

Figure 70A

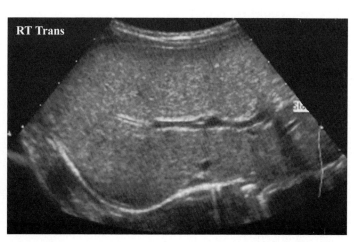

Figure 70B

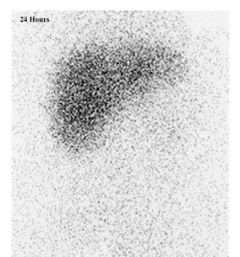

Figure 70C

Radiologic Findings

Small size of gallbladder (**Fig. 70A**, seen as *) and area of increased echogenicity at porta hepatis but no dilatation of bile ducts on ultrasonography (**Fig. 70B**). Hepatic iminodiacetic acid (HIDA) scan shows adequate hepatocyte uptake but no excretion in bowel by 24 hours (**Fig. 70C**).

Diagnosis

Biliary atresia

Differential Diagnosis

Neonatal cholestasis may result from a wide variety of etiologies. In up to 80% of the cases, the primary differential is idiopathic neonatal hepatitis versus biliary atresia.

- Anatomic anomalies:
  - Extrahepatic:
    - Biliary atresia
    - Choledochal cyst
  - Intrahepatic:
    - Idiopathic neonatal hepatitis
    - Bile duct paucity:
      - Syndromic (Alagille syndrome)
      - Nonsyndromic
- Metabolic diseases:
  - a1 antitrypsin deficiency
  - Tyrosinemia
  - Galactosemia
  - Cystic fibrosis
  - Glycogenosis type IV
- Hepatitis:
  - Septicemia
  - TORCH (toxoplasmosis, rubella, cytomegalovirus, herpes) infections
  - Total parenteral nutrition
- Miscellaneous:
  - Histiocytosis
  - Trisomy 8, 13, 21
  - Hemolysis

Discussion

Background

Biliary atresia is a condition that is initiated by the disruption of the normal extrahepatic biliary system. Biliary atresia is characterized by the destruction or absence of portions of the biliary system at a point(s) between the duodenum and the liver. Progressive damage of extra- and intrahepatic bile ducts secondary to inflammation may result in progressive sclerosis of biliary tissue, biliary cirrhosis, and eventual liver failure.

Biliary atresia is seen in 1 of 10,000 to 15,000 births in the United States with higher incidence in the Asian population. A slight female predominance is noted. Two distinct forms of biliary atresia are known: the fetal/embryonic form and the postnatal form. The *fetal form* presents in the first 2 weeks of life and accounts for 10 to 35% of cases. In this case, the ducts are discontinuous at birth, and 10 to 30% of affected children have associated congenital defects, including situs inversus, polysplenia, malrotation, intestinal atresia, and cardiac anomalies. The *postnatal form* presents in children 2 to 8 weeks of age and accounts for 65 to 90% of cases. These children may experience a short jaundice-free interval, and, unlike the fetal form, this form is not associated with congenital anomalies.

Although exact numbers may vary, overall survival of children post-surgical treatment for biliary atresia is ~60% at 5 years of age and 35% at 10 years of age.

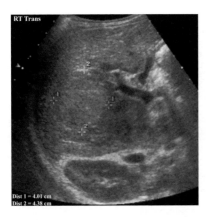

Figure 70D Ultrasound of regenerative liver nodule in a child with cirrhosis. This patient presented with hematemesis following failed Kasai operation for biliary atresia associated with malrotation and cat-eye syndrome.

Etiology

Its precise etiology is unknown. It is thought to result from inflammation of the hepatobiliary system. Obstruction to flow leads to secondary biliary cirrhosis. Many hypotheses have been proposed for its pathogenesis: antenatal infection with *Reovirus* type 3, biliary epithelial sloughing due to reflux of pancreatic juice because of abnormal connection between distal bile duct and pancreatic duct, and autoimmune destruction of the biliary epithelium.

Clinical Findings

- In early infancy, the clinical presentation is typically with hepatomegaly and persistent jaundice in a term baby.
- Cholestasis is associated with elevated gamma-glutamyl transferase (GT)
- Liver biopsy is essential for diagnosis following an algorithmic imaging approach often with a combination of ultrasonography, hepatobiliary scintigraphy, cholangiography, and biopsy.
- In view of surgical management, cholangiography can be intraoperative, percutaneous, or obtained as a preoperative MR cholangiopancreatography (MRCP).
- Later in infancy and childhood, either because of a delay in diagnosis or with failure of surgery there is a marked progression of hepatic disease with development of portal hypertension and cirrhosis.
- Failure to thrive, pruritus, and gastrointestinal hemorrhage are significant complications.

Pathology/Histology

- Proliferation of small intrahepatic ducts
- Absence of extrahepatic biliary duct
- Degeneration of duct epithelium or scarring in the extrahepatic biliary remnant

Anatomic Classification: There Are Three Types

- Type 1: focal atresia, rare
- Type 2: intrahepatic, with paucity of intrahepatic ducts, uncommon
- Type 3: extrahepatic biliary atresia involving common bile duct with patent intrahepatic bile tree
  ○ Subtype 1 or perinatal subtype with bile duct remnant at porta hepatis
  ○ Subtype 2 or fetal type without bile duct remnant at porta, associated with multiple congenital anomalies (malrotation, polysplenia, situs inversus, preduodenal portal vein)

Imaging Findings

ULTRASOUND

- Variable signs depending on type and severity

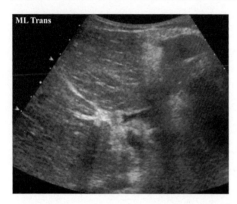

Figure 70E Increased periportal echogenicity on ultrasound, due to fibrosis in a 3-year-old boy with biliary atresia post–Kasai operation.

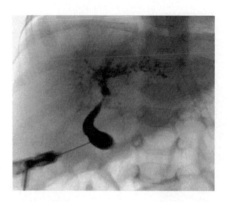

Figure 70F Preoperative cholangiography demonstrates atretic appearance of intra-hepatic biliary duct system, opacification of a small gallbladder, and no drainage into the bowel.

- Normal size or enlargement of liver
- Hepatic parenchyma is often inhomogeneous and increased in echogenicity with marked increase in periportal echoes due to fibrosis.
- Regenerative nodules of cirrhosis (**Fig. 70D**)
- Lack of visualization of the peripheral portal venous vasculature (related to fibrosis)
- No dilatation of intrahepatic bile ducts
- The "triangular cord" at porta hepatis: triangular or tubular echogenic area, which seems to be relatively specific for extrahepatic biliary atresia
- Gallbladder may be absent or small, <1.5 cm long (**Fig. 70A**). Gallbladder length <1.9 cm is more common, usually seen as thin or indistinct gallbladder wall and irregular, with lobular contour constituting the "gallbladder ghost triad" (literature suggests 97% sensitivity and 100% specificity for the diagnosis of biliary atresia).
- However, normal (≥1.5 cm in length) or large (>4 cm in length) gallbladder may be seen in up to 10% of patients.
- Late signs of portal hypertension with extensive periportal hyperechogenicity (**Fig. 70E**)
- Small central choledochal cysts may be present.
- If the diagnosis remains elusive following ultrasound, hepatobiliary scintigraphy and/or MR cholangiography, liver biopsy followed by operative or percutaneous cholangiography is recommended.
- Associated congenital anomalies:
  - Situs inversus
  - Polysplenia

SCINTIGRAPHY—HEPATOBILIARY

- Technetium (^{99m}Tc)—labeled iminodiacetic acid derivatives after 5 days of oral phenobarbital intake
- Normal hepatic extraction of tracer but no excretion into the gastrointestinal tract (**Fig. 70C**)
- This test is sensitive (100%) for biliary atresia but has low specificity (60%).
- Poor hepatic uptake and no excretion are seen in advanced cirrhosis.

CHOLANGIOGRAPHY

- Intraoperative or percutaneous cholangiography, via an identified gallbladder (**Fig. 70F**)
  - The pattern of biliary atresia is variable.
  - Assessment of the liver hilum determines if the atresia is correctable (12% of cases) with surgical anastomosis of intact bile ducts.
- Endoscopic retrograde cholangiopancreatography (ERCP)
  - Allows direct visualization of the extrahepatic biliary tree by injection of radiologic contrast agent

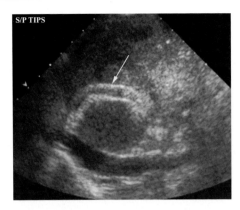

Figure 70G Ultrasonographic evidence of TIPS procedure with a stent (arrow) between portal vein and right hepatic vein.

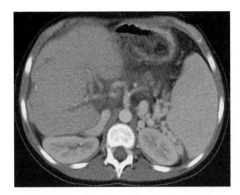

Figure 70H The CT image shows splenomegaly, extensive varices, splenorenal shunt, and liver cirrhosis in an 11-year-old-girl with prior Kasai operation and present signs of portal hypertension.

- ○ Obstruction of the common bile duct
- ○ Visualization of the extrahepatic biliary system distal to the common hepatic duct
- ○ Visualization of the extrahepatic biliary system with bile lakes at the porta hepatic

MRI

- MRCP
  - ○ Complete visualization of extrahepatic bile duct excludes biliary atresia.
  - ○ Incomplete visualization of the extrahepatic biliary system
- Periportal high signal intensity on T2-weighted images

DUODENAL INTUBATION

- Less commonly used in diagnosing biliary atresia
- A nasogastric tube is placed in the distal duodenum.
- Absence of bilirubin or bile acids in aspirated fluid is suggestive of obstruction.
- Literature suggests sensitivity of 92% and specificity of >90%.

Treatment

- Biliary atresia is a serious condition that may lead to liver cirrhosis, portal hypertension, hepatocellular cancer, or even death prior to 2 years of age; therefore, early diagnosis and treatment are essential.
- Nutritional management includes supply of easily absorbed forms of fat, essential fatty acids, and adequate protein and caloric intake.
- Operative management:
  - ○ Reconstructive Kasai portoenterostomy (primary complication is ascending cholangitis)
  - ○ Surgical venous shunts performed for treatment of portal hypertension and varices including the transjular intrahepatic portosystemic shunt (TIPS) procedure, (**Fig. 70G**) and portocaval, mesocaval, splenorenal shunt
  - ○ Liver transplantation, in which biliary atresia is the primary indication for transplant

Complications

- Progressive biliary cirrhosis
- Portal hypertension (**Fig. 70H**) and/or hemorrhage from esophageal varices is seen in 40% of children before 3 years of age.
- Postoperative complication after Kasai operation includes ascending cholangitis (in 50% of cases).

Prognosis

Multiple factors are important for prognosis.

- Age at surgery (the earlier the better; threshold is 60 to 80 days) following birth
- Anatomic pattern of extrahepatic bile ducts
- Size of ducts at porta hepatis
- Presence of cirrhosis, polysplenia
- Incidence of cholangitis
- Availability of transplantation

PEARLS

- Finding a gallbladder on ultrasound does not exclude biliary atresia.
- Biliary atresia is a progressive obliterative process of the bile ducts.
- Ascites is a relative contraindication for percutaneous liver biopsy.
- Extrahepatic biliary atresia is a misnomer because the disorder is of variable extent.
- Documenting a normal biliary system with MRCP excludes extrahepatic biliary atresia.

PITFALLS

- Mild hyperechogenicity in periportal area is related to inflammation, different from the "triangular cord."
- With poor hepatocytic function, differentiation of biliary atresia from hepatitis on hepatobiliary scan is impossible.

Suggested Readings

Gubernick JA, Rosenberg HK, Ilaslan H, Kessler A. US approach to jaundice in infants and children. Radiographics 2000;20:173–195

Ikeda S, Sera Y, Ohshiro H, et al. Gallbladder contraction in biliary atresia: a pitfall of ultrasound diagnosis. Pediatr Radiol 1998;28:451–453

McKiernan PJ. Neonatal cholestasis. Semin Neonatol 2002;7:153–165

Norton KI, Glass RB, Kogan D, et al. MR cholangiography in the evaluation of neonatal cholestasis: initial results. Radiology 2002;222:687–691

Tan Kendrick AP, Phua KB, Subramaniam R, et al. Making the diagnosis of biliary atresia using the triangular cord sign and gallbladder length. Pediatr Radiol 2000;30:69–73

CASE 71

Clinical Presentation

A 13-year-old boy presents with left chest pain following a snowboarding injury.

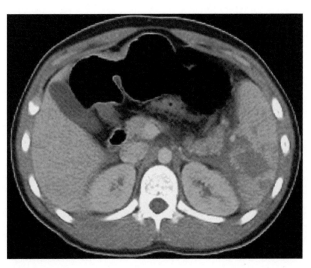

Figure 71A

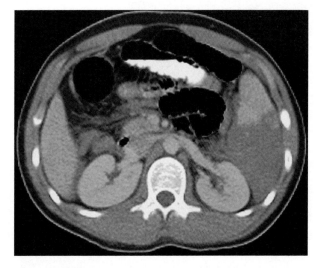

Figure 71B

Radiologic Findings

Selected abdominal CT images demonstrate hypodensity of the spleen in its mid (**Fig. 71A**) and lower portions (**Fig. 71B**) without fluid in the lateral paracolic gutter. Fluid is seen tracking medially along the pancreatic tail.

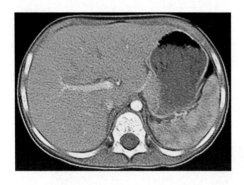

Figure 71C Normal CT pattern of early splenic enhancement following intravascular contrast administration.

Diagnosis

Splenic trauma

Differential Diagnosis

The following are the mimickers:
- Streak artifacts on CT related to beam hardening because of the ribs, air contrast interface in the stomach, or nasogastric tube or monitor device
- Early splenic enhancement with variable density (**Fig. 71C**)
- Splenic lobulated contour, a normal variant

Other causes of hypodense lesions in the spleen:
- Cyst, epidermoid
- Hydatid cyst
- Abscess
- Hamartoma/teratoma
- Lymphangioma
- Lymphoma

Discussion

Background

The spleen is commonly injured in children following blunt abdominal trauma, including motor vehicle accidents or child abuse. An underlying splenomegaly, which can occur, for example, in infectious mononucleosis, Gaucher's disease, or splenic epidermoid cyst, is a risk factor. The past decades have seen confirmation of nonoperative management, avoiding unnecessary laparotomy and the risk of postsplenectomy infection.

Etiology

Trauma to the left side of the abdomen is often associated with injury to the spleen and left lung contusion or laceration. Rib fractures are less commonly seen in children than in adults because of the greater pliability of the child's chest wall. Trauma to the left hemiabdomen is often associated with both splenic and renal trauma.

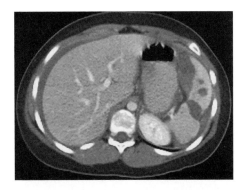

Figure 71D Delayed splenic rupture. Patient presented with acute abdominal pain and syncope. There was a history of skiing accident 4 weeks prior. CT demonstrates hemoperitoneum, subcapsular splenic hematoma, and splenic fracture.

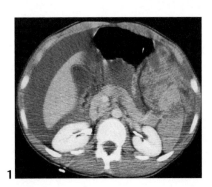

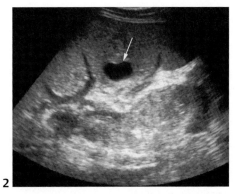

Figure 71E (1) Traumatic pseudoaneurysm of splenic artery. Initial CT of teenage boy after roller-blading injury shows splenic laceration, perisplenic hyperdense clots, and evidence of extensive hemoperitoneum. No contrast extravasation was seen on initial scans. **(2)** Follow-up ultrasound at day 8 identified a 2 cm splenic cystic area (arrow) with flow on color Doppler study. Angiogram confirmed the pseudoaneurysm, which was successfully embolized with coils.

Clinical Findings

It is important to assess and stabilize the hemodynamic status of an injured child before beginning any imaging. Conventional chest and trauma series radiographs are obtained initially with evaluation of the hemoglobin level and hematocrit, and presence of hematuria. CT scanning is generally the initial imaging test, having replaced peritoneal lavage in hemodynamically stable children. Ultrasonography of the abdomen also is used but is more operator dependent. Both are highly specific and sensitive for detection of hemoperitoneum. CT may better demonstrate the extent of splenic involvement.

Complications

- Resolution of splenic injury is the rule.
- Risk of delayed splenic rupture at any time (early or late) is low (**Fig. 71D**), and follow-up imaging is rarely beneficial to clinical follow-up.
- Splenectomy brings risk of serious complications of infection (abscess, pneumococcus +++).
- Splenosis can occur in case of severe splenic shattering or after splenectomy.

Pathology

- Parenchyma contusion
- Simple or complex laceration
- Devascularization of the spleen

- Hematoma formation may be intraperitoneal, subcapsular, or perisplenic.
- Hemoperitoneum usually reflects solid organ (liver/spleen/kidney) or small bowel injury.

Imaging Findings

PLAIN RADIOGRAPHY

- Diaphragmatic elevation
- Lower lung contusion
- Pneumothorax
- Rib fracture
- Hemoperitoneum

ULTRASOUND

- Hemoperitoneum +++
  - It implies a capsular involvement and disruption. Perisplenic fluid accumulates and may extend in left flank, around the liver, or in the pelvis. The fluid in the acute setting is anechoic and may have low-level echoes.
- Spleen
  - Risk of underestimation of acute injury by ultrasonography
  - Loss of normal echotexture of parenchyma
  - Laceration: hypoechoic zone
  - Hematoma: heterogeneous (clots)
  - Doppler examination may delineate the focal avascular area in the parenchyma or at the periphery (subcapsular).
  - Discrete heterogeneous splenomegaly may be the only sign.

CT

- Performed on a hemodynamically stable patient
- Higher sensitivity/specificity for solid viscous analysis and definition of extent of injury
- Comprehensive data on other viscera
- Intravenous contrast enhancement is essential in the examination. Use of oral contrast is controversial.
- Subcapsular hematoma
  - Hypo- or isodense to spleen, indenting the surface of spleen
- Central hematoma
  - Iso- or hypodense with hyperdense clots
- Laceration
  - Linear or radiating toward the hilum, hypodense or absent enhancement (**Figs. 71A** and **71B**)
- Perisplenic blood clots ("sentinel clots")
  - Hyperdense
- Hypoperfusion syndrome
  - Peritoneal fluid accumulation
  - Caliber of major vessels (inferior vena cava, aorta) decreases.
  - Bowel loops are dilated, and their walls show intense enhancement.
  - Spleen has a pseudoischemic appearance on enhanced CT (generalized hypodensity pattern).
- Contrast extravasation
  - Seen with active hemorrhage
- Traumatic pseudoaneurysm (predisposing to splenic rupture) (**Figs. 71E1** and **71E2**)
  - CT attenuation is similar to blood on enhanced CT.

Treatment

- Hemodynamic state stabilization
- Nonoperative management is now the standard for hemodynamically stable children.
- Clinical proactive guidelines for management include:
  - Organ injury grading
  - Admission with variable length of stay
  - Restriction of activity
  - Follow-up imaging may be used but is not routinely needed.
- Splenectomy required uncommonly with immunization (pneumococcus) needed post-splenectomy.

Prognosis

- In the United States, abdominal injuries are seen in 30% of pediatric blunt trauma and account for 10% of all trauma-related deaths.
- Usually: resolution of splenic injuries
- Correlation between initial grading of splenic injury (I–V) and rate of healing has been shown.
- The long-term risk, however, cannot be predicted.

PEARLS_____

- Initial grading of splenic injury does not influence the decision for laparotomy as the hemodynamic status of an injured child is the key factor in management.
- CT has resulted in decreased use of peritoneal lavage, scintigraphy, and angiography.

PITFALLS_____

- With helical CT imaging, inhomogeneous enhancement of spleen parenchyma due to rapid bolus contrast enhancement (**Fig. 71C**)
- Ultrasonography, which is operator dependent, may underestimate acute injury.
- Technical artifacts (CT beam hardening) are frequent.

Suggested Readings

Donnelly LF, Foss JN, Frush DP, Bisset GS III. Heterogeneous splenic enhancement patterns on spiral CT images in children: minimizing misinterpretation. Radiology 1999;493–497

Emery KH, Babcock DS, Borgman AC, Garcia VF. Splenic injury diagnosed with CT: US follow-up and healing rate in children and adolescents. Radiology 1999;212:515–518

Frumiento C, Sartorelli K, Vane D. Complications of splenic injuries: expansion of the nonoperative theorem. J Pediatr Surg 2000;35:788–791

Huebner S, Reed MH. Analysis of the value of imaging as part of the follow-up of splenic injury in children. Pediatr Radiol 2001;31:852–855

Sivit CJ. Detection of active intra-abdominal hemorrhage after blunt trauma: value of delayed CT scanning. Pediatr Radiol 2000;30:99–100

Tran CN, Oudjhane K, Sinsky AB, Laberge JM, Patenaude YG. Radiology for the surgeon. Case 12: Splenic laceration with pseudoaneurysm of the splenic artery. Can J Surg 1996;39:450–486

CASE 72

Clinical Presentation

A 14-year-old boy hit in a motor vehicle accident was brought to the emergency department. CT scan was performed with subsequent follow-up studies on days 12 and 26.

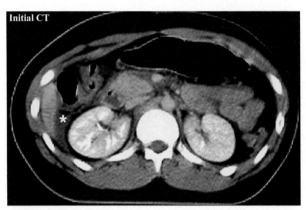

Figure 72A

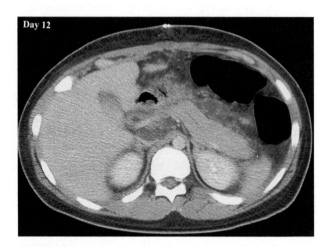

Figure 72B

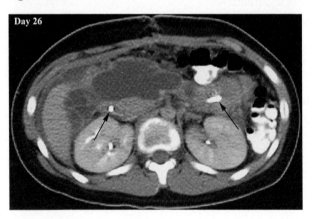

Figure 72C

Radiologic Findings

On the initial abdominal CT, there is free fluid in the subhepatic area and adjacent to the duodenum (**Fig. 72A**, asterisk). On day 12, the CT demonstrates injury to the anterior aspect of the head of the pancreas and a peripancreatic fluid collection (**Fig. 72B**). On day 26, a pseudocyst is noted next to the body and head of the pancreas (**Fig. 72C**), with persistent perihepatic fluid. A nasojejunal tube is present (**Fig. 72C**, arrows).

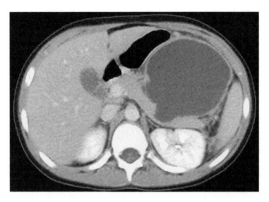

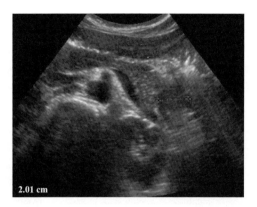

Figure 72D Traumatic pancreatic pseudocyst following a handlebar injury. CT shows transection of the tail of the pancreas with pseudocyst formation.

Figure 72E (Same patient as in **Fig. 72D**) Follow-up ultrasound 4 months later demonstrates significant reduction of size of pseudocyst, without interventional procedure.

Diagnosis

Pancreatic pseudocyst

Differential Diagnosis

Cystic lesions of pancreas include:
- Congenital cysts:
  - True cysts
  - Multiple cysts
  - Polycystic kidney disease
  - Von Hippel-Lindau disease
  - Gastrointestinal duplication cyst
- Acquired cysts:
  - Retention cyst of cystic fibrosis
  - Neoplastic cysts
  - Pancreatic pseudocysts (traumatic, inflammatory, or drug-related)
  - Tropical cysts (hydatid disease)

Discussion

Background

A pseudocyst is the most common type of pancreatic cyst in children. Granulation and fibrous tissue line the pseudocyst. They may be solitary or multiple, and of variable size (5–10 cm). Pseudocysts may be present within the pancreas or adjacent to the pancreas, or they can be found in the lesser sac or extending into the chest or pelvis. Infection of pseudocysts may occur with *Escherichia coli, Enterococcus,* or *Staphylococcus.*

Etiology

The epidemiology of pseudocysts is related to that of pancreatitis. Pediatric forms may be idiopathic or caused by trauma (**Figs. 72D** and **72E**) (bicycle accident, and direct impact), drug toxicity (steroids, tetracycline, L-asparaginase), or viral infection. Pancreatic injury leads to activation of precursor

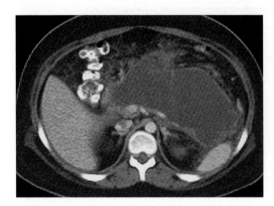

Figure 72F Pancreatitis with large pseudocyst and associated mesenteric fat stranding.

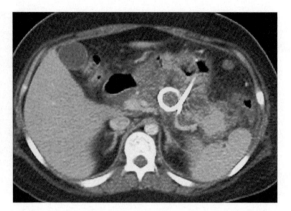

Figure 72G (Same patient as in **Fig. 72F**) A pigtail catheter has been placed with successful drainage of the pseudocyt.

enzymes causing pancreatic autodigestion with the end result being proteolysis, edema, necrosis, and hemorrhage. Pseudocyst is a complication of pancreatitis, with disruption of the pancreatic duct. Acute pseudocysts may develop within 6 weeks of injury, whereas chronic pseudocysts may occur months or years later.

Clinical Findings

Abdominal pain is always present. Other signs include weight loss, vomiting, fever, and/or jaundice. A mass is palpated in 50% of cases. An acute abdomen or intestinal hemorrhage occurs when a pseudocyst erodes a major blood vessel. Elevated white blood cell count and serum enzyme levels are commonly found. Spontaneous resolution of a pseudocyst may occur, especially within the first few weeks.

Complications

Rupture of pseudocyst can cause hemoperitonium or extensive gastrointestinal hemorrhage. Abscess formation may be iatrogenic and follow endoscopic retrograde cholangiopancreatography.

Pathology

A pancreatic pseudocyt is walled off by nonepithelialized granulation tissue. Its contents include loculated necrotic material, with pancreatic secretions with a high level of enzymes.

Imaging Findings

RADIOGRAPHY

- Elevated hemidiaphragm, pleural effusion
- Sentinel loop of localized reactive ileus
- Calcifications in the pancreas (chronic)
- Mass effect on the iliopsoas shadow, stomach, colon, or small bowel

ULTRASOUND

- High sensitivity and specificity for detection of pseudocyst
- Well-defined fluid collection with thin capsule
- Hypoechoic content (low echo debris)

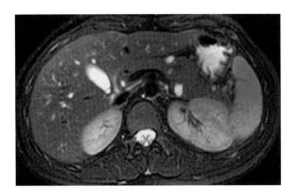

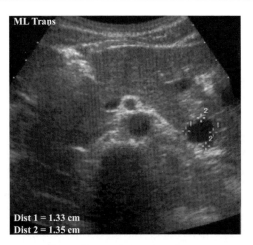

Figure 72H Differential diagnosis: von Hippel-Lindau disease. Small pancreatic cystic areas are delineated on axial T2-weighted MRI.

Figure 72I Differential diagnosis (Same patient as in **Fig. 72H**): von Hippel-Lindau disease in a 14-year-old girl with long-standing history of nausea/vomiting. Small pancreatic cystic areas are well defined on ultrasound.

- Topography of pseudocyst: peripancreatic, lesser sac, transverse mesocolon, and anterior pararenal space

CT

- Hypodense collection (20 HU) (**Figs. 72C, 72D,** and **72F**), unless hemorrhage/infection occur. Pancreatic necrosis is characterized by zones of nonviable, hypodense pancreatic parenchyma.
- Possible wall calcification, rare septations
- Gas bubbles caused by fistula to gastrointestinal tract

Treatment

- Drainage is the cornerstone for treatment (**Fig. 72G**).
- Excision of pseudocysts arising from pancreatic tail
- Cystogastrostomy or Roux-en-Y cyst jejunostomy for cysts of head/body of pancreas
- Percutaneous external drainage

Prognosis

- Long-term postsurgical prognosis varies according to the primary cause.
- If spontaneous resolution occurs, it is typically observed within 6 weeks of diagnosis.
- Urgent surgery for serious complications is associated with significant morbidity.

PEARLS

- Unexplained peripancreatic fluid is most likely related to pancreatic injury.
- Most cystic lesions of the pancreas are due to pancreatic pseudocysts.

PITFALLS

- Other cystic lesions in pancreas can be mistaken for pancreatic pseudocysts.
- Pancreatic involvement often accounts for the initial symptoms and presentation of von Hippel-Lindau disease (**Figs. 72H** and **72I**).

Suggested Readings

Boulanger SC, Borowitz DS, Fisher JF, Brisseau GF. Congenital pancreatic cysts in children. J Pediatr Surg 2003;38:1080–1082

Dutheil-Doco A, Ducou Le Pointe H, Larroquet M, Ben Lagha N, Montagne J. A case of perforated cystic duplication of the transverse colon. Pediatr Radiol 1998;28:20–22

Ferrucci JT III, Mueller PR. Interventional approach to pancreatic fluid collections. Radiol Clin North Am 2003;41:1217–1226

Hough DM, Stephens DH, Johnson CD, Binkovitz LA. Pancreatic lesions in von Hippel-Lindau disease: prevalence, clinical significance and CT findings. AJR Am J Roentgenol 1994;162:1091–1094

Johnson PR, Spitz L. Cysts and tumors of the pancreas. Semin Pediatr Surg 2000;9:209–215

King LJ, Scurr ED, Murugan N, et al. Hepatobiliary and pancreatic manifestations of cystic fibrosis: MR imaging appearances. Radiographics 2000;20:767–777

SECTION VI
Genitourinary

CASE 73

Clinical Presentation

A 2-year-old girl presents with a urinary tract infection. Renal ultrasound shows unilateral hydronephrosis.

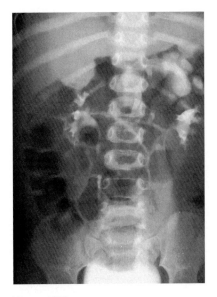

Figure 73A

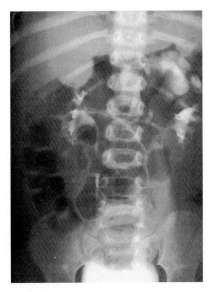

Figure 73B

Radiologic Findings

The intravenous urogram (IVU) 10 minutes (**Fig. 73A**) and 30 minutes (**Fig. 73B**) after contrast administration shows a normal right kidney and a duplicated left collecting system. The lower pole of the left kidney appears normal with no obvious scarring. There is dilatation of the upper moiety of the left kidney with delayed excretion of contrast into a dilated tortuous ureter draining the upper pole, which terminates as a filling defect in the left side of the bladder; that represents a ureterocele.

Diagnosis

Duplex left kidney with delayed excretion of contrast by the upper moiety, and a dilated upper moiety ureter ending in a ureterocele

Differential Diagnosis

- Bladder tumor (However, a ureterocele and dilated upper moiety ureter are very common in association with a duplex kidney.)
- Idiopathic megaureter (manifests as a dilated ureter in a single system)

Discussion

Background

Ureteroceles are congenital cystic dilatations of the distal ureter. A ureterocele is termed *simple* when it inserts normally into the bladder and *ectopic* when the orifice is away from the normal ureterovesical junction (UVJ) in the bladder trigone. Duplication of a collecting system may be partial or complete. In partial duplication, two ureters fuse at a variable level. With complete duplication, two renal pelves and two separate ureters drain the kidney and insert separately into the bladder. The lower pole collecting system inserts into the bladder at the normal site, although the intramural portion may be shorter than normal, and vesicoureteral reflux is commonly found in association. The upper pole ureter inserts in an ectopic position medial and inferior to the normal UVJ (Weigert-Meyer rule). The upper pole ureter may insert outside the bladder into the urethra or into the vagina in females: such ectopic drainage of the ureter is usually associated with dysplasia of the upper moiety. Ballooning of the submucosal aspect of the upper moiety distal ureter as it inserts into the bladder results in a ureterocele, which frequently causes partial or complete obstruction to drainage.

Clinical Findings

Duplicated kidneys systems without dilatation or obstruction are generally asymptomatic and have the same outlook as normal kidneys. Complicated renal duplications manifest with urinary tract infection, failure to thrive, hematuria, or symptoms of bladder outlet obstruction from a ureterocele. Increasingly, these lesions are picked up with prenatal ultrasonography. Females with insertion of the ectopic ureter below the external sphincter in the urethra or into the vagina will manifest later in childhood with dribbling, continuous wetting, or primary enuresis.

Imaging Findings

INTRAVENOUS UROGRAPHY (IVU)

- Diagnosis of an uncomplicated unilateral duplication on IVU is straightforward, with a larger kidney than the opposite normal kidney and two ureters.
- Occasionally, renal duplication is present bilaterally.
- A ureterocele frequently manifests simply as a faint rounded or elliptical filling defect in the bladder.
- A simple ureterocele may have a "cobra head" appearance on IVU when contrast opacifies a dilated distal ureter with a radiolucent halo produced by the ureterocele wall in the contrast-filled bladder.
- With increasing obstruction of the upper moiety, reduced function of the upper pole results, and delayed images may be necessary to visualize the upper moiety and its ureter.

- An obstructed upper moiety may not function and so not excrete contrast medium, but the hydronephrotic upper moiety may displace the orientation of the lower moiety leading to a "drooping flower" or "drooping lily" appearance to the lower moiety calices.
- Renal scarring of either moiety may be seen as reduced parenchymal thickening, often in association with distorted adjacent calices.
- Upper moiety dilatation is a result of obstruction.
- Lower moiety dilatation and scarring result from vesicoureteric reflux.

VOIDING CYSTOURETHROGRAPHY (VCUG)

- A ureterocele is best seen on early bladder filling.
- Eversion of the ureterocele with progressive bladder filling may mimic a bladder diverticulum.
- A large ureterocele may prevent reflux into the ipsilateral lower moiety ureter.
- Reflux is typically seen into the lower moiety system.
- Marked reflux into a very dilated lower moiety system may be mistaken for reflux into a single system.
- Reflux may occur simultaneously into both systems on one side, indicating that the ureteral openings in the bladder are close together or even common.

ULTRASOUND

- An unobstructed or uncomplicated duplex kidney may be difficult to diagnose with ultrasonography, although the kidney would typically be larger than a simplex kidney.
- Duplication of the renal collecting system is diagnosed when the central echo complex of the kidney appears separated by an area of normal renal parenchyma.
- Two separate renal pelves may be seen.
- When there is combined severe upper moiety dilatation and lower moiety reflux, it may be impossible to differentiate dilated lower from upper moiety ureters in the flanks.
- A ureterocele is seen as a cystic filling defect at the bladder base.
- The ureterocele is usually associated with a dilated ipsilateral ureter.
- Parenchymal thinning may be evident in the upper pole as a result of obstruction and in the lower pole secondary to reflux.
- An echogenic upper moiety with parenchymal thinning suggests dysplasia and reduced or nonfunction of the upper moiety.

MRI

- Magnetic resonance urography (MRU), with heavily T2-weighted imaging sequences, can also show a dilated ureter or ureterocele to good effect.
- MRU sequences are superior to ultrasound in identifying extravesical insertion of an ectopic ureter.

Treatment

- Uncomplicated, nondilated duplex systems require no treatment.
- Antibiotic prophylaxis is usually given to all diagnosed cases in early childhood.
- Ureterocele puncture may relieve upper moiety obstruction.
- Complete obstruction with nonfunction of the upper moiety, particularly when complicated by infection, may require upper pole nephroureterectomy

PEARLS

- A ureterocele frequently manifests simply as a faint rounded or elliptical filling defect in the bladder on IVU and/or VCUG.
- Lower pole reflux is the most common abnormality associated with a duplex kidney.
- Reflux nephropathy of the lower pole may be present at birth in the absence of urinary infection.

- Dilatation secondary to obstruction is commonly seen in the upper moiety.
- MRU sequences are superior to ultrasound in identifying extravesical insertion of an ectopic ureter.

PITFALLS_____

- A dilated, obstructed upper moiety may not function on IVU leading to a "drooping flower" appearance to the lower moiety calices.
- Ureterocele eversion with progressive bladder filling on VCUG may mimic a bladder diverticulum.
- Marked reflux into a very dilated lower moiety system may be mistaken for reflux into a single system.

Suggested Readings

Avni FE, Nicaise N, Hall M, et al. The role of MR imaging for the assessment of complicated duplex kidneys in children: preliminary report. Pediatr Radiol 2001;31:215–223

Berrocal T, Lopez-Perreira P, Arjonilla A, Gutierrez J. Anomalies of the distal ureter, bladder and urethra in children: embryologic, radiologic and pathologic features. Radiographics 2002;22:1139–1164

Bolduc S, Upadhyay J, Restrepo R, et al. The predictive value of diagnostic imaging for histological lesions of the upper poles in duplex systems with ureteroceles. BJU Int 2003;91:678–682

Staatz G, Rohrmann D, Nolte-Ernsting CC, et al. Magnetic resonance urography in children: evaluation of suspected ureteral ectopia in duplex systems. J Urol 2001;166:2346–2350

CASE 74

Clinical Presentation

Antenatal ultrasonography shows a large bladder and bilateral hydro-ureteronephrosis in a boy.

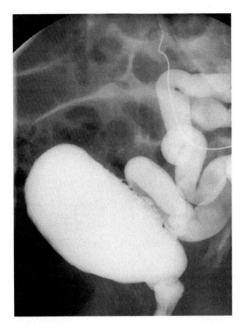

Figure 74A

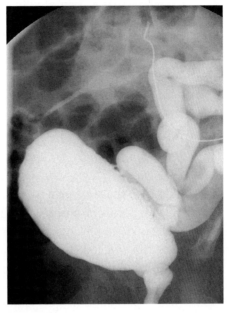

Figure 74B

Radiologic Findings

Images from voiding cystourethrography (VCUG) with a urethral catheter in place (**Fig. 74A**), and with the catheter removed (**Fig. 74B**), show a dilated posterior urethra with a sudden change in the caliber at the prostatic–penile junction and a narrow stream of contrast through the anterior urethra. There is bladder irregularity posteriorly, with reflux of contrast into a tortuous dilated left ureter, and into a hydronephrotic kidney with additional intrarenal reflux (international grade 5).

Diagnosis

Posterior urethral valves (PUVs) with unilateral vesicoureteral reflux

Differential Diagnosis

- Prune-belly syndrome, also known as abdominal muscular deficiency syndrome. The posterior urethra is frequently dilated but with a typical conical narrowing and the bladder wall is not trabeculated.
- Acquired urethral stricture (not seen in neonates); occurs secondary to severe perineal trauma or traumatic catheterization
- Megacystis: differential of enlarged posterior urethra, not spinning top

Discussion

Background

PUVs affect boys only, with an incidence of approximately 1 in 10,000. It is the commonest obstructive uropathy in male children. Typical prenatal ultrasonographic findings include bilateral hydronephrosis with a large bladder with or without progressive oligohydramnios. Many cases are now suspected from prenatal ultrasonography and are examined by VCUG soon after birth. PUV have been traditionally classified into three or four types, but in reality only two types are seen. Type 1 is the most common, seen in approximately 95% of cases, where two folds at the verumontanum have a ventral slitlike orifice. Type 3 has a pinpoint orifice that results in forward ballooning of the valve during VCUG, giving a so-called wind-in-the-sail appearance. In actual practice, it is usually impossible to tell type 1 from type 3 valves on VCUG. Type 3 valves have a higher association with renal dysplasia. Vesicoureteral reflux is commonly associated with PUV. Occasionally, bladder hypertrophy is such that reflux no longer occurs, but the ureters remain dilated.

Etiology

Although PUVs directly result from abnormal migration of mucosal folds (wolffian duct remnant) from the verumontanum to the membranous urethra, the etiology of PUVs is uncertain. Anomalous insertion of the mesonephric ducts into the cloaca has been suggested as a cause of type 1 valves. Incomplete dissolution of the urogenital membrane may result in type 3 valves.

Clinical Findings

Respiratory distress and pulmonary hypoplasia can be seen in the newborn period as a result of oligohydramnios. The neonate may present with retention of urine or dribbling. An occasional complication in the neonatal period is rupture of a calyx leading to a perinephric urinoma or a leak from the bladder resulting in urinary ascites. In the absence of prenatal or perinatal pick-up, boys may manifest with a weak urinary stream, recurrent urinary infection, or septicemia. Older boys may present later with only mild symptoms.

Complications

- Death from oligohydramnios resulting in lung hypoplasia may occur in the newborn period.
- In utero bladder outlet obstruction frequently results in renal dysplasia, which is irreversible.
- Renal failure in the neonatal period usually improves with bladder drainage.

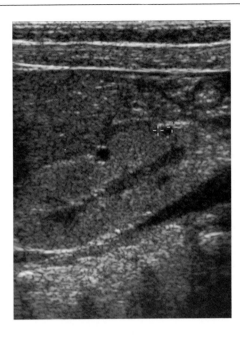

Figure 74C Longitudinal ultrasound image showing an echogenic kidney on the right side with loss of the normal corticomedullary differentiation, and peripheral cortical cysts. These findings, which occur in association with a small kidney, indicate in addition that the kidney is dysplastic.

- Continuing bladder dysfunction despite early treatment, however, with additional vesicoureteral reflux or intercurrent infections, may contribute to an inexorable decline in renal function and growth retardation.

Imaging Findings

VOIDING CYSTOURETHROGRAPHY(VCUG)

- Posterior urethral dilatation is invariable.
- Abrupt transition between dilated posterior urethra and nondilated penile urethra is typical.
- Actual membrane (valve) causing the obstruction is often difficult to identify.
- Narrowing of the bladder neck due to its hypertrophy is common.
- Poor stream and reduced caliber in the anterior urethra are seen.
- Bladder wall irregularity (trabeculation), often with multiple diverticula, is frequent.
- Vesicoureteric reflux into dilated ureters and hydronephrotic kidneys may be seen either unilaterally or bilaterally.
- Although it was common historical teaching that valves are best seen during voiding when the urethral catheter is removed, voiding with a catheter in situ can still lead to a reliable diagnosis of PUV when good urethral distension is achieved.

ULTRASOUND

- The bladder wall is usually markedly thickened with or without obvious diverticula.
- The bladder may be large or small in volume.
- One or both ureters and upper tracts may be dilated, but this is variable.
- Echogenic small dysplastic kidneys are often seen in association, but in a fortunate minority the kidneys may appear normal (**Fig. 74C**).
- Scanning the perineum during voiding can reveal an enlarged posterior urethra.
- Perinephric fluid collection (urinomas) or urinary ascites may be seen in the neonate.

Treatment

- Simple bladder catheterization via a suprapubic or urethral catheter is usually sufficient for drainage and relief of bladder outlet obstruction in the newborn period.

- The definitive treatment for PUVs is endoscopic valve ablation, which is performed a few weeks after bladder drainage has resulted in improved renal function.
- Intervention to drain perinephric urinomas or surgery to relieve bladder obstruction, for example, vesicostomy or other urinary diversion, may be deemed necessary on an individual basis.

Prognosis

- Depends on the degree of associated renal dysplasia and bladder abnormality
- Many boys need dialysis in childhood and undergo renal transplantation in adolescence.

PEARLS

- When hydronephrosis or hydroureter are seen antenatally in males, PUVs should always be considered
- Actual membrane (valve) causing the obstruction is often difficult to identify.
- Posterior urethral dilatation is reliably identified with VCUG.
- Narrowing of the bladder neck due to bladder neck hypertrophy is common.
- Bladder wall thickening is invariably seen on ultasonography.

PITFALLS

- Urethral catheterization prior to VCUG may destroy the valves causing the urethral obstruction, making the diagnosis less obvious (hence some urologists prefer suprapubic catheterization), but posterior urethral dilatation with bladder trabeculation will still be visible.
- Diagnosis may be missed with a small-volume bladder if the dilated posterior urethra is mistaken for the bladder and the valves misinterpreted as the bladder neck.

Suggested Readings

Bosio M, Manzoni GA. Detection of posterior urethral valves with voiding cystourethrosonography with echo contrast. J Urol 2002;168:1711–1715

Duel BP, Mogbo K, Barthold JS, Gonzalez R. Prognostic value of initial renal ultrasound in patients with posterior urethral valves. J Urol 1998;160:1198–1200

Lal R, Bhatnagar V, Mitra DK. Upper tract changes after treatment of posterior urethral valves. Pediatr Surg Int 1998;13:396–399

CASE 75

Clinical Presentation

An adolescent girl presents with intermittent abdominal pain and a lower abdominal mass.

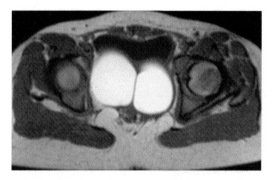

Figure 75A

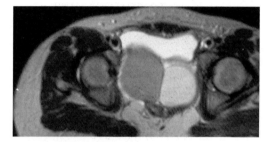

Figure 75B

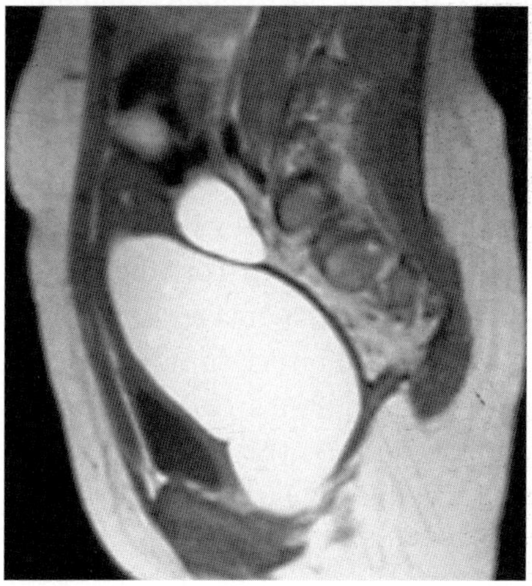

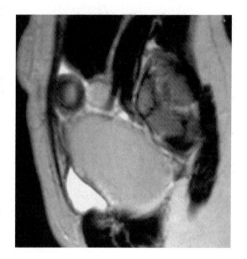

Figure 75C

Figure 75D

Radiologic Findings

On the axial T1-weighted image (**Fig. 75A**), two hyperintense structures, which represent a double vagina, are seen posterior to the bladder. On the axial T2-weighted image (**Fig. 75B**), the fluid collections in the vagina posterior to the bladder have varied signal, indicating subacute and more recent hemorrhage. (A second separate uterus not shown on these images was also present.) On the sagittal T1-weighted image (**Fig. 75C**), one vagina with very bright signal is seen to rise out of the pelvis. Another high-signal area seen posterior to the uterus, superior to the bright vaginal fluid in **Fig. 75C**, is a dilated fallopian tube. There is a small uterus anterosuperior to the vagina, which has similar signal to muscle on T1- and T2-weighted images (**Fig. 75D**).

Diagnosis

Hematocolpos, hematosalpinx, a double vagina with obstruction, and uterus didelphys

Differential Diagnosis

- Dilated rectum (A normal rectum is seen posterior to the double vagina on the axial images; rectal contents have intermediate to low signal on T1 sequences.)
- Large ovarian cyst (would not extend so inferiorly posterior to the bladder, nor would a midline septation be typical)
- Massively dilated ureters (should have similar signal as urine in the bladder)

Discussion

Background

Müllerian duct anomalies are often classified into five groups: (1) agenesis or hypoplasia, (2) unicornuate uterus, (3) uterus didelphys and septate vagina, (4) bicornuate uterus, and (5) septate uterus. Uterus didelphys describes total duplication of the uterus with two cervices and a double vagina, and this abnormality may be accompanied by unilateral or bilateral vaginal obstruction. Individual patients may not easily fit into one defined category. Diagnosis of the above anomalies in adolescent girls is by a combination of ultrasound and MRI. An imperforate hymen can also result in retained fluid (hydrocolpos/hydrometrocolpos) or retained menses (hematocolpos/hematometrocolpos) in the neonate or adolescent, respectively. In this circumstance, a prominent interlabial lump is found in association with a midline pelvic mass. Imperforate hymen is the most easily correctable of the vaginal obstructions and is not associated with other müllerian or renal anomalies. For other causes of vaginal obstruction, there is a strong association between müllerian duct anomalies and abnormalities of the urinary tract; thus every girl diagnosed with a genital malformation needs careful examination of the urinary tract. Ultrasonography may be sufficient for diagnosis in many cases, but MRI, particularly beyond infancy, often improves diagnostic accuracy. MRI has the ability to display the pelvic anatomy well and is able to distinguish the endometrium and myometrium of the uterine corpus and cervix.

Etiology

Duplication of the female reproductive system results from a lack of fusion of the paired müllerian ducts. The normal unfused cranial portions of the müllerian ducts form the paired fallopian tubes; the caudal fused ducts unite to form the uterus, cervix, and upper vagina. The lower vagina is formed by invagination of the urogenital sinus. Faults in the junction between the descending müllerian ducts and the ascending urogenital sinus result in complex disorders of vertical fusion, which also include transverse vaginal septa, imperforate cervix, or cervical agenesis. The hymen is a transverse perforate membrane where the caudal müllerian ducts meet the urogenital sinus. The hymen normally ruptures in the neonatal period and remains as a thin fold at the vaginal orifice.

Clinical Findings

Cases of simple imperforate hymen usually present with primary amenorrhea and are not associated with other congenital anomalies. Müllerian duct anomalies come to attention at two different stages of a girl's life. In neonates, a palpable abdominal mass may be seen in those with a urogenital sinus.

In adolescent girls, primary amenorrhea, delay in the onset of puberty, or recurrent abdominal pain are the common reasons for referral. Dysmenorrhea or vaginal discharge are other recognized presentations.

Complications

- Hematosalpinx may hinder fertility as the increased intraluminal pressure may affect ciliary motility and blood at the fimbriated ends of the fallopian tubes can cause adhesions.
- Retrograde menstrual flow into the peritoneal cavity can lead to endometriosis.
- Unrecognized genital or urinary tract malformations increase the risk of secondary infection.

Imaging Findings

ULTRASOUND

- Normal uterus (prominent endometrial stripe, and measures up to 3.5 cm in length) is easily visualized in neonates.
- The normal prepubertal uterus is smaller, tubular in shape, and lacks an echogenic endometrium.
- Mucoid material in a neonatal uterus or vagina may show low-level echoes or may be anechoic.
- Fluid–fluid levels or multiple internal echoes resembling a solid mass may be seen with a hematocolpos.
- Abdominal mass in a neonate or adolescent reflects a congenital hydrocolpos/hydrometrocolpos, or hematocolpos/hematometrocolpos (retained menses), respectively.
- With abnormal müllerian duct anatomy, despite uterine duplication, hematometrocolpos may be unilateral.
- Uterus didelphys manifests with two uteri, with two areas of thickened endometrium (in a neonate or postpubertal girl), and with two fluid-filled vaginas.
- In cases of vaginal obstruction, cystic dilatation of the vagina is usually more marked than endometrial distension.

MRI

- When the intrauterine contents have low T1 and high T2 signal intensity accumulation of mucoid material is likely.
- When intrauterine fluid has high signal on both T1 and T2 sequences, hemorrhagic fluid is likely because of the paramagnetic effects of methemoglobin.
- With high signal on T1- and intermediate signal on T2-weighted images, subacute hemorrhage is the usual explanation.
- Vaginal duplication is usually best seen on axial images.
- Normal endometrium is visible as a hyperintense stripe on T2 sequences.
- Zonal architecture with a hypointense inner myometrium (junctional zone) is seen on T2-weighted images.
- Myometrium and junctional zone are appreciable in the neonatal and postpubertal uterus.

Treatment

- Excision of a vaginal septum is curative in most cases.
- Hemihysterosalpingo-oophorectomy may be necessary in some instances.

Prognosis

- Delay in diagnosis, with long-standing hematosalpinx in particular, may hinder fertility by interfering with ciliary activity or causing adhesions in one or both fallopian tubes.

PEARLS

- Normal uterus (prominent endometrial stripe, and measures up to 3.5 cm in length) is easily visualized in neonates on ultrasound.
- Uterus didelphys manifests with two uteri and two fluid-filled vaginas, which may be asymmetric.
- In cases of vaginal obstruction, dilatation of the vagina is more marked than endometrial distension.
- On MRI, intravaginal and intrauterine contents with high signal on both T1 and T2 sequences are likely to be hemorrhagic fluid because of the paramagnetic effects of methemoglobin.

PITFALLS

- Dilated fallopian tube may be mistaken for a dilated ureter on ultrasound.
- Dilated vagina may be mistaken for the normal bladder in infants.

Suggested Readings

Buttram VC, Gibbons WE. Müllerian anomalies: a proposed classification (an analysis of 144 cases). Fertil Steril 1979;32:40–46

Carrington BM, Hricak H, Nuruddin RN, et al. Müllerian duct anomalies: MR imaging evaluation. Radiology 1990;176:715–720

Geley TE, Gassner I. Lower urinary tract anomalies of urogenital sinus and female genital anomalies. In: Fotter R, ed. Pediatric Uroradiology. Berlin, Germany: Springer; 2001:337–356

Li YW, Sheih CP, Chen WJ. Unilateral occlusion of duplicated uterus with ipsilateral renal anomaly in young girls: a study with MRI. Pediatr Radiol 1995;25:S54–S59

Scarsbrook AF, Moore NR. MRI appearances of Müllerian duct abnormalities. Clin Radiol 2003;58:747–754

CASE 76

Clinical Presentation

A 2-year-old boy presents having had a few episodes of urinary tract infection (UTI) 6 months earlier.

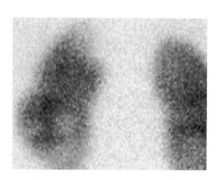
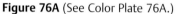

Figure 76A (See Color Plate 76A.)

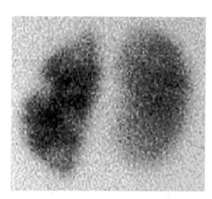

Figure 76B (See Color Plate 76B.)

Radiologic Findings

Posterior (**Fig. 76A**) and left posterior oblique (**Fig. 76B**) images from a technetium Tc 99m dimercaptosuccinic acid (DMSA) study show a photopenic defect at the upper pole of the left kidney. A suspicious area is also seen laterally in the mid-pole of the left kidney proven to be a real defect on the left oblique images. As this boy had had no UTI for 6 months, these photopenic areas on DMSA represent renal scarring. The right kidney is normal.

Diagnosis

Renal cortical scarring on ^{99m}Tc–DMSA scan

Differential Diagnosis

- Acute pyelonephritis (can cause an area of photopenia similar to scarring, hence the timing of the DMSA in relation to urinary infection is crucial)
- Renal masses

Discussion

Background

UTI is a common problem in pediatrics. It has been estimated that 8% of girls and 2% of boys will have a UTI during childhood. ^{99m}Tc–DMSA binds to the proximal convoluted tubules, resulting in fixation of the isotope and an unchanging image over many hours (hence the term *static* renal scan). Less than 10% of the injected dose is excreted in the urine. The delayed static images after intravenous injection represent functioning cortical mass and provide an accurate image of parenchymal outline. Posterior and oblique images are routinely obtained. Anterior views with the bladder empty are necessary when an ectopic or horseshoe kidney is suspected. Each image takes up to 5 minutes to acquire, and so sedation may be needed in a small number of children. DMSA studies are employed in some centers during an acute UTI to differentiate pyelonephritis from lower UTI. In many units, however, DMSA scans are reserved for assessing permanent renal scarring 3 to 6 months after a documented UTI.

Etiology

Pyelonephritis classically begins when bacteria enter the papilla. An inflammatory response with acute vasoconstriction results in regional ischemia and swelling. Depending on the organism's virulence and the rapidity of antibiotic treatment, a cascade of events with the release of destructive enzymes may result in renal parenchymal loss and, ultimately, renal scarring.

Clinical Findings

Urinary tract infection presents with a spectrum of illness. A severe acute pyelonephritis classically presents with pyrexia, flank pain, and septicemia. Low-grade cystitis may present with dysuria, hematuria, and/or frequency of urination. Unrecognized UTI may manifest as failure to thrive, vomiting, or diarrhea in small children.

Complications

- Mild lower urinary tract infection may have no later complications.
- Long-term consequences of small renal scars after a single episode of UTI are probably not significant.
- Data on the significance of renal scarring are derived from older studies that used excretory urography to detect scarring.
- Scars seen at urography are likely larger than those seen on DMSA or MRI.
- Later sequelae of scarring in severely affected children include hypertension (in 10–20% of patients), decreased glomerular filtration rate, and an increased incidence of toxemia during pregnancy.
- Although some authors suggest that the danger of end-stage renal failure has been overestimated, end-stage renal disease may occur in 5 to 10% of the most severely affected children

Imaging Findings

INTRAVENOUS UROGRAPHY

- Is less sensitive in detecting scarring than DMSA
- Carries a higher radiation burden than DMSA
- Scarring manifests as reduced parenchymal thickness and adjacent caliceal distortion.
- With upper or lower pole scarring, the calices of the affected kidney may appear to lie nearer to the vertebral pedicles than the calices of the contralateral normal kidney.

ULTRASOUND

- Cortical thinning at the upper or lower poles of the kidney may be diagnosed as renal scarring, but ultrasound, in general, is inferior to DMSA in detecting scars.
- Pyelonephritis in the acute phase may be demonstrable as a focal hyperechoic area in the kidney with reduced perfusion, but often no ultrasonographic abnormality is present.
- Significant echogenic debris in a dilated collecting system is suggestive of infection.
- Thickening of the uroepithelium may be seen with acute UTI but may also result from upper tract obstruction without infection.

NUCLEAR MEDICINE

- Mature scarring and acute pyelonephritis are both photopenic on DMSA.
- Complete photopenia with parenchymal retraction is typical of scarring.
- As acute pyelonephritis will also characteristically show a focal defect, to diagnose renal scarring DMSA scanning should be performed 3 to 6 months after an episode of UTI.
- Exclusion of a renal scar requires a normal DMSA study.
- DMSA allows an accurate estimate of differential renal function.

MRI

- Recently, fast imaging with gadolinium-enhanced inversion recovery sequences has shown high sensitivity and specificity for acute pyelonephritis.
- Standard T2- and T1-weighted images after gadolinium enhancement are not sensitive in the detection of pyelonephritis.
- Mature renal scarring is evident at MRI as loss of parenchyma often with an overlying contour defect.

Treatment

- Parenteral antibiotic therapy is required in any child with systemic symptoms from UTI.
- Long-term (for 1 year or more) prophylactic oral antibiotic therapy is used in many centers for all young children with proven UTI.

Prognosis

- Isolated small scars have probably little functional significance.
- The later sequelae of scarring in the most severely affected children include hypertension (in 10–20% of patients), decreased glomerular filtration rate, and an increased incidence of toxemia during pregnancy.

PEARLS

- The majority of renal scarring occurs in the first year of life, with few new renal scars acquired after the first 1 or 2 years of life.
- Complete photopenia with parenchymal retraction is the hallmark of renal scarring on DMSA.
- Exclusion of scarring requires a normal DMSA scan.

PITFALLS_____

- Ultrasonography is not sensitive in the detection of scarring.
- Acute pyelonephritis may mimic scarring on DMSA, hence a DMSA to detect scarring should be done 3 to 6 months after a UTI.

Suggested Readings

Ditchfield MR, Nadel HR. The DMSA scan in paediatric urinary tract infection. Australas Radiol 1998;42:318–320

Gordon I, Barkovics M, Pindoria S, et al. Primary vesico-ureteric reflux as a predictor of renal damage in children hospitalized with urinary tract infection: a systematic review and meta-analysis. J Am Soc Nephrol 2003;14:739–744

Hoberman A, Charron M, Hickey RW, et al. Imaging studies after a first febrile urinary tract infection in young children. N Engl J Med 2003;348:195–202

Lonergan GJ, Pennington DJ, Morrison JC, et al. Childhood pyelonephritis: comparison of gadolinium-enhanced MR imaging and renal cortical scintigraphy for diagnosis. Radiology 1998;207:377–384

Weiser AC, Amukele SA, Leonidas JC, Palmer LS. The role of gadolinium enhanced magnetic resonance imaging for children with suspected acute pyelonephritis. J Urol 2003;169:2308–2311

CASE 77

Clinical Presentation

A 6-year-old boy underwent abdominal ultrasonography because of a recent urinary tract infection (UTI). A positive family history of renal disease was present.

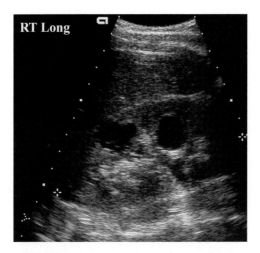

Figure 77A

Radiologic Findings

A longitudinal ultrasound image of the right kidney shows two anechoic lesions, both approximately 1.5 cm in diameter, with some posterior acoustic enhancement typical of renal cysts (**Fig. 77A**), which corresponded to the family history. The remaining right kidney and the left kidney were normal.

Diagnosis

Autosomal dominant polycystic kidney disease (ADPKD)

Differential Diagnosis

- Multiple simple renal cysts (An occasional simple renal cyst may be seen in childhood, but multiple cysts do not normally occur, and the positive family history mentioned above is conclusive.)
- Caliceal diverticula (Multiple diverticula would be very rare—one caliceal diverticulum may be indistinguishable from a simple renal cyst, but on IVU a caliceal diverticulum should opacify with contrast.)
- Multicystic dysplastic kidney (is a congenital unilateral disorder, usually without normal parenchyma on the affected side)
- Autosomal recessive polycystic kidney disease (manifests on ultrasound with bilateral large echogenic kidneys generally without resolvable cysts)
- Tuberous sclerosis (TS)

Discussion

Background

ADPKD is a multisystem disorder characterized by bilateral large (>2–3 cm) renal cysts, with cysts occasionally seen in other organs such as the liver or pancreas. The incidence in the general population is 1 in 1000. ADPKD is inherited, with nearly 100% penetrance. Up to 50% of patients, however, give no family history. ADPKD usually manifests between the third to fifth decades with hypertension, chronic renal failure, an abdominal mass, or hematuria. There is, however, great variation in the severity of the disease, with some cases being diagnosed in utero or in early childhood. TS may have identical renal manifestations to ADPKD, and in the absence of a family history of ADPKD, a thorough clinical examination and MRI of the brain to check for the lesions of TS is recommended in children. In addition to renal cysts, patients with TS frequently have foci of uniformly increased echogenicity in their kidneys due to angiomyolipomas. ADPKD may rarely manifest in infancy as bilateral enlarged echogenic kidneys without obvious cysts, mimicking autosomal recessive polycystic kidney disease (ARPKD). As the appearances of the hereditary polycystic kidney diseases may occasionally be identical in early childhood, some clinicians advocate biopsy in all patients.

Etiology

Two genes on chromosomes 16 and 4 have been identified as causal in this disorder. PKD1 is the gene on chromosome 16 and is responsible for 85% of detected cases. PKD2 is on chromosome 4, and a third gene is also likely. Proteins encoded by PKD1 and PKD2 have been named polycystin 1 and 2, respectively.

Pathology

- In ADPKD, the cysts and cystic dilatation involve the glomeruli and cortical tubules.

Clinical Findings

- Most young children with a family history of ADPKD will be asymptomatic and have a normal renal ultrasound study.

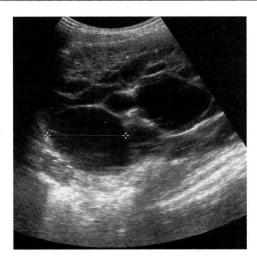

Figure 77B Longitudinal ultrasound image in an adolescent with a family history of ADPKD showing multiple anechoic cysts replacing most of the renal parenchyma.

- When cysts are seen in a young patient, the diagnosis of ADPKD is facilitated by a positive family history.
- Marked renal enlargement with numerous cysts may be seen in an occasional adolescent with ADPKD.
- Hepatic cysts are seen in a small number of patients in association with ADPKD, and the incidence of cysts in other organs depends on the stage and severity of the disease: the majority of young patients with ADPKD have cysts in the kidneys only.
- UTI is known to exacerbate kidney disease in adults.
- In children without known family history, routine ultrasound for intercurrent UTI brings some cases to attention. Vesicoureteral reflux (VUR), predisposing to UTI, may be more frequent in young patients with ADPKD than otherwise healthy age-matched children.

Complications

- Hypertension and renal insufficiency do not generally become a problem until adulthood.

Imaging Findings

ULTRASOUND

- Multiple, often large cysts with normal renal parenchyma are typical in young patients and are the ultrasound hallmark of ADPKD (**Fig. 77B**).
- Despite a positive family history, renal cysts may not be seen in early childhood.
- With a positive family history, if no cysts are seen by 20 years of age, the likelihood of developing ADPKD is small.
- Hepatic, pancreatic, or seminal vesicle cysts are evident in no more than 5% of young patients.
- Rarely, ADPKD may manifest in infancy as bilateral enlarged echogenic kidneys, mimicking ARPKD, and the typical large cysts appear over time.
- Hepatic cysts may be seen in association with ADPKD, but hepatic fibrosis is only seen in association with ARPKD.
- As ultrasonography may be normal in early childhood, screening may be better performed by gene probes than by imaging.

MRI

- Multiple bilateral renal cysts are easily identifiable.

Treatment

- Treatment is not usually necessary in childhood.
- Medical management of renal insufficiency and hypertension may be required in some older children.

Prognosis

- Often asymptomatic until adulthood
- Hypertension and chronic renal failure are inevitable.
- The clinical history tends to have a similar pattern in members of the same family.
- Up to 10% of adults with ADPKD die from rupture of an intracranial berry aneurysm.

PEARLS

- Hepatic cysts but not hepatic fibrosis may be seen in association with ADPKD.
- Despite a family history, when no cysts are seen by 20 years of age the likelihood of developing ADPKD is small.
- As the ultrasound appearances of ADPKD and ARPKD may occasionally be similar in young children, the parents of all children with suspected hereditary polycystic renal disease should undergo renal ultrasound.
- VUR and UTI may be more frequent in young patients with ADPKD than otherwise healthy age-matched children.

PITFALLS

- Renal cysts may not be visible in early childhood.
- Renal manifestations of TS may be identical to ADPKD.
- Hepatic cysts should not be mistaken for the biliary ectasia of Caroli's disease.

Suggested Readings

Avni FE, Guissard G, Hall M, et al. Hereditary polycystic kidney diseases in children: changing sonographic patterns through childhood. Pediatr Radiol 2002;32:169–174

Belet U, Danaci M, Sarikaya S, et al. Prevalence of epididymal, seminal vesicle, prostate and testicular cysts in autosomal dominant polycystic kidney disease. Urology 2002;60:138–141

Koslowe O, Frank R, Gauthier B, et al. Urinary tract infections, VUR and autosomal dominant polycystic kidney disease. Pediatr Nephrol 2003;18:823–825

CASE 78

Clinical Presentation

A female infant presents with palpable abdominal masses. Oligohydramnios had been noted in utero.

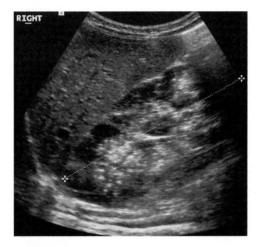

Figure 78A

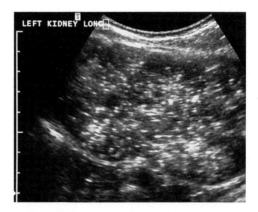

Figure 78B

Radiologic Findings

Longitudinal ultrasound images of the right (**Fig. 78A**) and left kidney (**Fig. 78B**), the latter from a prone position, show two enlarged hyperechoic kidneys with no corticomedullary differentiation. A relatively hypoechoic rim to the right kidney and prominent hyperechoic foci within the left kidney are noted. Both kidneys measured 9 cm in bipolar lengths, significantly above the 90th percentile for age.

Diagnosis

Autosomal recessive polycystic kidney disease (ARPKD)

Differential Diagnosis

- Autosomal dominant polycystic kidney disease (ADPKD) (Normal renal parenchyma with large renal cysts is characteristic.)
- Cystic dysplastic kidneys (small kidneys with small cysts)
- Renal vein thrombosis (is usually unilateral, but if bilateral is asymmetric and often associated with (inferior vena cava thrombus)
- Juvenile nephronophythisis

Discussion

Background

ARPKD has been termed *infantile polycystic kidney disease*. It is also known as hepatorenal cystic disease due to the association of renal cysts arising from the tubules and hepatic cysts from the bile ducts. The incidence is 1 in 20,000. Renal involvement is bilateral with normal collecting systems. Hepatic fibrosis with portal hypertension is the predominant clinical problem in patients presenting later in childhood.

Etiology

The ARPKD locus has been mapped to the short arm of chromosome 6. All phenotypic variants appear to result from mutations in a single gene.

Clinical Findings

ARPKD may be suspected on antenatal ultrasound when markedly enlarged echogenic kidneys, without visible cysts, are seen in the third trimester. Oligohydramnios may also be evident. In the absence of antenatal pick-up, the time of first manifestation of many cases of ARPKD depends on the severity of the disorder. Earlier clinical presentation is associated with a poorer prognosis. Presentation with respiratory distress from pulmonary hypoplasia is commonly seen in the neonatal period as a result of oligohydramnios. Chronic lung disease from prolonged ventilation is seen in 10% of patients. Of those who present in the neonatal period, up to 50% die in the first few days of life. Progressive renal dysfunction inevitably ensues in the survivors. Slightly older infants can present with large masses in both flanks. Hepatic fibrosis with hepatomegaly and splenomegaly from portal hypertension predominate in older children in whom the renal disease may be quite mild.

Complications

- Seventy to 80% of these patients develop renal hypertension.
- Varying degrees of renal impairment are seen in all patients.
- An increased incidence of urinary tract infections is seen.
- Bleeding esophageal or gastric varices, or hypersplenism can be problematic in older children.
- Hepatocellular function is usually preserved, but cholangitis can lead to hepatic failure.

Pathology

- The tubular abnormality primarily involves dilatation of the collecting tubules.

Imaging Findings

INTRAVENOUS UROGRAPHY

- No longer necessary for diagnosis
- Classic finding is a streaky radiating arrangement of contrast in the ectatic tubules.
- Delayed images (up to 24 hours postinjection) are needed to opacify the ectatic tubules.
- Is best done when the babies are a few weeks old—when the kidneys have "matured"—rather than in the immediate newborn period
- Little or no visualization of the pelvocaliceal system

ULTRASOUND

- Large symmetrical echogenic kidneys, without corticomedullary differentiation, are characteristic.
- Kidneys retain their reniform shape.
- No cysts are discernible in young children, although with high-resolution scanners small subcentimeter lesions may be seen, particularly in older children.
- Spectrum of findings change with the age of the patient.
- Prominent hyperechoic foci are characteristically seen in older children in association with renal failure.
- In older children, hepatic involvement manifests with hepatomegaly, increased periportal echogenicity, and ectatic cysts of the biliary system (Caroli's disease).
- Portal hypertension with splenomegaly and esophageal varices may be seen with advanced hepatic disease.

CT

- Shows massively enlarged kidneys, occasionally filling the abdomen
- In older children, splenic enlargement and intrahepatic biliary dilatation are seen.

MRI

- Marked heterogeneous renal enlargement is seen.
- Biliary ectasia is best evaluated by heavily T2-weighted imaging sequences.

Treatment

- Therapy is directed at respiratory distress in early life.
- Lifelong treatment consists of managing chronic renal failure, hypertension, and the consequences of hepatic fibrosis.
- Renal transplantation is necessary for end-stage renal failure.
- Control of portal hypertension by portal circulatory diversion or liver transplantation may be required.

Prognosis

- Perinatal mortality ranges from 30 to 50%.
- In survivors, the long-term prognosis has improved considerably in recent years.
- Of the survivors beyond infancy, approximately half develop end-stage renal failure in childhood.

PEARLS

- A streaky radiating arrangement to the contrast, on delayed images, in the ectatic tubules on intravenous urography is the classic appearance.
- Very large, symmetric, echogenic kidneys on ultrasound are characteristic.
- Hepatic fibrosis occurs in all cases.
- Relative degrees of kidney and liver disease tend to be inverse.
- Children with severe renal disease usually have milder hepatic disease, and those with severe hepatic disease have mild renal impairment.

PITFALLS

- Hepatic cysts, but not biliary duct dilatation, may be seen in ADPKD.
- In older children, hepatomegaly with portal hypertension may be so marked that subtle changes in the kidneys, typically in the renal medullae, may be overlooked.

Suggested Readings

Avni FE, Guissard G, Hall M, et al. Hereditary polycystic kidney diseases in children: changing sonographic patterns through childhood. Pediatr Radiol 2002;32:169–174

Guay-Woodford LM, Desmond RA. Autosomal recessive polycystic kidney disease: the clinical experience in North America. Pediatrics 2003;111:1072–1080

Lonergan GJ, Rice RR, Suarez ES. Autosomal recessive polycystic kidney disease: radiologic-pathologic correlation. Radiographics 2000;20:837–855

CASE 79

Clinical Presentation

A neonate presents with a history of abnormal antenatal ultrasound.

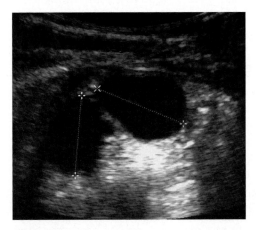

Figure 79A

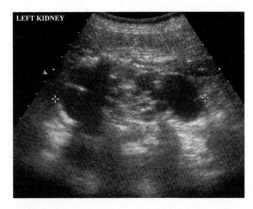

Figure 79B

Radiologic Findings

Only two cysts, marked with cursors, were visible in the left renal fossa (**Figs. 79A** and **79B**). No normal left renal parenchyma was seen. The right kidney was normal, albeit large, measuring 6 cm in bipolar length.

Diagnosis

Multicystic dysplastic kidney (MCDK)

Differential Diagnosis

- Cystic renal tumors, including mesoblastic nephroma or cystic Wilms' (typically, solid components are also present in these lesions)
- Autosomal dominant polycystic kidney disease (a bilateral disorder, only rarely manifests with identifiable cysts in infancy)
- Autosomal recessive polycystic kidney disease (large echogenic kidneys are seen, generally without resolvable cysts)

Discussion

Background

MCDK is a type of renal dysplasia characterized by multiple cysts of varying sizes, without identifiable normal renal parenchyma. MCDK typically occurs in association with a nonfunctioning kidney. There is loss of lobular organization, without the normal overall structural pattern characteristic of the kidney. With increasing sensitivity of renal scintigraphy, some minimal function has been described in some MCDK cases, but this is of no real clinical significance. Contralateral compensatory hypertrophy of the normal kidney is seen in most cases of MCDK. Partial renal involvement may be seen as MCDK may affect only part of a kidney; that is, the upper pole of a duplex or one side of a horseshoe kidney. MCDK disease is associated with contralateral urinary abnormalities in approximately one third of cases. When contralateral upper tract dilatation is seen, a voiding cystourethrogram (VCUG) is needed to evaluate for vesicoureteric reflux and a technetium Tc-99m MAG3 dynamic renogram (with diuretic challenge) to assess for ureteropelvic junction obstruction.

Etiology

In utero ureteral or pelviureteral atresia is the usual antecedent of MCDK. Less commonly, an obstructing ureterocele has been found in association. As in utero obstruction is common to both MCDK and (cystic) dysplastic kidney, some pathologists consider these entities as two ends of a spectum.

Clinical Findings

The diagnosis is usually made with antenatal or neonatal ultrasonography. Some cases manifest as an abdominal mass in the newborn period, although up to 50% of cases are not clinically detectable.

Complications

- Hypertension is a recognized, albeit unusual, complication.
- Vesicoureteral reflux to the contralateral kidney can usually be managed by antibiotic prophylaxis.
- Ureteropelvic junction obstruction in the contralateral kidney may require pyeloplasty.

Pathology

The microscopic appearance is characterized by large cysts lined by flattened cuboidal epithelium. No normal parenchyma is seen, but the tissue between the cysts is fibrotic and may contain cartilage. There is absence of a normal pelvicaliceal system.

Imaging Findings

RADIOGRAPHY

- No specific radiographic features of MCDK are found, which may rarely present with evidence of an abdominal mass.

ULTRASOUND

- Appearances range from a small single cyst to a large mass containing multiple, typically anechoic, cysts of varying sizes, often with a dominant large cyst situated peripherally.
- There is no identifiable normal renal parenchyma or collecting system.
- Hypertrophy of the contralateral kidney is characteristic.
- The condition must be distinguished from a severe ureteropelvic junction obstruction—occasionally isotope studies may be needed to differentiate.
- MCDK can generally be reliably diagnosed and monitored by serial ultrasound examinations.

VOIDING CYSTOURETHROGRAPHY (VCUG)

- Must be performed when a dilated contralateral ureter is seen on ultrasound to assess for vesicoureteric reflux

NUCLEAR MEDICINE

- MCDK typically shows no function on isotope studies.
- ^{99m}Tc–MAG3 renogram is indicated to assess drainage from the other kidney when ultrasound reveals a dilated renal pelvis without a dilated ureter.

Treatment

- Many undergo spontaneous involution
- Indications for surgery include a large mass that impedes normal breathing or feeding in infancy.
- Although approaches differ in different centers, many pediatric urologists will remove an enlarging MCDK mass, a mass >5 cm in diameter, or a mass that fails to involute after 2 years of follow-up.

Prognosis

- Long-term prognosis is excellent when the contralateral kidney is normal.
- Initial size of the MCDK is not a good predictor of eventual outcome.
- Albeit controversial, no convincing link with subsequent malignancy is proven.

PEARLS_____

- No normal renal parenchyma is visible in a MCDK.
- Unrecognized MCDK with involution during childhood is a likely cause of an apparent solitary kidney in an adult.
- Contralateral compensatory hypertrophy of the normal kidney is seen in most cases.
- Bilateral MCDK, or MCDK with contralateral renal agenesis, is incompatible with life.
- Diagnosis is often only possible in the third trimester in utero.

PITFALL_____

- Marked hydronephrosis may mimic an MCDK with one prominent cyst, but with true hydronephrosis some, albeit thin, renal parenchyma should be visible.

Suggested Readings

Metcalfe PD, Wright JR Jr, Anderson PA. MCDK not excluded by virtue of function on renal scan. Can J Urol 2002;9:1690–1693

Rottenberg GT, Gordon I, De Bruyn R. The natural history of multicystic dysplastic kidney in children. Br J Radiol 1997;70:347–350

Strife JL, Souza AS, Kirks DR, et al. Multicystic dysplastic kidney in children: US follow-up. Radiology 1993;186:785–788

CASE 80

Clinical Presentation

Initial abdominal sonogram in a male infant presenting with history of in utero oligohydramnios

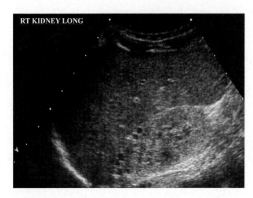

Figure 80A

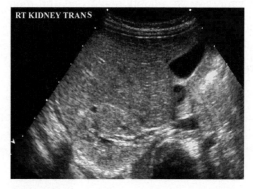

Figure 80B

Radiologic Findings

A highly echogenic kidney is evident on longitudinal (**Fig. 80A**) and transverse (**Fig. 80B**) ultrasound images with loss of the normal corticomedullary differentiation. Note the kidney is much more echogenic than the adjacent liver. A few small, peripheral, anechoic cysts are seen. Both kidneys have similar appearances and are small for age.

Diagnosis

Bilateral (cystic) renal dysplasia

Differential Diagnosis

- Autosomal dominant polycystic kidney disease (normal kidneys usually seen in early childhood and rarely manifest with identifiable cysts in infancy)
- Autosomal recessive polycystic kidney disease (large echogenic kidneys are seen without resolvable cysts)
- Multicystic dysplastic kidney (MCDK) (unilateral disorder with multiple large cysts without identifiable normal renal parenchyma in a nonfunctioning kidney)
- Acute tubular necrosis (causes enlarged kidneys without any cystic change)

Discussion

Background

Renal dysplasia is used to describe abnormal metanephric differentiation with the presence of primitive tubules and mesenchymal tissue in the kidney. Glomeruli, tubules, and collecting ducts are reduced in number. Although dyplasia is a histologic term, pediatric radiologists and nephrologists commonly apply this term as a generic description to several congenital conditions that result in small, echogenic kidneys with varying degrees of renal failure. Some functioning renal tissue is generally preserved within these abnormal kidneys. Cysts are not mandatory for this diagnosis but are often present. When present, these cysts are typically small (<1 cm) in contrast to the larger cysts seen in MCDK. Dysplastic kidneys are usually smaller than normal kidneys. Dysplasia is often seen in association with other urinary tract malformations such as a ureterocele obstructing the upper moiety of a duplex kidney, posterior urethral valves, or crossed fused ectopia. In addition, some syndromes have associated renal dysplasia, for example, Laurence-Moon and Opitz syndromes.

Etiology

True renal cystic disease and renal dysplasia are two distinct entities. Many dysplastic kidneys may develop cysts, however. Renal obstruction is the key determinant in the development of renal dysplasia. Although the pathologic features of renal dysplasia are considered to be the same whether the obstruction is at the level of the urethra, ureter, or ureteropelvic junction, the ultrasonographic findings vary significantly. In general, the more proximal the level of obstruction the more likely the cysts will be seen at ultrasonography. It is postulated that when the obstruction is at a higher level, the calices distend more and a more cystic form of dysplasia develops. If the obstruction is in the urethra, the pressure effects are more generalized, so the calices do not distend to the same degree but the kidney becomes dysplastic nevertheless. As in utero obstruction is common to both MCDK and (cystic) dyplastic kidney, some pathologists consider these entities as two ends of a spectrum.

Clinical Findings

Urinary tract dilatation that is secondary to an obstructing lesion, for example, posterior urethral valves, is frequently discovered prenatally. Clinical symptoms depend on the underlying disease and the degree of impairment of renal function. When bilateral dysplasia is present, chronic renal failure with failure to thrive and stunting of growth is inevitable. The onset of end-stage renal failure may not be until the second decade, however. An occult cause of enuresis, typically encountered in girls, is localized dysplasia of an upper moiety in a duplex kidney with ectopic drainage. The upper moiety kidney in this situation may be so small, and nonfunctioning, as to be undetectable on virtually all forms of imaging other than at retrograde pyelography, which is performed when an ectopic ureter is discovered at endoscopy.

Imaging Findings

INTRAVENOUS UROGRAPHY

- Dysplastic kidneys are small and poorly functioning (and are not well visualized at urography).
- Calices are blunted and often few in number.

ULTRASOUND

- Dysplastic kidneys are usually well below the 50th percentile for size for age.
- Dysplastic kidneys are echogenic with loss of corticomedullary differentiation.
- Cysts that are present tend to be small and peripherally located around the surface of the renal cortex.
- Upper-tract dilatation, when present, is usually secondary to reflux.

NUCLEAR MEDICINE

- When unilateral, the dysplastic kidney is seen to have reduced function on technetium Tc 99m dimercaptosuccinic acid (DMSA) and other isotope studies.
- If bilateral dysplasia is present, the kidneys are poorly visualized with ^{99m}Tc–DMSA.
- Focal defects in the dysplastic kidney are seen on ^{99m}Tc–DMSA studies in the absence of urinary infection (and so these defects are not strictly "scars").

Treatment

- Localized forms of dysplasia, particularly when resulting in enuresis or complicated by infection, may be treated by surgical removal.
- Treatment in cases of bilateral dysplasia centers on the management of chronic renal insufficiency.

Prognosis

- Children with bilateral dysplasia and chronic renal failure frequently undergo renal transplantation in childhood.

PEARLS

- Dysplastic kidneys are below the 50th percentile for size for age.
- Although several conditions, for example, acute tubular necrosis or ARPKD, may result in echogenic kidneys with loss of the normal corticomedullary differentiation, only renal dysplasia results in small kidneys.
- Cysts are not mandatory for the diagnosis of renal dysplasia but are often present.

PITFALLS

- Localized dysplasia of an upper moiety in a duplex kidney may result in a very small nonfunctioning moiety that is undetectable on virtually all forms of imaging other than at retrograde pyelography.

Suggested Readings

De Bruyn R, Gordon I, McHugh K. Imaging of the kidneys and urinary tract in children. In: Grainger RG, Allison DJ, Adam A, Dixon AK, eds. Diagnostic Radiology: A Textbook of Medical Imaging. 4th ed. Edinburgh, England: Churchill-Livingstone; 2001:1749–1751

Sanders RC, Nussbaum AR, Solez K. Renal dysplasia: sonographic findings. Radiology 1988; 167:623–626

Thomsen HS, Levine E, Meilstrup JW, et al. Renal cystic diseases. Eur Radiol 1997;7:1267–1275

CASE 81

Clinical Presentation

A 2-year-old girl presents with recurrent urinary tract infection (UTI), and a voiding cystourethrogram (VCUG) is performed.

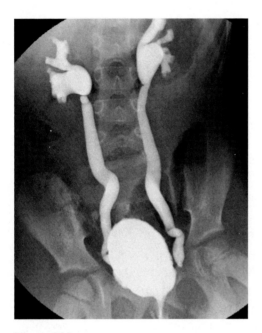

Figure 81A

Radiologic Findings

Bilateral vesicoureteric reflux (VUR) into mildly dilated ureters and renal pelves (international grade III–IV) is seen (**Fig. 81A**). Note the urethra is opacified, indicating the patient was actively voiding when the radiograph was taken.

Diagnosis

Bilateral VUR (international grade III–IV)

Differential Diagnosis

- Normal kidneys on intravenous urogram (But note the renal parenchyma is not opacified by contrast, and dense contrast is seen in the urethra.)
- Reflux into lower moieties of duplex kidneys (But note the normal orientation of calices and no ureterocele in the bladder.)

Discussion

Background

There is a well-recognized association between VUR, UTI, and consequent renal damage, so-called reflux nephropathy. In an individual patient, however, the significance of VUR is controversial. VUR, in general, is a weak predictor of pyelonephritis and subsequent renal impairment, although there does appear to be some association between higher grades of reflux and renal damage. Reflux is found in only one third of children with proven pyelonephritis. In addition, the development of a postpyelonephritic scar appears to be independent of demonstrable VUR. In children hospitalized with UTI, however, VUR is common. For this reason, the American Academy of Pediatrics recommends that infants and young children 2 months to 2 years of age with UTI should undergo ultrasound, with either VCUG or radionuclide cystography to detect dilatation secondary to obstruction or VUR. Ultrasound is routinely performed in the UTI setting to detect anatomic abnormalities of the urinary tract. Ultrasound findings are not, however, predictive of VUR. A VCUG is necessary to detect or exclude VUR regardless of the renal ultrasound findings.

Etiology

In primary reflux, there is abnormal function of the vesicoureteric junction thought to be due to a short submucosal tunnel of the distal ureter through the bladder with an incompetent orifice. The incidence of VUR is thought to be ~2% in asymptomatic young children, although the prevalence will vary with age. Sterile VUR has been shown to be associated with renal damage in studies investigating congenital uropathies. VUR occurs in a substantial proportion of kidneys with mild hydronephrosis (at least 20%), but VUR also occurs in normal kidneys investigated because of contralateral dilatation in infancy. Reflux is more common in kidneys associated with an ipsilateral hydroureter.

Clinical Findings

VUR is asymptomatic. Children come to attention because of associated UTIs. Prolonged neonatal jaundice is a classic association of bacteruria in the newborn. Infants with UTI may present with fever, diarrhea, vomiting, poor feeding, or failure to thrive. Cystitis-type symptoms such as frequency of urination or dysuria are seen in older children. The classic symptoms of pyelonephritis, manifesting with high fever, flank pain, and rigors, are an uncommon clinical presentation in children.

Complications

Many cases of VUR resolve without sequelae. The true incidence of children who go on to develop permanent renal scarring is unknown. A small percentage of the most severely affected children with bilateral scarring progress to chronic renal failure and/or hypertension.

Imaging Findings

VCUG

- VCUG is a highly sensitive and specific test for VUR.
- VCUG has the advantage over other tests for reflux in that bladder and urethral anatomy is also displayed.
- Double micturition or cyclic voiding should be performed in all patients to increase the sensitivity to VUR.

NUCLEAR MEDICINE

- Direct radionuclide cystography (DRC), which like VCUG requires catheterization, is more sensitive than VCUG for VUR as there is continuous monitoring rather than intermittent fluoroscopy.
- DRC, however, provides no anatomical information.
- Indirect radioisotope cystography (IRC) can be achieved following intravenous injection of technetium Tc-99m MAG3, with voiding after much of the isotope has reached the bladder.
- IRC is only possible in older toilet-trained children.
- IRC is contraindicated when there is a pelvic kidney; hydroureter or hydronephrosis as isotope in dilated systems, or in the bladder with a pelvic kidney, obscures reflux.
- No accurate grading of reflux is possible with any form of isotope cystography, as the anatomical definition is too poor to differentiate between similar grades of VUR.

ULTRASOUND

- Ultrasound is a poor predictor of VUR.
- Occasionally, normal kidneys may be seen at the start of an ultrasound examination whereupon a small child voids resulting in immediate hydroureter or hydronephrosis indicating VUR.
- Instillation of ultrasound contrast agent into the bladder greatly increases the sensitivity of ultrasound for VUR, but is not widely practiced at present.

Treatment

- Parenteral antibiotic therapy is required in a child with systemic symptoms from UTI.
- Discovery of VUR allows initiation of prophylactic antibiotics to prevent future episodes of UTI.
- Ureteric reimplantation is a known cure for VUR, but many studies have shown that there is no difference in the long-term outcome in children treated by surgery or medical antibiotic prophylaxis.
- In recent years the pendulum of treatment has swung to conservative medical management of VUR

Prognosis

- VUR resolves spontaneously in the vast majority of patients in early childhood.
- Dangers of end-stage renal failure from combined reflux and UTI have probably been overestimated.
- Up to 5 to 10% of the most severely affected children may develop postpyelonephritic hypertension or chronic renal failure.

PEARLS

- VUR is asymptomatic—these children are investigated because of associated UTIs.
- VCUG is necessary to rule out VUR, regardless of the renal ultrasound findings.
- VUR has been found in between 8 and 40% of children investigated for their first UTI.
- VUR is found in only one third of children with proven pyelonephritis.
- Development of a postpyelonephritic scar appears to be independent of demonstrable VUR.
- No anatomic information or grading of VUR is possible with isotope cystography.

PITFALLS_____

- Ultrasound findings are not predictive of VUR.
- VUR may be intermittent and so can be missed by all types of cystography.
- VCUG studies, due to bladder catheterization, run the risk of causing iatrogenic UTI in up to 1% of patients—antibiotic prophylaxis is used to prevent this.

Suggested Readings

American Academy of Pediatrics Committee on Quality Improvement Subcommittee on Urinary Tract Infection. Practice parameter: the diagnosis, treatment and evaluation of the initial urinary tract infection in febrile infants and young children. Pediatrics 1999;103:843–852

Mahant S, Friedman J, MacArthur C. Renal ultrasound findings and vesicoureteral reflux in children hospitalized with urinary tract infection. Arch Dis Child 2002;86:419–421

Pal CR, Tuson JRD, Lindsell DRM, et al. The role of micturating cystourethrography in antenatally detected mild hydronephrosis. Pediatr Radiol 1998;28:152–155

Piaggio G, Degl' Innocenti ML, Toma P, et al. Cystosonography and voiding cystourethrography in the diagnosis of vesicoureteral reflux. Pediatr Nephrol 2003;18:18–22

CASE 82

Clinical Presentation

A 7-year-old boy presents who had had previous bladder surgery. An intravenous urogram is performed.

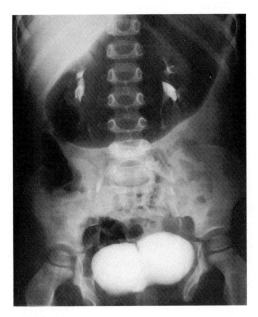

Figure 82A

Radiologic Findings

The kidneys are normal. The bladder appears wider than is usual with a midline septum seen superiorly from previous bladder reconstructive surgery (**Fig. 82A**). The pubic symphysis shows wide diastasis. (Note gaseous distension of the stomach, produced by a prior carbonated drink, in an attempt to improve visualization of the kidneys.)

Diagnosis

Bladder exstrophy (after bladder closure)

Differential Diagnosis

- Augmented bladder (But note also pubic symphysis diastasis.)
- Neuropathic bladder (classically leads to a cone-shaped bladder, is frequently associated with spinal dysraphism but not diastasis of the symphysis)
- Vesicoureteric reflux (**Fig. 82A** is an intravenous urogram with the renal parenchyma opacified by contrast, and note the urethra is not visible as the patient is not voiding.)
- Bladder duplication (extremely rare, is associated with urethral duplication but not pubic symphysis diastasis)

Discussion

Background

Bladder exstrophy is one of the anterior abdominal wall defects in which the bladder lies exposed on the lower abdominal surface. Males are affected three times as frequently as females. The incidence is 1 in 10,000 live births. It is often not diagnosed in utero as the lower abdominal area can be a difficult area to demonstrate in pregnancy and may be obscured by limbs during antenatal ultrasound. However, it is noteworthy nevertheless that in these patients a normal bladder is not identified on prenatal scanning. Epispadias is frequently associated. Indeed, exstrophy and epispadias represent a spectrum of anomalies. The pubic symphysis is always widened, being wider in cases of exstrophy than in epispadias, with diastasis also of the rectus muscles. Cases of exstrophy are more common than the milder variant epispadias. Vertebral anomalies are also sometimes seen in association with exstrophy. The genital structures are typically normal as are the upper urinary tracts prior to surgery.

Etiology

Abnormal mesodermal migration during development of the lower abdominal wall within the first 8 weeks of gestation is assumed to be causative. Whether the bony abnormality is the primary pathology or a consequence of another abnormality is unknown. Maternal age <20 years and one parent with exstrophy are known risk factors.

Clinical Findings

The diagnoses of exstrophy, and epispadias in a male, are clinically obvious with the bladder mucosa lying exposed on the lower abdominal surface. The umbilicus is low set, and an exomphalos may be observed. The penis is short. Inguinal hernias are present in up to 20% of patients. Epispadias in a female is rare and may result in an occult cause of enuresis.

Complications

VUR occurs after bladder repair in many cases. Ureterovesical junction obstruction also may result from surgery and may be clinically silent. There is an increased long-term risk of bladder adenocarcinoma.

Imaging Findings

RADIOGRAPHY

- Widened symphysis is seen where the width of the split symphysis increases with the size of the exstrophy.
- Pelvic girdle appears C-shaped rather than forming a ring.
- Pubic and iliac bones are rotated outward.

ULTRASOUND

- Prior to surgical repair no bladder is seen.
- Distal ureters may be seen to hook upward to reach the trigone as the bladder base is elevated.
- Surgical repair with or without bladder augmentation results in a bladder with an irregular outline.

SONOGRAPHY

- Normal kidneys are seen prior to bladder reconstruction.
- Upper tract dilation after surgery may be due to VUR or ureterovesical junction obstruction.

CT

- The iliac and pubic bones are externally rotated.

Treatment

- Surgical reconstruction involves closure of the exstrophy, bladder neck reconstruction, repair of epispadias, and, at times, additional bladder augmentation.
- Iliac osteotomies, in addition to approximating the pubic bones, facilitate the placement of all soft tissue structures closer to their normal anatomic position inside a reconstructed pelvic ring.
- Iliac osteotomies are known to improve continence.
- Bladder diversion procedures such as ureterosigmoidostomy are becoming obsolete.

Prognosis

- The majority of patients achieve long-term continence.

PEARLS

- Widening of the symphysis pubis results from outward rotation of the iliac and pubic bones.
- Width of the split in the symphysis pubis increases with the extent of the exstrophy.
- Kidneys are normal prior to bladder surgery.

PITFALL

- Occasionally, dysraphism with a meningocele may occur in association with exstrophy and result in a neuropathic bladder.

Suggested Readings

Ait-Ameur A, Wakim A, Dubousset J, et al. The AP diameter of the pelvis: a new criterion for continence in the exstrophy complex? Pediatr Radiol 2001;31:640–645

Currarino G, Wood B, Massoud M. The genitourinary tract and retroperitoneum: epispadias-exstrophy complex. In: FN Silverman, JP Kuhn, eds. Caffey's Pediatric X-ray Diagnosis. 9th ed. St. Louis, MO: Mosby; 1993:1298–1301

Corantin F. Epispadias-extrophy complex. In: Fotter, R, ed. Diagnostic Imaging: Pediatric Uroradiology. Berlin: Springer; 2001:111–120

CASE 83

Clinical Presentation

A 2-year-old girl presents with a palpable right-sided abdominal mass.

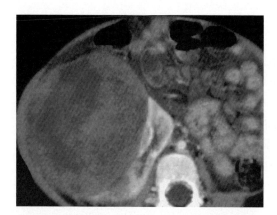

Figure 83A

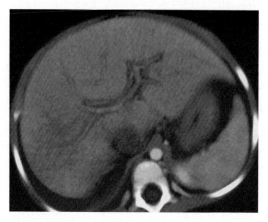

Figure 83B

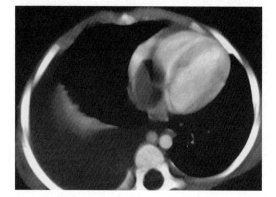

Figure 83C

Radiologic Findings

Axial CT images after intravenous contrast enhancement show a large heterogeneous mass arising from the right kidney (**Fig. 83A**). More superior sections through the liver (**Fig. 83B**) and heart (**Fig. 83C**) show distended but non-opacified inferior vena cava (IVC), a right pleural effusion, and a filling defect in the right atrium due to tumor thrombus extension along the IVC into the right side of the heart. Note the enlarged azygos vein adjacent to the aorta on **Fig. 83C**.

Diagnosis

Wilms' tumor with tumor thrombus in the IVC

Differential Diagnosis

- Hydronephrosis (Renal parenchymal distortion without excess intrarenal fluid and solid components to the mass exclude this from the differential diagnosis.)
- Mesoblastic nephroma (rare in a child >1 year of age)
- Other malignant renal tumors of childhood (such as a clear cell sarcoma or rhabdoid tumor) have similar appearances to a Wilms' tumor but are much less common.
- Renal cell carcinoma (occurs occasionally in children but uncommonly before 5 years of age)
- Neuroblastoma (typically is suprarenal in origin and displays encasement of the retroperitoneal vessels rather than simple displacement)

Discussion

Background

Wilms' tumor (nephroblastoma) is the most common renal malignancy in children. It accounts for ~10% of solid malignancies in childhood with a peak incidence around 3 years of age. There is an equal prevalence in boys and girls with the highest incidence being in African American children. Bilateral tumors are seen in 10% of patients at presentation. Associated anomalies occur in 15% of children. Genitourinary associations include cryptorchidism and a horseshoe kidney. One third of children with sporadic aniridia develop Wilms' tumors, frequently bilaterally. Other conditions predisposing to Wilms' tumor include Beckwith-Wiedemann (macroglossia, exomphalos, gigantism), hemihypertrophy, and Denys-Drash syndrome (pseudohermaphroditism). Clear cell sarcoma, which has a tendency to metastasize to bone, and rhabdoid tumor of the kidney, which has an association with posterior fossa neoplasms, used to be classified as variants of Wilms' tumor but are now regarded as separate entities. Tumor thrombus from a Wilms' tumor tends to be adherent within the IVC with little risk of embolization except at the time of surgery.

Etiology

Nephrogenic rests are areas of persistent embryonic renal parenchyma (metanephric blastema). Nephroblastomatosis, defined as the presence of multiple nephrogenic rests, is commonly found in bilateral tumors. Although foci of nephroblastomatosis may be variable in size and appearance, most lesions are small foci of homogeneous echogenicity on ultrasound and are uniformly hypovascular on contrast-enhanced CT and MRI, in contrast to the usually larger heterogeneous enhancing Wilms' tumor masses.

Clinical Findings

The most frequent presentation is with an asymptomatic abdominal mass. Hematuria, particularly after relatively minor trauma, is a recognized presentation, with microscopic hematuria being present in 25% of cases. Abdominal pain, fever, or hypertension is seen in a minority of children.

Pathology

Wilms' tumors may have either favorable or unfavorable histology. More than 90% of tumors have favorable triphasic histology comprising primitive blastema, stroma, and epithelial components. Tumors with foci of anaplasia, even if only in one small focus of the tumor, are deemed to have unfavorable histology and a worse prognosis.

Imaging Findings

RADIOGRAPHY

- Bowel displacement by a bulky abdominal mass is a nonspecific sign.
- Intravenous urography no longer has a role in the diagnosis of Wilms' tumor.
- Many international staging systems rely solely on the presence of lung nodules detectable on chest x-ray in Wilms' tumor patients to diagnose pulmonary metastases (omitting chest CT).

ULTRASOUND

- Large cystic, solid or mixed cystic, solid mass occupying much of the flank is characteristic.
- Normal native renal tissue can be difficult to detect but is typically present and stretched at the periphery of the tumor.
- Must carefully look for tumor thrombus in the renal vein, IVC, and right atrium
- Contralateral kidney should be evaluated for evidence of nephroblastomatosis and synchronous Wilms' tumor.

CT

- Calcification is uncommon.
- On contrast-enhanced CT, a portion of vividly enhancing normal kidney tissue can be seen stretched around the tumor.
- Most tumors are well-demarcated with a pseudo-capsule.
- Heterogeneous enhancement after contrast administration is typical of Wilms' tumors on CT, whereas foci of nephroblastomatosis tend to be uniformly hypovascular.

MRI

- Most tumors are of heterogeneous low-signal intensity on T1-weighted images and high-signal on T2.
- Heterogeneous enhancement after gadolinium administration is typical of Wilms' tumors on MRI, whereas foci of nephroblastomatosis tend to be uniformly hypovascular.
- IVC tumor thrombus may be seen to enhance after gadolinium administration, indicating viable tumor rather than simple intraluminal clot.

STAGING

National Wilms' Tumor Study Group (NWTSG) staging system is commonly used and depends on surgical findings and residual extent of disease.

- Stage 1: tumor confined to kidney without vascular or capsular invasion with complete resection
- Stage 2: tumor extends beyond renal capsule (but completely removed at surgery) with vessel infiltration
- Stage 3: positive lymph nodes in the abdomen or pelvis, peritoneal spill of tumor at surgery, residual tumor at surgical margins
- Stage 4: metastatic disease outside abdomen or pelvis
- Stage 5: bilateral tumors at diagnosis

Treatment

- Initial surgery followed by chemotherapy is the standard approach in North America.
- Chemotherapy prior to surgery can lead to tumor down-staging and potentially a decreased need for postoperative irradiation.
- Tumor thrombus in the IVC is usually regarded as a contraindication to surgery before chemotherapy.

Prognosis

- Localized stage 1 or 2 disease has a >90% cure rate.
- Four-year survival for stage 4 metastatic disease with favorable histology ranges from 60 to 80%.
- Metastatic stage 4 disease with unfavorable histology has a poor outlook.

PEARLS_____

- Contralateral tumor and renal vein extension of tumor must be looked for carefully.
- Ultrasound is the most reliable method to diagnose and exclude renal vein and IVC tumor thrombus.
- As some international staging protocols omit chest CT at diagnosis, a combination of chest x-ray, abdominal ultrasound, and MRI may be sufficient for diagnosis and initial staging.

PITFALLS_____

- Injection of contrast at CT into a foot vein may lead to streaming artifact (from non-opacified blood returning from the other leg) in the IVC mimicking thrombus and is to be avoided. Ultrasonography is very reliable in diagnosing IVC thrombus.
- Patients with lung nodules seen on CT, but not on chest radiographs, are classified according to the local abdominal stage of the tumor and not metastatic disease.
- Clear cell sarcoma and rhabdoid tumor may have identical appearances to Wilms' tumor on imaging.

Suggested Readings

Gylys-Morin V, Hoffer FA, Kozakewich H, Shamberger RC. Wilms' tumor and nephroblastomatosis: imaging characteristics at gadolinium-enhanced MR imaging. Radiology 1993;188:517–521

Meyer JS, Harty MP, Khademian Z. Imaging of neuroblastoma and Wilms' tumor. Magn Reson Imaging Clin N Am 2002;10:275–302

Neville H, Ritchey ML, Mayo UP, et al. The occurrence of Wilms' tumor in horseshoe kidneys: a report from the National Wilms' Tumor Study Group (NWTSG). J Pediatr Surg 2002;37:1134–1137

CASE 84

Clinical Presentation

A 3-year-old girl presents with a palpable hard lump in the buttock.

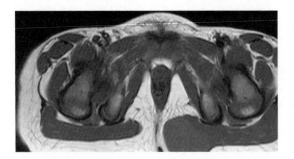

Figure 84A

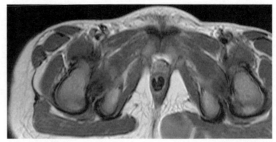

Figure 84B

Radiologic Findings

Axial T1-weighted MRI before (**Fig. 84A**) and after (**Fig. 84B**) gadolinium enhancement shows a solid mass merging with the medial aspect of the left gluteus maximus muscle. This mass shows moderate heterogeneous enhancement after gadolinium administration.

Diagnosis

Rhabdomyosarcoma

Differential Diagnosis

- Hemangioma (presents in infancy with a soft vascular mass)
- Sacrococcygeal teratoma (usually manifests in infancy as a mixed cystic-calcific presacral mass)
- Pelvic neuroblastoma (is often calcified and is also presacral in location)
- Lymphoma (rare <7 years of age, and seldom manifests as a focal lump)
- Pseudotumorous cystitis (an uncommon manifestation of bladder inflammation)

Discussion

Background

Rhabdomyosarcoma is the most common soft tissue sarcoma in children, representing 5 to 8% of all childhood cancers. Rhabdomyosarcoma is the most common malignant neoplasm of the pelvis in children, with a quarter of rhabdomyosarcoma cases affecting the genitourinary tract. These tumors can arise anywhere in the pelvis but in boys tend to occur predominantly in the bladder, prostate, and paratesticular sites (a so-called paratesticular location is applied to tumors arising in the spermatic cord, testis, epididymis, and penis). Paratesticular rhabdomyosarcoma accounts for 12% of scrotal tumors in childhood. The uterus and the vagina, in particular, are the more commonly affected organs in girls. Site of origin is critically important in determining prognosis in children with rhabdomyosarcoma. Tumors in the bladder/prostate area, for example, have a worse prognosis than the other genitourinary sites. Spread of disease is usually to regional lymph nodes initially, and it is important that these areas are scrutinized closely at all radiologic examinations. Routine staging at presentation with chest CT and technetium 99m methylene diphosphonate bone scans is recommended in all patients, as 10% of patients have metastatic disease at diagnosis. The goal of treatment is complete removal of tumor, with a residual soft tissue mass at the site of the original tumor being a known risk factor for later recurrence.

Etiology

- Etiology is unknown.
- Despite a superficial resemblance to skeletal muscle, the tumor frequently arises in sites lacking skeletal muscle.

Clinical Findings

The clinical presentation depends largely on the site of origin of the primary tumor. Vaginal masses in young girls frequently manifest as a polypoid lesion (sarcoma botryoides) at the introitus. Lesions in the bladder/prostate area present with urinary frequency or retention, whereas paratesticular masses typically present with a scrotal lump. A tumor in the dome of the bladder may result in hematuria or come to attention as an abdominal mass.

Pathology

- Rhabdomyosarcoma arises from primitive mesenchymal cells committed to skeletal muscle differentiation but does occur in sites that lack skeletal muscle.
- Two major histologic subtypes are embryonal and alveolar histology.

- Approximately 60% of newly diagnosed cases have embryonal histology, 20% alveolar histology, and the remainder may be undifferentiated or unclassifiable.
- Tumors with alveolar histology have a worse prognosis in general and tend to occur in unfavorable locations.

Imaging Findings

ULTRASOUND

- A solid, heterogeneous mass anywhere in the pelvis may be seen.
- In boys, a mass may be visible in the bladder base, arising from the dome of the bladder or in the scrotum.
- Obstruction of one or both ureters resulting in hydroureteronephrosis may occur.
- A hyperemic scrotal mass may mimic epididymoorchitis.
- Evaluation of the regional lymph nodes is mandatory, as nodal involvement alters treatment and prognosis.

CT

- CT clearly depicts most masses, but MRI is generally preferred for its better soft tissue resolution.
- Abdominal CT with careful examination for retroperitoneal adenopathy is recommended in all boys with paratesticular tumors.
- Routine staging chest CT detects pulmonary metastases in up to 10% of children at diagnosis.
- Calcification is seldom a feature of rhabdomyosarcoma tumors.
- Bladder/prostate tumors are visible on CT as bizarre filling defects in the contrast-filled bladder base.

MRI

- Multiplanar MRI, with coronal and sagittal planes, is particularly helpful in assessing for disease spread; for example, to assess bladder base invasion by a primary tumor arising in the prostate.
- At the end of treatment, MRI is the best modality to search for and evaluate small volume residual disease.
- Evaluation of the regional lymph nodes is mandatory, as nodal involvement alters treatment and prognosis.

Treatment

- Occasionally, surgery alone may be curative for vaginal rhabdomyosarcoma, but most cases undergo initial chemotherapy followed, where possible, by surgical resection.
- Radiotherapy is also more generally employed in the treatment of rhabdomyosarcoma than in most other pediatric tumors.

Prognosis

- Tumors in favorable sites such as the vagina, or paratesticular tumors in boys <10 years of age, have up to a 90% 5-year survival rate.
- Less favorable sites such as bladder/prostate tumors have a 70% 3-year survival rate.
- Despite some recent improvements in outcome, those with metastatic disease generally have a dismal prognosis.

- Rhabdomyosarcoma is the most common malignant tumor of the pelvis in children.
- Paratesticular rhabdomyosarcoma accounts for 12% of scrotal tumors in boys.
- Regional lymph node enlargement suggests disease spread and worsens the prognosis.
- Calcification is rarely seen in a rhabdomyosarcoma at diagnosis.
- Ten percent of patients have pulmonary metastases at diagnosis.

- Hyperemic scrotal mass may mimic epididymo-orchitis.
- Benign prostatic enlargement does not occur in boys: a prostatic mass in childhood is likely a rhabdomyosarcoma tumor.
- Residual soft tissue thickening at the end of treatment may be scarring, fibrosis, or tumor—biopsy is often needed to differentiate.

Suggested Readings

Lawrence W Jr, Anderson JR, Gehan EA, et al. Pretreatment TNM staging of childhood rhabdomyosarcoma: a report of the Intergroup Rhabdomyosarcoma Study group. Cancer 1997;80:1165–1170

McCarville MB, Spunt SL, Pappo AS. Rhabdomyosarcoma in pediatric patients: the good, the bad and the unusual. AJR Am J Roentgenol 2001;176:1563–1569

McHugh K, Boothroyd AE. The role of radiology in childhood rhabdomyosarcoma. Clin Radiol 1999;54:2–10

CASE 85

Clinical Presentation

A 14-month-old boy presents with a palpable abdominal mass.

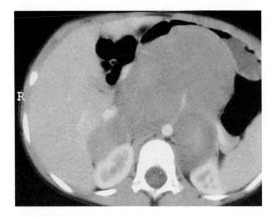

Figure 85A

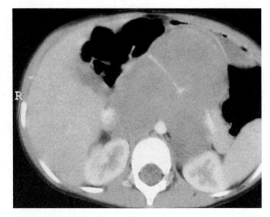

Figure 85B

Radiologic Findings

Two axial CT sections of the upper abdomen (**Figs. 85A** and **85B**) show a large solid mass without calcification extending across the midline anterior to both kidneys. The aorta is encased by tumor, and the celiac artery is also encased and stretched by the mass. The bowel and tail of the pancreas are displaced anteriorly, and no intraspinal extension of tumor is visible on these images.

Diagnosis

Neuroblastoma

Differential Diagnosis

- Wilms' tumor (is usually obviously renal in origin, is seldom calcified, and typically displaces the major retroperitoneal vessels rather than encasing them)
- Lymphoma (unusual before 4 years of age, seldom calcifies prior to treatment, bulky retroperitoneal disease is uncommon in childhood)
- Rhabdomyosarcoma (may occur anywhere in the abdomen, particularly in the pelvis, but uncommonly arises de novo in the retroperitoneum)

Discussion

Background

Neuroblastoma is the most common solid, extracranial malignancy in children, accounting for up to ~12% of all childhood cancers. It is a neurogenic tumor that can occur anywhere along the paravertebral sympathetic chain. The median age at diagnosis is 2 years. Seventy-five percent of tumors arise in the abdomen, the majority from the adrenal medulla. The remaining abdominal masses arise in the sympathetic ganglia or in the pelvis. Pelvic neuroblastoma manifests as a pre-sacral soft tissue mass with or without calcification. Intraspinal invasion and bone erosion are commonly seen with tumors arising from the sympathetic chain, although many masses are actually so large at diagnosis that their organ of origin is difficult to locate with any certainty. Common sites of metastatic spread include local and distant lymph nodes, cortical bone, bone marrow, and the liver. Increased urinary catecholamine metabolites (vanillylmandelic acid and homovanillic acid) are present in the majority of children >1 year of age. Unlike the usual stage 4 metastatic disease in slightly older children, stage 4S neuroblastoma occurs exclusively in the first year of life, and often undergoes spontaneous regression without treatment. (See page 409 for International Neuroblastoma Staging System.)

Clinical Findings

Most neuroblastoma presents as a palpable abdominal mass. Other clinical manifestations include skeletal pain, weight loss, anorexia, irritability, proptosis, periorbital ecchymoses ("raccoon eyes"), paraparesis, ataxia, or opsomyoclonus. Many of these symptoms and signs are due to metastatic spread of tumor, which is seen at presentation in up to two thirds of cases of abdominal neuroblastoma.

Pathology

Histologically, neuroblastoma consists of small round blue cells with fibrillary bundles, hemorrhage, necrosis, and attempts at rosette formation. A spectrum of malignancy is seen ranging from the most malignant type, neuroblastoma, through ganglioneuroblastoma to ganglioneuroma. Maturation to ganglion cells with fibrils may be patchy (ganglioneuroblastoma) or diffuse (ganglioneuroma). Amplification of the protooncogene *MycN* is associated with higher-stage tumors. Deletion of the short arm of chromosome 1, with its loss of a putative tumor suppressor gene, is also associated with more advanced disease.

Imaging Findings

RADIOGRAPHY

- A calcified upper abdominal mass with bowel displacement is typical.
- Skeletal metastases may be visible as ill-defined areas of osteolysis.
- Foci of abnormal uptake on radioisotope bone scan should have plain films of abnormal areas to confirm metastatic disease.
- Intravenous urography no longer has a role in the diagnosis of neuroblastoma.

ULTRASOUND

- Localized neuroblastoma may be confined to the suprarenal area.
- Most lesions are large heterogeneous masses with anterior displacement and encasement of the aorta and its branches and the inferior vena cava.
- Ultrasound tends to underestimate the extent of large masses.
- Suspected invasion of the adjacent liver, kidney, and other viscera is optimally assessed with ultrasound; separate movement of these organs and the mass indicates a lack of direct invasion.
- Congenital neuroblastoma, which usually has a very good prognosis, may be detected with antenatal ultrasound.
- Coarse hepatic echogenicity is a common finding with 4S metastatic involvement and may persist following treatment.

CT

- Neuroblastoma is frequently a large irregular mass without a definable capsule.
- Encasement of the major retroperitoneal vessels is very typical, with anterior displacement of the aorta away from the lumbar vertebral bodies.
- Primary tumor is usually heterogeneous, with areas of low attenuation and other areas displaying contrast enhancement.
- Calcification is present in ~85% of tumors on CT.
- Localized erosion of adjacent ribs and/or vertebral body by a large mass is a common feature and is not indicative of metastatic disease.
- Enlargement of intervertebral neural foramina is best seen with bone window settings.
- Skeletal metastases are optimally visualized on bone window settings.
- Spread into the chest may occur via the aortic or esophageal hiatus, or by direct invasion.
- Intraspinal invasion with displacement of the thecal sac is common.
- Stage 4S disease results in marked hepatomegaly with a diffuse infiltrative pattern in the liver.
- Focal discrete metastatic deposits in the liver are the typical metastatic lesions seen in stage 4 disease.

MRI

- Heterogeneous low T1 and high T2 signal in the primary mass is typical.
- Extradural extension by a dumbbell paravertebral tumor is best evaluated with MRI.
- Heterogeneous signal in the marrow of the vertebral bodies suggests metastatic involvement.
- Calcification within the tumor may not be discernible on MRI.

NUCLEAR MEDICINE

- Uptake of technetium 99m methylene diphosphonate (MDP) bone agent by the primary tumor occurs in one quarter of cases.
- Skeletal metastases are best detected by iodine 123 or iodine 131 metaiodobenzylguanidine (MIBG) scanning.
- Up to 10% of metastatic lesions, however, are not avid for MIBG, and some authors recommend both bone and MIBG scans in all proven neuroblastoma cases.
- Clearance of MIBG uptake after the completion of chemotherapy is a good prognostic factor in children >1 year of age with metastatic disease.

STAGING

International Neuroblastoma Staging System (INSS) is widely used:

- Stage 1: localized tumor with complete gross excision
- Stage 2: unilateral tumor with incomplete gross excision
- Stage 3: tumor infiltrating across the midline (defined as contralateral side of vertebral body)
- Stage 4: disseminated disease (except 4S)
- Stage 4S: localized primary tumor with dissemination limited to skin, liver, and/or bone marrow

Treatment

- Treatment varies with the stage of the disease.
- Chemotherapy is the mainstay of treatment, particularly in unresectable cases, that is, the majority.
- Surgery may be used initially for small localized tumors or delayed until unresectable tumors decrease sufficiently in volume.
- Radiotherapy is used occasionally for unresectable localized disease.
- Rarely, high-dose iodine 131 MIBG therapy may be used for refractory or recurrent metastatic disease.

Complications

- Hypertension is common at diagnosis due to excess catecholamines and often also renal arterial compromise.
- Massive hepatomegaly in stage 4S disease can compromise diaphragm motion and cause respiratory distress.
- Pelvic neuroblastoma frequently results in a neuropathic bladder.
- Intraspinal invasion of tumor leads to paraparesis in up to 50% of those affected.

Prognosis

- Prognosis is dependent on stage of disease at presentation.
- Presence of several biologic markers adversely affects prognosis including *MycN* amplification (>10 copies), diploid karyotype, and allelic loss of chromosome 1p.
- Resectable localized neuroblastoma with favorable biology has a 5-year survival rate of up to 80%.
- Survival of high-risk neuroblastoma (age >1 year, metastatic disease, *MycN* amplified) remains poor but has improved recently and reaches 30 to 40% at 3 years.

PEARLS

- Abdominal neuroblastoma is usually a large heterogeneous mass with anterior displacement and encasement of the aorta, aortic branches, and IVC.
- Suspected invasion of the adjacent liver, kidney, and other viscera is best assessed with ultrasound as separate movement of these organs and the mass indicate a lack of direct invasion.
- Bone window settings on CT should be evaluated in all patients to detect skeletal metastases.
- Heterogeneous signal in the marrow of the vertebral bodies on MRI is highly suspicious for metastatic involvement.
- Two thirds of abdominal neuroblatoma cases have metastatic disease at presentation.

PITFALLS

- Coarse hepatic echogenicity is a common finding after resolution of stage 4S liver involvement and should not be mistaken for continuing disease.
- Uptake of ^{99m}Tc–MDP bone agent by the abdominal primary tumor, in the absence of metastatic disease, occurs in a minority of cases.
- Up to 10% of metastatic lesions are not avid for MIBG.

Suggested Readings

Brodeur GM, Pritchard J, Berthold F, et al. Revisions in the international criteria for neuroblastoma diagnosis, staging and response to treatment. J Clin Oncol 1993;11:1466–1477

Frappaz D, Bonneu A, Chauvot P, et al. Metaiodobenzylguanidine assessment of metastatic neuroblastoma: observer dependency and chemosensitivity evaluation. Med Pediatr Oncol 2000;34:237–241

Matthay KK, Villablanca JG, Seeger RC, et al. Treatment of high-risk neuroblastoma with intensive chemotherapy, radiotherapy, autologous bone marrow transplantation, and 13-cis-retinoic acid. Children's Cancer Group. N Engl J Med 1999;341:1165–1173

CASE 86

Clinical Presentation

A 3-day-old newborn girl has abdominal ultrasonography for investigation of hematuria, which had been preceded by septicemia.

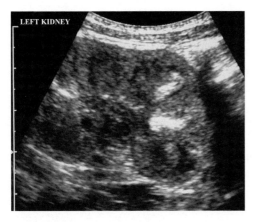

Figure 86A

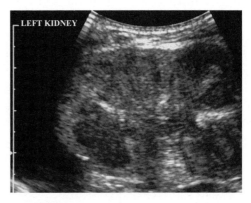

Figure 86B

Radiologic Findings

The left kidney is echogenic on these longitudinal ultrasound images with poor corticomedullary differentiation (**Figs. 86A** and **86B**). Within some of the medullary pyramids, linear areas of increased echogenicity are present, probably representing abnormal interlobar veins. Overall, the left kidney is enlarged. Venous signals from the left kidney were difficult to achieve on Doppler examination. The right kidney is normal.

Diagnosis

Neonatal left renal vein thrombosis (RVT)

Differential Diagnosis

- Autosomal recessive polycystic kidney disease (causes bilateral enlarged echogenic kidneys with symmetrical appearance)
- Acute tubular necrosis (usually bilateral and symmetrical without echogenic streaks in the kidneys)
- Tamm-Horsfall proteinuria (transient bilateral hyperechogenicity of the tips of the medullary pyramids, seen in otherwise well neonates, occasionally precipitated by dehydration)
- Mesoblastic nephroma (results in a unilateral cystic renal mass, is often exophytic, and is usually associated with some normal preserved renal parenchyma)
- Multicystic dysplastic kidney (causes unilateral "renal" enlargement, but no normal renal tissue is seen, merely multiple anechoic cysts of varying size)
- Renal lymphoma (would be a consideration in older children, but is usually bilateral in association with non-Hodgkin's lymphoma elsewhere)

Discussion

Background

Thrombus in the renal vein may be seen in children with Wilms' tumor (where it most often represents tumor extension along the renal vein), in the postrenal transplantation setting, or, occasionally, due to nephrotic syndrome. RVT is more commonly seen, however, in the neonatal period as a complication of central venous catheters, perinatal asphyxia, polycythemia, dehydration, septicemia, thrombophilia, or maternal diabetes. Ultrasonography is the best modality to depict RVT. The ultrasonographic findings depend on the severity of thrombosis and the stage of evolution of the process. Lack of venous flow and reversed arterial diastolic flow are the classic Doppler signs of RVT in transplanted kidneys. In early neonatal thrombosis, an enlarged echogenic kidney is seen with loss of the normal corticomedullary differentiation. In addition, intermedullary echogenic streaks are recognized as early signs of RVT and probably represent intravascular thrombotic material and perivascular hemorrhage. Reduced arterial diastolic forward flow and absent venous flow at the renal hilum on Doppler interrogation are often also seen with established thrombosis. Extension of clot into the inferior vena cava (IVC) is a recognized further complication.

Etiology

Recently, thrombophilia, a genetically determined tendency toward thrombosis, has been associated with RVT in infancy. It is believed that an episode of perinatal infection or dehydration may be the triggering factor for the thrombotic event in the susceptible infant with prothrombotic risk factors. In noncatheter-induced neonatal RVT, the thrombotic process starts in the arcuate and interlobular veins, spreading subsequently via the larger interlobar and segmental veins to the main renal veins and inferior vena cava. By contrast, in situ thrombosis at the catheter tip near the main renal vein is the assumed mechanism in those cases occurring in association with prolonged central venous catheterization.

Clinical Findings

RVT may present with hematuria, hypertension, or renal failure, or as a palpable flank mass from renal enlargement.

Imaging Findings

ULTRASOUND

- Ultrasonographic findings depend on the severity and stage of the thrombotic process.
- Kidney is typically enlarged with loss of corticomedullary differentiation.
- Prominent interlobar veins may be seen as echogenic stripes.
- In the acute phase, high arterial resistance with reversed diastolic flow may be seen on Doppler examination.
- Hilar and intrarenal venous flow may be reduced or absent.
- Prominent capsular venous collaterals may be seen.
- In catheter-related cases, in particular, thrombus may be seen in the main renal vein and IVC.
- In cases of left RVT, an associated adrenal hemorrhage is common as the left adrenal vein usually drains via the left renal vein, whereas the right adrenal vein typically drains directly into the IVC.

CT

- CT is not indicated in neonates in whom ultrasonography is diagnostic.
- In cases of Wilms' tumor, tumor thrombus extension up the IVC into the right atrium may be observed.

MRI

- Not usually necessary as ultrasonography is diagnostic
- A swollen kidney with low T2 signal is characteristic.
- Loss of corticomedullary differentiation is evident on T1 images.
- Poor function after gadolinium administration is seen with persistent cortical enhancement.

Treatment

- Anticoagulation may be indicated with low molecular weight heparin.

Prognosis

- With treatment, the IVC clot typically retracts and calcifies.
- Despite anticoagulation, normalization of arterial flow, and apparent improvement in venous flow, renal atrophy, and loss of function result in many cases.
- In some children the affected kidney may actually involute and disappear.

PEARLS

- Unilateral enlarged echogenic kidney on ultrasonography is characteristic.
- Reduced or absent venous flow may be a late finding.
- Renal function is often permanently impaired.
- Later atrophy of the affected kidney is common.
- RVT may be a bilateral process, but the kidneys are affected asymmetrically.

PITFALLS

- Highly reflective medullary pyramids and echogenic intermedullary streaks seen in RVT need to be differentiated from the normal, early neonatal findings of Tamm-Horsfall proteinuria (where transient echogenic medullary pyramids may be seen in non-enlarged kidneys).
- Acute tubular necrosis, which may also result in acute renal failure in the neonate, may coexist with RVT.

Suggested Readings

Argyropoulou MI, Giapros VI, Papadopolou F, et al. Renal vein thrombosis in an infant with predisposing thrombotic factors: colour Doppler ultrasound and MR evaluation. Eur Radiol 2003;13:2027–2030

Hibbert J, Howlett DC, Greenwood KL, et al. The ultrasound appearances of neonatal renal vein thrombosis. Br J Radiol 1997;70:1191–1194

Wilkinson AG, Murphy AV, Stewart G. Renal vein thrombosis with calcification and preservation of function. Pediatr Radiol 2001;31:140–143

SECTION VII

Musculoskeletal

CASE 87

Clinical Presentation

An otherwise healthy newborn male presents with left foot deformity.

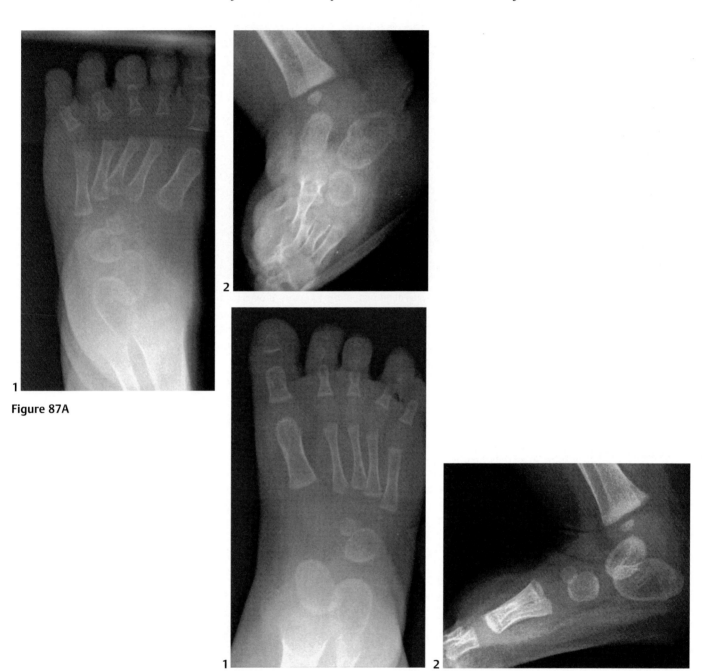

Figure 87A

Figure 87B

Radiologic Findings

The long axis of the left talus points lateral to the base of the first metatarsal on the frontal film. There is a horizontal alignment of talus and calcaneus on both frontal and lateral radiographs (**Fig. 87A**). The calcaneus is in an equinus position. The forefoot is inverted resulting in a stepladder appearance to the metatarsals on the lateral view. The normal right foot is shown for comparison (**Fig. 87B**).

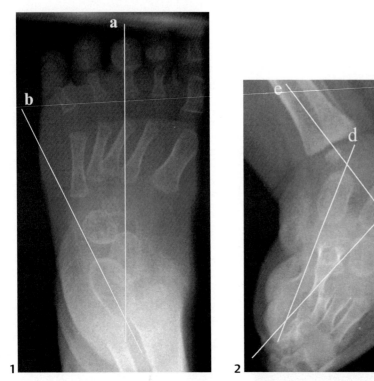

Figure 87C (**1**) Frontal radiograph of foot demonstrates alignment of the long axis of talus with the base of second metatarsal (line a). Metatarsals are adducted. Cuboid ossification appear shifted medially on calcaneus. Long axis of calcaneus (line b) lies lateral to base of fifth metatarsal with cuboid shifted medially. (**2**) Lateral foot radiograph demonstrates a stepladder appearance to the metatarsals with the 1st metatarsal most superior. The talus and calcaneus have a more parallel alignment (angle formed by lines d and c). The calcaneus is in equinus position relative to long axis of tibia (angle formed by lines e and c).

Diagnosis

Left congenital equinovarus or clubfoot with normal right foot for comparison

Discussion

Background

Clubfoot is commonly subdivided into four types: congenital, teratogenic, syndromic, and positional. The congenital variety is the most common, with an incidence of 1 in 1000. This usually isolated deformity is more common in males (2:1) and is bilateral in up to 50% of cases. First-degree relatives are estimated to have a 30× increased incidence compared with the general population.

Etiology

The etiology for the congenital form is uncertain. Defective connective tissues with ligamentous laxity, abnormal types and number of muscle fibers, vascular hypoplasia, and defective anterior horn cells have been reported in pathologic studies. A resulting deformity of the talus is suspected to lead to the altered angular relationships of the foot. The teratogenic type is found in children with underlying disorders such as arthrogryposis. The positional variety is the result of a normally formed foot held in an abnormal intrauterine position as in oligohydramnios.

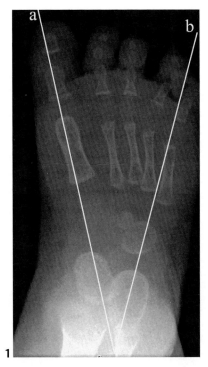
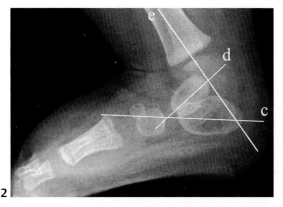

Figure 87D (**1**) Frontal radiograph demonstrates normal angular relationship of bone structures. Long axis of talus (line a) points to base of first metatarsal. Long axis of calcaneus (line b) points to base of fourth through fifth metatarsals. (**2**) Lateral radiograph depicts normal angular relationship of bone structures of foot. Normal dorsiflexion of calcaneus, as depicted by angle formed by the long axis of tibia (line e), intersecting long axis of calcaneus (line c). Normal angular relationship of talus (line d) with calcaneus (line c).

Clinical Findings

On clinical examination the infant with clubfoot displays a variable degree of foot inflexibility. The hindfoot varus and equinus with forefoot adduction seen on imaging is apparent on physical exam. There may be mild calf atrophy and hypoplasia of the bony structures of the lower leg and foot. There is cavus with relative pronation of the first ray (compared with second to fifth).

Imaging Findings

RADIOGRAPHY

- The talus and calcaneus show a more parallel alignment (**Figs. 87C1** and **87C2**). Normally, the angle on the AP view is between 20 to 40 degrees and 35 to 50 degrees on the lateral view (**Figs. 87D1** and **87D2**). With clubfoot, both angles (formed by a and b on the frontal view, and c and d on the lateral view) are reduced.
- A line (**Fig. 87C1**, line a) drawn along the long axis of the talus will pass lateral to the base of the first metatarsal.
- The calcaneus is less dorsiflexed and is usually in the equinus on the lateral view in relation to the long axis of tibia (**Fig. 87C2**, angle formed by lines c and e).
- The forefoot is in adduction or inversion with superimposition of the metatarsal bases, resulting in narrowing of the forefoot on the AP view (**Fig. 87C1**).
- The inverted forefoot results in a stepladder appearance of the metatarsals on the lateral view, with the first metatarsal highest on lateral view (**Fig. 87C2**).

Medial Projection

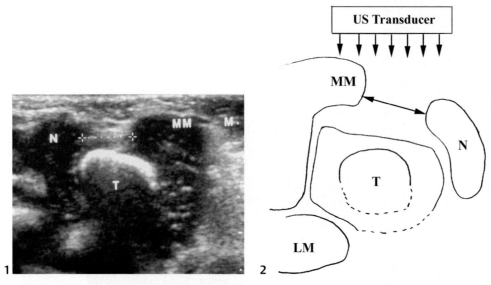

Figure 87E **(1)** Coronal oblique ultrasonographic image of the medial foot depicts caliper markings for measurement of distance between cartilaginous medial malleolus (MM) and cartilaginous navicular (N). Talar ossification is labeled (T). **(2)** Illustration depicting scan plane for ultrasonographic evaluation of foot talus (T), lateral maleolus (LM), medial malleolus (MM), and navicular (N). Distance between medial malleolus and navicular (arrow) is decreased with clubfoot.

ULTRASOUND

- Scanning along the long axis of the medial foot border will show the cartilaginous navicular (N) medially subluxed on the talar head (T) leading to a decrease in distance to the medial malleolus (MM) (**Figs. 87E1** and **87E2**).
- Scanning along the long axis of the lateral foot margin will demonstrate an increase in distance to the cuboid (CU) from a line drawn parallel to the calcaneus (CA) (lateral margin) (**Figs. 87F1** and **87F2**).

MRI

MRI demonstrates abnormal angular relationships as on plain radiographs but also see:

- Tibiotalar plantar flexion resulting in only the posterior body of talus articulating with mortise
- Medial talar neck inclination
- A wedge-shaped talar head, navicular and distal calcaneal articular surface
- Medial displacement and inversion of navicular so that it articulates only with medial tuberosity of talar head
- An adducted and inverted calcaneus resulting in the anterior tuberosity of the calcaneus lying under the talar dome as opposed to lateral to it
- Cuboid is medially displaced and inverted in front of calcaneus.

TREATMENT

Treatment usually begins with physiotherapy, splinting, and casting. The Ponseti method of nonoperative treatment now replaces earlier traditional regimens. If inadequate correction is achieved by 6 to 12 months of age, surgery is indicated. If casting is unsuccessful, then soft tissue releases are usually performed at 6 to 12 months of age. Young children (<3 years) may require tendon transfer, while older children (<5 years) may require bony operations.

Lateral Projection

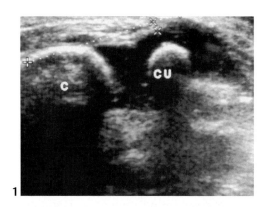

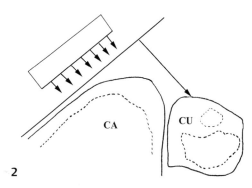

Figure 87F (**1**) Axial oblique sonogram of the lateral foot depicts caliper markings parallel to the long axis of calcaneus (CA). Distance between this line and cuboid (CU) is measured to assess degree of medial shifting of cuboid on calcaneus, which is increased with clubfoot. (**2**) Illustration depicting scan plane to determine the degree of medial off-setting of cuboid (CU) on calcaneus (CA). Normal lateral margin of cuboid should align with long axis of calcaneus.

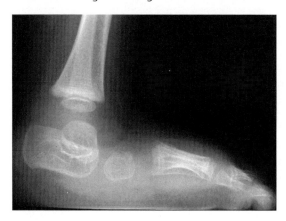

Figure 87G Lateral radiograph of foot demonstrates a convex plantar arch, often referred to as "rocker-bottom." This can be related to early application of dorsiflexion to a clubfoot before correction of the equinus and varus.

PROGNOSIS

The Ponseti method of treatment, often combined with percutaneous achilles tenotomy, has a reported good or excellent result success rate of >78%. This method also obviates the need for a posterior medial release in up to 95% of cases (previously 11–58% of patients were spared this procedure). Conservative management of clubfoot after 3 months has been successful in only 5% of patients. This success rate has improved since newer Ponseti methods have been introduced. Satisfactory outcomes from surgical management are achieved in 72 to 88% of repairs, although some longer-term studies are less favorable, with pain, stiffness, and recurrent deformity being problematic.

COMPLICATIONS

Untreated, incompletely treated, or relapsed clubfoot results in a decreased range of motion/flexibility, decreased strength, and pain. Abnormal weight-bearing on the side of the inverted foot can result in stress fractures of the metatarsals. Following repair of clubfoot, the most common problem is a fixed or dynamic cavovarus deformity, which can be corrected by a soft tissue release ± osteotomy. A "rocker-bottom" foot (**Fig. 87G**) is a severe, less common complication of treatment often requiring surgery. Calf atrophy, leg-length discrepancy, and small foot size may result. Avascular necrosis of the talus and, less commonly, the navicular, talar dome flattening, and sustenaculum hypoplasia are further long-term complications.

PEARLS_____

- Standing views provide most reliable alignment assessment. (In infants, simulated weight-bearing is required.)
- Stressed dorsiflexed lateral view is needed to determine the degree of correctable equinus.
- Talus is the bone of reference in evaluation of hindfoot valgus/varus.
- Ponseti method treatment response can be monitored via ultrasonography.
- Clubfoot often is diagnosed on fetal ultrasound or fetal MRI.

PITFALLS_____

- Difficulties in positioning lead to erroneous measurements and observations (flattening of talar dome) on radiographs. The ankle and not forefoot should be in lateral position on radiograph.
- Lack of ossification limits radiographic assessment of angular relationships of foot components.
- Multi-planar reformat (MPR) techniques with MRI can be useful; however, long postprocessing time may be required.
- Ponseti treatment relapse rate is ~20% (develop forefoot supination and require tibialis anterior tendon transfer after 2 years of age).

Suggested Readings

Cummings RJ, Davidson RS, Armstrong PF, Lehman WB. Congenital clubfoot. Instr Course Lect 2002;51:385–400

Hamel J, Becker W. Sonographic assessment of clubfoot deformity in young children. J Pediatr Orthop B 1996;5:279–286

Herbsthofer B, Eckardt A, Rompe JD, Kullmer K. Significance of radiographic angle measurements in evaluation of congenital clubfoot. Arch Orthop Trauma Surg 1998;117:324–329

Herzenberg JE. Radler C, Bor N. Ponseti versus traditional methods of casting for idiopathic clubfoot. J Pediatr Orthop 2002;22:517–521

Pirani S, Zeznik L, Hodges D. Magnetic resonance imaging study of the congenital clubfoot treated with the Ponseti method. J Pediatr Orthop 2001;21:719–726

Sobel E, Giorgini RJ, Michel R, Cohen SI. The natural history and longitudinal study of the surgically corrected clubfoot. J Foot Ankle Surg 2000;39:305–320

CASE 88

Clinical Presentation

A 3-year-old female presents with leg-length discrepancy (LLD).

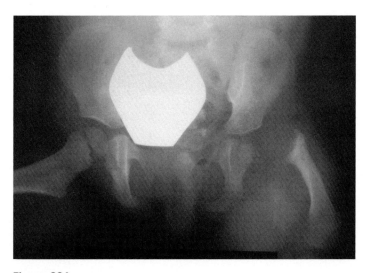

Figure 88A

Radiologic Findings

A frontal view of the pelvis demonstrates shortening with proximal deformity of the left femur (**Fig. 88A**). A small, left femoral head epiphyseal ossification center is present within a dysplastic acetabulum, and this epiphysis shows no bony continuity with the superolaterally displaced femoral shaft. The proximal end of the ossified femoral shaft is irregular with bone inhomogeneity and sclerosis.

Table 88-1   Aitken Classification

Type	Femoral Head	Acetabulum	Shape of Proximal Femur at Maturity
A	Present	Normal	Short, with bone continuity of head and neck ± subtrochanteric pseudoarthrosis
B	Present	Dysplastic	Short, lack of bone continuity between head and neck, proximal ossified tuft, subtrochanteric pseudoarthrosis (**Figs. 88B1** and **88B2**)
C	Absent	Severely dysplastic	Bulbous proximal end of femur, proximal tuft (**Fig. 88C**)
D	Absent	Absent (if bilateral, box-shaped pelvis with wide obturator foramen)	Pointed appearance of proximal femur, no tuft

Diagnosis

Proximal focal femoral deficiency (PFFD)

Differential Diagnosis

- Radiographically: infantile coxa vara (This entity has a femoral diaphysis of normal length.)
- Femoral hypoplasia
- Salter injury of the proximal femoral physis
- Clinically: developmental hip dysplasia and hip dislocation can mimic

Discussion

Background

PFFD, also known as longitudinal deficiency of the femur, is defined as a deficiency of iliofemoral articulation associated with limb malrotation and leg-length discrepancy (LLD). This rare anomaly (incidence 1 in 52,000) presents as a spectrum of defects ranging from mild femoral hypoplasia with varus bowing to complete absence of the proximal femur and acetabulum. Most observers consider PFFD as a sporadic condition; however, several hereditary case reports have been reported. Associated anomalies are seen in ~65% of patients, the most common being ipsilateral fibular hemimelia, which is seen in 50%. Numerous hip, knee, ankle, and foot anomalies have been described, including abnormalities of the contralateral extremity in 25% and bilateral involvement in 15%.

Etiology

Given the wide spectrum of deformities, it is unlikely that there is a single etiologic factor producing PFFD. A developmental insult between 4 and 6 weeks' gestation is suspected with anoxia, ischemia, trauma, infection, irradiation, or thermal injury all proposed as possible agents. Thalidomide is the only agent proven to cause PFFD.

Clinical Findings

Patients have a characteristic appearance with the hip flexed, abducted, and externally rotated. The thigh is short and bulky and tapers to the knee resulting in a shape described as a "ship's funnel." Most patients can walk; however, they have an abnormal gait (abductor lurch).

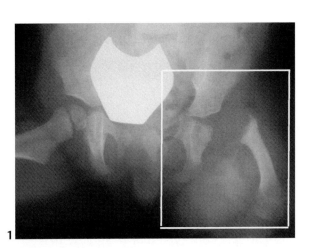
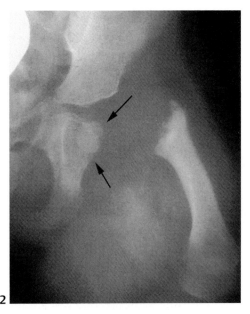

Figure 88B (**1**) Frontal view of pelvis depicts a shortened left femur with proximal deformity and tufting. There is lack of continuity between femoral shaft and a femoral head ossification center, which lies within the acetabulum. (**2**) Coned view of left hip depicts a shortened left femur with proximal deformity and tufting. There is lack of continuity between femoral shaft and a femoral head ossification center (arrows), which lies within the acetabulum.

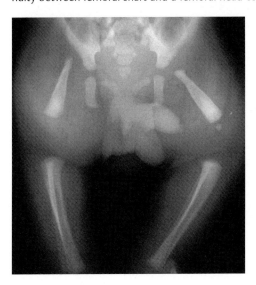

Figure 88C Frontal view of pelvis demonstrates short deformed femurs with proximal tapering and mild tufting. Acetabuli are dysplastic with no femoral head ossification centers apparent. Right femur is superolaterally placed with subtle pseudoacetabular formation.

Complications

Discrepancy in leg-length ranges from 35 to 50%. All patients will have a prominent varus deformity. Flexion contractures and instability of both hip and knee are common. At maturity, subtrochanteric pseudoarthrosis is common with type B (less with type A).

Imaging Findings

Various radiologic and surgical classifications exist, with that described by Aitken being perhaps the most commonly used. This classification is based on the presence or absence, and location, of the femoral head on plain radiographs (**Table 88-1**, **Figs. 88B1, 88B2,** and **88C**).

ULTRASOUND

- Can determine the presence or absence of the cartilaginous femoral head and its continuity with the femoral shaft, separating types A/B from C/D

MRI

- Increasingly is the preferred method to provide early and more accurate classification and assessment of adjacent musculature

Treatment

The majority of patients need a rotation plasty and nonstandard prosthesis (considered nonstandard because the patient's extremity end is not a typical stump). The principal aim of surgical management is to provide an optimal stump for a prosthesis. Intervention most commonly involves a Syme's amputation (ankle disarticulation) or a Boyd's amputation with fitting of a prosthesis incorporating a prosthetic knee. Leg lengthening using the Ilizarov method holds promise for children with a projected LLD of <15 cm. The Van Ness procedure is another option for LLD >15 cm. Valgus osteotomies are reserved for patients with type A or B. Surgery to correct the bony discontinuity for type B PFFD can be performed; however, nonoperative management has resulted in satisfactory long-term outcomes. For types C and D, surgery to increase hip stability is generally not advocated.

Prognosis

Most patients with PFFD can walk; however, they will have an abnormal gait. Surgery to correct LLD and the use of prostheses allow children to ambulate in a more cosmetically appealing manner and helps achieve stature closer to their peers. The benefits of surgery to increase hip stability must be balanced against the possibility of potentially increasing hip pain and decrease in range of motion for types A and B.

PEARLS

- A radiograph at 2 years of age is more accurate in staging PFFD than earlier radiographs as the femoral head should be ossified by 2 years.
- Four major biomechanical problems to address with PFFD:
  - Unstable hip
  - Malrotation of thigh with flexed knee
  - Inadequate proximal musculature
  - Inequality in leg length
- The goals of classification systems are to aid in predicting potential function and for planning surgery.
- MRI is increasingly used for characterization of type.

PITFALLS

- What is seen on radiograph in the infant may not predict what is found at skeletal maturity, and children may move from one Aitken type to another.
- A cartilaginous structure reflecting the unossified tuft (greater trochanter) may be confused with the presence of a femoral head on ultrasonography.

Suggested Readings

Aitken GT. Proximal femoral focal deficiency: definition, classification, and management. In: Aitken GT, ed. Proximal Femoral Focal Deficiency, a Congenital Anomaly: A Symposium. Washington, DC: National Academy of Science; 1968:1–22

Anton CG, Applegate KE, Kuivila TE, Wilkes DC. Proximal femoral focal deficiency (PFFD): more than an abnormal hip. Semin Musculoskelet Radiol 1999;3:215–226

Bryant DD III, Epps CH Jr. Proximal femoral focal deficiency: evaluation and management. Orthopedics 1991;14:775–784

Court C, Carlioz H. Radiological study of severe proximal femoral focal deficiency. J Pediatr Orthop 1997;17:520–524

Kant P, Koh SHY, Neumann V, Elliot C, Cotter D. Treatment of longitudinal deficiency affecting the femur: comparing patient mobility and satisfaction outcomes of Syme amputation against extension prosthesis. J Pediatr Orthop 2003;23:236–242

Sanpera I, Sparks LT. Proximal femoral focal deficiency: does a radiologic classification exist? J Pediatr Orthop 1994;14:34–38

Schatz S, Kopits SE. Proximal femoral focal deficiency. AJR Am J Roentgenol 1978;131:289–295

CASE 89

Clinical Presentation

A 12-year-old obese boy presents with bilateral hip pain, worse on the left.

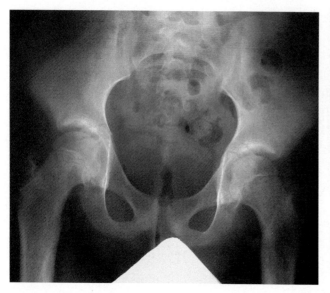

Figure 89A

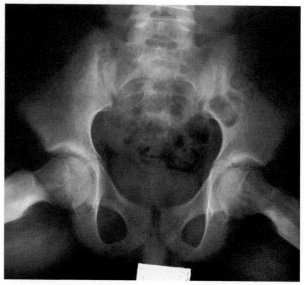

Figure 89B

Radiologic Findings

The frontal film of the pelvis demonstrates widening of the femoral physeal plate on the left compared with the right (**Fig. 89A**). No portion of the left femoral epiphyseal center lies lateral to a line drawn tangential to the lateral border of the femoral neck. The "frog-leg" view demonstrates slight medial offsetting of the epiphyseal margins on underlying metaphyses (**Fig. 89B**), left greater than right.

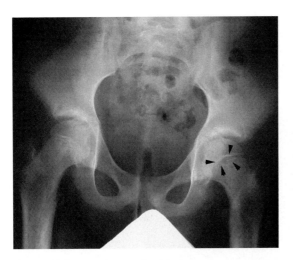

Figure 89C Frontal view of pelvis demonstrates relative equal size, configuration, and bone density of femoral head epiphyseal centers. The left physeal plate (arrowheads) is slightly more prominent than the right.

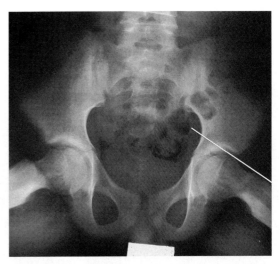

Figure 89D A line drawn along the left lateral femoral neck does not intersect any portion of the femoral epiphyseal center, confirming the presence of "slip."

Diagnosis

Slipped capital femoral epiphyses (SCFE)

Differential Diagnosis/Considerations

- Traumatic Salter 1 fracture
- Secondary causes:
  - Association with rickets
  - Pseudohypoparathyroidism
  - Hypogonadism
  - Pituitary gigantism
  - Radiation treatment
  - Development hip dysplasia
  - Osteomyelitis

Discussion

Background

SCFE is the result of a fracture involving the proximal femoral physis. The apparent posterior and medial displacement of the epiphysis relative to the proximal metaphysis is the result of the lateral hip musculature pulling the femoral shaft anteriorly and laterally, giving a varus relationship. Rarely, a valgus slip is produced with superior and posterior displacement of epiphysis. SCFE is most often seen in adolescent males (2–4 male:female) who are often overweight. The age range is typically between 10 and 15 years, with the median age of males 2 years greater than females. SCFE occurs more commonly in African Americans than in whites and usually presents during a growth spurt. Bilateral epiphyseal slips are demonstrated 25% of the time. Approximately 60% of affected children have a skeletal maturity below the mean.

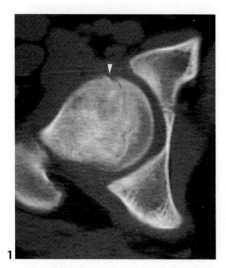 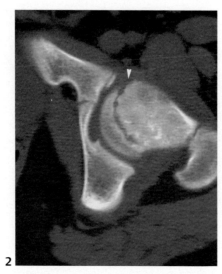

Figure 89E (**1**) Axial CT scan through right hip depicts minimal inferior offsetting of epiphyseal center (arrowhead). (**2**) Axial CT scan through the left hip depicts more prominent inferior offsetting of epiphyseal center (arrowhead) on metaphysis with a widened physeal plate.

Etiology

Changes to femoral neck orientation during rapid growth spurts (from valgus to varus) resulting in an increase in shear stress across the physeal plate may be a factor in pathogenesis. Given the usual history of minimal trauma, various predisposing factors have been implicated including chronic stress, biochemical and genetic abnormality, hormonal imbalance, and radiation therapy.

Clinical Findings

Approximately 50% of children will have a history of significant trauma and a similar percentage complain of hip pain. The SCFE will be clinically classified as stable or unstable with the ability to weight bear with or without crutches the differentiating feature. If the onset of symptoms is <2 weeks previous, the slip is regarded as acute. Chronic slipped femoral epiphyses may have a history of medial thigh pain for months to years.

Imaging Findings

FRONTAL PELVIC RADIOGRAPHY

- May see widening of physeal plate (**Fig. 89C**, arrowheads).
- A line drawn tangential to the lateral margin of femoral neck does not intersect a portion of epiphyseal ossification center (**Fig. 89D**).
- The frog-leg, or lateral view of hip, better demonstrates the offsetting of the epiphyseal margins relative to the underlying metaphysis.
- Head and neck demineralization may be seen.
- Foreshortening of femoral head with increased density inferior to growth plate due to superimposed base of epiphysis or reactive sclerosis
- If chronic, see buttressing of femoral neck posteriorly and medially or sclerosis of subphyseal metaphysis.

CT

- Better delineates (but not usually needed) the epiphyseal offsetting with posterior and medial displacement of epiphyses relative to the proximal metaphyses (**Fig. 89E**)

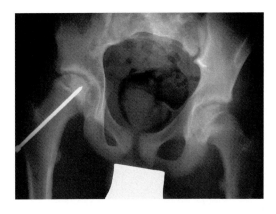

Figure 89F AP radiograph of pelvis demonstrates a solitary screw stabilizing a mild, right-slipped capital epiphysis. The epiphysis appears sclerotic compared with the left side; physeal plate is wide on right compared with left.

MRI

- Not usually performed acutely, helpful if suspect avascular necrosis (AVN).
- Physeal plate widening can be appreciated on T1-weighted images.
- T2-weighted images demonstrate synovitis and bone marrow edema as increased signal.

Treatment

The objective of treatment is to stabilize the hip not to reduce the slip. Treatment should prevent further slippage of epiphysis and promote physeal plate closure. Usual treatment involves threaded pins, which are removed after physeal plate fusion. Biplane or basal neck osteotomies may be required for severe SCFE or coxa vara and increase the chances of AVN.

Complications

- AVN, recognized as fragmentation, collapse, and inhomogeneity of epiphyseal center seen on hip radiographs, develops following treatment (**Fig. 89F**).
- Chondrolysis, a decrease in hip joint space, is seen by 1 year following treatment for SCFE and may be preceded by premature closure of greater trochanteric physis. Chondrolysis may be associated with intra-articular position of the fixation pin.
- Premature osteoarthritis—estimated to occur in 50% of African American patients.
- Premature fusion of growth plate with resulting femoral shortening

Prognosis

AVN of the femoral head is more likely to occur with severe slips and in cases where open reduction and repositioning have been performed. The incidence is highest in unstable slips, occurring in up to 45% of cases in this group and overall in ~10% of patients.

PEARLS_____

- SCFE is the most common hip abnormality in young adolescents.
- The fracture cleft extends through the hypertrophic/degenerative zone and the cartilage-bone junction.
- One quarter of patients will present with knee pain.
- Tip of fixation pin to subchondral bone should be >15 mm to reduce risk of penetration, or tip of fixation to peripheral cortex should be >15% of overall bone diameter.

- Following treatment, always look for contralateral slips and complications of pin position.
- Chondrolysis complication is clinically significant in 10% of patients.

PITFALLS_____

- Frontal radiographs may appear normal (therefore a lateral or frog-leg view is required).
- Fixation pin tip penetrating subarticular cortex may lead to chondrolysis.
- SCFE may present as thigh pain in ~20% of cases.

Suggested Readings

Gordon JE, Abrahams MS, Dobbs MB, Luhmann SJ, Schoenecker PL. Early reduction, arthrotomy, and cannulated screw fixation in unstable slipped capital femoral epiphysis treatment. J Pediatr Orthop 2002;22:352–358

Kumm DA, Schmidt J, Eisenburger SH, Rutt J, Hackenbrock M. Prophylactic dynamic screw fixation of the asymptomatic hip in slipped capital femoral epiphysis. J Pediatr Orthop 1996;16: 249–253

Lubicky JP. Chondrolysis and avascular necrosis: complications of slipped capital femoral epiphysis. J Pediatr Orthop B 1996;5:162–167

Ozonoff MB. The hip: slipped capital femoral epiphysis: epidemiology, etiology, and clinical findings. Chapter 3. Pediatric Orthopedic Radiology. 2nd ed. Philadelphia: W.B. Saunders; 1992:293–300

Tokmakova KP, Stanton RP, Mason DE. Factors influencing the development of osteonecrosis in patients treated for slipped capital femoral epiphysis. J Bone Joint Surg Am 2003;85-A:798–801

CASE 90

Clinical Presentation

A 17-year-old presents with an acutely swollen tender ankle.

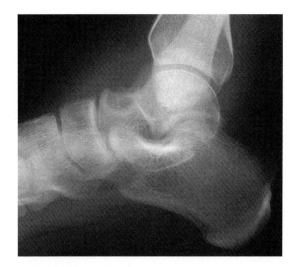

Figure 90A

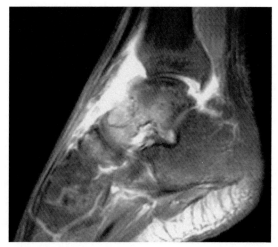

Figure 90B

Radiographic Findings

Lateral radiograph demonstrates evidence of a tibiotalar joint effusion with a large erosion showing marginal indistinct sclerosis at the talar neck (**Fig. 90A**). Corresponding sagittal fat-suppressed enhanced T1-weighted MRI depicts a joint effusion with diffuse increased signal intensity within talus and navicular (**Fig. 90B**). There is a focal area of higher signal intensity with a low-intensity margin within the talar neck with loss of adjacent anterior cortex.

Diagnosis

Septic arthritis

Differential Diagnosis

- Inflammatory arthritis (usually has a more gradual onset and commonly polyarticular)
- Pauciarticular form of Lyme disease (seen in endemic areas)
- Trauma

Discussion

Background

Septic arthritis, defined clinically as joint inflammation, is an infection of the joint space. It is diagnosed with a positive synovial or blood culture, an antigen detection test, or a standard tube agglutination titer of 160 or greater for *Brucella* species. Approximately 7% of childhood arthritis is septic in origin with the vast majority of these patients being previously healthy. The incidence varies with age (ranging from 5 to 37 per 100,000), being most common in patients <2 years old (one third to one half of cases). Septic arthritis is most commonly seen in the hip and knee joints, followed by ankle and shoulder.

Etiology

Hematogenous seeding during a bacteremic episode is the most common etiology in children. Less commonly, the infectious joint is the result of direct extension from an adjacent cellulitis/myositis. Spread from an adjacent osteomyelitis is seen more often in infants <8 months or >18 months of age, particularly in the hip, where the physis is intra-articular. Traumatic penetration of the joint is a less common etiology but can be seen with plant-thorn synovitis.

Clinical Findings

- Fever, motion exacerbated joint pain, erythema, and swelling are typical in older children.
- Mild signs and symptoms can be present in patients <2 years of age.
- Infants are more likely to present with fever, pseudoparalysis, irritability, and poor feeding.

Complications

- Destruction of cartilage and underlying bone can lead to ankylosis/fibrosis/contractures.
- Subluxation, dislocation, epiphyseal separation, and osteonecrosis have been reported.
- Growth disturbance leading to limb-length discrepancy and ambulatory disorder
- Can progress to osteomyelitis
- Infrequently, heterotopic ossification develops.
- Subsequent degenerative changes

Pathophysiology

Bacterial seeding into the highly vascular synovium during the course of a bacteremia initiates an inflammatory reaction. Release of cytokine and proteolytic enzymes by neutrophils, synovial cells, and bacteria at the site subsequently leads to cartilage destruction. A loose periosteum and epiphyseal cartilage easily transversed by capillaries promotes infectious spread from adjacent osteomyelitis in

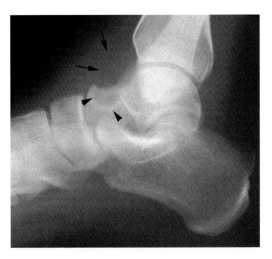

Figure 90C Lateral radiograph of the foot shows a focal lucency with ill-marginated sclerotic borders involving superior talar neck (arrowheads). Overlying cortical margins are not visualized. Joint effusion displaced soft tissue facial planes (arrow).

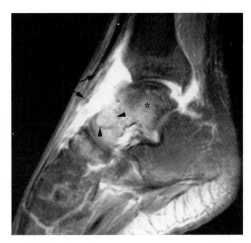

Figure 90D Lateral T2-weighted image depicts joint effusion with a focal area of increased signal intensity within talar neck (arrowheads). There is low signal margin and more diffuse ill-marginated increased signal (*) in adjacent marrow. There is loss of overlying cortical margin and increased signal intensity within adjacent soft tissues (arrows).

the neonate and infant. Increased pressure within the joint due to pus accumulation can compromise vasculature, subsequently leading to necrosis.

Laboratory/Microbiology

- Synovial fluid white blood cell count >50,000 with at least 75% polymorphonuclear leukocytes is usually used as benchmark in diagnosis.
- An etiology agent is found in 30 to 74% of patients through blood or synovial fluid culture.
- *Staphylococcus aureus* most common pathogen in patients >2 years of age.
- In the neonate, *S. aureus, Streptococcus agalactiae* (group B), enterobacteriaceae, and *Neisseria gonorrhoeae* are more commonly found.
- Between neonate and child <2 years old, the likely pathogen varies with immunization status.
- Since the advent of the *Haemophilus influenzae* B immunization program, the incidence of *H. influenzae* B pathogen has dropped from ~34 to ~4% in some geographic locations. *Kingella kingae* is now more commonly recognized, and is often associated with a mild benign course of illness.
- Salmonella is commonly identified if underlying hemoglobinopathy, systemic lupus erythromatosus, or previous trauma.

Imaging Findings

RADIOGRAPHY

- Soft tissue swelling (as depicted by indistinctness of adjacent tissue fascial planes) and joint effusion (as depicted by displacement of tissue planes/subluxation/dislocation) are earliest changes (**Fig. 90C**, arrows).
- Osteopenia
- Joint space widening followed by joint space loss due to effusion and subsequent cartilage destruction
- Erosion into adjacent bony structures (**Fig. 90C**, arrowheads)

ULTRASOUND

- Sensitive in identifying joint effusions, particularly at the hip, for potential aspiration (not specific for septic versus aseptic collections)

MRI

- Best identifies synovial thickening, enhancement, and joint effusions (**Fig. 90D**, arrows)
- Depicts adjacent reactive bone marrow edema (**Fig. 90D**, asterisk) (not often seen with transient synovitis)
- Delineates extent of cartilaginous erosion and cortical penetration (**Fig. 90D**, arrowheads)

Treatment

- Initial regimen usually begun before identification of pathogen is available, oxacillin covers most common pathogens. Antibiotic treatment lasts ~28 days (on average: 19 days intravenous course).
- Surgical drainage with irrigation and debridement
- Immediate arthrotomy and open drainage with septic hip

Prognosis

- Vast majority respond to treatment with return of full range of motion.
- Less than 5% have enduring complications, but significant joint destruction is possible if diagnosis is delayed.
- Higher occurrence of sequelae if hip or shoulder involved (up to 60%)
- Increased sequelae:
  - If delay or inadequate treatment (>4 days)
  - If *S. aureus* pathogen present
  - In neonates

PEARLS_____

- In the absence of a joint effusion, septic arthritis is unlikely, and bone scintigraphy or MRI is recommended to exclude osteomyelitis or pyomyositis.
- Imaging is not reliable to distinguish septic from aseptic arthritis.
- Hip dislocation often is seen in neonate secondary to effusion.
- Femoral metaphyseal osteomyelitis is seen in ~15% of patients with septic hip arthritis (increased with neonates).
- Negative Gram's stain does not exclude a septic process.

PITFALLS_____

- Takes ~10 days for osseous changes to be seen on plain radiographs
- Septic arthritis can cause reactive bone marrow edema mimicking osteomyelitis.
- MRI appearance is often nonspecific and can be seen with reactive arthritis, transient synovitis, trauma, and juvenile chronic arthritis.
- Displacement of hip fat pads on pelvic radiographs can be related to positioning of patient/limb.
- Normal radiograph does not exclude septic joint.

Suggested Readings

Barton LL, Dunkle LM, Habib FH. Septic arthritis in childhood: a 13-year review. Am J Dis Child 1987;141:898–900

Gylys-Morin VM. MR imaging of pediatric musculoskeletal inflammatory and infectious disorders. Magn Reson Imaging Clin N Am 1998;6(3):537–559

Kothari NA, Pelchovitz DJ, Meyer JS. Imaging of musculoskeletal infections. Radiol Clin North Am 2001;39:663–671

Luhmann JD, Luhmann SJ. Etiology of septic arthritis in children: an update for the 1990's. Pediatr Emerg Care 1999;15:40–42

Lyon RM, Evanich DJ. Culture-negative septic arthritis in children. J Pediatr Orthop 1999;19:655–659

Ma LD, Frassica FJ, Bluemke DA, Fishman EK. CT and MRI evaluation of musculoskeletal infection. Crit Rev Diagn Imaging 1997;38:535–568

Wang CL, Wang SM, Yang YJ, Tsai CH, Liu CC. Septic arthritis in children: relationship of causative pathogens, complications, and outcome. J Microbiol Immunol Infect 2003;36:41–46

Yagupsky P, Bar-Ziv Y, Howard CB, Dagan R. Epidemiology, etiology and clinical features of septic arthritis in children younger than 24 months. Arch Pediatr Adolesc Med 1995;149:537–540

CASE 91

Clinical Presentation

A 6-year-old male presents with a painless limp.

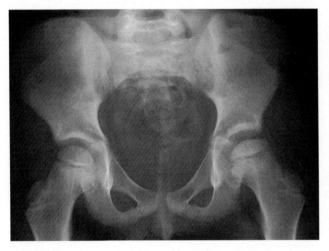

Figure 91A

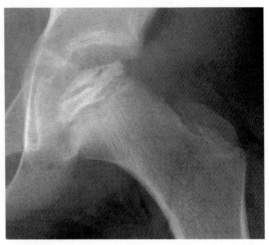

Figure 91B

Radiologic Findings

A frontal view of the pelvis demonstrates a flattened inhomogeneous left femoral epiphyseal ossification center (**Fig. 91A**). A follow-up coned view of the left hip depicts an inhomogeneous flattened epiphyseal ossification center with areas of sclerosis and a large subchondral fissure (**Fig. 91B**) There is apparent widening of the medial joint space compartment.

Diagnosis

Legg-Calvé-Perthes disease (LCP)

Differential Diagnosis/Consideration

- Meyer's dysplasia
- Multiple epiphyseal dysplasia
- Spondyloepiphyseal dysplasia
- Hypothyroidism
- Avascular necrosis secondary to:
  - Sickle-cell disease
  - Gaucher's disease
  - Trauma
  - Steroid use

Discussion

Background

LCP is an osteochondrosis affecting the femoral head. The process is generally seen in Caucasian children 3 to 12 years of age, with a peak incidence between 4 and 8 years. Males are afflicted 5 times more frequently than females, with both hips involved in 10 to 15% of patients. Decreased birth weight, low socioeconomic class, attention-deficit disorder, delayed bone maturation, exposure to passive smoke, and abnormal birth presentation are all associated with an increased risk of LCP. A family history is seen in ~6% of cases.

Etiology

The origin remains uncertain; however, clotting abnormalities with resulting episodes of vascular thrombosis may play a role. Toxic synovitis, noted as a precursor for LCP in 1 to 3% of cases, however, is probably not a cause.

Clinical Findings

Children classically present with a painless limp, although in the "synovitis phase" pain can be present, which may be referred to the knee. The pain is typically worse with activity and lessened with rest. Limitation of abduction and internal rotation of the hip, with resistance of "to and fro" rolling motion (+ log roll test) is found on physical examination. Atrophy of buttock, calf, and thigh musculature can be seen with long-standing disease. Leg-length discrepancy may be noted in more severe cases.

Complications

Premature hip osteoarthritis may develop in the fourth or fifth decade, often necessitating hip arthroplasty. Osteochondritis dessicans develops in <5% of patients, often after a long symptom-free interval. Lateral extrusion of epiphysis can lead to "hinge" abduction, the result of failure of the femoral head to rotate medial with hip abduction due to blocking of the flattened femoral head on the lateral acetabular margin.

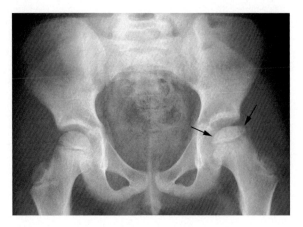

Figure 91C AP radiograph of pelvis demonstrates a slightly flattened, sclerotic left femoral head epiphyseal center (arrows), which shows apparent mild lateral subluxation.

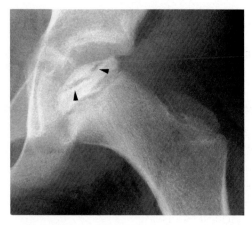

Figure 91D Coned AP view of left hip depicts a subchondral fissure (arrowheads) spanning >50% of a slightly small, flattened sclerotic epiphyseal center.

Pathology

Four stages are typically described with all the osteochondroses:

- Initial stage: osteocytic death
- Second stage: revascularization of the bone with fissuring of necrotic segments; articular cartilage continues to grow because nutrient supply is from the synovial fluid
- Third stage: resorption of necrotic bone and new bone formation
- Final stage: development of mature haversian systems

Imaging Findings

RADIOGRAPHY

- Radiographs remain the mainstay of diagnosis, classification, and treatment selection.
- Changes are also often characterized into four stages mimicking the pathologic stages.
  - Initial stage: no plain radiographic features found.
  - Second stage: see decreased size of epiphyseal ossification center from diminished growth, an increase in bone density (**Fig. 91C**, arrow); may see a crescent sign (**Fig. 91D**, arrowheads) due to subchondral fissuring/fracture as well as an apparent increase in joint space related to continued cartilaginous growth.
  - Third stage: classically demonstrates variable areas of sclerosis and lucency within femoral head due to resorption of bone and new bone formation. The new bone formation will ultimately predominate, with decreasing areas of lucency over time.
  - Final stage: radiographs depict bone remodeling with formation of mature cancellous bone. An ovoid femoral head, coxa magna, and trochanteric overgrowth may be identified.
- The three common classification systems that are based on radiographs and used in clinical practice are as follows.
  - The Catterall system is divided into four groups:
    - **Group 1** shows mineralization changes in the anterolateral segment of the femoral head in the "frog-leg" projection.
    - **Group 2** is characterized by partial involvement of femoral head with collapse/resorption, possibly resulting in mild deformity.
    - **Group 3** shows more complete femoral head involvement with resulting deformity of femoral head and neck.
    - **Group 4** shows widening of physis, total collapse and loss of height of head, and extensive metaphyseal changes.

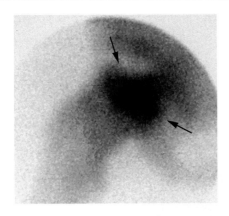

Figure 91E Delayed-phase scintigraphic scan coned to hip depicts increased activity within epiphyseal center (arrows).

- ○ The Salter-Thompson classification divides the hips into two groups:
  - **Group 1** is based on whether a subchondral fissure involves <50% of the femoral head.
  - **Group 2** is based on whether a subchondral fissure involves >50% of the femoral head.
- ○ The Herring system divides the hips into three groups:
  - **Group A** has no reduction in the lateral pillar height of the femoral head.
  - **Group B** has >50% of lateral pillar height maintained.
  - **Group C** has <50% of lateral pillar height.

BONE SCINTIGRAPHY

- Demonstrates decreased activity early in course of LCP.
- Later stages show normal or increased uptake/activity due to revascularization (**Fig. 91E**, arrows).

MRI

- At an early stage, may show decreased enhancement with gadolinium on dynamic study.
- Late findings include low-signal peripheral rim with underlying bright signal margin "double line sign" on T2-weighted images, which is specific for necrosis (**Figs. 91F** and **91G**).
- Better delineates cartilaginous components for extent of femoral head containment and loss of head sphericity.

Treatment

Treatment is based on control of symptoms, restoration of hip range of motion, and maintenance and containment of a spherical femoral head. Nonoperative treatment consisting of traction, crutches, Petrie casts, abduction bracing, and physical therapy is generally indicated in children who maintain good hip motion and are Herring group A or B (if bone age <6 years). Several studies have shown value for surgical management in the more severe cases of LCP. Herring group B (bone age >6 years) and all group C patients >6 years of age should be considered for surgical containment. Surgical options include soft tissue releases of adductors and medial capsule to restore motion. The most frequent acetabular procedures are innominate osteotomy and shelf acetabuloplasty. Some centers perform a "triple" acetabular osteotomy to improve coverage of femoral head in severe cases/older children. Femoral varus osteotomy to improve containment and valgus osteotomy to treat hinge abduction are also commonly used. Distraction and external fixation is being used in some centers to offload and contain the femoral head.

Prognosis

The majority of patients with LCP (~70%) heal spontaneously without functional impairment at maturity. A significant number without surgery will experience pain in the fifth decade and will ultimately

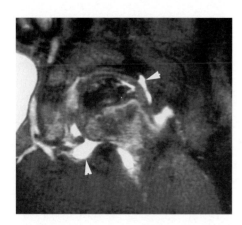

Figure 91F Coronal T2-weighted imaging of hip depicts joint effusion (arrowheads). Femoral head epiphyseal center shows decreased signal intensity with small, bright subchondral linear fissure laterally.

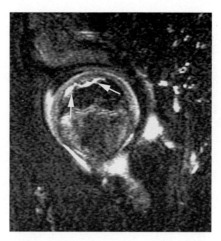

Figure 91G Sagittal T2-weighted imaging of hip depicts subchondral fissure of high-signal intensity (arrows) within epiphyseal center.

require arthroplasty. Prognosis is ultimately dependent on the final shape of the femoral head, which is affected by the age at presentation, extent of epiphyseal involvement, duration of disease, amount of femoral head containment, and premature closure of the physeal plate. Children <6 years of age tend to have less severe disease. Prognosis is improved if the lateral pillar of epiphysis is spared.

PEARLS_____

- Bilateral Perthes disease usually presents in different stages for each hip.
- Symmetric involvement of hips should raise suspicion of underlying systemic disorder.
- Revascularization pattern on gadolinium-dynamic MRI or scintigraphy is a useful prognostic feature.
  - Increased dynamic enhancement (best seen at 2 minutes) or increased activity in lateral column means better prognosis.
- Poor prognostic features:
  - Subchondral fissure involving >50% of the epiphysis
  - Center-edge angle <20 degrees
  - Acetabular index >20
  - Loss of femoral head sphericity with increased collapse of lateral pillar (Herring group C)
  - Metaphyseal lesion
  - Bone age >6 years
- Majority of epiphyseal collapse happens in first 7 months of symptoms.
- MRI best performed at 4 to 6 months after symptoms to delineate revascularization pattern.

PITFALLS_____

- LCP may be radiographically occult for first 3 to 6 months.
- Early findings may just be asymmetry in femoral head size.
- Classifications for grading/prognosis based on radiographs are limited.
  - Herring method using lateral pillar height is difficult in very young and not possible with bilateral cases.

- ○ Catterall method using extent of head involvement in fragmentation stage lacks interobserver reliability.
- ○ Salter-Thompson method based on extent of subchondral fissure is limited due to lack of fissuring in early and late stages of LCP.

Suggested Readings

Cho TJ, Lee SH, Choi IH, et al. Femoral head deformity in Catterall groups III and IV Legg-Calve-Perthes disease: magnetic resonance image analysis in coronal and sagittal planes. J Pediatr Orthop 2002;22:601–606

de Sanctis N, Rondinella F. Prognostic evaluation of Legg-Calve-Perthes disease by MRI, II: pathomorphogenesis and new classification. J Pediatr Orthop 2000;20:463–470

Doria AS, Guarniero R, Molnar LJ, et al. Three-dimensional (3D) contrast-enhanced power Doppler imaging in Legg-Calve-Perthes disease. Pediatr Radiol 2000;30:871–874

Lamer S, Dorgeret S, Khairouni A, et al. Femoral head vascularisation in Legg-Calve-Perthes disease: comparison of dynamic gadolinium-enhanced subtraction MRI with bone scintigraphy. Pediatr Radiol 2002;32:580–585

Lappin K, Kealey D, Cosgrove A. Herring classification: how useful is the initial radiograph? J Pediatr Orthop 2002;22:479–482

Roy DR. Current concepts in Legg-Calve-Perthes disease. Pediatr Ann 1999;28:748–752

Song HR, Dhar S, Na JB, et al. Classification of metaphyseal change with magnetic resonance imaging in Legg-Calve-Perthes disease. J Pediatr Orthop 2000;20:557–561

Weishaupt D, Exner GU, Hilfiker PR, Hodler J. Dynamic MR imaging of the hip in Legg-Calve-Perthes disease: comparison with arthrography. AJR Am J Roentgenol 2000;174:1635–1637

Wiig O, Terjesen T, Svenningsen S. Inter-observer reliability of radiographic classifications and measurements in the assessment of Perthes' disease. Acta Orthop Scand 2002;73:523–530

CASE 92

Clinical Presentation

A 1-week-old female is referred with a positive Ortolani test.

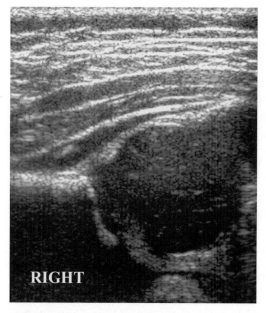

Figure 92A

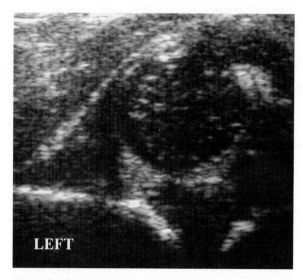

Figure 92B

Imaging Findings

Standard coronal ultrasonographic exam of both hips shows a shallow acetabulum on the left (**Fig. 92B**) compared with the normal right (**Fig. 92A**). The left femoral head epiphyseal center is dislocated superolaterally with an elevated echogenic labrum.

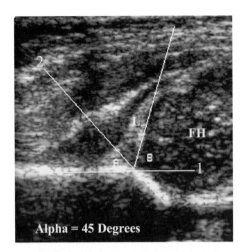

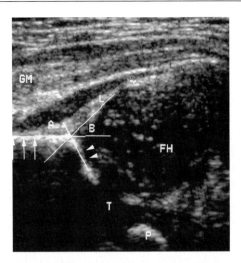

Figure 92C Coronal sonogram of the hip depicts superolateral subluxation of the femoral head (FH). There is uplifting of labrum (L). The α angle (A) is formed by a line drawn parallel to the straight iliac echo (line 1) and a crossing line (line 2) drawn parallel to acetabular echogenic margin.

Figure 92D Coronal hip sonogram depicts femoral head (FH) well covered by echogenic labrum (L). Alpha (A) and β (B) angles are within normal limits. The deepest portion of the acetabulum is demonstrated based on visualization of triradiate cartilage. Gluteus medius (GM) spans hip joint in coronal plane. Arrows depict echogenic iliac margin. Arrowheads depict cartilaginous acetabulum.

Diagnosis

Developmental dysplasia of the hip (DDH) with dislocation

Differential Diagnosis

Dislocation related to:

- Trauma
- Neonatal sepsis (usually clinical findings)

Discussion

Background

DDH constitutes a spectrum of abnormalities ranging from minor neonatal instability to frank irreducible dislocation. The disorder is dynamic, with the potential to improve or worsen over time, and evolves prenatally (36–40 weeks) or postnatally (98%). The remaining cases are teratogenic, initiating early in development of the fetal hip. The incidence of hip instability detected at birth is 1 to 2%; however, the vast majority of these cases reflect transient instability and resolve. The quoted incidence of DDH is ~1 in 1000. Girls have a significantly higher incidence compared with boys (5:1). Lack of fetal mobility as seen in breech presentations has associated DDH in up to 23%. Two thirds of cases involve first-born children, with an overall familial incidence of 20%.

Etiology

The cause of DDH appears multifactorial with a combination of genetic, hormonal, and positional factors playing a role. A lack of congruent mutual development of the femoral head and acetabulum can lead to insufficient coverage of the femoral head by the acetabulum with resulting altered mechanics

Table 92-1   Classification of Developmental Dysplasia of the Hip

Type	Description	a Angle (degrees)	b Angle (degrees)
1	Normal	>60	
2A	Physiological immature <3 months	50–59	
2B	Delayed ossification >3 months	50–59	
2C	Deficient bony acetabulum, but femoral head still concentric	43–49	<77
2D	Femoral head subluxed	43–49	>77
3	Dislocated	<43	>77
4	Severe dysplasia/dislocation	Not measurable; flat, shallow, bony acetabulum	

with the application of stress/movement. This may be the result of ligamentous laxity or underlying acetabular dysplastic changes. The natural history of DDH is variable. More than 90% of these hips stabilize over the first 2 to 3 weeks after birth, whereas a minority will go on to either sublux or dislocate. Others will remain located in an abnormally shaped acetabulum termed *acetabular dysplasia*.

Clinical Findings

The mainstays of clinical diagnosis are the Ortolani maneuver and Barlow test routinely performed on the newborn. The "clunk" felt during the Ortolani exam reflects relocation of the initially displaced femoral head across the posterior acetabular lip (ischium) during flexion and abduction of the hip. This may be obtained only in the first few weeks of life. Limited abduction, unequal creases, limb shortening, and Trendelenburg gait are further signs.

Complications

The major complications of treated patients with DDH are residual dysplasia and proximal growth disturbance also known as avascular necrosis. The overall reported rate of avascular necrosis is between 0 and 12%. This complication is related to the degree of abduction used during treatment to achieve reduction. Inadequate treatment or residual deformity will result in premature degenerative disease and for the more severe cases, pseudoacetabulum formation with limb shortening.

Imaging Findings

ULTRASOUND

- Ultrasonography, with a combined dynamic and morphologic evaluation, is the modality of choice for patients up to 6 to 9 months of age (unless a teratogenic nature is suspected).
- It is recommended that a plain radiograph of the pelvis be obtained to confirm successful outcome and when other underlying conditions may be present.
- The α and β angles using Graf's method based on the coronal image is of value (**Figs. 92C** and **92D**).
- **Table 92–1** reflects the well-accepted classification.
- A dynamic ultrasonographic study with the patient supine in a transverse plane with monitoring during the Ortolani and Barlow maneuvers is also recommended. The degree of movement of the femoral head with the maneuvers can help determine instability.

RADIOGRAPHY

For older children, once ossification of the femoral heads occurs, plain frontal radiographs can be used in diagnosis. Multiple lines and angles are used as illustrated in **Fig. 92E.**

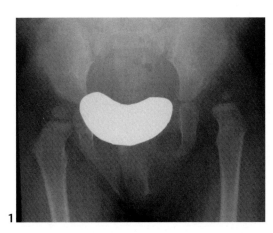 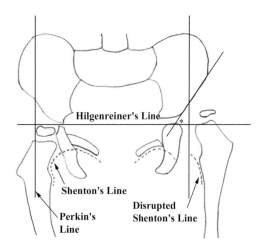

Figure 92E (**1**) Frontal pelvis depicts superolateral dislocation of the left hip and mild lateral subluxation on the right. Note the small left femoral head epiphyseal center and dysplastic (steep) left acetabulum. (**2**) Illustration depicting orientation of Hilgenreiner's, Shenton's, and Perkin's lines used for determination of hip subluxation and dislocation. The femoral head ossification centers should lie medial to Perkin's line. Shenton's line should be a smooth arc. Acetabular angle (*) is measured from a line drawn along the acetabular margin intersecting Hilgenreiner's line and should measure ~30 degrees.

- Acetabular index or angle increases with dysplasia (normal = 28 degrees in newborn).
- Femoral head ossification center should be medial to Perkins' line and inferior to Hilgenreiner's line.
- Shenton's line should be a smooth arc.
- A decrease in size or delay in appearance of ossification of femoral head epiphyseal center is a common sign of DDH.

Treatment

If the patient is diagnosed before 6 months of age, then Pavlik bracing is used. One should see improvement after 3 weeks of treatment.

Closed reduction (with casting) or open reduction is needed for patients who fail Pavlik bracing or who are >6 months of age. Open reduction with osteotomy, acetabuloplasty, limbectomy, or adductor/ iliosoas releases to remove obstructing soft tissue preventing reduction or to improve coverage of femoral head by acetabulum are methods used to treat DDH.

Prognosis

If diagnosed before 6 months of age and treated with a Pavlik harness, the success of treatment is ~85 to 95%. This decreases to <50% if treatment is delayed beyond 6 months to 2 years of age. Untreated bilateral complete dislocations may do remarkably well with good range of motion if there is no false acetabula formation. Back pain from excess lumbar lordosis can occur. In unilateral cases, there may be leg-length discrepancy with gait disturbance. In comparison to the dislocated hip, the subluxed hip has a poor prognosis with osteoarthritis and clinical disability in nearly all patients. The more severely affected having onset of symptoms in the second decade of life.

PEARLS

- Increase in acetabular cartilage thickness, >3.5 mm, may be the first ultrasonographic feature of DDH.
- It is estimated that 20 to 50% of osteoarthritis in adults is caused by subluxation or residual dysplasia.

- The "safe zone" for the degree of abduction for bracing/casting is 30 to 40 degrees.
- The development of acetabular internal concavity, the "teardrop" configuration, and the remodeling of the superolateral acetabular margin are indicators of concentric reduction used to monitor treatment on radiographs.
- Failure of the epiphysis to ossify during the first year after reduction generally indicates proximal femoral growth disturbance.
- An adequate coronal sonogram to classify DDH requires visualization of:
  - A straight iliac echogenic bony margin parallel to transducer
  - A cartilaginous acetabular roof with echogenic labrum at tip
  - A deep bony acetabulum seen through to triradiate cartilage
  - A spherical femoral head (FH)

PITFALLS

- Capsular laxity decreases and muscle tightness increases by 8 to 12 weeks, limiting maneuvers for clinical diagnosis. By 12 weeks the most reliable sign of DDH is limitation of abduction.
- Up to 6 mm of posterior displacement (physiologic laxity) can be produced in normal newborns on dynamic ultrasonography. This decreases to 1 mm by 5 months of age.
- A normal neonatal radiograph does not exclude DDH.

Suggested Readings

Babcock DS, Hernandez RJ, Kushner DC, et al. Developmental dysplasia of the hip. American College of Radiology. ACR Appropriateness Criteria. Radiology 2000;215(suppl):819–827

Eastwood DM. Neonatal hip screening. Lancet 2003;361:595–597

Graf R. New possibilities for the diagnosis of congenital hip dislocation by ultrasonography. J Pediatr Orthop 1983;3:354–359

Graf R. Guide to Sonography of the Infant Hip. New York: Thieme; 1987

Holen KJ, Tegnander A, Bredland T, et al. Universal or selective screening of the neonatal hip using ultrasound? A prospective randomised trial of 15,529 newborn infants. J Bone Joint Surg Br 2002;84:886–890

Lorente Molto F, Gregori AM, Casas LM, Perales VM. Three-year prospective study of developmental dysplasia of the hip at birth: should all dislocated or dislocatable hips be treated? J Pediatr Orthop 2002;22:613–621

Murray KA, Crim JR. Radiographic imaging for treatment and follow-up of developmental dysplasia of the hip. Semin Ultrasound CT MR 2001;22:306–340

Paton RW, Hossain S, Eccles K. Eight-year prospective targeted ultrasound screening program for instability and at-risk hip joints in developmental dysplasia of the hip. J Pediatr Orthop 2002;22:338–341

Rosenberg N, Bialik V. The effectiveness of combined clinical-sonographic screening in the treatment of neonatal hip instability. Eur J Ultrasound 2002;15:55–60

Soboleski DA, Babyn PS. Sonographic diagnosis of developmental dysplasia of the hip: importance of increased thickness of acetabular cartilage. AJR Am J Roentgenol 1993;161:839–842

CASE 93

Clinical Presentation

A 14-year-old male with a previous history of Salter–Harris type 2 fracture of the distal femur presents with leg-length discrepancy (LLD).

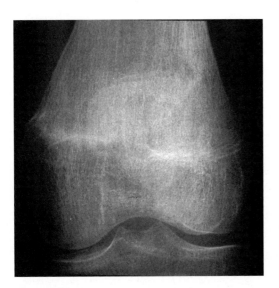

Figure 93A

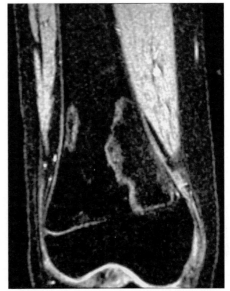

Figure 93B

Radiologic Findings

Frontal radiograph of distal femur demonstrates loss of lucent physeal plate visualization centrally (**Fig. 93A**). Coronal spoiled gradient echo (SPGR) MRI demonstrates loss of normal high-signal intensity physeal plate visualization centrally with spanning bridge of isointense signal between metaphysis and epiphysis (**Fig. 93B**).

Classification of fractures affecting the physis

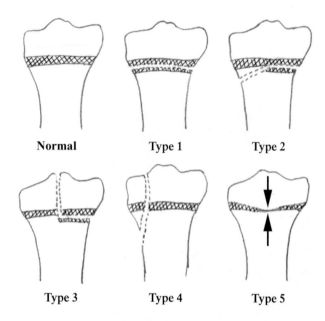

Figure 93C Illustration of five types of Salter–Harris injury with damage to physeal plate depicted.

Diagnosis

Traumatic bone bridge formation with growth plate arrest

Discussion

Background

Physeal plate injury in children is common, and when associated with bony bridge formation and/or subsequent growth arrest can result in lifelong disability. The vast majority of cases are post-traumatic with an estimated incidence of physeal fracture of 3 in 1000. Seventy-five percent of these injuries occur between the ages of 10 and 16 years. The Salter-Harris classification of physeal plate fractures described more than 40 years ago is still widely used today, with higher grades showing increasing likelihood of growth plate injury (**Fig. 93C**). The risk of physeal plate dysfunction depends on the fracture type, underlying growth potential, anatomic site, and severity of injury. Significant displacement, comminution, or loss of a segment of germinal or proliferative layer of physeal cartilage increases the risk of future growth arrest. Independent of cause, growth plate arrest and bone bar/bridge formation are more common in the lower extremities. Posttraumatic bone bars usually involve the distal physeal plates, whereas bridges from other causes are more common at proximal physeal centers. Although the distal radius and phalanges are the most common sites for physeal plate fractures, the distal femur and tibial physeal plates are more likely (16 to 35%) to undergo growth arrest post-trauma.

Etiology

Physeal plate arrest is most often the result of previous trauma. Fifteen percent of all pediatric fractures involve a physis, and ~15% of these fractures will subsequently suffer growth plate dysfunction. Infection, tumor, irradiation, burns, frostbite, electrical trauma, vitamin A toxicity, surgical procedures and underlying sensory neuropathy, sickle-cell disease, and metabolic abnormalities have all been documented to occasionally result in growth plate disturbance. Some patients with poliomyelitis and multiple dysplasias, including osteopetrosis, are associated with physeal dysfunction and secondary metaphyseal dysfunction.

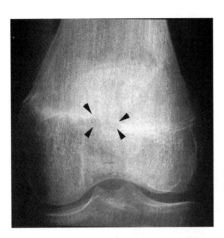

Figure 93D Frontal radiograph of distal femur depicts loss of visualization of physeal plate centrally (arrowheads) with bone continuity across physis from metaphysis to epiphysis at this site.

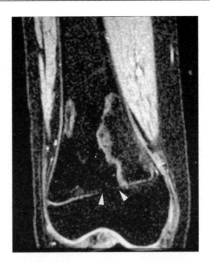

Figure 93E Coronal SPGR demonstrates loss of normal high-signal physeal plate centrally (arrowheads) with a bridge isointense to bone connecting metaphysis and epiphysis.

Clinical Findings

A child with physeal trauma will generally present with symptoms of a fracture, including local pain and limitation of motion. Subsequent growth plate arrest presents as length discrepancy or angular deformity.

Pathogenesis

The physis is responsible for longitudinal growth of the bone and is composed of three main cartilage zones: germinal, proliferative, and hypertrophic. The perichondral groove of Ranvier, which is a band of osteoblasts, chondrocytes, and fibrous cells found at the periphery of the germinal zone, is responsible for latitudinal growth. Physeal plate dysfunction can be seen from epiphyseal, physeal, and/or metaphyseal injuries.

Epiphyseal injuries are more commonly seen in patients with developmental dysplasia of the hip undergoing abduction treatment, in Legg-Calvé-Perthes disease, or in patients with joint effusions that result in subluxation. Focal ischemia of the germinal and proliferative zones of the growth plate results in chondrocytic death followed by bone bridge formation in these patients.

Direct physeal injury is usually traumatic in nature (Salter–Harris type fracture) but is also seen with infections and tumors that span the physis. The significant force required to cause injury, and the undulating nature of the physis at the distal femur and proximal tibia particularly predispose these sites to growth arrest. With physeal disruption there is resultant communication between metaphyseal and epiphyseal vasculature. These vessels are accompanied by osteoprogenator cells that can deposit bone, resulting in a bridge forming at the site.

Metaphyseal injury does not usually lead to bone bridge formation and growth arrest, as the metaphyseal vasculature does not contribute to the physeal blood supply. Injury to this site is more prone to alteration in enchondral ossification, resulting in physeal plate widening.

Imaging Findings

RADIOGRAPHY

- A growth recovery line if visible, will not parallel the physeal plate, but it will run into the tethered site.

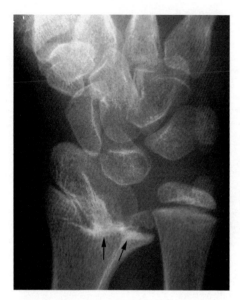

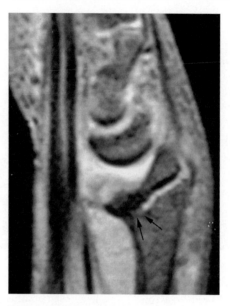

Figure 93F Frontal radiograph of wrist depicts loss of physeal plate visualization (arrows) with resulting tethering and shortening of medial radius. There is resulting angular deformity of articular surface.

Figure 93G Sagittal T2-weighted image depicts loss of bright signal physeal plate anteriorly (arrows) with resulting tethering angular deformity of articular surface.

- May see limb shortening, metaphyseal cupping, or angulation
- May see a bony bridge (**Fig. 93D**, arrowheads) crossing the more lucent physeal plate

MRI

- On T1-weighted images, bone bridges are of variable signal with smaller bone bridges seen as hypointense, whereas larger ones are iso- or hyperintense.
- On gradient echo (GRE), the bone bridge will appear as a low-signal zone crossing the high-signal physeal plate (**Fig. 93E**, arrowheads).
- A maximum intensity projection physeal map can be obtained from reformatted coronal fat-suppressed 3D SPGR images to aid surgical approach and determine extent of bridge.
- A devascularized metaphyseal fracture fragment (high-signal marrow on T1-weighted image with surrounding low-signal periphery) is identified in up to 15% of cases of growth arrest.

Treatment

- Physeal bar excision (Langenskiold's procedure), with interposition of fat, Silastic, or methylmethacrylate, is considered if <50% of the physeal plate is involved and the patient has a bone age of <12 years for girls and <14 years for boys (i.e., at least 2 years of growth remaining).
- Ipsilateral epiphysiodesis or osteotomies can be used to correct angular deformity, and contralateral epiphysiodesis can be used to correct LLD.

Complications

- If the physis is affected centrally, continued growth at its periphery will lead to metaphyseal cupping and bone shortening.
- If eccentric physeal plate damage is present, localized tethering may result in a progressive deformity leading to altered joint mechanics and early degenerative changes as seen on radiograph (**Fig. 93F**) and MRI (**Fig. 93G**).

Prognosis

- Excision of bony bridges/bars can be beneficial; however, 15 to 38% of patients end up with poor or fair result usually due to insufficient growth remaining, large bony bar (>40%), or retethering ± dislocation of graft.
- Bar resection for congenital abnormality, osteomyelitis, Legg-Calvé-Perthes disease, and central or multiple bars generally have poor result.

PEARLS

- Ligaments and joint capsule 2 to 5 times stronger than physis.
- Younger patients have poorer prognosis.
- Only bony bridges with a peripheral component are associated with tethered growth arrest lines, and these are usually small (<25%).
- The tenuous vascular supply to center of physis makes it more vulnerable to injury.
- If growth arrest line parallels entire physis, then a bony bar is unlikely to form.
- Physeal widening implies dysfunction without bony bar formation.
- Physeal fractures of the distal femur have the highest incidence of subsequent growth arrest at 40%.
- Early postoperative MRI can give information on completeness of resection, validity of graft, and recurrence of bar or premature fusion.

PITFALLS

- Interposed fat, placed during epiphysiolysis, is prone to bone formation after bleeding at graft site, fibrous degeneration, shrinking, and dislocation.
- Fat may also grow resulting in increased radiolucency at surgical site over time, mimicking infection.
- At the earliest, a bone bar is detected on imaging 2 to 3 months post-injury.
- Transphyseal signal abnormalities on MRI may be transient and resolve.

Suggested Readings

Borsa JJ, Peterson HA, Ehman RL. MR imaging of physeal bars. Radiology 1996;199:683–687

Carey J, Spence L, Blickman H, Eustace S. MRI of pediatric growth plate injury: correlation with plain film radiographs and clinical outcome. Skeletal Radiol 1998;27:250–255

Craig JG, Cramer KE, Cody DD, et al. Premature partial closure and other deformities of the growth plate: MR imaging and three-dimensional modeling. Radiology 1999;210:835–843

Ecklund K, Jaramillo D. Patterns of premature physeal arrest: MR imaging of 111 children. AJR Am J Roentgenol 2002;178:967–972

Hasler CC, Foster BK. Secondary tethers after physeal bar resection: a common source of failure? Clin Orthop 2002;405:242–249

Laor T, Jaramillo D, Ostreich AE. Chapter 5, Musculoskeletal. In Kirks DR, Griscom NT, eds. Practical Pediatric Imaging. 3rd ed. Philadelphia: Lippincott-Raven; 1998:421–426

Lohman M, Kivisaari A, Vehmas T, et al. MRI in the assessment of growth arrest. Pediatr Radiol 2002;32:41–45

CASE 94

Clinical Presentation

An infant presents with irritability and overlying bruising of one knee.

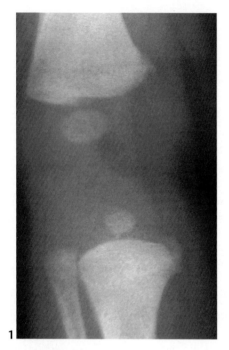 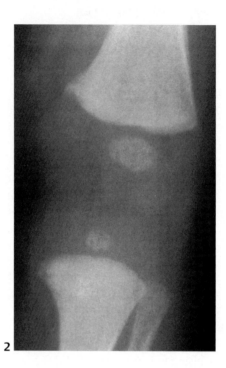

Figure 94A

Radiologic Findings

The frontal radiographs of the right (**Fig. 94A1**) and left (**Fig. 94A2**) knees demonstrate metaphyseal lesions classically described as "corner" and "bucket handle" fractures involving the distal metaphyses of the femurs and adjacent proximal tibial metaphyses. The overall bone density and configuration are normal.

Diagnosis

Non-accidental injury

Differential Diagnosis/Considerations

Processes that predispose to fracture:

- Congenital insensitivity to pain (lack of pain and occasionally temperature sensation)
- Metabolic bone disease (usually osteopenic), including Menkes, or kinky-hair syndrome
- Myelodysplasia (has spinal dysraphism)
- Rickets (has osteopenia leading to insufficiency fractures)
- Methotrexate treatment (osteopenia, unlikely with current treatment protocols)
- Osteogenesis imperfecta (only type IV difficult to exclude clinically; estimated incidence 1 in 1–3 million)

Discussion

Background

There are close to 1 million confirmed and >2.8 million estimated cases of child abuse in the United States each year. Risk factors identified for abuse are low-income socioeconomic status, children with disabilities, males, twins, stepchildren, and low birth weight/premature infants. It is estimated that ~2000 of these children will die from the inflicted injury, with infants representing 40% of the victims. One third of abused children will suffer fractures indistinguishable from the typical accidental injuries encountered in children. Fractures of higher specificity for abuse include the classic metaphyseal lesions (CMLs), posterior rib fractures, and sternal, scapular, and spinous process fractures in the infant.

Mechanisms

Excessive shaking is often the mechanism of injury for both skeletal and cerebral trauma in these cases. Anterior-posterior compression/squeezing of the thorax, often during shaking of the infant, results in focal stress points to the posterior ribs where the tubercle articulates with the transverse process of the vertebral body. Further stress sites are present laterally and at the anterior rib end.

CMLs are thought to be the result of extensive torsional (twisting) and tractional (pulling) forces to the extremity causing disruption of the primary spongiosa of the metaphysis. These appear as either corner or bucket-handle fracture fragments on radiographs.

Clinical Findings

Abused children/infants can present to the family or emergency physician with a variety of complaints ranging from limp, lack of extremity motion, irritability, and failure to thrive to more ominous symptoms of altered mental status, seizures, coma, and death. A thorough search for bruising, burns, and retinal hemorrhages (due to shaking) is vital. Any findings must be viewed in context to the purported mechanism of injury. Often the findings of suspicious fractures or the presence of multiple fractures in varying stages of healing on radiographs raise the initial warning flag to alert the unsuspecting referring physician.

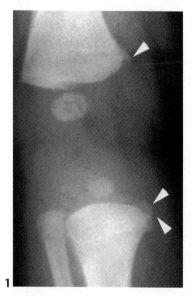
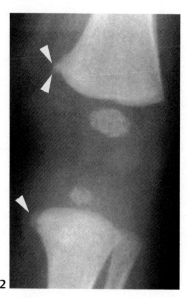

Figure 94B (1) Frontal radiograph of knee depicts small metaphyseal fragment adjacent to distal femur medially and proximal tibia medially (arrowheads). (2) Frontal radiograph of infant knee depicts subtle metaphyseal fragment along distal medial femur and proximal tibia medially (arrowheads).

Imaging Findings

RADIOGRAPHY

- With suspected abuse in infants and in young children, a skeletal survey is recommended. Further, dedicated orthogonal views may be necessary depending on the finding. The suggested skeletal survey includes:
  - Antero-posterior skull
  - Lateral skull
  - Lateral cervical spine
  - AP thorax
  - Lateral thorax
  - AP pelvis
  - Lateral lumber spine
  - AP humeri
  - AP forearms
  - AP femora
  - Oblique hands
  - AP femora
  - AP tibias
  - AP feet
- Patterns of injury more typical of abuse include:
  - Within the skull: often complex, depressed, diastased, or multiple fractures
  - Long bones: Most common is a diaphyseal fracture, but CMLs are highly specific (**Fig. 94B**, arrowheads).
  - Ribs: Fractures are highly specific for abuse, especially posteriorly (**Fig. 94C**).
  - Salter-Harris fractures: uncommon in abuse apart from epiphyseal separation in infants
  - Hands/Feet: typically torus type involving metatarsal/metacarpals
  - Clavicle: mid and distal fractures common with birth trauma, if medial location, suspicious for abuse

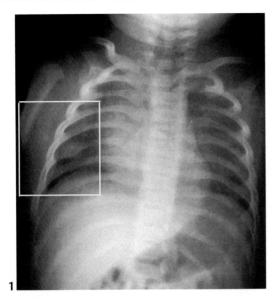
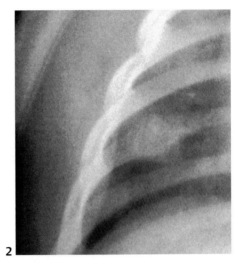

Figure 94C (**1**) Frontal chest radiograph demonstrating fracture with focal expansion and bone inhomogeneity of sixth right posterolateral rib. (**2**) Coned view of chest radiograph better depicts focal rib expansion related to healing with new bone formation being incorporated into the underlying cortex.

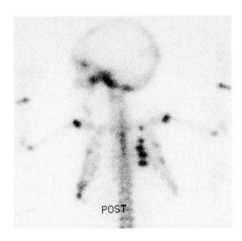

Figure 94D Bone scintigraphy of posterior view showing multiple areas of increased activity within posterior right ribs and more subtle areas of increased activity in lower lateral left ribs and laterally within right midribs.

- ○ Scapula: usually acromian, high-specificity
- ○ Sternum, spinous processes: due to excessive hyperextension/flexion, high specificity in children <2 years of age

CT/MRI

- Frequently used in the evaluation of suspected head injury but may also be used to better define specific injuries
- Direct trauma will result in fractures, subdural/epidural hematomas, and parenchymal contusions.
- Shaking mechanism results in superficial contusions, subarachnoid hemorrhage (SAH), and white matter shear injury/diffuse axonal injury.

BONE SCINTIGRAPHY

- Often primary screen in patients >1 year of age
- Can complement skeletal surveys where there is strong clinical suspicion or questionable finding on radiographs
- May help identify fractures missed on radiographs, particularly if acute (**Fig. 94D**), and demonstrate the typical linear alignment of traumatic injuries

Table 94-1   ACR/AAP Imaging Recommendations in Work-up for Non-accidental Abuse

Age	Imaging Recommendation
0 to 12 months	Skeletal survey
	Follow-up skeletal survey (2 weeks)
	CT/MRI of head for intracranial injury
12 month to 2 years	Skeletal survey or scintigraphy
	CT/MRI of head for intracranial injury as needed
2 to 5 years	Skeletal survey or scintigraphy in selected cases where physical abuse is strongly suspected
	CT/MRI of head for intracranial injury as needed
5 to <17 years	Radiographs of affected areas
	CT/MRI of head for intracranial injury as needed

Treatment

Suspicion of child abuse by any health care worker warrants contact with a child protective agency and is required by law in most jurisdictions to ensure protection of the child. A concern of abuse by the physician should result in appropriate imaging as recommended by the American College of Radiology and American Association of Pediatrics. The imaging recommendations for skeletal injury are shown in **Table 94–1**.

Prognosis

- Primarily depends on the extent of intracranial injury

PEARLS

- Rib fractures make up 5 to 27% of the skeletal injuries in abuse and are often bilateral and at multiple levels; they frequently involve middle ribs.
- Birth rib fractures are rare. Of 15,435 consecutive term deliveries in one study no infant sustained rib fractures.
- In preterm infants, ~2% incidence of rib fractures in infancy
- Several studies have found that cardiopulmonary resuscitation is extremely unlikely to cause rib fractures.
- Absence of callus/periosteal reaction at a fracture site in an infant >11 to 14 days old rules against birth injury as a cause.
- Follow-up radiographs within 2 weeks to show healing response is valuable in confirming and dating a subtle CML and in distinguishing it from a normal variant and demonstrating additional lesions.

PITFALLS

- Rib fractures secondary to birth trauma are often posterior in location, similar to abuse site.
- After 2 years of age, long bone fractures are more commonly the result of an accidental trauma.
- Acute rib fractures may be difficult to detect and are often not radiographically apparent (CT or scintigraphy may help delineate). Look for subtle bowing and soft tissue swelling.
- Absence of fractures does not exclude abuse.
- Diagnosis of child abuse often depends on the technical quality of the skeletal survey.
- AP and lateral skull radiographs are required if screening with bone scintigraphy

Suggested Readings

Bulloch B, Schubert CJ, Brophy PD, et al. Cause and clinical characteristics of rib fractures in infants. Pediatrics 2000;105:1–5

Cadzow SP, Armstrong KL. Rib fractures in infants: Red alert! the clinical features, investigations and child protection outcomes. J Paediatr Child Health 2000;36:322–326

Kleinman PK, ed. Diagnostic Imaging of Child Abuse. 2nd ed. St. Louis, MO: Mosby, 1998

Kleinman PK, Marks SC Jr. A regional approach to the classic metaphyseal lesion in abused infants: the distal femur. AJR Am J Roentgenol 1998;170:43–47

Lysack JT, Soboleski D. Classic metaphyseal lesion following external cephalic version and cesarean section. Pediatr Radiol 2003;33:422–424

McGraw EP, Pless JE, Pennington DJ, White SJ. Postmortem radiography after unexpected death in neonates, infants, and children: should imaging be routine? AJR Am J Roentgenol 2002;178:1517–1521

Nimkin K, Kleinman PK. Imaging of child abuse. Radiol Clin North Am 2001;39:843–864

Rubin A. Birth injuries incidence, mechanisms and end results. J Obstet Gynecol 1964;23:218–221

CASE 95

Clinical Presentation

A 14-year-old athletic male presents with a swollen painful ankle after forced external version of foot.

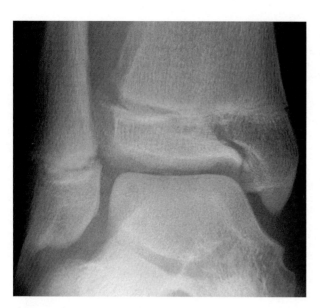

Figure 95A

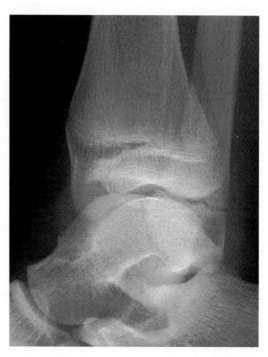

Figure 95B

Radiologic Findings

The frontal oblique radiograph shows a faint vertical lucent line, which extends through the distal tibial epiphysis (**Fig. 95A**). The lateral view shows an oblique fracture line extending through the distal tibial metaphysis posteriorly (**Fig. 95B**). Widening of the anterior and lateral physeal plate is also seen.

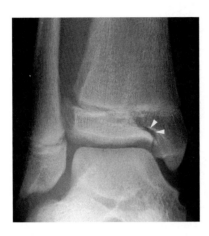

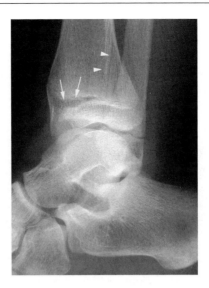

Figure 95C Frontal oblique radiograph of the ankle demonstrates a lucent cleft (arrowheads) spanning the distal tibial epiphysis. There is widening of the lateral physeal plate.

Figure 95D Lateral radiograph of ankle depicts widening of anterior physeal plate (arrows). A fracture line spans the distal tibial metaphysis posteriorly (arrowheads) with mild dorsal displacement of the metaphyseal fragment.

Diagnosis

Triplane fracture

Differential Diagnosis

Tillaux fracture (no metaphyseal component)

Discussion

Background

The distal tibial epiphysis is the second most common site for fractures involving the physeal plate with an estimated incidence of 60 in 10,000. The degree of skeletal maturity at the time of trauma plays the major role in the resulting fracture/injury pattern. Marmor in 1970 first described the complex nature and coronal, sagittal, and axial fracture components of the triplane fracture, which encompasses ~7% of ankle fractures in girls and ~15% in boys. There are several anatomic variants for triplane fractures consisting of two to four principle fragments. Triplane fractures occur in children between 11 and 16 years of age with a mean age in boys of 14.8 years and in girls 12.8 years.

Etiology

The triplane fracture and its variants are primarily the result of excessive external rotational forces placed on the ankle/foot. A degree of forced plantar flexion can also contribute to the pattern.

Pathogenesis

The partially fused growth plate is a prerequisite for sustaining a triplanar fracture, given that the open growth plate is weaker than the adjacent ligaments and bone. Closure of the growth plate

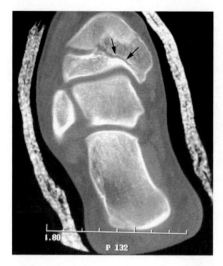

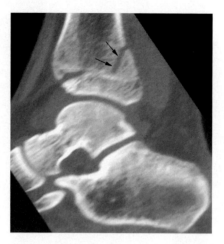

Figure 95E Coronal CT of ankle depicts widening of lateral physeal plate and vertical epiphyseal fracture cleft (arrows) extending into medial malleolus. No articular step is evident.

Figure 95F Sagittal reconstructed CT of ankle depicts distal tibial metaphyseal fracture extending to physeal plate (arrows). There is widening of physeal plate anteriorly.

begins in the central portion and proceeds medially then posteriorly. The anterolateral portion fuses last and is therefore a potential weak spot over an ~18-month span when the remainder of the plate is closed. With external rotational force the anterior tibiofibular ligament exerts tension on the anterolateral margin of the epiphysis. This force results in separation from the remainder of the epiphysis/growth plate and associated posterior metaphyseal fragment. Two- or three-part fractures are the most common types, each having fracture lines extending in sagittal, coronal, and axial planes. The sagittal plane fracture may extend into the medial malleolus rather than to the joint surface.

Clinical Findings

As with other traumatic fractures, symptoms of pain, swelling, tenderness, and loss of range of motion occur.

Imaging Findings

RADIOGRAPHY

Radiographs remain the primary means of diagnosis.
- Oblique view of ankle often depicts vertical (sagittal) fracture component (**Fig. 95C**, arrowheads) through epiphysis providing the best depiction of displacement.
- Lateral view demonstrates the metaphyseal (coronal) fracture component (**Fig. 95D**, arrowheads) and widening of physeal plate anteriorly (**Fig. 95D**, arrows) in the axial component.

CT

- With reformatting, better delineates the exact fracture type and direction of fracture lines (**Figs. 95E** and **95F**, arrows) to aid in placement of screws
- Better delineates degree of displacement at articular surface in determining treatment (~40% of fractures get CT scans before open reduction.)

MRI

- Gradient-echo sequences best visualize the course of fracture lines.

Treatment

- Based on the amount of articular surface affected
- Approximately one third of patients are treated with immobilization (nondisplaced) for 3 weeks of long casting followed by 3 weeks of short casting
- One third are treated with closed reduction using internal rotation (>3 mm of displacement at articular surface).
- One third are treated with open reduction with internal fixation.
- Arthroscopic reduction has been accomplished by manipulation of lateral epiphyseal fragment with Steinmann pins.

Complications

- If articular surface step deformity or incongruity persists, early degenerative changes and pain may result.
- Inadequate reduction or loss of reduction can result in deformity.
- Because the physeal plate is close to fusing completely, there is generally little risk for subsequent limb-length discrepancy or angulation.

Prognosis

- Excellent results in ~80%; uninfluenced by sex, age, or treatment.
- Free of symptoms, generally in 6 months.
- Sixteen percent of patients have minor symptoms of reduced joint mobility, tenderness, and swelling.
- Approximately 4% of patients show degenerative changes ± pain and deformity.

PEARLS_____

- The same mechanism of injury that causes ligamentous disruption in adults causes epiphyseal injury in children.
- Variants of injury including four-part and medial triplane fractures have increased adduction as a contributing mechanism.
- Metaphyseal fragment is always posterior.
- Physeal plate component always involves varying degrees of anterior portion.
- Always suspect an intra-articular fracture if there is a posterior tibial metaphyseal fragment.

PITFALLS_____

- Thin cortical avulsed fragments easily missed on MRI.
- Bone bruises generally begin to resolve around 3 months post-trauma but can take many months to disappear.
- If there is a separate anterolateral corner fragment off epiphysis, conservative treatment won't stabilize (argument for more routine use of CT).

Suggested Readings

Dailiana ZH, Malizos KN, Zacharis K, et al. Distal tibial epiphyseal fractures in adolescents. Am J Orthop 1999;28:309–312

Jones S, Phillips N, Ali F, et al. Triplane fractures of the distal tibia requiring open reduction and internal fixation: pre-operative planning using computed tomography. Injury 2003;34:293–298

Karrholm J. The triplane fracture: four years of follow-up of 21 cases and review of the literature. J Pediatr Orthop B 1997;6:91–102

Lohman M, Kivisaari A, Kallio P, et al. Acute paediatric ankle trauma: MRI versus plain radiography. Skeletal Radiol 2001;30:504–511

Marmor L. An unusual fracture of the tibial epiphyses. Clin Orthop 1970;73:132–135

O'Connor DK, Mulligan ME. Extra-articular triplane fracture of the distal tibia: a case report. Pediatr Radiol 1998;28:332–333

Petit P, Panuel M, Faure F, et al. Acute fracture of the distal tibial physis: role of gradient-echo MR imaging versus plain film examination. AJR Am J Roentgenol 1996;166:1203–1206

CASE 96

Clinical Presentation

A short, lethargic 2½-year-old boy presents with enlarged wrists and knees.

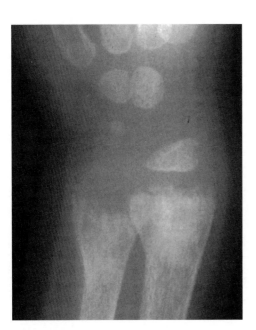

Figure 96A

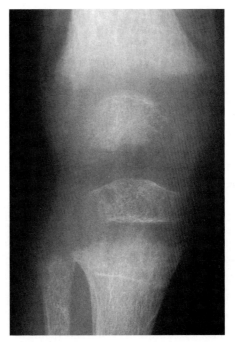

Figure 96B

Radiologic Findings

A frontal view of the wrist (**Fig. 96A**) and knee (**Fig. 96B**) depicts widened physeal plates with cupping and fraying of subphyseal metaphysis.

Diagnosis

Rickets

Differential Diagnosis

- Hypophosphatasia (often has prominent lucent extensions into metaphysis and craniosynostosis; wormian bones)
- Metaphyseal chondrodysplasia, Schmid type (short stature, metaphysis is well mineralized, and generally has benign course)

Discussion

Background

Rickets can be described as an alteration in the orderly mineralization and development of the growing skeleton generally related to defective vitamin D metabolism. The disease process was first recognized in the 1600s during the industrial revolution. Lack of sun exposure due to the smog, high buildings, and crowded streets in urbanized centers was the primary initiating factor at that time. In 1900 it was estimated that ~80% of children <2 years of age had evidence of rickets in the Boston area. The availability of synthesized vitamin D in the 1920s nearly eradicated vitamin D-deficiency rickets. The most common causes of rickets in the United States today are vitamin D-resistant or vitamin D-dependent disorders and renal osteodystrophy. In regions of Asia and Africa, the prevalence of vitamin D-dependent rickets is ~40%. There are >50 disease processes, with a vast spectrum of etiologies and clinical presentations, that can result in rickets.

Etiology

The causes of rickets can be categorized into the following groups:
- Abnormalities of vitamin D metabolism, which are divided into:
  ○ Deficiency of intake (nutritional) or gastrointestinal malabsorption
  ○ Liver disease (prevents normal 25-hydroxylation of vitamin D): anticonvulsant treatment, biliary atresia, total parenteral nutrition, tyrosinemia
  ○ Renal disease (prevents 1-hydroxylation of vitamin D): renal osteodystrophy, vitamin D-dependent rickets, tumor-associated rickets, and parathyroid disorders (hypo-, hyper-, and pseudohypoparathyroidism)
- Alterations in phosphorus or calcium metabolism due to renal tubular disorders:
  ○ X-linked hypophosphatasia rickets
  ○ Fanconi's syndrome
  ○ Tumor-associated rickets

Histology/Pathology

The primary histologic changes occur at the physis. The normal physeal plate can be divided into germinal (resting), proliferative, hypertrophic, and primary/secondary spongiosa layers. The hypertrophic layer is further divided into zones of maturation, degeneration, and provisional calcification. In rickets, the zone of maturation is abnormal with a disorganized increase in the number of cells and a loss in columnar arrangement leading to widening of the physeal plate. Diminished calcification/hydroxyapatite deposition of cartilage with continuing osteoid production by osteoblasts and a decrease in resorption of osteiod due to altered osteoclast function at the zone of provisional calcification also

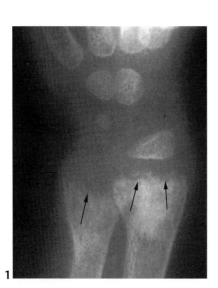 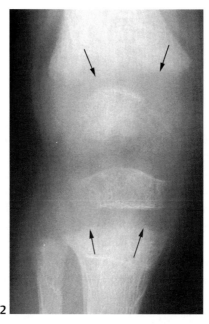

Figure 96C (**1**) Frontal view of the wrist demonstrates physeal plate widening with arrows pointing to frayed subphyseal metaphyseal margins. There is a coarse trabecular pattern. (**2**) Frontal view of the knee demonstrates widened physeal plates with arrows pointing to frayed subphyseal metaphyseal margins. There is a generalized coarse trabecular pattern.

contributes to the widening, fraying/blurring of margins and bone softening. Mechanical stresses placed at these weakened sites can result in the metaphyseal cupping/splaying seen on radiographs.

The primary function of vitamin D is in calcium and phosphate homeostasis, which is required for organized skeletal growth. To be active, vitamin D must undergo two hydroxylations, first in the liver, then in the kidney. The multitude of disease processes causing rickets generally alter either gut absorption, 25-hydroxylation, or 1-hydroxylation resulting in a lack of "active" vitamin D. Laboratory analysis usually shows decreased serum and urine calcium and phosphate with increased alkaline phosphatase.

Clinical Findings

Abnormalities of vitamin D metabolism present differently depending on the child's age.
- Infants and young child:
  - Enlarged wrists, knees, rib ends (rachitic rosary), stunted growth
  - Lethargy, irritability, weakness
  - Skull is rapidly expanding due to brain growth in the first few months; therefore, see rachitic changes reflected as a squared configuration due to accumulation of osteoid in frontal region (craniotabes).
- Older child:
  - With ambulation, lower extremities are prone to bowing.
  - As child gets older, see tendency for scoliosis/kyphosis.
  - "Saber" shin deformity can result from pull of Achilles on tibia.

Complications

- Bone softening leads to bowing deformities, protrusion, cranial molding, basilar invagination, and vertebral end-plate indentation.

- Scoliosis, kyphosis, genu valgum, coax vara, and fractures can result.
- Slipped capital femoral epiphysis

Imaging Findings

- Early radiographic feature is axial widening of physis (metaphyseal cupping) followed by a decrease in radiodensity at zone of provisional calcification.
- Widening of physis with irregularity/fraying of margins (**Fig. 96C**, arrows)
- If associated hyperparathyroidism, may see resorption of subphyseal metaphyseal bone and osteitis fibrosa cystica (often indistinguishable from rickets).
- Prominent costochondral rib ends, craniotabes in infants
- Some syndromes may show characteristic features in addition to the rickets.
  - In renal osteodytrophy, secondary hyperparathyroidism may result in osteosclerotic foci and Rugger-Jersey appearance to vertebra, vascular calcification, periarticular amorphous CA deposits, and aluminum toxicity changes.
  - In X-linked hypophosphatasia an overall increase in bony density in adults with prominent paravertebral ossification may be noted.

Treatment

- Dependent on etiology
- Most cases respond to vitamin D therapy ± calcium supplements.
- If lack of response (with no chronic renal disease), consider renal tubular disorder, tumor, hypophosphatasia, or metaphyseal dysplasia.

Prognosis

- Generally, see response in 2 to 3 weeks, with bone lesions healing in 8 to 12 weeks.

PEARLS_____

- Radiographs are useful in detecting response to treatment as zone of provisional calcification becomes dense metaphyseal band as early as 2 to 3 weeks after treatment.
- Breast-fed infants, vegetarians, and African Americans (due to melanin pigment in the skin that absorbs UV radiation, therefore less available for vitamin D production) are at risk.
- Progressive bowing of lower extremities >18 months of age is most common presentation of vitamin D–resistant rickets.
- Vitamin D–dependent rickets is hereditary with symptoms of hypophosphatasia generally before 2 years of age.
- If rickets occurs at <6 months of age, think of biliary atresia, hypophosphatasia, or a maternal disorder (vitamin D deficiency, uncontrolled hyperparathyroidism, or renal insufficiency during pregnancy).
- Marginal rim of ossified epiphyseal center is similar to zone of provisional calcification; therefore it becomes indistinct with rickets.
- Tumors associated with oncogenic rickets are usually benign non-ossifying fibromas, hemangiopericytoma, giant cell, osteoblastoma, or fibrous dysplasia. After removal of tumor, rapid improvement is observed.
- If Fanconi's syndrome, child presents with metabolic acidosis, aminoaciduria, glycosuria, and galactosemia with renal tubular insufficiency leading to rickets.

PITFALLS

- Nutritional rickets is not usually clinically apparent before 6 months of age due to prenatal stores.
- Inadequate/incomplete treatment can result in visualization of both lucent and dense subphyseal bands ("Afghan–turban" sign).

Suggested Readings

Fukumoto S, Takeuchi Y, Nagano A, Fujita T. Diagnostic utility of magnetic resonance imaging skeletal survey in a patient with oncogenic osteomalacia. Bone 1999;25:375–377

Griscom NT, Jaramillo D. Osteoporosis, osteomalacia and osteopenia: proper terminology in childhood. AJR Am J Roentgenol 2000;175:268–269

Lenchik L, Sartoris DJ. Orthopedic aspects of metabolic bone disease. Orthop Clin North Am 1998; 29:103–134

Pitt MJ. Rickets and osteomalacia are still around. Radiol Clin North Am 1991;29:97–118

Renton P. Radiology of rickets, osteomalacia and hyperparathyroidism. Hosp Med 1998;59:399–403

States LJ. Imaging of metabolic bone disease and marrow disorders in children. Radiol Clin North Am 2001;39:749–772

Teotia M, Teotia SPS. Nutritional and metabolic rickets. Indian J Pediatr 1997;64:153–157

Tortolani PJ, McCarthy EF, Sponseller PD. Bone mineral density deficiency in children. J Am Acad Orthop Surg 2002;10:57–66

CASE 97

Clinical Presentation

A 12-year-old female presents with a 2-month history of a dull ache in the left knee.

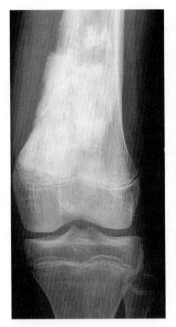

Figure 97A

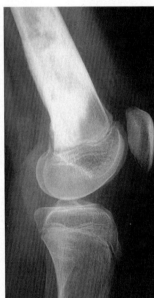

Figure 97B

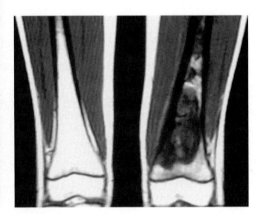

Figure 97C

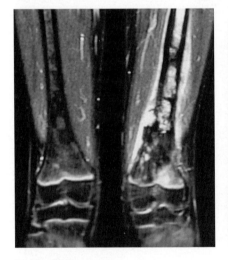

Figure 97D

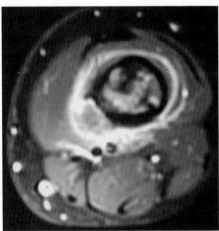

Figure 97E

Radiologic Findings

Frontal (**Fig. 97A**) and lateral (**Fig. 97B**) plain radiographs of the left knee demonstrate a destructive and poorly marginated lesion within the distal femoral metaphysis (**Figs. 97A** and **97B**). The lesion shows extensive areas of sclerosis. Interrupted periosteal new bone is present proximally with demonstration of a Codman's triangle. MRI depicts abnormal inhomogeneous low signal intensity within the left metaphyseal and diaphyseal marrow on T1-weighted imaging and inhomogeneous signal increase on T2-weighted imaging (**Figs. 97C, 97D,** and **97E**). There is cortical disruption with loss of segments of cortical bone. Following gadolinium administration, there was an inhomogeneous enhancement throughout the region and within a circumferential soft tissue mass. Areas of very low signal intensity remain unchanged between sequences.

Diagnosis

Osteosarcoma (OS)

Differential Diagnosis

- Ewing's tumor: usually diaphyseal and lytic, less commonly can be sclerotic
- Metastatic deposit: usually multiple sites and not as extensive
- Osteomyelitis: increased erythrocyte sedimentation rate, temperature, and white blood cell count

Discussion

Background

OS accounts for ~60% of the primary malignant bone tumors found in children and adolescents, generally occurring in the appendicular skeleton (80%) and arising in the metaphyseal region (90%). The peak incidence is in the second decade, with boys affected twice as often as girls. Overall incidence of OS is 2 to 3 per million.

Etiology

Etiologically, OS can be divided into primary (predominating in the metaphyses) and secondary (arising in underlying disease; Paget's, fibrous dysplasia, and multiple enchondromas). Radiation is a well-documented causal agent in OS development usually seen 7 to 15 years after radiation treatment. Loss of function of the p53 and Rb tumor suppressor genes is believed to play a role in tumorgenesis. The incidence of OS is increased among patients with retinoblastoma, likely due to germline mutations of the Rb gene, and ~3% of OS patients have a mutation of the p53 gene.

Clinical Findings

The typical patient presents with a few months' history of dull aching pain within an extremity. An increase in pain severity can reflect cortical penetration by tumor or pathologic fracture. Approximately 50% of OS are found about the knee, most commonly in distal femoral metaphysis with the second most common site being the proximal humerus. Eighty percent of patients have no clinically detected metastatic disease at presentation. Pallor, fever, and weight loss suggest dissemination and are rare at presentation.

Complications

- Approximately 20% of patients will have evidence of metastatic disease, usually lung deposits.
- Death often results from respiratory failure.
- Less commonly, bony metastases or skip lesions are present.
- OS may present as a pathologic fracture, particularly with the more lytic types.
- Neurovascular bundle compromise due to tumor invasion is a rare complication (<4%).
- Complications of prosthetic reconstruction include loosening, infection, and mechanical failure.

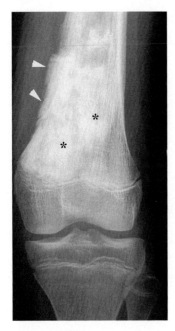

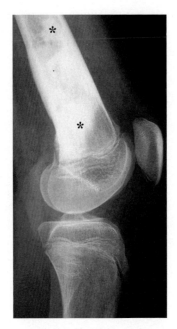

Figure 97F Frontal view of femur depicts areas of sclerosis (*) involving diaphysis and metaphysis. Interrupted periosteal new bone formation with a Codman's triangle or a sunburst appearance is evident medially (arrowheads). Distal diaphyseal cortex is destroyed in segments medially.

Figure 97G Lateral view of femur demonstrates patchy areas of sclerosis (*) throughout visualized diaphysis and metaphysis extending to posterior physeal plate. There is periosteal new bone formation that is not incorporated into cortex.

Pathology/Histology

Microscopically, osteosarcoma is a pleomorphic spindle-cell tumor that forms an extracellular osteoid matrix. The tumor can be categorized by:

- The predominant histologic components (osteoblastic ~50%, chondroblastic ~25%, fibroblastic ~20%, and telangiectatic ~5%)
- By the degree of cellular differentiation (high versus low grades)
- By the location in a bone (intramedullary-single site ~75%, intramedullary-multiple sites 14.8%, intracortical ~0.2%, and juxtacortical ~10%). The juxtacortical types are further divided into parosteal ~65%, periosteal ~25%, and high-grade surface subtypes 10%.

Pathologically, osteoid production by the tumor is characteristic of each type. Given the increased bone activity, alkaline phosphatase may be elevated. Serum lactate dehydrogenase also is elevated.

Imaging Findings

RADIOGRAPHY

- Most commonly, an eccentric destructive mixed lytic and sclerotic metaphyseal lesion with associated soft tissue mass. Periosteal new bone is typically interrupted with resulting Codman's triangle or "sunburst" appearance (**Fig. 97F**, arrowheads).
- Osteoid production (**Figs. 97F**, asterisks; and **97G**, asterisks) by tumor may appear amorphous/cloudy or irregular and is seen in 90%.

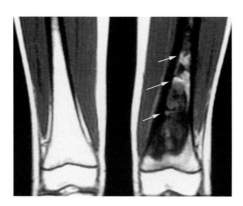

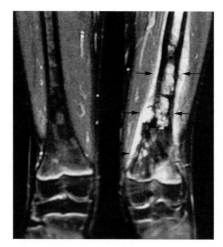

Figure 97H T1-weighted coronal MRI depicts abnormal marrow signal involving left diaphysis and metaphysis. Low signal intensity soft tissue and sclerotic deposits (arrows) occupy a large portion of the medullary space with extension through medial cortex.

Figure 97I Coronal STIR MRI better depicts cortical destruction and inhomogeneous soft tissue and sclerotic medullary deposits throughout diaphysis and metaphysis. There is increased signal paralleling femoral shaft with interrupted periosteal new bone formation (arrows).

- Parosteal type on radiographs typically is a lobulated juxtacortical mass with a broad base that is separated from underlying cortex by a radiolucent cleft reflecting periosteum or fibrous capsule. The lesion is more heavily calcified centrally and at its base of attachment.

MRI

- Homogeneous to markedly heterogeneous signal intensity dependent on the predominant cell type and presence or absence of hemorrhage, necrosis, or sclerotic bone formation (**Figs. 97H** and **97I**, arrows).
- Generally low signal on T1-weighted imaging and high on T2-weighted imaging and short tau inversion recovery (STIR)
- Areas of sclerosis will be low signal on T1- and T2-weighted imaging.
- Gadolinium enhancement may help delineate synovial spread and aid in predicting response to chemotherapy.
- Need to image the whole limb for "skip" lesions and across the proximal joint.
- Extension across physes is seen in one third of cases.

CT

- Typically see mixed sclerotic and lytic lesion with interrupted periosteal new bone and ossification of areas of matrix.

BONE SCINTIGRAPHY

- Depicted as an area of increased activity
- May see bone metastases and ossified pulmonary metastases.

THALLIUM-201

- See increased uptake in tumor.
- Useful for monitoring therapeutic response and recurrence

PET-F18-FDG (FLUORINE-18-2-DEOXY-2-FLUORO-3-GLUCOSE)

- Increased uptake at more active tumor sites, therefore may help guide biopsy
- May be useful for predicting outcome and tumor response to neoadjuvant chemotherapy

- Useful for determining if residual soft tissue after treatment is tumor/relapse or postsurgical change
- May help determine which lung nodules are metastatic deposits

Treatment

- Most patients are enrolled into international neoadjuvant chemotherapy trials prior to surgery.
- Chemotherapy regimens both inductive (preoperative) and adjuvant (postoperative) are vital.
- Doxorubicin, cisplatin, and isosfamide with mesna and methotrexate are most effective.
- Limb-salvaging surgery is possible in >90% of extremity lesions with a 3 cm surgical resection margin for best results.
- Radiation is generally not used in primary therapy unless nonresectable tumor.

Prognosis

- Best long-term survival is in patients with >90% to 95% tumor necrosis on histology of resected specimen after neoadjuvant chemotherapy.
- Long-term survival rates are 60 to 80% in patients with localized disease.
- If local relapse, 5-year survival drops to 21%; relapses usually occur in first 2 years.
- Worse prognosis if pulmonary metastasis; however, cure still possible in a small number of patients if they can undergo successful metastatectomy
- Only 11% disease free at 5 years if pulmonary metastasis
- Without chemotherapy, 90% of patients develop recurrence after surgery.

Follow-up

- CT thorax and radiograph of reconstructed extremity recommended every 3 months for 2 years then every 6 months for 2 years to 5 post-treatment.
- Bone scintigraphy recommended annually for first 2 years.

PEARLS_____

- Include an anatomic reference point on at least one MRI sequence so accurate measurements can be obtained.
- Forty to 50% of trabecular bone must be destroyed to see a discrete lucency on radiographs.
- Rare telangiectatic type of OS is highly vascular and mainly lytic on radiographs and can mimic an aneurysmal bone cyst with fluid–fluid levels on MRI.
- Rare pathologic variant is small-cell OS.
- Periosteal OS is cortically based and does not involve medullary space initially; typically diaphyseal location.
- If OS is centered in diaphysis, suspect chondroblastic cell type.
- Cortical desmoid can mimic OS but can help distinguish by typical location at posterior aspect of medial femoral condyle.
- Multicentric OS lesions are referred to as osteosarcomatosis.
- Biopsy tract should be excised during limb-salvage surgery.
- Seventy-five percent of patients are clinically staged as IIB (histologically poorly differentiated/ undifferentiated with tumor extension to periosteum without lymph node or distant metastasis).
- Almost all patients are considered to have subclinical microscopic metastatic disease.
- Parosteal OS is a low-grade malignancy occurring in an older age group, generally with a much better prognosis than other types.

PITFALLS_____

- Osseous OS rarely changes in size after chemotherapy; therefore, it is difficult to assess response by radiography.
- Stress fractures and chronic avulsions can mimic malignancy on radiographs and on pathology.
- Normal high activity in physes may obscure small OS on bone scans.
- Treatment of OS includes granulocyte colony stimulating factor, which alters the marrow signal making tumor margins difficult to assess accurately with MRI.
- The prominent marrow and soft tissue edema seen with OS on MRI also is common with osteoid osteoma, osteoblastoma, stress fractures, and chondroblastomas.
- Post-traumatic myositis ossificans at 4 to 8 weeks may stimulate OS on radiography (amorphous sclerosis in soft tissue mass, underlying periosteal reaction) and pseudosarcomatous appearance centrally on histology.
- Osteoid osteoma and osteoblastoma also may resemble OS on histologic analysis.

Suggested Readings

Brenner W, Bohuslavizki KH, Eary JF. PET imaging of osteosarcoma. J Nucl Med 2003;44:930–942

Davies AM. Imaging in skeletal paediatric oncology. Eur J Radiol 2001;37:79–94

Fletcher BD. Imaging pediatric bone sarcomas. Radiol Clin North Am 1997;35:1477–1494

Hoffer FA. Primary skeletal neoplasms: osteosarcoma and Ewing sarcoma. Top Magn Reson Imaging 2002;13:231–240

Mazumdar A, Siegel MJ, Narra V, Luchtman-Jones L. Whole-body fast inversion recovery MR imaging of small cell neoplasms in pediatric patients: a pilot study. AJR Am J Roentgenol 2002;179:1261–1266

Meyers PA, Gorlick R. Osteosarcoma. Pediatr Clin North Am 1997;44:973–989

Miller SL, Hoffer FA. Malignant and benign bone tumors. Radiol Clin North Am 2001;39:673–699

Russell EC, Dunn NL, Massey GV. Lymphomas and bone tumors: clinical presentation, management, and potential late effects of current treatment strategies. Adolesc Med 1999;10:419–435

Stokkel MPM, Linthorst MFG, Borm JJJ, Taminiau AH, Pauwels, EKJ. A reassessment of bone scintigraphy and commonly tested pretreatment biochemical parameters in newly diagnosed osteosarcoma. J Cancer Res Clin Oncol 2002;128:393–399

Wittig JC, Bickels J, Priebat D, et al. Osteosarcoma: a multidisciplinary approach to diagnosis and treatment. Am Fam Physician 2002;65:1123–1132

CASE 98

Clinical Presentation

A lethargic 7-year-old boy presents with painful knees/shins.

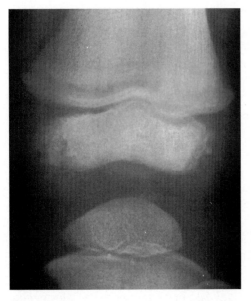

Figure 98A

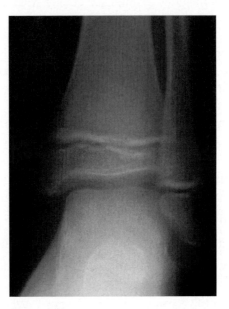

Figure 98B

Radiologic Findings

Coned-down frontal views centered on the knee and ankle demonstrates subphyseal metaphyseal lucent bands involving distal femur as well as proximal and distal tibia (**Figs. 98A** and **98B**). The bone configuration/modeling appears normal.

Diagnosis

Acute lymphoblastic leukemia (ALL)

Differential Diagnosis

The differential diagnosis of lucent metaphyseal bands are:
- Infection (congenital)
- Neuroblastoma
- Rickets, hypophosphatasia
- Scurvy, nutritional deficiency
- Juvenile idiopathic arthritis

Discussion

Background

Of all pediatric malignancies, leukemia is the most common, accounting for 30 to 40% of all child-hood cancers. ALL is the most common form, comprising up to 85% of patients. The disease is most frequent in children 2 to 5 years of age. Skeletal manifestations may be the initial presentation in up to 20% of cases. Between 70 and 90% of children with leukemia will manifest skeletal radiographic changes during their course of illness and treatment. Long bones (usually lower limbs) are more often affected than axial bones.

Etiology

Radiation exposure has been linked with the development of ALL; patients with ataxia telangiectasia, Down syndrome, and Fanconi's anemia are also predisposed.

Oncogenic mechanisms include enhanced expression of protooncogenes (*MYC, TAL-1, LYL-1, HOX-11*), the expression of translocation-generated fusion oncogenes (*BCR-ABL, TEL-AML-1, E2A-PBX-1,* and *MLL* fusions), and alterations in chromosomal number (decrease or increase). The majority of these mechanisms are insufficient on their own to generate a full leukemic phenotype. The nature and number of mutations needed to induce leukemia appear to vary, depending on unknown initiation lesions, some of which may be acquired in utero.

Clinical Findings

- Fever, lethargy, irritability, pallor, loss of appetite, petechiae, bleeding
- Testicular enlargement
- Headaches and cranial nerve palsies if central nervous system (CNS) involvement
- Inability or reluctance to walk/move limb, pain (27 to 50%), tenderness, swelling
- Lymphadenopathy, hepatosplenomegaly

Complications

- Infiltration of marrow results in thrombocytopenia and anemia.
- Osteopenia predisposes to pathologic fractures (~2% of patients have vertebral body compression).
- Rarely, see bone marrow necrosis prior to treatment
- Pulmonary complications include infection, edema, hemorrhage, cryptogenic organizing pneumonia, and malignant infiltration.
- Subsequent learning difficulties and decreased cognitive function described on some long-term follow up studies

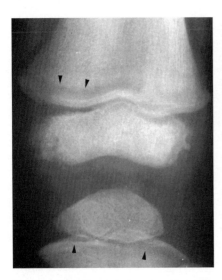

Figure 98C Frontal knee radiograph depicts subphyseal distal femoral metaphyseal lucent band paralleling growth plate. Similar, less prominent lucency spans subphyseal metaphysis of proximal tibia (arrowheads).

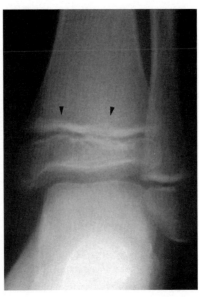

Figure 98D Frontal radiograph of ankle depicts a distal metaphyseal lucent band paralleling the normal subphyseal sclerosis of tibia (arrowheads) and fibula.

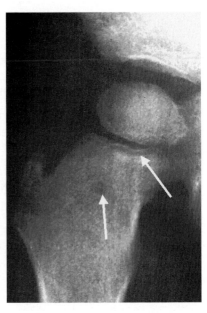

Figure 98E Frontal radiograph of the left hip depicts a subphyseal lucent band and more focal radiolucency within femoral neck (arrows).

Pathogenesis/Histology/Laboratory

- Most bone lesions are due to proliferation of leukemic cells.
- Subperiosteal infiltration by malignant cells leads to periosteal uplifting and new bone formation resulting in pain/tenderness.
- Lucent metaphyseal bands are usually the result of "stress" reaction as opposed to infiltration.
- Alteration in mineral homeostasis is the mechanism for decreased bone mass, which predisposes to fractures.
- Initial blood counts: anemia, abnormal leukocyte and differential counts (60% elevated, 35% depressed), and thrombocytopenia (10% have normal peripheral blood counts)
- Definitive diagnosis rests on bone marrow exam: usually completely replaced by leukemic lymphoblasts; if bone marrow biopsy does not lead to diagnosis, then minimally invasive radiologic intervention is effective method.

Imaging Findings

RADIOGRAPHY

- Diffuse osteopenia is the most common finding.
- Periostitis present in up to 35% cases.
- Subphyseal lucent metaphyseal bands with a normal zone of provisional calcification (**Figs. 98C** and **98D**, arrowheads)
- Metaphyseal erosions, osteolysis, osteosclerosis (**Fig. 98E**), vertebral body compression (**Fig. 98F**)

SCINTIGRAPHY

- Symmetric increased activity in metaphyses (usually lower limbs)
- Less commonly, see photopenic areas due to vascular compromise.

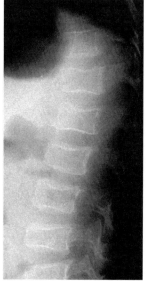

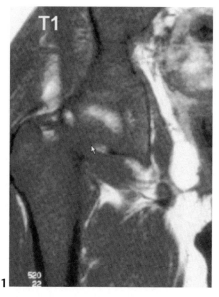

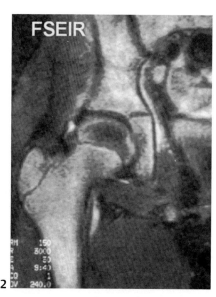

Figure 98F Lateral thoracolumbar spine radiograph demonstrates decrease in height of multiple vertebra with prominent end-plate indentation and diffused osteopenia.

Figure 98G Coronal T1-weighted MRI of hip (**1**) showing extensive low-signal replacement of fatty marrow. Coronal STIR MRI (**2**) shows corresponding high-signal in fatty marrow.

MRI

- Leukemic infiltration of marrow usually iso- or low signal intensity on T1-weighted image (lower than adjacent muscle or disk signal for vertebra) and increased signal on T2-weighted image, fat-saturated, and short tau inversion recovery (STIR) images (**Fig. 98G**)
- Cortical infiltration and adjacent soft tissue edema common
- Abnormal marrow signal can be shown on long-term studies, consisting of patchy inhomogeneity believed due to fibrosis and/or osteonecrosis, which may be asymptomatic (up to 32% of patients).

Treatment

- Most induction regimens include: vincristine, prednisone, L-asparginase, and intrathecal methotrexate (MTX) for standard-risk patients; add anthracycline for high-risk patients
- Consolidation therapy (after induction): intermediate dose intravenous MTX, vincristine, and every 2 weeks intrathecal MTX
- Maintenance protocols include daily oral 6-mercaptopurine, weekly intramuscular MTX, and pulses of vincristine every 1 to 2 months; prednisone and intrathecal MTX every 2 to 3 months.
- Bone marrow transplantation used for patients with relapse or predicted poor response to chemotherapy agents

Prognosis

- Approximately 80% of children with ALL are cured.
- Children are placed in a risk group based on following:
  - High risk (HR)
    - White blood cell count (WBC) >50 × 10^9/L
    - CNS involvement

- • Mediastinal mass
- • T or B cell ALL
- • Chromosomal translocation
- ◦ Intermediate risk (IR)
  - • No HR criteria
  - • Age 2 to 10 years and white blood cells (WBC) 10 to 50 $\times$ 10^9/L or
  - • Age 1 to 2 years and WBC <50 $\times$ 10^9/L
- ◦ Standard risk
  - • No IR or HR criteria
  - • Age 2 to 10 years and WBC ≤10 $\times$ 10^9/L
- • Leukemic remission correlates with disappearance of pain and return to normal function.
- • Most relapses occur during treatment or within first 2 years post-treatment and have poor prognosis.

PEARLS

- • Delay in diagnosis on average is 7 weeks.
- • Treated leukemia with resulting aplastic anemia does not manifest as low-signal marrow on T1-weighted MRI (if low signal, consider relapse or hemosiderosis).
- • Imaging marrow may help identify sites for more successful aspiration/biopsy in patients with necrosis.
- • Patients in blast crisis may show diffuse increased activity on scintigraphy.
- • Rebound thymic hyperplasia seen on radiographs is common after chemotherapy.

PITFALLS

- • Marrow signal intensity alone is not reliable to diagnose and determine extent of leukemic disease (remission versus relapse).
- • Reconversion to red marrow may occur with resolution of "stress" and if asymmetric may require biopsy to exclude infiltration.
- • Radiographic changes do not always correlate with sites of abnormal bone activity on scintigraphy scans.

Suggested Readings

Abbas AAH, Husain AH, Abdelaal MA, et al. Acute lymphoblastic leukemia presenting with extensive skeletal lesions and bone marrow necrosis. Med Pediatr Oncol 2001;37:64–66

Bernard EJ, Nicholls WD, Howman-Giles RB, Kellie SJ, Uren RF. Patterns of abnormality on bone scans in acute childhood leukemia. J Nucl Med 1998;39:1983–1986

Carriere B, Cummins-Mcmanus B. Vertebral fractures as initial signs for acute lymphoblastic leukemia. Pediatr Emerg Care 2001;17:258–261

Downing JR, Shannon KM. Acute leukemia: a pediatric perspective. Cancer Cell 2002;2:437–445

Iuvone L, Mariotti P, Colosimo C, et al. Long-term cognitive outcome, brain computed tomography scan, and magnetic resonance imaging in children cured for acute lymphoblastic leukemia. Cancer 2002;95:2562–2570

Kayser R, Mahlfeld K, Nebelung W, GraBhoff H. Vertebral collapse and normal peripheral blood cell count at the onset of acute lymphatic leukemia in childhood. J Pediatr Orthop B 2000;9:55–57

Lorand-Metze I, Santiago GF, Lima CSP, Zanardi VA, Torriani M. Magnetic resonance imaging of femoral marrow cellularity in hypocellular haemopoietic disorders. Clin Radiol 2001;56:107–110

Ojala AE, Paakko E, Lanning FP, Harila-Saari AH, Lanning BM. Bone marrow changes on MRI in children with acute lymphoblastic leukemia 5-years after treatment. Clin Radiol 1998;53:131–136

Paredes-Aguilera R, Romero-Guzman L, Lopez-Santiago N, Trejo RA. Biology, clinical, and hematologic features of acute megakaryoblastic leukemia in children. Am J Hematol 2003;73:71–80

Razzouk BI. Minimally invasive radiological diagnosis of pediatric hematological malignancies. Pediatr Radiol 2002;32:652

States LJ. Imaging of metabolic bone disease and marrow disorders in children. Radiol Clin North Am 2001;39:749–772

Winer-Muram HT, Arheart KL, Jennings SG, et al. Pulmonary complications in children with hematologic malignancies: accuracy of diagnosis with chest radiography and CT. Radiology 1997;204:643–649

CASE 99

Clinical Presentation

An 11-year-old boy presents with chronic heel pain and mild fever.

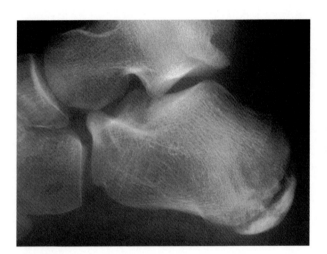

Figure 99A

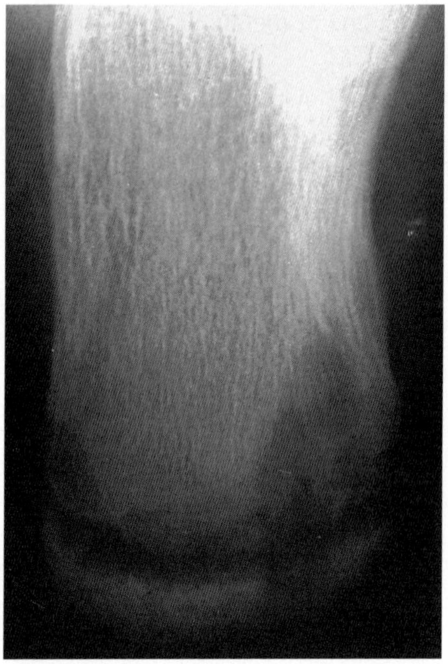

Figure 99B

Radiographic Findings

Lateral radiograph of calcaneus demonstrates inhomogeneous bone density with areas of both patchy sclerosis and increased lucency posteriorly (**Fig. 99A**). The calcaneal view better defines the lytic component extending into adjacent apophyseal center (**Fig. 99B**).

Diagnosis

Chronic osteomyelitis (OM)

Differential Diagnosis

Langerhans' cell histiocytosis

Discussion

Background

OM is an infection of bone and bone marrow clinically divided into acute, subacute, and chronic entities. Host resistance, virulence of the organism, and the response to treatment with antimicrobials are the major factors contributing to the development of one entity over another. OM is polyostotic in ~6% of cases and has a predilection for rapidly growing sites in the immature skeleton such as the metaphyses (or metaphyseal equivalent) of the distal femur and radius as well as proximal tibia and humerus. Neonatal OM has an incidence of 1 to 3 per 1000 hospital admissions, often involving the hips, and is multifocal in 23 to 47% of cases.

Etiology

Routes for infection include hematogenous seeding infection (most common form in children), contiguous spread from adjacent soft tissue or joint, and direct inoculation due to trauma. Approximately 2% of all orthopedic procedures are complicated by infection.

Clinical Findings

Infection in the neonate and young infant is often clinically silent. Toddlers and children present with pain in limb with passive motion, pseudoparalysis, or a limp. The area may be red, swollen, and warm on examination.

Complications

- Extension of infection into joint with resulting destruction, subluxation/dislocation, or ischemic necrosis (one third of hip OM has septic joint)
- Slipped epiphysis
- Premature closure of growth plate due to destruction of proliferating cartilage cells
- Overgrowth of limb due to chronic hyperemia
- Squamous cell carcinoma develops in 0.5% of patients with long-standing draining OM (very rare before 20 years of age)

Pathophysiology

Acute infection via hematogenous seeding results in marrow edema and cellular infiltration usually in the metaphysis of a long bone. The physeal plate in infants and children between ~8 and 18 months of age acts as a relative barrier, localizing the disease process, whereas in both younger infants and older children the infection is more likely to spread to the epiphysis via transphyseal vascular pathways and may extend into the joint space. Progression of infiltrate within the marrow cavity results in an increase in intraosseous pressure leading to extension of the inflammatory process through the cortex and into subperiosteal space via haversian and Volkmann's canals.

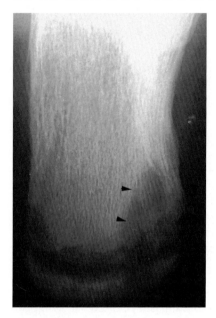

Figure 99C Calcaneal view depicts area of ill-marginated lucency (arrowheads).

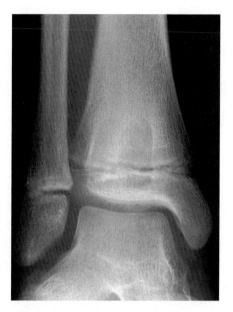

Figure 99D Frontal radiograph of ankle depicts a lytic lesion within distal tibial metaphysis crossing the physis and extending into epiphysis. Margins are ill defined in some segments and well demarcated in others. There is a faint central area of increased bone density.

The process may then continue to spread into periosteum and overlying soft tissues. The increased intraosseous pressure can impair blood flow leading to ischemic necrosis of bone resulting in devascularized fragments called sequestra. A subacute OM is a more localized pyogenic process in which the term *Brodie's abscess* is used when complicated by surrounding granulation tissue and sclerotic bone. Chronic OM is a low-grade continuing infection classified as active or inactive. The process may be indolent for long periods before re-activation. The clinical diagnosis of chronic osteomyelitis can be made if symptoms have been present for >1 month, if there has been inadequate treatment, or if the infection arose >1 month after surgery for trauma.

Laboratory

- Serial blood cultures are positive in 30 to 60%.
- Cultures from aspiration are positive in up to 90% of acute cases.
- Increased erythrocyte sedimentation rate and leukocytosis are nonspecific and may not be present.

Microbiology

- Causative organism found in ~75% of acute OM overall.
- Most common organism isolated in hematogenous OM is *Staphylococcus aureus*, followed by b-hemolytic streptococci. *Kingella kingae* (a gram-negative coccobacillus) is increasing in frequency.
- With chronic OM usually no bacteria found on culture of aspirate.
- Fifty percent of Brodie's abscesses are sterile.
- *Pseudomonas* more common with penetrating injuries to foot.
- *Salmonella* is found more often in patients with sickle-cell disease, but *S. aureus* is still more common.

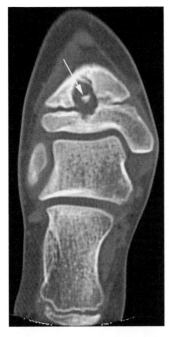

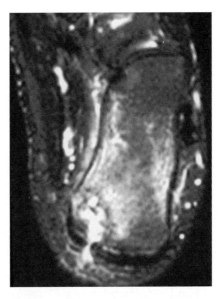

Figure 99E Coronal CT image better demonstrates the lytic metaphyseal lesion extending into central epiphysis. A small bone fragment lies centrally within the lesion.

Figure 99F Fat-suppressed, contrast-enhanced axial oblique MRI of calcaneus depicts an irregular high-signal intensity lesion extending through to the apophyseal ossification center. Less prominent ill-marginated increased signal is evident within adjacent marrow.

Imaging Findings

RADIOGRAPHY

- **Acute (hematogenous)**
  - Soft tissue swelling or indistinctness of soft tissue fascial planes
  - Ill-marginated ± permeative lytic pattern in cortex/medullary space
  - May see marginal sclerosis, serpiginous tract, sequestrum (a devitalized bony fragment), or involucrum (sheath of new bone developing around a sequestra)
- **Subacute**
  - Often better marginated lytic lesion with sclerotic margin (**Fig. 99C**)
  - Serpiginous tract often seen and highly suggestive of OM
  - Periosteal reaction present and often "onion skin" in character
- **Chronic**
  - Generally mixed lytic and sclerotic process (**Fig. 99D**)
  - Cortical thickening
  - Sinus tracts/sequestrum/involucrum, and cloaca
  - Chronic recurrent multifocal OM (CRMO): multifocal lytic or mixed lytic/sclerotic lesions ± sclerotic rim

BONE SCINTIGRAPHY

- Increased activity on all three phases of technetium bone scan Tc 99m methylene diphosphate (MDP) scan has a sensitivity of 75 to 100%; positive by 24 to 48 hours after onset of symptoms.

GALLIUM SCAN

- Increased activity at site of OM; sensitivity 25 to 80%, specificity 67%

WHITE BLOOD CELL SCANS

- ^{99m}Tc–labeled murine immunoglobulin M monoclonal antigranulocyte antibody, and infection labeled with ^{99m}Tc have been used to establish diagnosis.

ULTRASOUND

- See soft tissue thickening in acute stage
- See elevation of thickened periosteum with hypoechoic deep and superficial layers resulting in a "sandwich" appearance
- If elevation of periosteum by >2 mm by hypoechoic or anechoic collection, collection may be echogenic.

CT

- Best method to show foci of gas, cortical erosion, and sequestra (**Fig. 99E**)/involucra formation
- See increased attenuation in marrow, increased soft tissue ± abscess and cortical destruction
- May also depict sinus tracts and marginal sclerosis

MRI

- **Acute phase**
  - An area of decreased signal intensity that has an indistinct margin with adjacent normal marrow on T1-weighted images that becomes bright on T2-weighted and STIR images
  - See enhancement of region with gadolinium.
- **Subacute phase**
  - May see a classic target appearance of Brodie's abscess
  - Central abscess is low signal on T1-weighted and high on T2-weighted and STIR images.
  - This is surrounded by granulation tissue that is isointense on T1-weighted and increased on T2-weighted/STIR sequences showing contrast enhancement.
  - A peripheral fibrotic layer results in a low-intensity rim on all sequences.
  - This low-intensity rim is surrounded by a peripheral endosteal reaction that is low signal intensity on T1- and high on T2-weighted images.
- **Chronic phase**
  - Observe more distinct interface with marrow, cortical thickening; sequestra will appear as low signal intensity on all sequences and without enhancement following contrast.
  - Active areas of inflammation in soft tissue and bone marrow will enhance following gadolinium enhancement (**Fig. 99F**).

Treatment

- Acute osteomyelitis:
  - Appropriate antimicrobials using intravenous route until clinical response and improvement then switch to oral overall course of treatment ~6 weeks in total
  - If clinical suspicion of OM, needle aspiration of potential subperiosteal fluid
  - Presence of pus on aspiration often warrants incision and drainage.
- Subacute/chronic osteomyelitis:
  - Presence of abscess on imaging, sequestrum, involucrum/cloaca necessitates surgical debridement and drainage followed by antimicrobial treatment.

Prognosis

- Depends on underlying health condition, rapidity of appropriate treatment
- Overall good prognosis with appropriate antimicrobials
- CMRO often has exacerbations/remissions over 2 to 7 years.

PEARLS_____

- Consider "active" OM if change from previous study, ill-defined lucency, thin/fine or fluffy periosteal reaction, or presence of sequestra (most specific).
- If multifocal OM foci, consider sickle-cell disease, chronic granulomatous disease, or underlying diabetes.
- CRMO is found primarily in metaphyses of long bones and in medial clavicles and may be part of SAPHO syndrome (synovitis, acne, pustulosis, hyperstosis, osteosis).
- In neonates, sequestra are rare, but involucrum formation is more common.
- Increased signal on T1-weighted imaging due to regenerating marrow fat is a sign of healing on MRI.
- Central closing of physeal plate resulting in tethering often seen with meningococcal septicemia and seeding
- Sequences that suppress signal of bone marrow fat increase conspicuity of lesions; sensitivity of MRI for OM is 82 to 100%, specificity quoted at 77 to 96%.
- Garre's sclerosing OM is a form of chronic infection with prominent cortical thickening and sclerosis.
- Brodie's abscess found most frequently in tibial metaphysis, may also be centered in cortex

PITFALLS_____

- Radiographic changes of OM lag 10 to 14 days after onset of symptoms.
- Sensitivity of radiographs 43 to 75% for OM, specificity 75 to 83%.
- Trauma with bone bruise, infarction, fracture, and neoplasm can all mimic acute OM on MRI.
- Scarring in postoperative bone defects leads to false-positive diagnosis of OM on MRI for up to 13 months.
- In 60% of septic joints, may see increased signal in adjacent marrow on T2-weighted imaging that can mimic OM.
- White blood cell scan sensitivity is 90% with acute OM but ~50 to 60% with chronic OM.

Suggested Readings

Boutin RD, Brossmann J, Sartoris DJ, Reilly D, Resnick D. Update on imaging of orthopedic infections. Orthop Clin North Am 1998;29:41–66

Gylys-Morin VM. MR imaging of pediatric musculoskeletal inflammatory and infectious disorders. Magn Reson Imaging Clin N Am 1998;6:537–559

Kothari NA, Pelchovitz DJ, Meyer JS. Imaging of musculoskeletal infections. Radiol Clin North Am 2001;39:653–671

Lane-O'Kelly A, Moloney AC. Acute haematogenous osteomyelitis: evaluation of management in the 1990's. Ir J Med Sci 1995;164:285–288

Ledermann HP, Kaim A, Bongartz G, Steinbrich W. Pitfalls and limitations of magnetic resonance imaging in chronic posttraumatic osteomyelitis. Eur Radiol 2000;10:1815–1823

Ma LD, Frassica FJ, Bluemke DA, Fishman EK. CT and MRI evaluation of musculoskeletal infection. Crit Rev Diagn Imaging 1997;38:535–568

Mazur JM, Ross G, Cummings RJ, Hahn GA, McCluskey WP. Usefulness of magnetic resonance imaging for the diagnosis of acute musculoskeletal infections of children. J Pediatr Orthop 1995;15:144–147

Oudjhane K, Azouz EM. Imaging of osteomyelitis in children. Radiol Clin North Am 2001;39:251–266

Poyhia T, Azouz EM. MR imaging evaluation of subacute and chronic bone abscesses in children. Pediatr Radiol 2000;30:763–768

Santiago-Restrepo CS, Gimenez CR, McCarthy K. Imaging of osteomyelitis and musculoskeletal soft tissue infections: current concepts. Rheum Dis Clin North Am 2003;29:89–109

CASE 100

Clinical Presentation

A 5-year-old boy presents with back pain and fever.

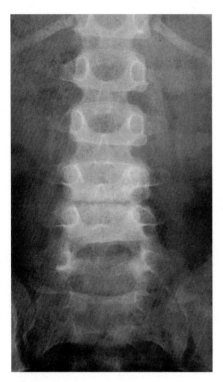

Figure 100A

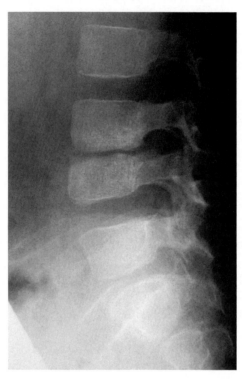

Figure 100B

Radiologic Findings

Frontal and lateral radiographs of the lumbar spine demonstrate decreased intervertebral disk space height at L3-L4. The adjacent vertebral body end-plate margins are indistinct and irregular with underlying areas of sclerosis and erosions (**Figs. 100A** to **100B**). Corresponding sagittal MRI show inhomogeneous decreased signal in the L3 and L4 vertebral bodies on T1-weighted imaging (**Fig. 100C**) with increased signal on T2-weighted imaging (**Fig. 100D**). There is narrowing of the L3-L4 disc space and retrograde protrusion of a portion of disc or fluid from inflammation.

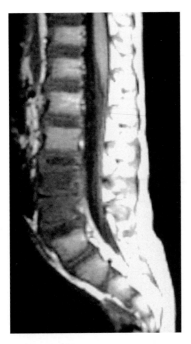

Figure 100C

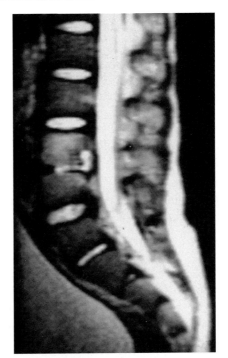

Figure 100D

Diagnosis

Diskitis with vertebral osteomyelitis.

Differential Diagnosis

- Traumatic disk herniation (usually localized impaction to anterior portion of superior end plate with more distinct end-plate margins)
- Scheuermann's disease (multiple levels usually between T3-T12; loss of disk height more prominent anteriorly with anterior vertebral body wedging)

Discussion

Background

Diskitis and vertebral osteomyelitis are disease processes with distinct epidemiologic, clinical, and radiographic features. Diskitis is an inflammatory process of the disk space, more common in children than adults, especially in girls (2×). The disease affects the lumbar spine predominantly. The mean age at presentation is 2.8 years with bimodal age peaks at 6 months to 4 years and 10 to 14 years. Vertebral osteomyelitis most commonly also affects the lumbosacral region (64%) but can be seen in the thoracic spine (29%) and occasionally in the cervical location. The mean age at presentation for vertebral osteomyelitis is 7.5 years with the duration of symptoms longer on average than diskitis (33 days vs 22 days). Whether diskitis and vertebral osteomyelitis are distinct processes or reflect a spectrum of a single disease is controversial. Early in the course of the disease, differentiation

Table 100-1   Comparison of Typical Features of Diskitis and Vertebral Osteomyelitis

Diagnosis	Mean Age	Typical Findings			
		Fever	Disk Space	Destruction Vertebra	Hx URTI*
Diskitis	2.8 years	<101°F	+	−	+
Vertebral osteomyelitis	7.5 years	>102°F	±	+	−

* Hx URTI, history of upper respiratory tract infection.

clinically can be difficult. The imaging modality of choice in a patient with possible vertebral osteomyelitis is MRI, which has high sensitivity and specificity.

Etiology

The pathophysiology of diskitis and vertebral osteomyelitis remains unclear. The cartilaginous regions of the disk in children have vascular channels with abundant intraosseous arterial anastomoses that may promote clearance of microorganisms or entrap emboli resulting in hematogenous seeding. In contrast, vertebral osteomyelitis is thought to occur when microorganisms lodge in the low-flow end-organ vasculature adjacent to the end plates. Vascular communications from this region, also known as the vertebral metaphysis, to the periphery of the disk may allow an inflammatory process to spread. The venous plexus of Batson located within the spinal canal allows direct communication between the veins in the pelvis and the thoracolumbar spine.

Clinical Findings

The presenting symptoms in children with diskitis are dictated by the child's verbal skills. Children <3 years of age often present with a limp or refusal to walk, whereas the older child may present with back pain. Children with vertebral osteomyelitis most often present with back pain (60%) and are significantly more likely to have a fever than those with diskitis (79% vs 28%) with temperature exceeding 102°F in the majority (**Table 100-1**). Mean white blood cell counts and erythrocyte sedimentation rates are elevated in both conditions and provide nonspecific information. Needle aspiration or biopsy is not warranted in patients with noncomplicated diskitis and is negative in nearly all cases. In patients with vertebral osteomyelitis, aspiration/biopsy yields positive results in ~60%, with *Staphylococcus aureus* the most common pathogen isolated.

Imaging Findings

RADIOGRAPHY

- Disk space narrowing (diskitis) (**Fig. 100E**, arrowheads)
- Loss of end-plate margins with reactive sclerosis (diskitis) (**Fig. 100E**, arrowheads)
- Destruction and erosion of end plates with extension into vertebral body (**Fig. 100E**, arrowheads)
- Soft tissue/paraspinal mass
- Vertebral body inhomogeneity ± compression

CT

- End-plate erosion
- Disk space loss
- Enhancement of disk and inflammatory soft tissue
- Paravertebral soft tissue mass/abscess

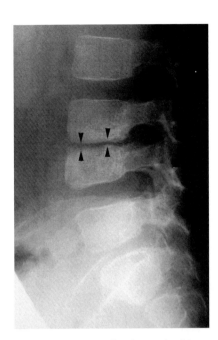

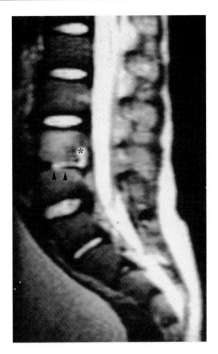

Figure 100E Lateral radiograph of lumbar spine shows decreased disk space height at L3–L4. Adjacent end-plate margins are irregular (arrowheads) with ill-marginated areas of lucency and sclerosis.

Figure 100F Sagittal T2-weighted image of T2 spine shows abnormal high signal within L3 vertebral body and superiorly within L4 body. The L3–L4 disk space is narrowed (arrowheads) with herniation of disk material posteriorly (asterisk).

MRI

- Decrease in disk space height (**Fig. 100F**, arrowheads)
- Decrease in signal in disk and vertebral body on T1-weighted images with loss of distinctness of end-plate margins
- Increase in signal in vertebral body on T2-weighted images (**Fig. 100F**)
- On T2-weighted images, disk centrally and in periphery may be hypointense.
- May be extension of enhancing soft tissue into paraspinal and epidural spaces with subsequent abscess formation identified by rim-enhancement post gadolinium
- May see herniation of nucleus pulposis through eroded end-plate (**Fig. 100F**, asterisk)

Treatment

- Diskitis: Antimicrobials, nonsteroidals, and spine immobilization have all been used successfully.
  - Duration of treatment ranging from 10 days to 4 weeks
- Vetebral osteomyelitis: antimicrobials dependent on culture and response
  - Drainage/intervention for abscess/soft tissue mass complications

Complications and Prognosis

Diskitis in children is generally a benign self-limiting process with full symptomatic recovery in 2 to 3 months. Complications of vertebral osteomyelitis include vertebral body compression, and paraspinal and epidural soft tissue inflammation with potential abscess formation and mass effect on spinal cord and nerves. After appropriate treatment or drainage, disk space narrowing often partially resolves with occasional disk calcification. Vertebral body fusion is a late sequela seen in up to 20%. Protrusion of the disk can lead to nerve entrapment.

PEARLS_____

- Most common organism isolated is *S. aureus.*
- Aspiration/biopsy not warranted for uncomplicated diskitis
- Early MRI has reduced the delay between presentation to hospital and diagnosis by >50%.
- Consider tuberculosis if:
  - Multilevel involvement
  - Prominent paraspinal mass or calcification present
  - Increasing vertebral body destruction with preserved disk space

PITFALLS_____

- Plain radiographic changes may not be seen for 2 to 4 weeks into illness.
- Only ~55% of vertebral osteomyelitis have abnormal plain radiographs at presentation.
- Aspiration/biopsy positive in only ~50% of cases of vertebral osteomyelitis

Suggested Readings

Brown R, Hussain M, McHugh K, Novelli V, Jones D. Diskitis in young children. J Bone Joint Surg Br 2001;83:106–111

du Lac P, Panuel M, Devred P, Bollini G, Padovani J. MRI of disc space infection in infants and children: report of 12 cases. Pediatr Radiol 1990;20:175–178

Fernandez M, Carrol CL, Baker CJ. Diskitis and vertebral osteomyelitis in children: an 18-year review. Pediatrics 2000;105:1299–1304

Payne WK III, Ogilvie JW. Back pain in children and adolescents. Pediatr Clin North Am 1996;43:899–917

Szalay EA, Green NE, Heller RM, Horev G, Kirchner SD. Magnetic resonance imaging in the diagnosis of childhood diskitis. J Pediatr Orthop 1987;7:164–167

Ventura N, Gonzalez E, Terricabras L, Salvador A, Cabrera M. Intervetebral diskitis in children: a review of 12 cases. Int Orthop 1996;20:32–34

CASE 101

Clinical Presentation

A 4-year-old girl presents with back pain.

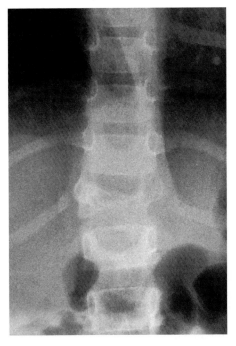

Figure 101A

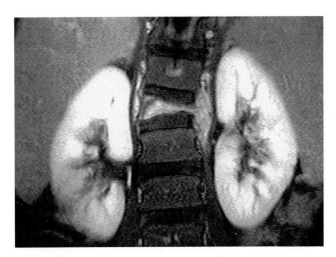

Figure 101B

Radiologic Findings

Frontal radiograph (**Fig. 101A**) demonstrates marked loss of T12 vertebral body height (vertebra plane) with preservation of adjacent disk spaces and posterior elements. Coronal enhanced MRI (**Fig. 101B**) depicts asymmetrically marked collapse of the vertebral body and a left paraspinal enhanced soft tissue mass.

Diagnosis

Langerhans' cell histiocytosis (LCH)

Differential Diagnosis

- Leukemia
- Hodgkin's lymphoma
- Metastatic disease: neuroblastoma
- Hemangioma
- Osteopenia: steroid treatment
- Gaucher's disease

Discussion

Background

LCH is a spectrum of disease processes resulting from the abnormal clonal proliferation of the Langerhans' cell histiocyte (and its precursors), and the resultant infiltration of these cells into normal tissues. Bone, skin, and lymph nodes are the most common sites for infiltration, with 80 to 95% of patients demonstrating bone lesions at some time during the course of illness. LCH was previously known as histiocytosis X and grouped into three forms based on clinical manifestations. What was previously labeled eosinophilic granuloma, Hand-Schüller-Christian disease, and Letterer-Siwe disease are now referred to as localized, chronic recurring, and acute/subacute disseminated LCH, respectively. The disease process occurs during the first 3 decades of life, with a peak between 5 to 10 years. Males are more often affected, and the disease is less prominent outside the Caucasian population. Overall, the disease is rare, representing <1 to 2% of biopsied bone lesions. The disseminated form is found primarily in infants, whereas isolated bone lesions are seen in the 5- to 10-year-old age group.

Etiology

The cause of LCH is unknown. Spontaneous resolution in some cases and a response to steroids in others has suggested a possible infectious (viral) etiology. Immunologic alterations in various patients support the concept of a disorder of immune regulation. The disease is usually sporadic; however, an autosomal recessive inheritance has been proposed by some researchers.

Clinical Findings

The clinical presentation will be dependent on the site, tissue, and extent of infiltration. The localized form of LCH is the mildest form usually presenting with pain and tenderness at the involved bone site. These patients are between 5 and 15 years of age and make up ~75% of cases of LCH. Skull, mandible, ribs, and pelvis account for >50% of involved sites. Approximately one third of lesions involve the long bones, usually the femur. The chronic-recurring form of LCH makes up ~20% of the patient population, with otitis media being the most common presentation. Bone pain, dermatitis, and growth retardation are further symptoms. The classic triad of diabetes insipidus, exophthalmos, and destructive skeletal lesions (90% in skull) is seen in 10 to 15% of patients with this form of LCH. The acute disseminated or fulminant form of LCH presents in infants and children generally <2 years of age. Hepatosplenomegaly, lymphadenopathy, anemia, diffuse bone marrow infiltration, and hemorrhage are the typical clinical findings.

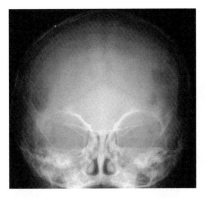 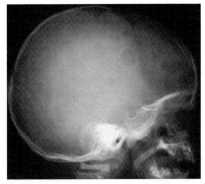

Figure 101C Frontal skull radiograph depicts multiple, mostly ill-marginated lytic lesions.

Figure 101D Lateral skull radiograph better depicts the multiple lytic lesions. Subtle marginal sclerosis is evident at a few of the lesions.

Complications

The larger bone lesions are susceptible to pathologic fractures. Although marked vertebral body collapse is seen, subsequent neurologic compromise is unusual. Diabetes insipidus develops in <50% of patients with the chronic recurrent form of LCH and is due to secondary compression from skull-base involvement or from direct infiltration of hypothalmus. Patients with the acute disseminated disease are extremely vulnerable to infection and often succumb to the illness. LCH can involve the lung, resulting in interstitial disease with cyst formation, which can present with pneumothorax.

Pathology

The cytoplasm of the Langerhans' cells in the lesions of LCH contains inclusion bodies identical to the Birbeck's granules in normal Langerhans' cells. Demonstration of these granules by electron microscopy or staining for S-100 antigens by immunohistochemistry helps establish the diagnosis. On occasion, prominent eosinophils are found in LCH lesions, which led to the previous labeling of eosinophilic granuloma.

Imaging Findings

RADIOGRAPHY

- In general, the skeletal findings consist of geographic, lytic lesions without matrix mineralization (**Figs. 101C** and **101D**).
- The margins will vary depending on the activity of the lesion. Early on in the course of disease a more aggressive appearance with ill-defined margination and lamellated periosteal reaction is typical, whereas more chronic lesions tend to have better-defined sclerotic margins. Periosteal reaction in these cases tends to be continuous and solid.
- Common locations for the disease have led to more characteristic descriptions such as the "beveled-edge" appearance of skull lesions related to uneven lysis of inner and outer tables, vertebra "plana" related to marked compression of vertebral body with sparing of disk spaces/posterior elements (**Fig. 101A**) and "floating teeth" due to extensive infiltration of mandible or maxilla. A "button" sequestrum is a further radiographic appearance described with LCH lesions involving the skull.

BONE SCINTIGRAPHY

- Generally show increased activity within lesions; however, a significant number do not accumulate a radiopharmaceutical.
- Skeletal surveys at time of diagnosis are suggested.

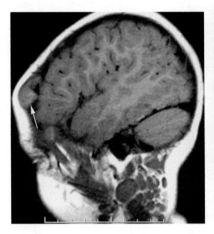

Figure 101E Sagittal T1-weighted MRI depicts a soft tissue mass within the diploic space of frontal bone with focal expansion (arrow) resulting in a palpable mass.

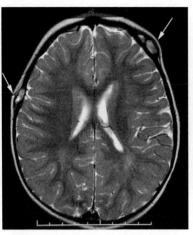

Figure 101F Axial T2-weighted MRI shows multiple inhomogeneous soft tissue masses (arrows) resulting in expansion of inner and outer tables.

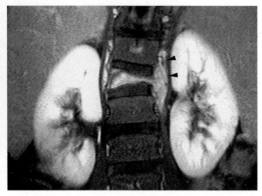

Figure 101G Coronal gradient, contrast enhanced image of spine better depicts left paraspinal soft tissue (arrowheads) spanning T11 to L1. The T12 vertebral shows asymmetric vertebral collapse with an increase in inhomogeneous signal intensity.

MRI

- Typically, the lesions are low signal intensity on T1-weighted imaging and high on T2-weighted imaging. Bone and soft tissue abnormality may be present (**Figs. 101E** and **101F**).
- Lesions typically show prominent enhancement with gadolinium (**Fig. 101G**).
- Often adjacent soft tissue enhancement believed due to associated edema
- Approximately one half of the lesions show a rim of low signal intensity on T2-weighted imaging (flare phenomenon), which has also been described with Ewing's, osteomyelitis, osteoid osteoma, and osteoblastoma.

Treatment

The majority of patients with localized LCH require no treatment unless there is a concern of a subsequent pathologic fracture (weight-bearing location), unremitting pain, or compromise on adjacent vital structure such as spinal cord or optic nerve. Often biopsy and currettage result in healing of the localized lesion. Low-dose radiation (300–600 cGy) has been used successfully as well as intra-lesion injection of steroids. Vertebral body lesions often respond to bed rest, bracing, and nonsteroidal anti-inflammatory medications. Patients with systemic symptoms and organ dysfunction require chemotherapy. Corticosteroids, etoposide, vinblastine, methotrexate, and interferon have been used in this regard. If there are >3 bone lesions, recurrent lesions, or diabetes insipidus, chemotherapy utilizing vinblastine and prednisone is the first-line treatment protocol. Healing response is generally apparent by 4 months but may take many months to complete.

Prognosis

Patients with localized disease have a >90% favorable outcome regardless of treatment regimen. There may be mild residual sclerosis or deformity. Recurrence is seen in ~10%, some of which become multifocal or have extraosseous disease. The chronic recurrent form of LCH has a variable course. The disease worsens with the involvement of multiple sites and has a fatal outcome in 10 to 30% of cases. The disseminated or fulminant form of LCH tends to be rapidly progressive with extensive multiorgan dysfunction and failure resulting in death within 2 years.

PEARLS_____

- Medical student Paul Langerhans was the first to describe the unique cell in 1868.
- LCH is the most common cause of a vertebra plana in children.
- The skull is the most frequent site of LCH.
- In general, the younger the patient, the worse the prognosis.
- Skin lesions, when present, are the easiest site for tissue biopsy diagnosis.
- Enhanced MRI, bone scintigraphy, and fluorine-18,2-deoxy-Z-fluoro-D-glucose PET may help determine active from inactive lesions and guide treatment.
- A skeletal survey should be done once at 6 months when a monostotic lesion is found.

PITFALLS_____

- Bone scans are negative in ~35% of lesions.
- A low-grade temperature, elevated erythrocyte sedimentation rate, and leukocytosis may result in LCH mimicking osteomyelitis.
- Half of all bone lesions are asymptomatic.
- Secondary malignancy from radiation treatment is estimated at 5%.
- Two percent of long bone lesions are epiphyseal.
- Vertebral biopsy can result in growth disturbance.

Suggested Readings

Azouz EM. Magnetic resonance imaging of benign bone lesions: cysts and tumor. Top Magn Reson Imaging 2002;13:219–230

Buckwalter JA, Brandser E, Robinson RA. The variable presentation and natural history of Langerhans' cell histiocytosis. Iowa Orthop J 1999;19:99–105

Kransdorf MJ, Smith SE. Lesions of unknown histogenesis: Langerhans' cell histiocytosis and Ewing sarcoma. Semin Musculoskelet Radiol 2000;4:113–125

Meyer JS, Camargo BD. The role of radiology in the diagnosis and follow-up of Langerhans' cell histiocytosis. Hematol Oncol Clin North Am 1998;12:307–326

Raab P, Hohmann F, Kuhl J, Krauspe R. Vertebral remodeling in eosinophilic granuloma of the spine. Spine 1998;23:1351–1354

Van Nieuwenhuyse JP, Clapuyt P, Malghem J, et al. Radiographic skeletal survey and radionuclide bone scan in Langerhans' cell histiocytosis of bone. Pediatr Radiol 1996;26:734–738

Yanagawa T, Watanabe H, Shinozaki T, et al. The natural history of disappearing bone tumours and tumour-like condition. Clin Radiol 2001;56:877–886

Yeom JS, Lee CK, Shin HY, et al. Langerhans' cell histiocytosis of the spine. Spine 1999;24(16):1740–1749

SECTION VIII
Interventional

CASE 102

Clinical Presentation

Patient presented with a peripherally inserted central catheter (PICC) that did not give blood return and was flushing with some difficulty. During flushing the pressure suddenly improved. On further examination there was swelling over the PICC insertion site.

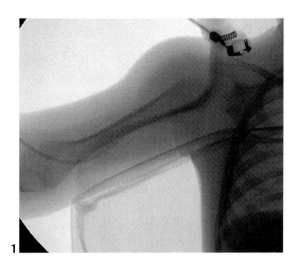 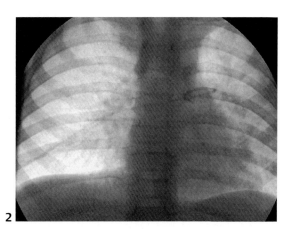

Figure 102A

Radiologic Findings

The fluoroscopic image of the right arm demonstrates PICC line above the elbow (**Fig. 102A1**) with a detached fragment in the main pulmonary artery extending to the right side (**Fig. 102A2**).

Diagnosis

Fractured PICC line

Differential Diagnosis

- Partially fractured line
- Tip thrombus/fibrin sheath
- Malpositioned catheter

Discussion

Background

Reliable vascular access is an integral part of pediatric care. A peripherally inserted central catheter provides stable access to a central vein and allows for regular blood work. PICC lines are indicated for administrating medications that are damaging or irritating, have high osmolality, or a nonphysiologic pH. They can also allow for aggressive parenteral nutrition. A PICC line eliminates the need for repeated peripheral access with its associated pain and trauma.

PICC lines are made of either silicone or polyurethane. They come in sizes from no. 2 to 7 French. They are available in single and double lumens. They are fixed in position with dressings and tape, sutured to the skin, or have a polyethelene terephthalate (e.g., Dacron) cuff that is placed just below the skin, with the exit site sutured tight with resorbable sutures. We use the cuffed silicone catheters for children, as we feel that the catheter is more secure, and there are no sutures to remove.

Etiology

The etiology of catheter fractures is uncertain; however, it probably results from an incomplete occlusion with attempt to unblock the line (with a small volume syringe) resulting in significant pressure rise and fracture at the junction between the thicker proximal part of the catheter and the smaller internal portion. Incidence of PICC fracture and embolization is estimated to be 6.7 per 1000 PICCs inserted.

Clinical Findings

- A history of at least one of the following:
  - Difficulty flushing the line or withdrawing blood
  - Leakage of the administered fluid around the skin entry site
- Cardiac or pulmonary symptoms may not be present.
- Also, there may not be any clinical evidence of line infection or thrombus.

Complications

- The catheter fragments migrate distally along the bloodstream, finally lodging in the vena cava, right atrium, right ventricle, or main pulmonary artery or one of its branches.
- Possible complications include:
  - Myocardial perforation or necrosis culminating in tamponade
  - Myocardial infarction
  - Valvular perforation
  - Arrhythmia
  - Cardiac arrest

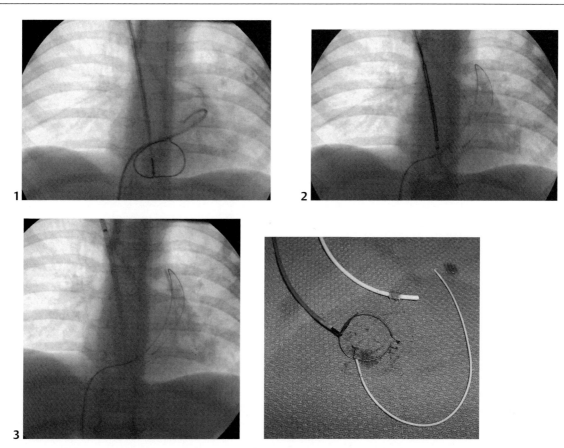

Figure 102B (**1**) Oblique fluoroscopic view of the heart with the snare open and the delivery catheter with the fractured fragment close by. (**2**) Fractured catheter is captured by the snare and is being pulled out via the jugular vein. (**3**) Catheter fragment is seen within the delivery catheter.

Figure 102C The proximal section and the fractured fragment of the PICC line as well as the snare are seen.

- The foreign body can act as a nidus for thrombus formation with resultant pulmonary embolism.
- Infectious complications include:
  - Arrhythmia endocarditis
  - Secondary infection of thrombus
  - Mycotic aneurysm
  - Pulmonary abscesses
- However, in one large-scale study conducted in our institution there were no long-term complications in any of the fractured PICCs over a 6-year period.

Technique

- Depending on the position of the fragment, access may be obtained from either the jugular or the femoral vein. In certain occasions there may be a need to access both simultaneously.
- A sheath is placed to allow a loop snare with a guiding catheter to be placed.
- The catheter is directed to either end of the fragment, which is captured within the snare (**Fig. 102B**). This requires fluoroscopy from multiple angles, especially when the fractured fragment is located within the heart.
- The fragment is retrieved and extracted under fluoroscopic guidance so that it does not fracture on removal. The extracted fragment is examined to confirm that the entire fragment has been removed (**Fig. 102C**).

Treatment

- Prompt investigation should be done due to potentially life-threatening complications.
- A chest x-ray with a view of the insertion site in the arm should be ordered initially.
- Before attempting percutaneous removal, venography may be considered to exclude thrombus.
- Percutaneous retrieval may be performed using loop snares, hooked guide wires, Fogarty balloon catheters, and Dormia baskets.
- Percutaneous extraction may be performed at a relatively low risk.
- If extraction fails, surgical retrieval may be necessary.
- Caregivers should be warned against flushing with a small volume syringe (1 or 3 mL) and instead should use a 5 or 10 mL syringe.

Prognosis

- Additional long-term studies are required; however, long-term outcomes are good in studies reported thus far.
- A replacement PICC or central line may be placed immediately following removal if venous access is still required.

PEARLS_____

- A history of blockage, difficulty flushing or withdrawing from the line with repeated attempts at clearing the line, or of a leakage at the site of insertion should increase suspicion.
- Only use 5 or 10 mL syringes when flushing a PICC line. Small-volume catheters increase the risk of fracture.
- Prompt diagnosis is key.

PITFALL_____

- The absence of cardiac or pulmonary signs does not exclude a PICC fracture.

Suggested Readings

Chow LM, Friedman JN, Macarthur C, et al. Peripherally inserted central catheter (PICC) fracture and embolization in the pediatric population. J Pediatr 2003;142:141–144

Crowley JJ. Vascular access. Tech Vasc Interv Radiol 2003;6:176–181

Pettit J. Assessment of infants with peripherally inserted central catheters, I: Detecting the most frequently occurring complications. Adv Neonatal Care 2002;2:304–315

Smith JR, Friedell ML, Cheatham ML, et al. Peripherally inserted central catheters revisited. Am J Surg 1998;176:208–211

Thanigaraj S, Panneerselvam A, Yanos J. Retrieval of an IV catheter fragment from the pulmonary artery 11 years after embolization. Chest 2000;117:1209–1211

Thiagarajan RR, Ramamoorthy C, Gettmann T, Bratton SL. Survey of the use of peripherally inserted central venous catheters in children. Pediatrics 1997;99:E4

CASE 103

Clinical Presentation

A 12-year-old female presents to the emergency department with persistent abdominal pain, fever, and tachycardia. She had several episodes of vomiting, diarrhea, and dysuria. Seven days earlier she had experienced abdominal pain followed by sudden improvement and then gradual worsening prior to admission. On examination she had a firm abdomen with involuntary rebound and absent bowel sounds.

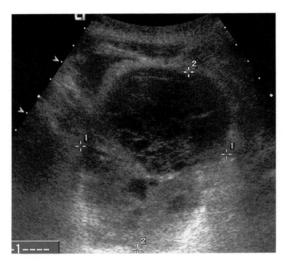

Figure 103A

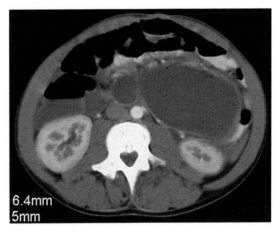

Figure 103B

Radiologic Findings

Radiographs of the abdomen demonstrated no appendicolith, free air, or obvious masses. An ultrasound was performed that demonstrated some complex fluid collections deep in the abdomen (**Fig. 103A**). The appendix was not visualized. CT of the abdomen, at the level of the abscess, demonstrates interposed bowel with fluid collections deep in the abdomen, making a standard percutaneous approach difficult (**Fig. 103B**).

Diagnosis

Deep intra-abdominal abscess (most likely secondary to a ruptured appendix)

Differential Diagnosis

- Sterile abscess (white blood cells but no bacteria)
- Urinomas (have elevated creatinine)
- Lymphoceles (contains lymphocytes and fat globules)
- Pseudocysts (characterized by amylase)
- Bile collections (contain bilirubin)
- Seromas (typically a clear yellowish fluid)
- Fluid-filled loops of bowel
- Aneurysm

Discussion

Background

Intra-abdominal abscess is an important and serious problem in pediatric patients. The variety of possible clinical presentations makes the diagnosis and localization of an abscess difficult. This may result in delayed treatment, increased morbidity, and even mortality; therefore, a high index of suspicion must be maintained.

Over the past 2 decades percutaneous abscess drainage (PAD) has emerged as the treatment of choice. Even in cases where surgery is indicated, PAD may still be used preoperatively for its temporizing effect.

Clinical Findings

Intra-abdominal abscesses can have highly variable presentations depending on the location of the abscess. Symptoms may include persistent dull abdominal pain, focal tenderness, fever, weight loss, impaired function of nearby structures (e.g., ileus), leukocytosis, or leucopenia (in immunocompromised patients).

A deep abdominal abscess represents a diagnostic challenge. Many of the classic features may be absent. There may only be persistent fever with mild liver and gastrointestinal dysfunction.

The symptoms of a postoperative abdominal abscess may be masked by analgesics and incisional pain. In addition, the administration of prophylactic antibiotics may decrease signs of tenderness and leukocytosis.

Pelvic abscesses may present with urinary frequency, diarrhea, or tenesmus, whereas subphrenic abscesses may present with pulmonary manifestations such as pneumonia, pleural effusion, or atelectasis. Irritation of the diaphragm may also produce shoulder pain.

Late findings are multiple organ failures, primarily the lungs, kidneys, or liver. Gastrointestinal bleeding with disseminated intravascular coagulopathy may also occur if the abscess is not treated.

The most common sites for abscesses are in the lower abdominal quadrants followed by pelvic, subhepatic, and subdiaphragmatic spaces. As well, intra-abdominal abscesses appear to present three times more often on the right side (upper and lower) compared with the left.

Pathology and Laboratory

- Microbiology includes a mixture of aerobic and anaerobic organisms.
- The most commonly encountered aerobic organism is *Escherichia coli.*

- The most commonly encountered anaerobic organism is *Bacteroides fragilis.*
- Abscess fluid from patients on prolonged antibiotic therapy may yield yeast colonies (e.g., *Candida*).
- Skin flora may be responsible for abscesses following a penetrating abdominal injury.
- *Neisseria gonorrhoeae* and *Chlamydia* are commonly present in pelvic abscesses in females as part of pelvic inflammatory disease.
- Hematologic signs of infection (e.g., leukocytosis, anemia, abnormal liver function) are frequently present.
- Blood cultures indicating persistent polymicrobial bacteremias strongly suggest the presence of an intra-abdominal abscess.

Imaging Findings

- Initial investigations should be with ultrasonography and/or CT.

ULTRASOUND

- On ultrasound, a sonolucent area with well-defined walls containing fluid/debris of variable density is typically seen. Ultrasonography is better at characterizing the collection than CT.
- Ultrasonography is very useful when locating an abscess in the right upper quadrant, the paracolic, and pelvic areas.
- Ultrasonography may miss small collections and interloop abscesses and can be difficult in patients with an ileus.
- Ultrasonography is the most commonly used primary modality for abscess drainage.

CT

- CT is highly sensitive and specific for identifying abscesses. It is considered the best imaging and diagnostic modality.
- On CT, abscesses will appear as hypodense collections with density measurements between 0 and 15 Hounsfield units.
- The abscess wall enhances with intravenous contrast media administration and may be distinguished from an adjacent loop of bowel by the administration of oral or rectal contrast.
- CT is used for guidance of pancreatic, interloop, complex abscesses, and abscesses not adequately visualized with ultrasonography.
- CT is valuable for characterizing abscesses, as well as identifying multiple collections.
- CT can image the entire abdomen despite the presence of distended bowel, which can decrease the sensitivity of an ultrasonography examination.

MRI

- MRI currently has no clinical role in PAD.

Treatment

- Broad-spectrum antibiotic therapy covering both aerobic and anaerobic bacteria should be initiated prior to drainage and maintained until all systemic signs of sepsis resolve.
- Antibiotic therapy should be altered according to the results of cultures from the abscess.
- In immunocompromised patients, antifungal medications may be indicated for treatment of candidal infections.
- If the abscess is located in the upper abdominal area, then caution should be taken in avoiding the pleura during drainage. In general, an access site anteriorly should be below the 8th rib and posteriorly below the 12th rib.
- Real-time ultrasonography followed by fluoroscopy is used for needle guidance in most patients.
- The size and type of puncture needle are determined by the size, location, and anticipated fluid viscosity of the abscess. For large collections a single-wall, 19-gauge needle can be advanced into the lesion.

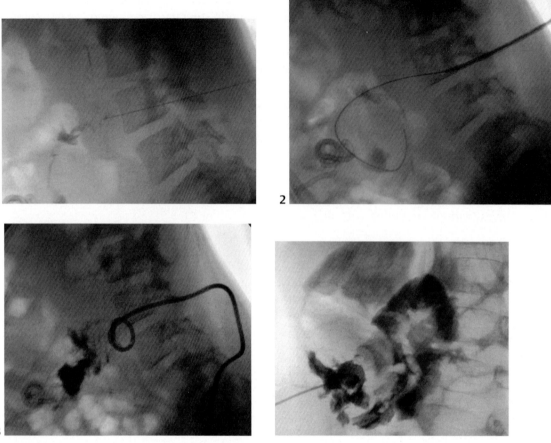

Figure 103C (**1**) Patient in the decubitus position with needle access from a posterior approach under ultrasonographic and fluoroscopic guidance. (**2**) Wire and dilator seen on fluoroscopy. (**3**) Catheter placed in the abscess with some contrast seen within the collection.

Figure 103D Tubogram demonstrating communication with bowel.

- A fine needle (22 gauge) is used to define a safe access route for the catheter. It is also used to aspirate a small amount of fluid, which is sent for laboratory evaluation (**Fig. 103C1**).
- If pure pus is aspirated, a catheter may be placed immediately. If there is doubt, a Gram's stain is performed.
- To place the catheter, a guide wire is passed through the needle into the collection. This is followed by dilating the tract using a dilator(s) (**Fig. 103C2**) and eventual placement of a drainage catheter into the abscess.
- A no. 8, 10, or 12 French locking pigtail catheter with side holes is commonly used for simple, nonviscous fluid drainage. For larger or more viscous fluid collections, a tissue plasminogen activator (alteplase) may be introduced into the collection to break down fibrin and locules.
- After the placement of the drainage catheter into the lesion, the catheter is secured into position. Correct positioning is confirmed with contrast media and fluoroscopy (**Fig. 103C3**).
- A tubogram with diluted contrast should be performed if a fistula to bowel or other structure is suspected (**Fig. 103D**). It can also be used to outline the walls of the cavity. The final step is securing the catheter externally either by suturing or taping it to the skin.

Complications

- Percutaneous drainage has a relatively low complication rate (usually <5%).
- Fever shortly after the procedure may be due to bacteremia as a result of manipulation or lavage of an abscess cavity.

- Hemorrhage from various etiologies such as laceration of a vessel or unsuspected coagulopathy may occur.
- Disruption of the pleura from upper abdominal abscess drainage may result in pneumothorax, hemothorax, or empyema.
- Other complications are peritonitis, septic shock, and bowel perforation, all of which have a very low incidence.

Prognosis

- Abscess complexity influences drainage success rate and can be divided into three groups based on complexity:
  - A simple unilocular and discrete abscess is cured in >90% of cases.
  - A moderate complexity abscess with associated gastrointestinal communications is cured in ~80 to 90% and may require a surgical correction.
  - The most complex collections, such as intermixed pancreatic abscess/necrosis or an infected tumor, may have a cure rate of 30 to 80%.
- Bad prognosticators include collections, which are associated with malignancy, phlegmon, and necrotic tissue.

PEARLS_____

- Image-guided abscess drainage is the first line of treatment even in postoperative patients.
- A combination of ultrasonography and CT is often needed for visualizing and characterizing the collection. CT demonstrates the extent of the disease, other collections, and associated pathology.
- If multiple collections are present, drainage with as many catheters as is needed, and aspiration of smaller collections should be performed during the initial procedure.

PITFALLS_____

- Postoperative abscess may be masked by analgesics and antibiotics; therefore, maintain a high index of suspicion.
- Pulmonary symptoms may be secondary to an abdominal cause. Consider subphrenic abscess in the differential diagnosis.
- Deep pelvic abscesses may be very difficult to drain percutaneously. Consider other guided approaches such as transrectal drainage.

Suggested Readings

Jamieson DH, Chait PG, Filler R. Interventional drainage of appendiceal abscesses in children. AJR Am J Roentgenol 1997;169:1619–1622

Lorber B, Swenson RM. The bacteriology of intra-abdominal infections. Surg Clin North Am 1975;55:1349–1354

Specht NT, Russo RD, eds. Practical Guide to Diagnostic Imaging. New York: Mosby-Year Book; 1998:89–177,568–612

van Sonnenberg E, Wittich GR, Goodacre BW, Casola G, D'Agostino HB. Percutaneous abscess drainage: update. World J Surg 2001;25:362–372

van Sonnenberg E, Wittich GR, Casola G, et al. Periappendiceal abscesses: percutaneous drainage. Radiology 1987;163:23–26

CASE 104

Clinical Presentation

A 5-year-old male presents with a history of tracheoesophageal fistula, having had several surgical attempts at repair, which were unsuccessful. The final surgery was a gastric pull-up that resulted in a stricture at the anastomosis. Endoscopic attempts at repairing or dilating the stricture were unsuccessful and resulted in a fistula to the skin surface. Image-guided dilatations were performed, with recurrence of the stricture soon after. A decision was made to place a stent.

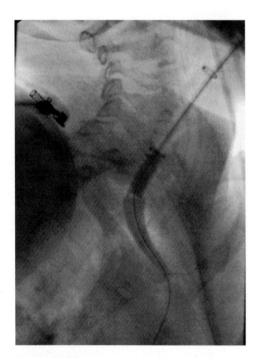

Figure 104A

Radiologic Findings

Contrast esophageal study demonstrates a complete stricture with a small sinus to outer skin in the area of the upper chest and shows the catheter and dilator with wire at the site of the stricture (**Fig. 104A**).

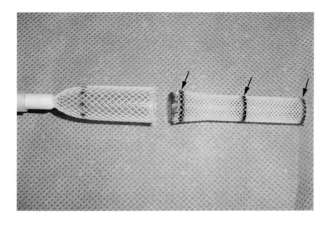

Figure 104B Rusch polyflex silicone-coated stent.

Diagnosis

Recurrent stricture at the site of anastomosis

Discussion

Background

Tracheoesophageal strictures in the pediatric population can occur through a variety of causes and may result in major airway collapse. Stents are used to establish and maintain luminal continuity and have become an extremely valuable technique in the management of these patients. A variety of stent designs are available for both the trachea and esophagus, each with distinct advantages and drawbacks. Generally, there are two subtypes of stent design: metallic and silicone (**Fig. 104B**). The arrows show radiopaque markers. In the pediatric population, metallic stents are used more often than silicone. Improvements in silicone stent technology including a decrease in wall thickness will likely increase their use in the pediatric population. A major advantage of silicone stents, as compared with metallic stents, is their ease of removal. Rare erosions, fistulizations, and even death during attempted removal have been reported with metallic stents. Most silicone stents are designed as a solid cylinder, as opposed to the perforated or honeycombed design of the metallic stents. Metallic stents are more appropriate for placement over airway branch orifices that would otherwise be blocked by the solid silicone stent. As stent technology continues to improve, it will likely become the primary treatment option for many pediatric conditions that affect the lumen of the tracheobronchial tree and esophagus.

Etiology

Several conditions may result in a decrease in tracheal or esophageal luminal area. In such patients, stenting may be required to maintain patency.

The most common cause of tracheal collapse in the pediatric age group is primary or secondary tracheobronchial malacia. Stricture of the trachea or the esophagus may often result from attempted reconstruction of a congenital malformation, whereas caustic ingestion still accounts for many severe esophageal strictures. Stents are also increasingly used as a palliative treatment for malignant obstruction. Other consideration includes posttraumatic (e.g., intubation), post-anastomosis (e.g., lung transplant), or post-inflammatory strictures.

Clinical Findings

Decreases in luminal cross-sectional area may result in significant dyspnea or dysphagia.

Complications

- Potential complications of stent placement include stent malposition, displacement, or fracture causing respiratory distress, mucous impaction, and granulation tissue formation.
- A tracheal stent may result in erosion leading to hemoptysis, including a reported case of erosion into the pulmonary artery causing death.
- Complication rates vary slightly between the various stent designs.

Indications

- Tracheal stenting is indicated for symptomatic relief of life-threatening dyspnea. Stenting is usually used as a last resort for severe conditions that may result in prolonged periods of apnea such as tracheal collapse.
- Esophageal stenting is indicated for relief of dysphagia, including that caused by malignant esophageal obstruction.
- Recurrent tracheoesophageal fistula

Relative Contraindications

- Infection
- Inflammation
- Vascular malformations in the trachea or the esophagus
- Patients who are medically unstable and unable to undergo general anesthesia
- Allergy to the stent material

It should be emphasized, however, that tracheal stents are usually used as a last resort to prevent asphyxiation when other measures have failed. Therefore, a decision may be made to place a stent despite the patient having one or more of these contraindications.

- Contraindications for esophageal stenting include:
  - Patients with a very high stricture (<2 cm from the upper esophageal sphincter).
  - Patients with mild noncircumferetial strictures in whom anchoring the stent may be a problem.
  - Patients who are still candidates for chemotherapy or radiation in which tumor shrinkage may lead to stent migration.

Imaging Findings

- The primary imaging for evaluating the trachea is direct bronchoscopy.
- Fluoroscopy can be used to help define tracheal narrowing; however, bronchoscopy is preferred.
- Contrast studies or endoscopy can be used to evaluate the esophagus.
- Occasionally, an imaging study such as MRI, CT scan, or plain x-ray film helps in defining the length of stenosis, wall thickening, or extrinsic disease.

Technique

- Esophageal stenting:
  - The patient is placed in the supine position.
  - The procedure may be performed under conscious sedation or general anesthesia.
  - The stent may be placed under fluoroscopic guidance only or in combination with endoscopy.

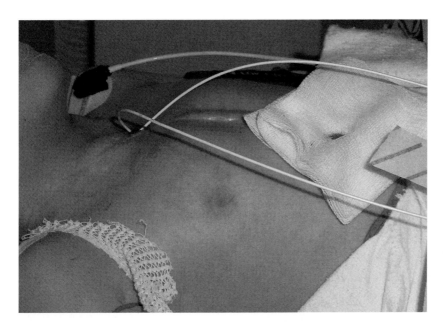

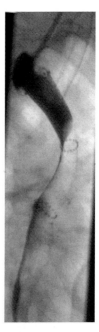

Figure 104C Access to the stricture via the cutaneous sinus tract.

Figure 104D Contrast study shows patent esophageal lumen.

- ○ Dilatation of the stricture prior to stent placement is usually not required, unless dilatation inhibits the access of the delivery system. Dilatation may increase the risk of stent migration or perforation.
- ○ When there is a fistula to the skin, access may be acquired via this route (**Fig. 104C**).
- ○ In patients with proximal esophageal malignancy, a chest CT is mandatory to estimate the risk for tracheal compression.
- ○ For stent insertion, a guide wire is placed through the stricture, and the delivery system is introduced over the wire.
- ○ Radiopaque markers on the stent allow for accurate positioning (**Fig. 104B**, arrows).
- ○ Care should be taken when removing the delivery system after deploying the stent to avoid accidental dislodgment.
- ○ Following placement, contrast study is performed to confirm stent position and patency (**Fig. 104D**).
- ○ If the stent is placed across the esophagogastric junction, the patient should be placed on proton pump inhibitors. Antiemetics should also be used to prevent vomiting, which may result in catheter migration.
- • Tracheal stenting:
  - ○ Usually performed with endoscopy and fluoroscopy.
  - ○ In children, it is mostly used for benign disease and as a last resort.
  - ○ Stainless-steel fenestrated balloon expandable stents are most commonly used.
  - ○ There is a significant risk of complications at time of removal due to the tendency of epithelial and granulation tissue to overgrow the stent.

PEARLS_____

- • If possible, stenting in the pediatric population should be temporary.
- • Stenting is one of a few treatment modalities. Cooperation with ear, nose, and throat and general surgery will improve patient care.

PITFALLS_____

- Stenting esophageal strictures may result in tracheal compression.
- In patients with proximal esophageal malignancy, a chest CT must be performed to evaluate the risk of tracheal compression as a result of esophageal stenting.

Suggested Readings

Filler RM, Forte V, Chait P. Tracheobronchial stenting for treatment of airway obstruction. J Pediatr Surg 1998;3:306–311

Forte V, Chait P, Sommer D. Endoscopic management of tracheal and esophageal strictures. Semin Pediatr Surg 2003;12:71–79

Mergener K, Kozarek RA. Stenting of the gastrointestinal tract. Dig Dis 2002;20:173–181

Nashef SAM, Dromer C, Velly FJ, et al. Expanding wire stents in benign tracheobronchial disease: indications and complications. Ann Thorac Surg 1992;54:937–940

Rafanan AL, Mehta AC. Stenting of the tracheobronchial tree. Radiol Clin North Am 2000;38:395–408

CASE 105

Clinical Presentation

A 4-year-old female presents with high fever, cough, increased respiratory rate, bronchial breathing, and decreased breath sounds on the right side. Her pediatrician had treated her with antibiotics. She continued to deteriorate, and after a chest radiograph was performed she was referred to a pediatric tertiary care center. After admission she was further imaged with CT and ultrasonography. What interventional procedure should be performed?

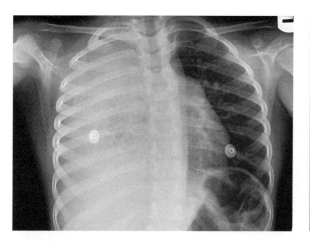

Figure 105A

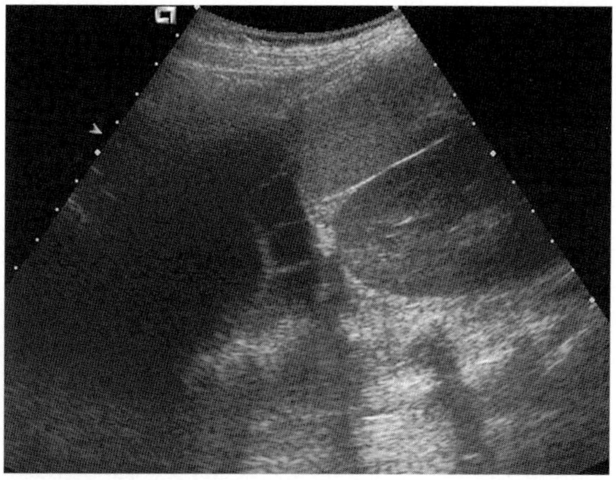

Figure 105B

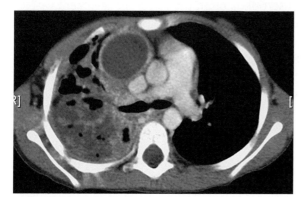

Figure 105C

Radiologic Findings

The chest radiograph demonstrates complete opacification of the right hemithorax (**Fig. 105A**). Ultrasound shows a complex collection (**Fig. 105B**), whereas CT provides evidence of empyema with underlying lung inflammation, abscess, and likely necrosis. In addition, there is a medial enhancing fluid collection that represents either a medial loculated empyema or a mediastinal abscess (**Fig. 105C**).

Diagnosis

Necrotizing or aggressive pneumonia with empyema, and possible mediastinal abscess requiring chest tube placement

Discussion

Background

Chest tubes (or thoracostomy tubes) are placed in the pleura space for the drainage of air and/or fluids in the thoracic region. Chest drainage techniques have been used since the early 1900s for the treatment of postpneumonic empyema. In recent years, the traditional technique has been replaced by an image-guided technique and adjunctive intracavitary fibrinolytic therapy. The image-guided technique has the potential of reducing many of the complications associated with a "blind" placement technique, including accidental damage to the internal thoracic arteries.

Etiology/Indications for Drainage

Chest drainage is used in situations where a loss of pleural negative pressure is noted. This may have the following causes:

- Persistent or recurrent pneumothorax: The first occurrence of a pneumothorax in a patient should initially be aspirated. Chest drainage should be initiated if aspiration is unsuccessful. With recurrent pneumothoraces, the associated adhesions will likely necessitate chest tube placement because aspiration is often unsuccessful in such situations.
- Tension pneumothorax: Decompression and chest tube placement are usually performed blindly due to the acuity and severity of the situation.
- Traumatic pneumothorax: This is an unpredictable situation, which may rapidly evolve into a tension pneumothorax. Therefore, a chest tube insertion is often the safest management.
- Pneumothorax in a patient in need of positive pressure ventilation
- Bilateral pneumothoraces
- Hemothorax: Lack of drainage may result in empyema or a fibrothorax.
- Empyema: An image-guided approach allows for a precise targeting of the collection and is especially vital in cases of a loculated empyema.
- Malignant pleural effusions
- Chylothorax

Clinical Findings

Clinical findings are usually related to the underlying pathology. Some common symptoms may include:

- Dyspnea, the most common clinical finding
- Chest pain, includes sharp pain that worsens with deep inspiration and may refer to upper abdomen or ipsilateral shoulder
- Tachypnea and hypoxia
- Diminished breath sounds on affected side
- Hypo- or hyperresonance to percussion

Complications

- The complication rates of indwelling chest tubes have been reported to range from 9 to 30%.
- Forceful use of a trocar to penetrate the pleura is the most common reason for complications.
- Other possible complications include:
  - Traumatic perforation of lung, heart chambers, inferior vena cava, pulmonary artery, diaphragm, and intra-abdominal organs (usually seen when a blind technique is used and unlikely if image guidance is used)
  - Trauma to the intercostal neurovascular bundle, which may lead to hemothorax or intercostal neuralgia
  - Re-expansion pulmonary edema
  - Infection, possibly resulting in empyema
  - Subcutaneous emphysema
  - Minor complications may include dislodgement, kinking, disconnection, and failure to drain.

Pathology and Laboratory Findings

- If pleural effusion is present, at least 20 mL of fluid should initially be aspirated and sent for laboratory analysis.
- The initial step in the analysis of the pleural fluid should be to determine whether the effusion is a transudate or an exudate. Tests include:
  - Pleural fluid protein, lactate dehydrogenase (LDH), and albumin levels in relation to serum levels
- Exudative effusions require further tests: cell count with differential; glucose, LDH, and amylase levels; total protein level; pH; cytologic analysis (especially recommended for patients with a history of exudative effusions, or suspected malignancy); Gram, acid-fast, and fungal staining, including culture and sensitivity; in addition, white and red blood cell counts should be performed.
- Additional studies can be ordered in the event that a specific condition is suspected. For example:
  - A yellow or whitish turbid fluid (possible chylothorax) should undergo lipoprotein analysis, which may show chylomicrons in the pleural fluid.
  - A blood-tinged fluid color should raise the suspicion of a hemothorax; however, color alone is not diagnostic.
  - To diagnose hemothorax, the pleural fluid hematocrit level should be at least 50% of the serum hematocrit level.
  - If rheumatoid arthritis or systemic lupus erythematosus is suspected, the fluid may be tested for rheumatoid factor and antinuclear antibody levels.

Evolution

Empyema progresses through three major stages:
- Acute phase: The fluid is sterile and nonviscous, and the collection is not loculated.
- Subacute phase: The collection in the chest cavity may be loculated, and the fluid is usually fibrinous or purulent.
- Chronic (organizing) phase: Adhesions form between the visceral and parietal pleura (pleural peel).

Imaging Findings

- Chest tubes are usually placed under ultrasonographic and fluoroscopic guidance.
- To ensure accurate placement, CT guidance may be required if the collections are loculated, small, or located deep in the chest.

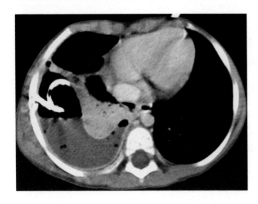

Figure 105D CT with right chest tube and complex fluid.

Treatment

Technique

- Coagulation factors including international normalized ratio, partial thromboplastin time, and platelets should be investigated and corrected if abnormal.
- Prior to the procedure, patients are prepared using sterile techniques and provided with appropriate sedation as well as local anesthesia.
- In the pediatric population, a 16-gauge angiocatheter is advanced into the pleural fluid under ultrasonographic guidance.
- Fluid is aspirated and sent for laboratory analysis.
- The puncture site is imaged, and the locations of the internal thoracic and other vessels in the area are noted and avoided.
- The needle is removed, and through the plastic cannula a guide wire is inserted into the pleural space.
- The tract is dilated to the appropriate size and followed by placement of a no. 8 to no. 12 French pigtail locking catheter (**Fig. 105D**).
- Selection of appropriate catheter size is based on the viscosity of the fluid drained:
  - Larger catheter sizes may be needed to ensure effective drainage of pus and debris commonly associated with empyema.
  - However, recent evidence suggests that smaller-size catheters may be equally effective and may be associated with fewer complications.
- Children with complicated parapneumonic effusions (effusion with multiple loculations and/or pleural glucose <2.2 mmol/L) can be treated with tissue plasminogen activator (tPA), which is introduced through the catheter into the fluid collection (4 mg of tPA in 30 to 50 mL of normal saline). Evidence for the effectiveness of tPA treatment is still somewhat inconclusive, although the data suggest that it holds the potential to reduce the duration of drainage.
- A three-way stopcock is attached to the catheter to seal it and to allow easy aspiration and flushing or administration of thrombolytic therapy.
- The catheter and stopcock are connected to an underwater drainage unit set at 20 cm of water, and then they are unclamped.
- The catheter is fixed to the chest with clear Tegaderm dressing (3M Healthcare Corporation, St Paul, MN), a sterile transparent dressing, and the three-way stopcock is held with a Mefix (a tape apertured, nonwoven, synthetic adhesive) and gauze against the patient's flank so that it is easily accessible and does not cause patient discomfort.
- All connections are taped and checked to avoid accidental disconnection.
- The drainage unit should always be kept below the level of the drainage site.
- A drainage unit without additional suction is usually sufficient; however, low-pressure suction may expedite drainage and lung re-expansion.

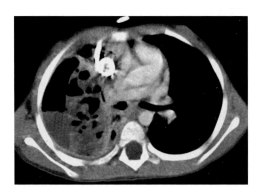

Figure 105E CT with medial collection drained.

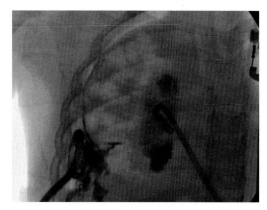

Figure 105F Contrast study through catheters showing absence of communication to the bronchial tree.

- When draining a large pleural effusion, a rare complication of re-expansion pulmonary edema may occur. To prevent this, if 500 mL of fluid is drained in a short amount of time (1 hour), the tube should be temporarily clamped for 1 to 2 hours before further drainage is resumed.
- Nondraining medial collections should be drained separately (**Fig. 105E**).
- Contrast study through the catheters can be performed to exclude bronchopleural fistulae (**Fig. 105F**).
- Drain removal:
  - Prior to drain removal the patient must be symptomatically improved, and:
    - For pneumothorax: Imaging should indicate that the lungs are fully expanded and the air leak has been stopped for at least 24 hours.
    - For pleural effusion: Imaging should indicate that the effusion has resolved and the tube has stopped draining for at least 24 hours.
  - The tube is then clamped for a further 24 hours, and imaging is repeated. If the effusion or pneumothorax does not recur, the tube can be removed.
  - To prevent air from entering the chest cavity during removal of the catheter, the patient should be instructed to take a full inspiration and perform Valsalva's maneuver.
  - A chest radiograph should be obtained following removal.

Contraindications

- Infection at planned entry site
- Uncorrectable bleeding diathesis

Prognosis

- The complication rates of indwelling chest tubes have been reported to range from 9 to 30%.
- Although direct comparative studies are unavailable, it is likely that image-guided techniques have a lower complication rate due to the ability to avoid local vessels, improved ability to optimally place the catheter with respect to the target collection, and the insertion of a smaller diameter catheter.
- Intrapleural tPA in children with complicated parapneumotic effusions may be associated with improved drainage and shorter drainage time. Further studies are required to fully elucidate the role of tPA in the treatment of pleural collections.
- Proper positioning of the catheter is vital to a successful treatment. tPA should not be used in attempts to correct for a malpositioned catheter.

- Early treatment is essential. An effusion older than 6 weeks is more likely to be associated with a pleural peel. In such cases drainage is usually unsuccessful and surgery may be required.

PEARLS

- Start treatment early.
- tPA treatment is less effective when started in the later stages of an empyema.
- Imaging studies performed immediately after full drainage are often abnormal, but this does not mean that drainage has failed.
- The residual pulmonary abnormalities will usually gradually resolve within 2 to 4 months.

PITFALLS

- Re-expansion pulmonary edema is a rare and serious complication that is associated with rapid drainage of a large collection and can be avoided with controlled drainage.
- Initial puncture and catheter placement should be performed adjacent to the upper border of the rib to avoid damage to the intercostal neurovascular bundle.

Suggested Readings

Tang ATM, Velissaris TJ, Weeden DF. An evidence-based approach to drainage of the pleural cavity: evaluation of best practice. J Eval Clin Pract 2002;8:333–340

Tattersall DJ, Traill ZC, Gleeson FV. Chest drains: does size matter? Clin Radiol 2000;55:415–421

Valji K, ed. Vascular and Interventional Radiology. Philadelphia: WB Saunders; 1999

Weinstein M, Restrepo R, Chait PG, Connolly B, Temple M, Macarthur C. Effectiveness and safety of tissue plasminogen activator in the management of complicated parapneumonic effusions. Pediatrics 2004;113:e182–e185

CASE 106

Clinical Presentation

A 15-year-old male returns to the hospital 7 days following surgery for appendicitis with lower abdominal pain, diarrhea, dysuria, and fever. On examination, he has a tender lower abdomen with faint bowel sounds. On rectal examination, a mass is felt anterior to the rectum. Ultrasonographic examination reveals a collection deep in the pelvis. The patient is referred to a tertiary care center for further management. How should the collection be drained?

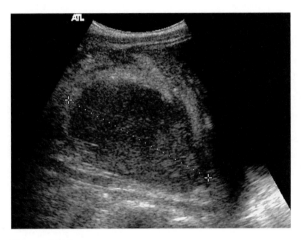

Figure 106A

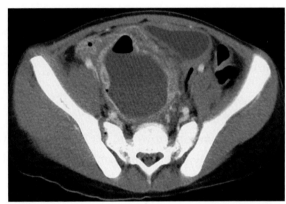

Figure 106B

Radiologic Findings

Ultrasonography demonstrated a hypoechoic collection posterior to the bladder and anterior to the rectum with some debris within it (**Fig. 106A**). CT confirmed a deep pelvic abscess with an enhancing rim and small anterior air/fluid level. No other collections were identified (**Fig. 106B**).

Diagnosis

Postsurgical deep pelvic abscess requiring transrectal abcess drainage

Discussion

Background

Pelvic abscesses are often located deep within the pelvis and are surrounded by overlying bowel, urinary bladder, pelvic vessels, and bones, thus preventing a safe percutaneous transabdominal approach. The main advantage of a transrectal approach is that it provides a shorter and more direct path to the collection. The risk of injuring or contaminating adjacent structures is therefore reduced.

Etiology

The most common causes of a pelvic abscess include appendicitis and following surgery, often postappendectomy (the appendix may or may not have ruptured). Other less common causes may include underlying inflammatory bowel disease, pelvic inflammatory disease, or perforation as a consequence of neoplasm.

Clinical Findings

The typical postoperative abscess occurs in a patient who had an appendectomy 7 to 10 days prior and now has abdominal pain and fever. This scenario is the most common cause of pelvic abscess in the pediatric population.

Indications

- A deep pelvic collection that does not have a safe percutaneous transabdominal access route as assessed by pre-procedural imaging
- This can be due to a collection that is obscured by overlying bowel, pelvic vessels, and organs.
- This technique can also be used to drain multiple collections.

Contraindications

- Clinical triage is important.
- Patients with diffuse peritonitis should undergo surgery.

Technique

- All patients undergo CT and ultrasonography examination prior to the procedure to assess the location, size, and nature of all collections.
- Prophylactic triple antibiotic coverage is given prior to the procedure (typically gentamycin, ampicillin, and metronidazole).
- Patients are usually sedated; if sedation fails, the procedure may be done under general anesthesia.
- The patient is placed in a lateral decubitus position lying on the left side. A pillow may be placed between the patient's knees.
- The left index finger can be used to guide the trocar needle toward the anterior rectal wall. If the collection is out of reach, a plastic enema tip is inserted rectally and is guided using transabdominal ultrasonography until indentation of the abscess is visualized (**Fig. 106C**).

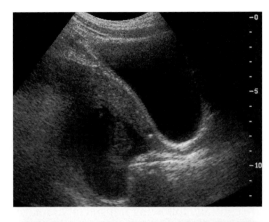

Figure 106C Transabdominal sonogram with index finger in rectum seen against the abscess.

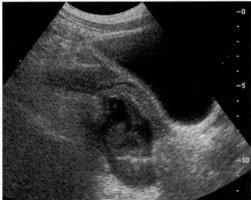

Figure 106D Needle seen in collection with the finger in the rectum.

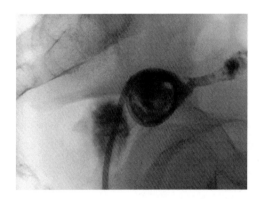

Figure 106E Drainage catheters with contrast injected into the drained collection with no fistula.

- An 18-gauge trocar needle is advanced through the lumen of the enema tip or along the index finger and is used to puncture the abscess (**Fig. 106D**).
- The needle is advanced under ultrasonographic guidance. The stylet is removed, and a specimen of the collection is obtained and sent for culture and sensitivity.
- If pus is obtained, contrast is then injected to outline the abscess.
- An Amplatz stiff wire is introduced under fluoroscopic guidance followed by a Coons dilator and usually a no. 10 French all-purpose drain (**Fig. 106E**).
- The drain is connected to a three-way stopcock and a closed drainage system.
- A 50 mL Luer-lock is used to aspirate the collection until it is dry. The contents of the syringe are injected directly back to the drainage bag.
- The catheter is taped to the patient's inner thigh, and the patient is sent to recovery and later back to the ward.
- Postprocedure analgesics are ordered, and the catheter is flushed twice daily with 5 cc of normal saline.
- The drainage catheter can be removed when:
  ○ Patient's symptoms resolve.
  ○ There is no significant drainage from the catheter over a 24-hour period.
  ○ Ultrasonographic imaging shows resolution of the collection.
- The catheter is removed on the ward without sedation by the interventional radiologist.

Complications

- Catheter malplacement
- Incomplete drainage due to loculations

- Peritoneal spread of infection due to wire, dilator, or catheter perforation through the collection resulting in peritonitis
- Bleeding
- Injury to bladder and ureter
- Colonic or bowel fistula
- Accidental tube removal
- Early catheter expulsion

Prognosis

- Drainage is successful in the vast majority of patients.
- Surgery may be indicated if the patient does not improve clinically following transrectal drainage.
- The catheter remains in place for ~4 to 7 days.
- If the collections recur or if additional collections develop, there may be a need for additional drainage procedures.

PEARLS

- For deep pelvic abscesses, the transrectal route is preferable over the transabdominal route because the location of the tube is in the deepest part of the collection, and this allows good drainage.
- If many collections are present, multiple drains can be placed.

PITFALLS

- There is a potential for a fistula track to develop from the collection to the rectum.
- A poorly echoic or hypodense mass may simulate a fluid collection, and this would require a biopsy and not a drain.
- Thorough imaging and careful planning of needle trajectory are required when choosing a drainage approach.

Suggested Readings

Alexander AA, Eschelman DJ, Nazarian LN, Bonn J. Transrectal sonographically guided drainage of deep pelvic abscesses. AJR Am J Roentgenol 1994;162:1227–1230

Chung T, Hoffer FA, Lund DP. Transrectal drainage of deep pelvic abscesses in children using a combined transrectal sonographic and fluoroscopic guidance. Pediatr Radiol 1996;26:874–887

Jamieson DH, Chait PG, Filler R. Interventional drainage of appendiceal abscesses in children. AJR Am J Roentgenol 1997;169:1619–1622

Lorén I, Lasson A, Lundagards J, Nilsson A, Nilsson PE. Transrectal catheter drainage of deep abdominal and pelvic abscesses using combined ultrasonography and fluoroscopy. Eur J Surg 2001;167:535–539

Pereira JK, Chait PG, Miller SF. Deep pelvic abscesses in children: transrectal drainage under radiologic guidance. Radiology 1996;198:393–396

CASE 107

Clinical Presentation

A newborn presents with respiratory distress and fluid return from the nose and mouth following the first few attempts at swallowing. The abdomen is noted to appear small. Attempts at placing a nasogastric tube failed, and the patient is sent for chest and abdominal radiographs. What should be done for this neonate?

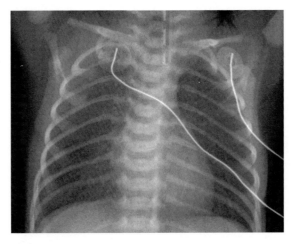

Figure 107A

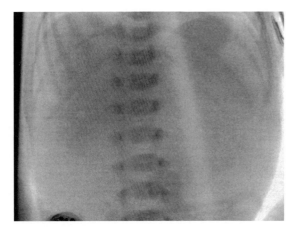

Figure 107B

Radiologic Findings

Chest radiograph shows the nasogastric tube coiled in the upper esophagus (**Fig. 107A**). Abdominal radiograph demonstrates a gasless abdomen (**Fig. 107B**).

Diagnosis

Esophageal atresia without evidence of a tracheoesophageal fistula (TEF), requiring definitive repair or gastrostomy tube prior to definitive repair

Differential Diagnosis

- Upper small bowel atresia
- Esophageal stenosis

Discussion

Background

Neonates with esophageal atresia may require a gastrostomy tube prior to definitive repair. Traditionally, the tube has been inserted via an open surgical approach. Recently, less invasive techniques for gastrostomy tube insertion, including the percutaneous image-guided gastrostomy, has been used in the pediatric population. The main advantage of this technique is the avoidance of a laparotomy.

In patients with esophageal atresia without TEF, percutaneous gastrostomy tube insertion is problematic. The stomach is small and gasless, and it cannot be inflated as is usually done with a nasogastric tube. Access to the abdomen under radiologic guidance is therefore risky. A novel transhepatic approach is used to instill air into the stomach, which can then permit percutaneous gastrostomy tube insertion under fluoroscopic guidance.

Indications

- Placing a gastrostomy tube is indicated for enteral nutrition to allow the child to receive appropriate nutrition; therefore, making a primary esophageal repair more successful.

Imaging Findings

- Ultrasonographic and fluoroscopic guidance are used in this procedure.

Technique

- Children with esophageal atresia and TEF, in whom the stomach is full of air, undergo gastrostomy insertion using the standard Seldinger technique under fluoroscopic guidance but without a nasogastric tube (because the patient has esophageal atresia).
- In patients with pure esophageal atresia, a transhepatic approach is used.
- A preliminary contrast enema is done to identify the location of the colon (**Fig. 107C**), and ultrasonography is used to demarcate the positions of the liver and spleen.
- The procedure is done under general anesthesia or under sedation with local anesthesia.
- The location of the stomach is found using ultrasonographic guidance by starting at the gastroesophageal junction and following it caudally.
- Because the stomach characteristically is small and nondistended in this group of patients, it initially is accessed transhepatically by inserting a 25-gauge spinal needle using ultrasonographic guidance (**Fig. 107D**).
- Once the needle is in place, its location in the stomach is confirmed by injecting water-soluble, non-ionic contrast through the needle (**Fig. 107E**).
- This is followed by the injection of air to distend the stomach.

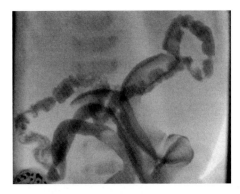

Figure 107C Contrast enema outlining a microcolon.

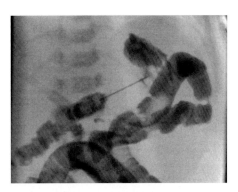

Figure 107D Twenty-seven-gauge needle accessing the small stomach with contrast and some air injected.

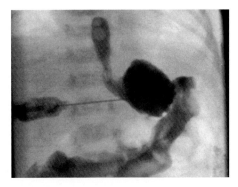

Figure 107E Further contrast injection with reflux up the distal esophagus.

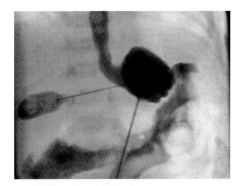

Figure 107F Second needle in the stomach prior to gastrostomy tube insertion.

- If the stomach is distended sufficiently so that it extended below the liver, a needle is inserted into the stomach under fluoroscopic guidance.
- If the stomach is not sufficiently distended, ultrasonographic and fluoroscopic guidance are used to advance the needle from below the liver, being careful not to perforate bowel.
- An 18-gauge single-wall puncture needle loaded with a retention suture (the pediatric cope gastrointestinal suture anchor) is used for this procedure.
- Once the needle is in place, its location within the stomach is confirmed by injecting contrast through the needle (**Fig. 107F**).
- A 0.035-inch wire is inserted, and the retention suture is deployed into the stomach.
- The needle is subsequently withdrawn, leaving the wire in place.
- The tract is then dilated, the catheter is inserted, and its location is confirmed.
- The anchor suture is cut 14 days after the procedure, and the small metal fragment is left to pass through the bowel.

Complications

- Postoperative complications are rare and often minor, not requiring surgical intervention
- Possible complications may include:
  - Minor leaks at the site of the insertion
  - Infection
  - Tube displacement or dislodgement
  - Tube blockage or mechanical complications
  - Stomal prolapse
  - Persistent gastrocutaneous fistula after removal of the tube

Prognosis

- Few studies are available regarding the use of gastrostomy tubes in patients with esophageal atresia.
- The technical success rate for this procedure appears to be high with few minor complications usually not requiring surgical intervention.
- The tubes remain in situ until surgical repair of the esophagus is possible.

PEARLS_____

- Percutaneous gastrostomy placement is possible in neonates with pure esophageal atresia.
- Esophageal atresia is commonly associated with a TEF.

PITFALLS_____

- Be aware of any associated duodenal or small bowel atresias.
- The procedure requires significant experience in ultrasonographic and fluoroscopic guidance.
- The procedure should only be performed by someone with extensive experience with ultrasonographic guidance and percutaneous gastrostomy placement.

Suggested Readings

Aziz D, Chait P, Kreichman F, Langer JC. Image-guided percutaneous gastrostomy in neonates with esophageal atresia. J Pediatr Surg 2004;39:1648–1650

Cahill AM, Kaye RD, Fitz CR, Towbin RB. "Push-pull" gastrostomy: a new technique for percutaneous gastrostomy tube insertion in the neonate and young infant. Pediatr Radiol 2001;31:550–554

Chait PG, Weinberg J, Connolly BL, et al. Retrograde percutaneous gastrostomy and gastrojejunostomy in 505 children: a 4½-year experience. Radiology 1996;201:691–695

Giuliano AW, Yoon HC, Lomis NN, Miller FJ. Fluoroscopically guided percutaneous placement of large-bore gastrostomy and gastrojejunostomy tubes: review of 109 cases. J Vasc Interv Radiol 2000;11:239–246

Moore KL, Persaud TVN. The Developing Human: Clinically Oriented Embryology. 6th ed. Philadelphia: WB Saunders; 1998

Wilson L, Oliva-Hemker M. Percutaneous endoscopic gastrostomy in small medically complex infants. Endoscopy 2001;33:433–436

CASE 108

Clinical Presentation

Prenatal ultrasonography demonstrated hydronephrosis and oligohydramnios. Immediate postnatal ultrasonography confirms the hydronephrosis and shows posterior urethral valves and a thickened bladder wall.

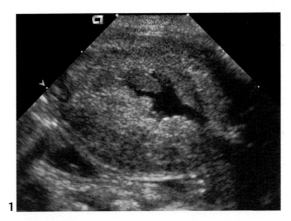 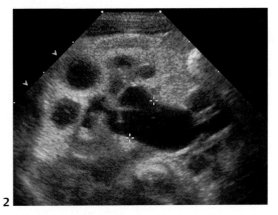

Figure 108A

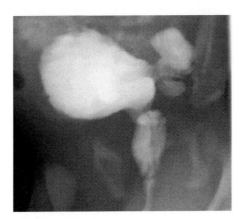

Figure 108B

Radiologic Findings

Ultrasonography of the abdomen and pelvis demonstrates a markedly thickened bladder wall (**Fig. 108A1**), hydroureter, hydronephrosis (**Fig. 108A2**), and distended posterior urethra. Voiding cystourethrogram shows posterior urethral valves with thickened bladder and diverticulae (**Fig. 108B**).

Diagnosis

Posterior urethral valves with thickened bladder wall, hydroureter, and hydronephrosis. A percutaneous nephrostomy was requested.

Differential Diagnosis

- Bilateral ureterovesical junction (UVJ) obstruction
- Bilateral ureteropelvic junction (UPJ) obstruction

Discussion

Background

Percutaneous nephrostomy is a well-established procedure for the treatment of obstructive uropathy in the pediatric population. The neonatal population presents some additional difficulties, which are not seen in older children. Placing catheters in neonates may therefore be challenging even when the collecting systems are severely dilated.

Etiology

Congenital malformations are the predominant cause of urinary tract obstruction in the pediatric population. These include:

- Ureteral malformations:
  - UPJ narrowing or obstruction
  - UVJ narrowing or obstruction
  - Ureterocele
  - Retrocaval ureter
- Bladder outlet malformations:
  - Bladder neck obstruction
  - Ureterocele
- Urethra malformations:
  - Posterior urethral valves
  - Anterior urethral valves
  - Stricture
  - Meatal stenosis
  - Phimosis

Indications

Percutaneous nephrostomy is often used for temporary urinary diversion until permanent treatment can be performed. Common indications for the percutaneous nephrostomy procedure include:

- Bilateral UPJ obstruction or narrowing
- Unilateral UPJ with a single functional kidney
- Obstruction after pyeloplasty
- UVJ obstruction or narrowing
- Posterior urethral valves
- Primary obstructing megaureter
- Urinary diversion for postoperative urine leak or fistula

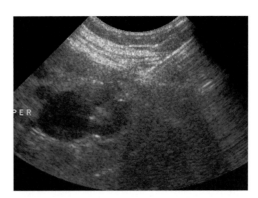

Figure 108C Sonogram of access to the dilated pelvicaliceal system.

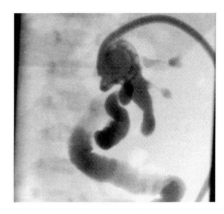

Figure 108D Left collecting system accessed with a no. 8 French Dawson-Mueller Mac-Loc catheter.

- Functional evaluation of a hydronephrotic kidney
- Severely compromised renal function or infection (pyonephrosis)

Contraindicatons

- Uncorrectable severe coagulopathy

Imaging Findings

- Ultrasonographic and fluoroscopic guidance are used in this procedure.

Technique

- Patient is placed in the prone or in the decubitus position.
- General anesthetic is used, with a sterile technique.
- Ultrasonographic guidance is used to access the dilated pelvicaliceal system.
- Procedure is performed with either a 22-gauge Chiba needle or a 22-gauge angiocatheter (**Fig. 108C**).
- The neonatal kidney is very mobile, and access to the caliceal system requires a sharp jab or else the kidney can rotate anteriorly and make access extremely difficult.
- Urine is aspirated and sent for culture and microbiology.
- Contrast is introduced to visualize the collecting system.
- A 0.018-inch Terumo guide wire is advanced and, if possible, is guided down the ureter.
- A Neff introducer system is then advanced, followed by a 0.035-inch wire and a no. 8 French dilator. A no. 8 French Dawson-Mueller Mac-Loc catheter is introduced and fixed with clear dressing and is connected to a drainage bag (**Fig. 108D**).
- The same procedure is repeated on the other side as needed (**Fig. 108E**).

Complications

- Overall complication rate, including both major and minor complications, is ~6.5 to 10%.
- Possible complications include:
  - Bleeding
  - Infection and sepsis
  - Mechanical problems including tube blockage

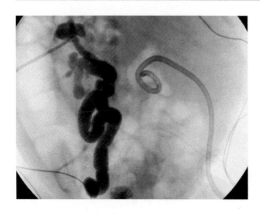

Figure 108E Bilateral nephrostomies with tortuous ureters.

- ○ Inadvertent puncture of adjacent organs
- ○ Pneumothorax
- ○ Catheter dislodgement

Prognosis

- The success rate of the percutaneous nephrostomy procedure is ~98 to 99% in the adult population.
- Few data are available concerning the success rate in the neonatal population; however, it likely is somewhat lower.
- Residual renal dysfunction depends on the extent of the obstruction and length of time before treatment was initiated.

PEARLS

- Nephrostomies can be performed in the decubitus position.
- Attempt to place the wire down the ureter for better security.

PITFALLS

- It is easy to lose access to the collecting system during either guide wire insertion or dilator or catheter placement.
- A dilated collecting system can easily decompress during this procedure, therefore making positioning of this catheter difficult.

Suggested Readings

Koral K, Saker MC, Morello FP, Rigsby CK, Donaldson JS. Conventional versus modified technique for percutaneous nephrostomy in newborns and young infants. J Vasc Interv Radiol 2003;14:113–116

Millward SF. Percutaneous nephrostomy: a practical approach. J Vasc Interv Radiol 2000;11:955–964

Ramchandani P, Cardella JF, Grassi CJ, et al. Quality improvement guidelines for percutaneous nephrostomy. J Vasc Interv Radiol 2003;14:S277–S281

Riccabona M, Sorantin E, Hausegger K. Imaging guided interventional procedures in paediatric uroradiology: a case based overview. Eur J Radiol 2002;43:167–179

Seifter JL, Brenner BM. Urinary tract obstruction. Chapter 270. In: Kasper DL et al, eds. Harrison's Principles of Internal Medicine. 16th ed. New York: McGraw-Hill Medical Publishing Division; 2005:1222–1224

Farrell TA, Hicks ME. A review of radiologically guided percutaneous nephrostomies in 303 patients. J Vasc Interv Radiol 1997;8:769–774

CASE 109

Clinical Presentation

A 9-year-old male presents to his family physician with a cough lasting a few days, shortness of breath with minimal exercise (worse when lying down), lethargy, chest pain, and intermittent fever. Patient is given antibiotics for possible pneumonia and is sent home. The child returns with persisting symptoms. A chest x-ray is ordered, which reveals a mediastinal mass.

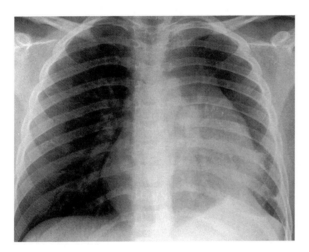

Figure 109A

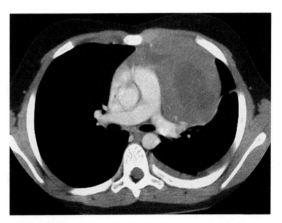

Figure 109B

Radiologic Findings

Chest radiograph demonstrates a left-sided mediastinal mass overlying the heart border (**Fig. 109A**). Chest CT shows a mass in the anterior mediastinum adjacent to the left cardiac border. The mass is of soft tissue density with central areas of hypodensity (**Fig. 109B**).

Diagnosis

Mediastinal mass requiring biopsy subsequently confirmed lymphoblastic lymphoma.

Differential Diagnosis

The diagnosis of mediastinal masses in children may present a challenge. They are a heterogeneous group and may be of congenital, infectious, or neoplastic origin:

- Mediastinal lymph nodes are the most common source of mediastinal masses (including Hodgkin's and non-Hodgkin's lymphoma).
- Fatty masses: herniation of omental fat, mediastinal diffuse lipomatosis, lipoma, liposarcoma, and thymolipoma
- Cystic masses: usually congenital (foregut cysts), pericardial cysts, thymic cysts, lymphangiomas, intrathoracic meningocele
- Solid tissue masses: goiter (look for tracheal deviation in the upper mediastinum), hemangioma, parathyroid mass, Castleman disease, medullary cancer of the thyroid, thymic carcinoid, and metastasis of sarcomas and melanomas
- Germ cell tumor: benign teratomas (60%); malignant germ cell tumors are more common in males (teratocarcinoma, embryonic carcinoma, seminoma, endodernal sinus tumor, choricarcinoma, and mixed germ cell tumors).
- Neurogenic tumors are of three main types:
  - Nerve sheath tumors (common with neurofibromatosis): schwannoma and neurofibroma
  - Ganglion cell tumors (common in the pediatric population): neuroblastoma and ganglioneuroma
  - Paraganglionic cell tumors: paraganglioma and chemodectoma
- Post-transplant lymphoproliferative disease: children seem to be more susceptible; usually develops within 1 year of transplant.

Discussion

Background

A percutaneous core biopsy is a valuable tool in the diagnosis and pathologic characterization of a mediastinal mass. It is especially indicated if imaging suggests that the mass is invasive or unresectable. Four approaches have been used traditionally to biopsy mediastinal masses: parasternal, suprasternal, transpulmonary, and paraspinal. A transsternal approach also can be used in certain cases to biopsy mediastinal masses.

Etiology

Thymoma, neurogenic tumors, and benign cysts represent ~60% of mediastinal masses. Some differences exist between the adult and the pediatric populations. In adults, the most frequent lesions include primary thymic neoplasms, thyroid masses, and lymphomas. In the pediatric population, however, neurogenic tumors, germ cell tumors, and foregut cysts represent ~80% of all cases.

Clinical Findings

The majority of cases are asymptomatic and are discovered incidentally on chest radiographs. Symptoms are often the result of the mediastinal mass compressing adjacent structures. Symptoms may include dyspnea, dysphagia, cough, superior vena cava syndrome, and hoarseness due to laryngeal nerve involvement. Occasionally, myasthenia gravis or Cushing's syndrome may be the first signs of a mediastinal mass.

Pathology

The accuracy of percutaneous biopsy is limited by the nature of the tumor. In cases of non-Hodgkin's lymphomas, thymomas, and Hodgkin's disease, a core biopsy has been shown to be more valuable than a fine-needle aspiration for ensuring an accurate diagnosis. Biopsy sampling should be obtained in non-necrotic tissue, most commonly using a coaxial technique. This allows multiple passes and the option of embolization of the tract at the end of the procedure.

Imaging Findings

RADIOGRAPHY

- First line in the diagnosis
- Many masses are discovered incidentally on routine radiographs.
- Posteroanterior and lateral views may exhibit deformations in the contours of the mediastinum and trachea and may allow for a focused differential based on age, gender, location, and clinical findings.

CT

- CT is the next imaging step and may be sufficient.
- Both noncontrast and contrast-enhanced slices may be needed.
- Used to localize a mass to the lungs, pleural space, or mediastinum

MRI

- Often used in cases where contrast cannot be given or if CT imaging is equivocal
- Excellent soft tissue contrast and multiplanar imaging allows for the preoperative assessment of the mass's location with respect to the pericardium and spinal cord.

ULTRASOUND

- Has only a limited role; may be useful in children with masses adjacent to the chest wall
- Transesophageal ultrasonography can be useful in the evaluation of posterior mediastinal masses.

Technique

- The approach to mediastinal biopsy can be transsternal, parasternal, paraspinal, transpulmonary, or suprasternal.
- A parasternal approach is appropriate for lesions in the anterior mediastinum, which have a component lateral to the sternum. It is usually performed under ultrasonographic guidance, which limits the risk of puncturing the internal thoracic arteries.
  - The biopsy can be performed under limited sedation and even with local anesthetic alone. This is helpful particularly in patients with large masses and possible airway compromise.
  - If the patient is symptomatic in the supine position, the biopsy may be performed in the decubitus position.
  - Normal saline can be introduced to widen the mediastinal space in patients with narrow mediastina. This may help avoid transgressing lung tissue and decrease the risk of postbiopsy pneumothorax.

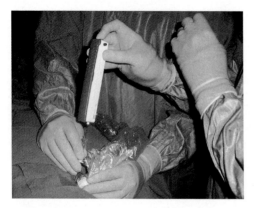

Figure 109C Coaxial biopsy with a 17-gauge needle and an 18-gauge Biopince needle, a full-core biopsy instrument.

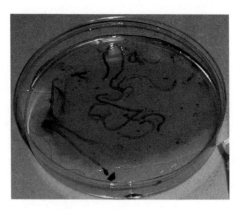

Figure 109D Numerous specimens obtained for adequate pathologic analysis.

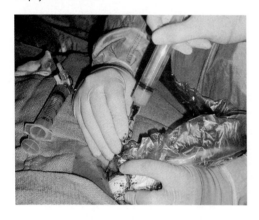

Figure 109E The biopsy needle has been removed, and Gelfoam slurry is injected through the coaxial needle.

- A coaxial technique can be performed so that many cores can be obtained and the tract embolized to reduce the risk of bleeding (**Fig. 109C**).
- Numerous specimens are obtained via the coaxial needle to give sufficient material for pathologic assessment (**Fig. 109D**).
- The biopsy needle is removed, and then through the coaxial needle an absorbable gelatin (e.g., Gelfoam) slurry is injected under ultrasonographic guidance to reduce the risk of hemorrhage (**Fig. 109E**).
- A suprasternal approach is valuable when the mass extends above the level of the aortic arch.
- A paraspinal approach is performed under CT guidance to obtain tissue from a posterior mediastinal mass.
- A transsternal approach has the advantage of reducing the risk for both hemorrhage and pneumothorax and is performed under CT guidance.
- A transpulmonary approach can access most mediastinal masses. However, the needle path crosses the lung and pleura thereby increasing the risk for pneumothorax and limiting the amount of tissue that can be obtained (usually performed via a bronchoscope).

Complications

- Hemorrhage may result due to puncture of the internal thoracic arteries during a parasternal approach. When using image guidance these vessels can be visualized and avoided, thus greatly reducing the risk of hemorrhage.
- Pneumothorax (especially using a transpulmonary approach)

Prognosis

- Biopsy of mediastinal mass is a safe and well-tolerated procedure that provides extremely useful diagnostic information.
- Complications can be reduced by using ultrasonographic guidance. Its main advantages are that it is real time and vessels can be avoided with the use of color Doppler.
- Overall diagnostic accuracy is ~94% for core biopsies but does vary according to the type of neoplasm.

PEARLS_____

- Ultrasonographic guidance has the advantage of decreasing the risk of pneumothorax and accidental injury to the internal mammary vessels, and it allows for real-time imaging and multiple cores to be obtained.
- Bone marrow biopsy and aspiration are often done at the same time under the same anesthetic as well as placement of a chest port for therapy.

PITFALLS_____

- Large mediastinal masses carry a significant risk for airway compromise when the patient is in the supine position. This represents a significant risk for anesthesia and must be considered when planning this procedure. To minimize the risk of airway compromise, the procedure may be performed in a sitting or decubitus position. Appropriate anesthesia assistance must be obtained to avoid airway compromise.
- Vascular abnormalities such as aneurysms are uncommon in the pediatric population; however, they may represent up to 10% of mediastinal masses in adults. These must be ruled out before any interventional procedure is planned.

Suggested Readings

Gupta S, Wallace MJ, Morello FA Jr, Ahrar K, Hicks ME. CT-guided percutaneous needle biopsy of intrathoracic lesions by using the transsternal approach: experience in 37 patients. Radiology 2002;222:57–62

Laurent F, Latrabe V, Lecesne R, et al. Mediastinal masses: diagnostic approach. Eur Radiol 1998;8:1148–1159

Morrissey B, Adams H, Gibbs AR, Crane MD. Percutaneous needle biopsy of the mediastinum: review of 94 procedures. Thorax 1993;48:632–637

CASE 110

Clinical Presentation

A 28-week (1.2 kg) premature neonate presented soon after birth with a distended abdomen, and appeared clinically to be septic. The patient required intubation and ventilation. On examination, there was paucity of bowel sounds. Patient was transferred to a tertiary care center. Abdominal radiography and ultrasonography were performed. Conservative management with total parenteral nutrition and antibiotics were prescribed, which required secure central venous access. What would you use?

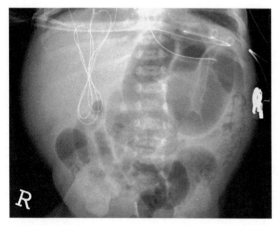

Figure 110A

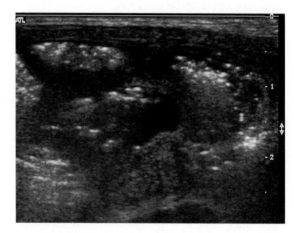

Figure 110B

Radiologic Findings

A radiograph of the abdomen shows pneumatosis in the right lower quadrant and air in the portal veins (**Fig. 110A**). The air in the portal veins was confirmed on ultrasonography. The bowel demonstrates poor peristalsis, decreased vascularity, and pneumatosis (**Fig. 110B**); all features consistent with necrotizing enterocolitis.

Diagnosis

Necrotizing enterocolitis requiring initial conservative therapy and probable surgery. A peripherally inserted central catheter was placed.

Discussion

Background

Peripherally inserted central catheters (PICCs) are an increasingly used modality in the neonatal intensive care unit. PICCs are inserted into a peripheral vein, usually in the upper arm, and are threaded into the central circulation. This provides stable access to a central vein, eliminating the need for repeated peripheral intravenous punctures, which are associated with pain and complications. It has been suggested that a PICC line is more cost effective than a central venous line (CVL) when venous access is required for up to 21 days. If one compares an image-guided PICC line placement and an image-guided CVL placement, the risks and benefits are a little more complicated to determine, and the PICC line may actually be associated with increased risk for venous complications. A CVL should be used when more long-term access is required. PICC designs include single and double lumen varieties. They are constructed from silicone or polyurethane and are radiopaque. We use cuffed silicone catheters for children and neonates, as we feel that these catheters are more secure, and there are no sutures to remove. The catheters are available in various lumen sizes, the most commonly used being the no. 3 French, followed by the no. 2 French. The placement of these catheters is increasingly performed by pediatric interventional radiologists because imaging guidance increases the options and success rate of placement.

Indications

- Reduction of the number of venipuncture procedures during prolonged treatment course as peripheral intravenous lines have a very short life span. Repeated venipuncture is recognized as one of the greatest stresses for a hospitalized child. A PICC line can remain in situ for months, dramatically reducing the number of required needle sticks; a stable vascular access is maintained, and home treatment may be possible in certain cases.
- Total parenteral nutrition: PICC lines allow for the administration of a high-calorie, dense, and concentrated parenteral nutrition with little venous irritation. This is especially important when managing premature and low birth weight babies.
- Administration of irritant medications: the ability to deliver medications with a low or high pH (<6 or >8) or hyperosmolar or vesicant properties. Such medications include many chemotherapeutic and antibiotic agents.
- Obtaining repeated blood samples

Contraindications

- Bacteremia or septicemia is known or suspected.
- Anatomy will not permit introduction of the catheter into a vessel.
- Uncorrected coagulopathy or hypercoagulable state
- Local infection or burns at insertion sites
- Vascular insufficiency of an extremity

Imaging Findings

- Ultrasonography is used to access the basilic vein in the upper arm.
- Fluoroscopic guidance is used to advance the wire, peel away the sheath, and finally place the catheter into position with its tip in the superior vena cava–right atrial junction.

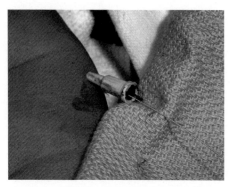

Figure 110C Ultrasonographic-guided access to the basilic vein with a 22-gauge angio-catheter and a 0.014 wire in place.

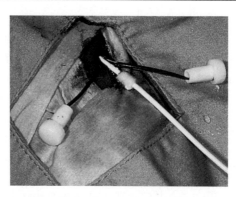

Figure 110D Peel-away sheath and cuffed PICC line prior to burying of the cuff.

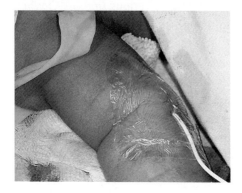

Figure 110E Catheter in place with clear sterile Tegaderm dressing.

Technique

- The neonate is placed in the supine position, and the arm is prepped with Germi-Stat prep gel 0.5% (Germiphene Corporation, Brantford, ON Canada) from the antecubital fossa to the lower neck region.
- Following this, a tourniquet is placed in the axilla.
- The basilic vein is the preferred choice; alternative sites include axillary, scalp, cephalic, and superficial temporal veins. In the lower extremities, greater and lesser saphenous and popliteal veins can be used.
- Ultrasonographic guidance is usually used for the initial puncture. Unlike adults, both arteries and veins may be compressible in neonates.
- A small injection dose of 1% lidocaine is used for local anesthetic.
- Doppler is used to help distinguish between the artery and vein. A pulsatile waveform indicates arterial blood flow, and the vessel is thus avoided. Once the entry site has been determined it should be marked.
- Once the correct vessel has been determined, a 24- or 22-gauge needle intravenous cannula is used for the initial entry.
- On entry, a guide wire is inserted through the cannula and placed near the superior vena cava–right atrium junction (**Fig. 110C**).
- The guide wire insertion length is used to estimate the distance from the insertion site to the superior vena cava–right atrium junction. This estimate is used to trim the length of the catheter.
- A peel-away sheath is subsequently placed over the guide wire, followed by insertion of the catheter into the sheath. The polyethylene terephthalate (e.g., Dacron) cuff is advanced just under the skin (**Fig. 110D**). The entry site is sutured with 2–0 Vicryl resorbable sutures and is dressed with clear sterile Tegaderm dressing (3M Healthcare Corporation, St Paul, MN) (**Fig. 110E**).

- Confirmation of catheter placement is done by fluoroscopy with contrast injection. The catheter is then covered with a transparent sterile dressing and heparin locked.
- If the PICC procedure fails bilaterally in the upper extremities, a CVL can be inserted as long as the neonate has no contraindications (i.e., jugular vein thrombosis).

Complications

- The overall complication rate for indwelling PICCs is reported at 20 to 30%.
- The majority of complications are minor and usually only require catheter replacement.
- The most common complications include:
  - Catheter occlusion
  - Mechanical problems: tears, leaks, dislodgement, and fractures
  - Infection or suspected infection: Incidence rate increases with duration of catheter placement.
  - Venous thrombosis
  - Catheter migration
- Some less frequent complications may include:
  - Effusions and arrhythmias: rare complications that may in some cases be due to catheter breakage and migration
  - Bleeding
  - Vein damage or injury
  - Brachial plexus injury/nerve damage
  - Drug extravasations
  - Erosion of catheter through skin and/or blood vessel
  - Fibrin sheath formation around the catheter and its tip
  - Hemothorax/pneumothorax
  - Phlebitis
  - Pulmonary embolism

Prognosis

- Technical success rate for the insertion of a PICC line under image guidance is >95%.
- In ~70% of cases, therapy is completed using the original device.
- In the other 30% of cases, the catheter must be removed or revised due to complications.

PEARLS_____

- A PICC line should be used when therapy is expected to be required for up to 2 or 3 weeks. Longer-term therapies are often completed with a PICC line but may occasionally necessitate the insertion of a CVL. Outcome studies are needed to determine which treatment option (PICC or CVL) is associated with fewer long-term complications.
- PICC line occlusion is a common complication. Attempts at unblocking a PICC line should never be performed with a small volume syringe as this may result in catheter fracture. Ideally, a 10 mL syringe filled with saline should be used when attempting to unblock the catheter. Chest radiograph should first be performed to confirm catheter tip position, and then a linogram should be performed. Placing a wire may also be used to unblock the catheter. Depending on the cause, a blocked catheter potentially may be unblocked using hydrochloric acid or tissue plasminogen activator. Catheter revision may be necessary if the line cannot be cleared by such means.
- Line-related infections may be treated with a catheter left in place; however, if the infection is coagulase negative *Staphylococcus*, *Pseudomonas*, or fungal infection (or other difficult-to-treat infections), the catheter must be removed and a new line placed only after blood cultures are clear for 24 hours.

PITFALL_____

- If a patient presents with a PICC that did not give blood return and was flushing with some difficulty that then suddenly improved, a PICC line fracture should be suspected.

Suggested Readings

Bakal CW, Silberzweig JE, Cynimon J, Sprayegen S, eds. Vascular and Interventional Radiology: Principles and Practice. New York: Thieme; 2002:109–123

Foo R, Fujii A, Harris JA, LaMorte W, Moulton S. Complications in tunneled CVL versus PICC lines in very low birth weight infants. J Perinatol 2001;21:525–530

Petitt J. Assessment of infants with peripherally inserted central catheters, I: Detecting the most frequently occurring complications. Adv Neonatal Care 2002;2:304–315

Hogan MJ. Neonatal vascular catheters and their complications. Radiol Clin North Am 1999; 37:1109–1125

Smith JR, Friedell ML, Cheatham ML, Martin SP, Cohen MJ, Horowitz JD. Peripherally inserted central catheters revisited. Am J Surg 1998;176:208–211

Sofocleous CT, Schur I, Cooper SG, Quintas JC, Brody L, Shelin R. Sonographically guided placement of peripherally inserted central venous catheters: review of 355 procedures. Am J Roentgenol 1998;170:1613–1616

Thiagarajan RR, Ramamoorthy C, Gettmann T, Bratton SL. Survey of the use of peripherally inserted central venous catheters in children. Pediatrics 1997;99:E4

Valk WJC, Liem KD, Geven WB. Seldinger technique as an alternative approach for percutaneous insertion of hydrophilic polyurethane central venous catheters in newborns. J Parenter Enteral Nutr 1995;19:151–155

CASE 111

Clinical Presentation

A 5-year-old boy presents with abdominal mass, malaise, and a history of intermittent fever over the previous few months. Biopsy of the abdominal mass showed Burkitt's lymphoma. To begin chemotherapy, placement of a subcutaneous chest port was ordered.

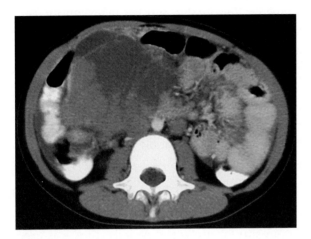

Figure 111A

Radiologic Findings

CT demonstrated the large lower abdominal mass (**Fig. 111A**). Biopsy under ultrasonographic guidance was ordered, as well as a bone marrow biopsy, lumbar puncture, and port placement.

Diagnosis

Burkitt's lymphoma

Discussion

Background

Long-term placement of subcutaneous, implantable chest ports in adults and children is now widely accepted. A chest port is ideal when stable access to a central vein will likely be required on an intermittent basis for longer than 6 months. A subcutaneous implantable port has many advantages; there is no skin entry site that must be constantly maintained, it is more cosmetically appealing, there are no external components that can be pulled or accidentally dislodged by the child, and, finally, there are no limitations on the child's daily activities. A tunneled catheter may be more suitable if daily access will likely be required. Pediatric interventional radiologists are now increasingly performing the procedure, which was previously performed by pediatric surgeons. There are three sizes of single lumen ports available (mini, petite, and adult) and two sizes of double lumen ports (petite and adult). A double lumen port is used when two incompatible drugs must be given simultaneously (e.g., for the treatment of osteosarcomas).

Indications

- A chest port for central venous access can remain in situ for prolonged periods; thus it is used when a stable long-term access is required.
- Administration of irritant medications: the ability to deliver medications with a low or high pH (<6 or >8) or hyperosmolar or vesicant properties. Such medications include chemotherapeutic and antibiotic agents.
- Hemophiliac patients requiring weekly factor replacement and transfusions.

Contraindications

- Bacteremia or septicemia is known or suspected.
- Anatomy will not permit introduction of the catheter into a vessel.
- Past irradiation of the upper chest area or diffuse skin disease over the chest area (e.g., epidermolysis bulossa)
- Hypercoagulable state

Technique

- The procedure is performed under general anesthetic using a sterile technique.
- Pre-procedure dose of a first generation cephalosporin is given prior to the procedure.
- The right internal jugular vein (**Fig. 111B**) is the most preferred access site, followed by the left internal jugular, the external right or left jugular, and, finally, the right subclavian vein.
- The right internal jugular vein is approached under ultrasonographic and Doppler guidance. The ultrasonography probe is placed parallel to the internal jugular vein, and the needle is inserted using the lateral margin of the transducer as reference mark.
- When the tip of the needle reaches the anterior wall of the vein, a push on its surface will cause the vein to collapse temporarily before the needle pierces the wall.
- A guide wire is advanced under fluoroscopic guidance into the superior vena cava, the right atrium, and, preferably, into the inferior vena cava.

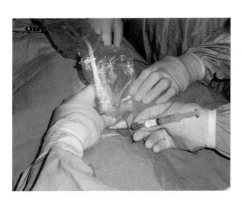

Figure 111B Access to the right jugular under ultrasonographic guidance.

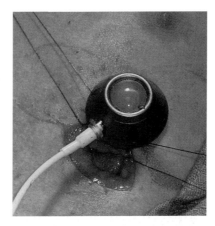

Figure 111C Port pocket created with Prolene sutures into the pectoralis fascia and attached to the port.

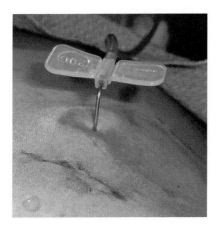

Figure 111D Percutaneous access to the port with a Huber needle.

- An appropriate size peel-away sheath is introduced.
- A subcutaneous pocket is created in the right upper chest using cautery and blunt dissection.
- The port is sutured to the fascia of the pectoralis muscle (**Fig. 111C**). The catheter that is attached to the port is tunneled to the neck access site.
- Using fluoroscopy, the catheter is cut to the appropriate length (tip at the superior vena cava–right atrial junction).
- The dilator and wire are removed from the sheath, and the sheath is clamped. The catheter is advanced into the sheath until the sheath has been completely removed.
- The port pocket is closed with three layers of resorbable sutures, and the neck access site is closed with one suture.
- A Huber needle is introduced into the port, and a contrast study is performed to confirm the catheter's position and to check for leaks (**Fig. 111D**).

Complications

- Overall complication rate for a chest port is reported at up to 20%.
- The most common complications include:
  - Infection of the port chamber and catheter or a port pocket infection
  - Mechanical malfunction including:
    - Occlusion of the catheter (most common)
    - Malposition and kinking
    - Leaks, tears, and fractures

- • Venous thrombosis
- • Catheter migration
- Some less frequent complications may include:
  - ○ Effusions and arrhythmias: Rare complications that may in some cases be due to catheter breakage and migration
  - ○ Bleeding
  - ○ Vein damage or injury
  - ○ Drug extravasations
  - ○ Erosion of catheter through skin and/or blood vessel
  - ○ Fibrin sheath formation around the catheter and its tip
  - ○ Hemothorax/pneumothorax
  - ○ Phlebitis

Prognosis

- • Technical success rate for the insertion of a chest port is extremely high.
- • Early removal of port may be necessary in some circumstances (catheter-related infection or thrombosis).

PEARLS_____

- • A chest port should be implanted when therapy is expected to last >6 months.
- • A PICC line may be sufficient for short-term therapies.
- • To reduce the difficulty in accessing low-profile ports, educating the health care staff on how to access chest ports may be necessary.

PITFALLS_____

- • When accessing the jugular vein, anatomic landmarks alone should not be used.
- • The use of ultrasonography with Doppler greatly reduces the risk of an accidental arterial puncture.

Suggested Readings

Bodner LJ, Nosher JL, Patel KM, et al. Peripheral venous access ports: outcomes analysis in 109 patients. Cardiovasc Intervent Radiol 2000;23:187–193

Funaki B, Szymski GX, Hackworth CA, et al. Radiologic placement of subcutaneous infusion chest ports for long-term central venous access. AJR Am J Roentgenol 1997;169:1431–1434

Kurul S, Saip P, Aydin T. Totally implantable venous-access ports: local problems and extravasation injury. Lancet Oncol 2002;3:684–692

Lorenz JM, Funaki B, Van Ha T, Leef JA. Radiologic placement of implantable chest ports in pediatric patients. AJR Am J Roentgenol 2001;176:991–994

Nosher JL, Bodner LJ, Ettinger LJ, et al. Radiologic placement of a low profile implantable venous access port in a pediatric population. Cardiovasc Intervent Radiol 2001;24:395–399

SECTION IX

Dysplasias

CASE 112

Clinical Presentation

A healthy, active child presents with height well below fifth percentile for age. He demonstrates frontal bossing, generalized limb shortening with a relatively normal trunk, a mild "swayback" deformity, and spatulate hands.

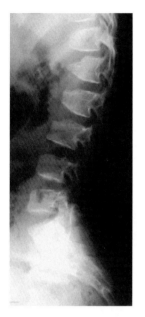

Figure 112A

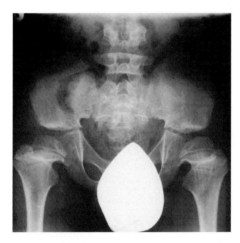

Figure 112B

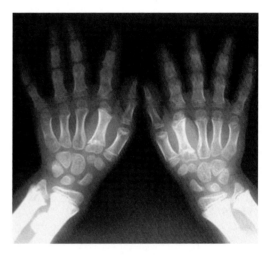

Figure 112C

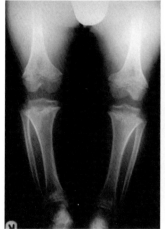

Figure 112D

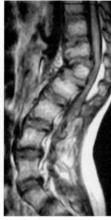

Figure 112E

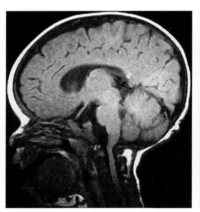

Figure 112F

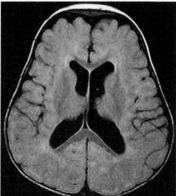

Figure 112G

Radiologic Findings

Lateral radiograph of lumbosacral spine (**Fig. 112A**) demonstrates anteroinferior beaking at L1 and L2, resulting in a mild gibbus. Distal lumbar lordosis is slightly exaggerated. The lumbar pedicles are quite short, resulting in spinal stenosis. Frontal radiograph of the pelvis (**Fig. 112B**) demonstrates short, squared iliac wings ("elephant ear" appearance), with horizontal acetabular roofs. The femoral necks are quite short, but the femoral heads are well developed. Note progressive narrowing of the distal lumbar interpediculate space.

The hands (**Fig. 112C**) show mild generalized shortening of metacarpals and phalanges. Note the divergence of the fingers from one another ("trident hand"). Frontal view of the knees (**Fig. 112D**) demonstrates relative broadened distal femoral and proximal tibial metaphyses, with narrowing of the femoral intercondylar notch. The femora and tibiae are short and broad, and the fibulae are relatively elongated.

Sagittal T2-weighted MRI of the lumbar spine (**Fig. 112E**) clearly demonstrates anterior upper lumbar beaking, with resultant gibbus deformity. Note compression of the conus medullaris at the T12-L1 disk interspace. Severe distal central lumbar canal stenosis is present; the lumbar cistern is not visible. Sagittal T1-weighted MRI of the brain just to the right of midline (**Fig. 112F**) demonstrates severe narrowing of the foramen magnum, with compression of the cervical cord at this level. Note mild frontal bossing. Axial short tau inversion recovery (STIR) weighted image demonstrates minimal prominence of the lateral ventricles (**Fig. 112G**).

Diagnosis

Achondroplasia

Differential Diagnosis

- Hypochondroplasia
- Metaphyseal chondrodysplasias
- Pseudoachondroplasia

Discussion

Background

Achondroplasia is the most common nonlethal skeletal dysplasia, seen in 1 in 26,000 live births. This condition has been long recognized and is represented in paintings from the Renaissance.

Etiology

Achondroplasia is an autosomal dominant condition caused by one of four distinct point mutations in the transmembrane domain region of fibroblast growth factor receptor 3 (FGFR3). This region is quite close to the defects seen in thanatophoric dysplasia type 1 and hypochondroplasia, both of which share many phenotypic and radiographic similarities with achondroplasia. Although most cases are the result of new mutations, vertical transmission is occasionally seen. Homozygous achondroplasia may be seen in children of two affected adults, demonstrating phenotypic severity between that of achondroplasia and thanatophoric dysplasia.

Clinical Findings

- Generalized shortening and broadening of limbs
- Relatively large head, often with frontal bossing and mild midface constriction
- Normal to near-normal trunk length
- Gibbus deformity of spine
- Excessive lumbosacral lordosis (swayback)
- Genu varum in younger patients
- Short fingers with divergence (trident hand)
- Spinal stenosis in some produces paresthesias, paresis, paralysis
- Proximal cervical canal and foramen magnum stenosis may result in sudden death.
- Some patients develop hydrocephalus.
- Patients are of normal intelligence.

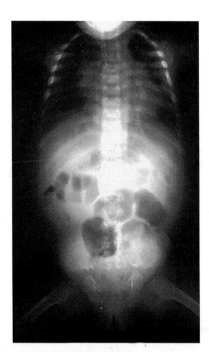

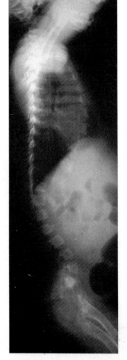

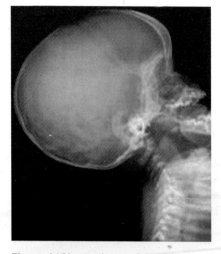

Figure 112H Frontal chest and abdomen radiograph of a patient with achondroplasia demonstrate short, squared iliac wings with narrowed sacrosciatic notches and mild shortening of the ribs with anterior cupping. Progressive interpediculate narrowing at lumbar level is seen.

Figure 112I Lateral chest and abdomen radiograph in the same patient as **Fig. 112H** show mild platyspondyly, and anteroposterior shortening of the vertebrae. Note the short lumbar pedicles.

Figure 112J Lateral view of the skull showing frontal bossing.

Pathology

Short, widened cartilage columns with decreased enchondral ossification

Imaging Findings

RADIOGRAPHY

- Newborns
  - Mildly shortened ribs with anterior cupping (**Figs. 112H** and **112I**)
  - Short, squared iliac wings with narrowed sacrosciatic notches and medial and lateral acetabular spikes (**Fig. 112H**)
  - Mild platyspondyly, with vertebrae demonstrating shortening on lateral view (**Fig. 112I**)
  - Variable anteroinferior beaking at L1 through L3
  - Progressive interpediculate narrowing at lumbar level on frontal view (**Fig. 112H**)
  - Progressive shortening of vertebral pedicles on lateral view
  - Variable frontal bossing (**Fig. 112J**)
  - "V" or cup-shaped physes at shoulder, hip, and knees, with metaphyseal widening (**Fig. 112K**)
  - Generalized shortening and thickening of long bones
  - Generalized shortening of metacarpals, metatarsals, and phalanges. The fingers diverge from one another, resulting in the classic trident hand appearance (**Fig. 112L**)
- Older children
  - Persistent shortening and broadening of long bones
  - Progressive frontal bossing

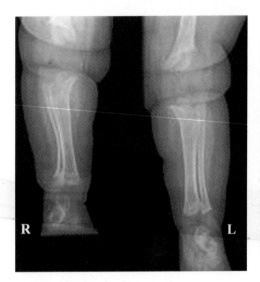

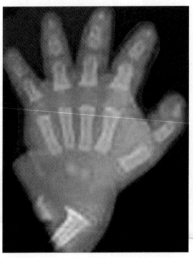

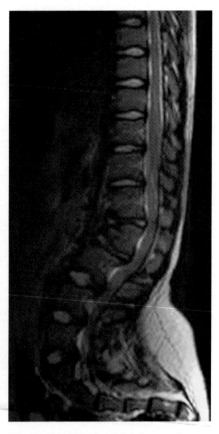

Figure 112K Anteroposterior lower extremity radiograph of the of patient demonstrates a "V" or cup-shaped physes at knees.

Figure 112L Frontal view of hand in patient with achondroplasia shows classic "trident hand" appearance with fingers diverge from one another. Shortening of metacarpals, metatarsals, and phalanges is also seen.

Figure 112M Lateral lumbosacral spine MRI demonstrating lumbosacral lordosis ("swayback") and/or a progressive upper lumbar gibbus. The degree of spinal stenosis and the significance of gibbus deformity is best evaluated with MRI.

- ○ Persistent trident hand appearance
- ○ Often develop a progressively accentuated lumbosacral lordosis (swayback) and/or a progressive upper lumbar gibbus
- ○ Older children and adults predisposed to accelerated degenerative disk disease
- ○ Pelvis retains a "champagne glass" appearance, with narrowed sacrosciatic notches and iliac wing hypoplasia.
- ○ Relative metaphyseal broadening, especially at shoulders and knees

CT/MRI

- Patients usually have normal ventricles but may develop hydrocephalus.
- Foramen magnum and proximal cervical canal stenosis is well seen on these modalities.
- The degree of spinal stenosis and the significance of gibbus deformity are best evaluated with MRI (**Fig. 112M**).

Treatment

- Limb lengthening has been performed on many patients but remains controversial within the community.
- Foramen magnum/proximal cervical decompression with dorsal fusion is required in some patients to relieve proximal cord compression.
- Lumbar decompressive laminectomy is required in some to relieve symptoms of distal spinal canal stenosis.

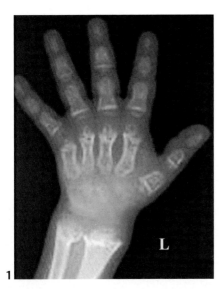
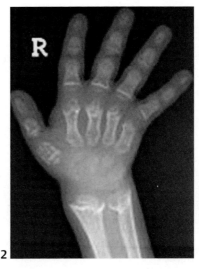
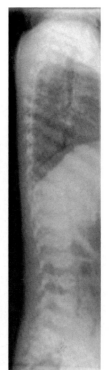

Figure 112N Frontal view of hands (**1,2**) in a patient with pseudoachondroplasia. Note generalized shortening of metacarpals and phalanges, with hypoplastic epiphyses. Metaphyses are broad and cupped.

Figure 112O Lateral view of spine in a patient with pseudoachondroplasia, showing characteristic superior and inferior end-plate humps, with anterior tonguelike projections. The appearances of the spine are quite different from achondroplasia.

Complications

- Hydrocephalus in a minority of patients, usually due to foramen magnum/skull base hypoplasia.
- Severe foramen magnum/proximal cervical canal stenosis can cause sudden death due to cord compression.
- Some patients develop progressive distal neuropathies due to progressive lumbar canal stenosis and/or compression at the level of the conus medullaris due to gibbus deformity.

Prognosis

- Provided that foramen magnum/proximal cervical spinal canal stenosis is not severe or progressive, these patients live a normal, productive life.
- Distal neuropathies and degenerative disk disease, as well as osteoarthritis, are seen in some adult patients. These conditions cause variable physical limitations.

PEARLS

- This is the most common nonlethal skeletal dysplasia.
- Trident hand appearance is suggestive of achondroplasia.

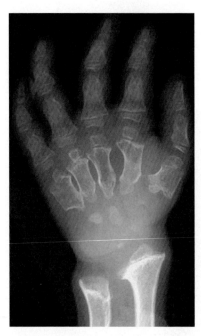

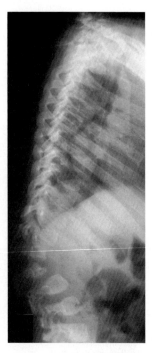

Figure 112P Frontal radiograph of the hand in a patient with Hurler syndrome (see Case 118). Note the "trident" appearance of the hand, with characteristic proximal metacarpal tapering and epiphyseal irregularity. The appearances of the hand are quite different from achondroplasia.

Figure 112Q Lateral radiograph of spine in a patient with Hurler syndrome. Appearances are not similar to achondroplasia.

PITFALLS

- Not all short limb dysplasias are achondroplasia. Achondroplasia is overdiagnosed, usually due to unfamiliarity with other dysplasias (**Figs. 112N** and **112O**).
- A slightly milder phenotype may represent hypochondroplasia, another condition caused by a fibroblast growth factor receptor 3 (FGFR3) mutation.
- Trident or spatulate hand may be seen in other disorders (**Fig. 112P**).
- Gibbus deformities may be seen in many other conditions, particularly in mucopolysaccharidoses and mucolipidoses (**Fig. 112Q**).

Suggested Readings

Cohen MM Jr. Short-limb skeletal dysplasias and craniosynostosis: what do they have in common? Pediatr Radiol 1997;27:442–446

Taybi H, Lachman RS. Radiology of Syndromes, Metabolic Disorders, and Skeletal Dysplasias. 4th ed. Chicago: Mosby Year Book Medical Publishers; 2001

Tsai F-J, Tsai C-H, Chang J-G, Wu J-Y. Mutations in the fibroblast growth factor receptor 3 (FGFR3) cause achondroplasia, hypochondroplasia, and thanatophoric dysplasia. Taiwanese data. Am J Med Genet 1999;86:300–301

CASE 113

Clinical Presentation

Two stillborn term infants present with similar short-limbed dwarfism.

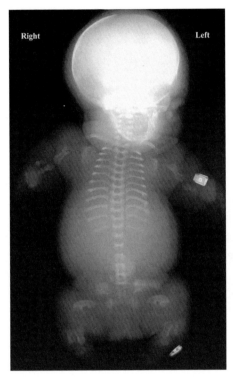

Figure 113A

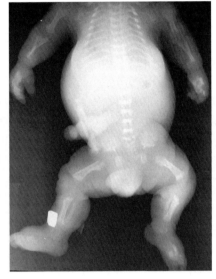

Figure 113B

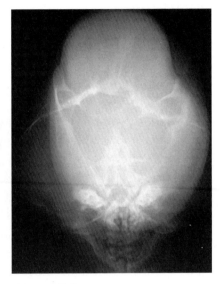

Figure 113C

Radiologic Findings

The stillborn neonate in **Fig. 113A** demonstrates dramatic platyspondyly with markedly shortened ribs and severe micromelia with markedly curved humeri and femora, with the latter showing characteristic "telephone receiver" appearance. Marked shortening of digits and metacarpals (brachydactyly and brachymetacarpalia) of hands is noted without evidence of craniosynostosis. The stillborn neonate in **Figs. 113B** and **113C** shows dramatic platyspondyly with markedly shortened ribs, severe micromelia with straight long bones, marked brachydactyly and brachymetacarpalia, and "cloverleaf" or kleebattschädel skull, indicative of universal craniosynostosis.

Diagnosis

Thanatophoric dysplasia (TD), type 1 (**Fig. 113A**) and type 2 (**Figs. 113B** and **113C**)

Differential Diagnosis

- Osteogenesis imperfecta
- Campomelic dysplasia
- Crouzon disease
- Apert syndrome

Discussion

Background

Although many skeletal dysplasias are compatible with a normal life span, lethal dysplasias do exist. Aside, perhaps, from type 2 osteogenesis imperfecta, the most common lethal skeletal dysplasia is TD. The term *thanatophoric* is from the Greek, meaning "death bearing." Most patients are stillborn, with the vast majority of affected live-born neonates succumbing within the first week. It is important to accurately diagnose the lethal skeletal dysplasias in order to tailor supportive care and to counsel parents regarding the relative risk for recurrence in subsequent pregnancies.

TD occurs as two major, distinct subtypes, with several additional "thanatophoric variants" also recognized. Classic TD occurs in 1 in 35,000 to 1 in 50,000 births. TD type 1 (TD1) is characterized by severe micromelia, with curved long bones (especially the femora) having a "telephone receiver" appearance. Craniosynostosis is seen in 27.6% of patients with TD1, and it is mild in many cases. TD type 2 (TD2) is characterized by relatively straight but short long bones; however, craniosynostosis is almost universal (>93%) and is severe, resulting in a cloverleaf appearance of the calvarium (kleebattschädel) in 53%.

Etiology

Both major subtypes of TD are the result of distinct mutations in fibroblast growth factor receptor type 3 (FGFR3), a receptor tyrosine kinase that spans the cellular membrane and is found in several tissue types, primarily cartilage and central nervous system. FGFR3 consists of an extracellular ligand-binding domain, a transmembrane portion, and a split intracellular tyrosine kinase domain. Activation occurs when a heparan sulfate proteoglycan and FGF bind to FGFR3, to form a trimolecular complex. FGFR3 regulates endochondral ossification, and it essentially acts as a "brake" on growth. The FGFR3 defect seen in TD causes loss of this function, resulting in premature, excessive growth and maturation at sites of maximal cartilage growth at the physes and sutures.

Because FGFR3 plays a vital role in regulating cartilaginous growth and development, defects or loss of function would be expected to result in characteristic growth abnormalities. In fact, achondroplasia (the most common skeletal dysplasia), hypochondroplasia, and TD are all caused by distinct mutations in FGFR3.

The TD1 phenotype is caused by at least two separate amino acid substitutions in FGFR3, whereas all patients with TD2 studied to date have had a single, identical FGFR3 amino acid substitution. Therefore, there is a mild spectrum in the severity of TD1, whereas all patients with TD2 share an almost identical phenotype.

Histology

Decreased, abnormal chondrocyte proliferation results in disorganized, shortened chondrocyte columns at the physes. Relative metaphyseal overgrowth occurs, with bands of mesenchymal tissue projecting inward from the perichondrium at the physeal periphery.

Clinical Findings

Most affected patients are stillborn, whereas live-born infants usually do not survive their first week. TD1 and TD2 are characterized by severe micromelia, narrow thorax, brachydactyly, brachymetacarpalia/brachymetatarsalia, and a relatively large head. The extremely narrow thorax and narrowed foramen magnum are associated with severe respiratory difficulty, the usual cause of death in live-born infants. Affected surviving infants usually have redundant skin about the neck, frontal bossing, moderate to severe exophthalmos, hypertelorism, and a flattened nasal bridge. The few reported long-term survivors have suffered from severe respiratory insufficiency and severe developmental delay. CNS anomalies reported in TD1 and TD2 include polymicrogyria, gray matter heterotopias, and gyral disorganization. Acanthosis nigricans, a disorder consisting of thickened, redundant skin, is also usually present.

Complications

Thanatophoric dysplasia is a lethal skeletal dysplasia.

Imaging Findings

RADIOGRAPHY

- TD1 and TD2 are best separated by the presence (TD1) or absence (TD2) of curved femora:
  - TD1: Femora are quite short and curved (telephone receiver appearance), with other long bones also affected.
    - Twenty-seven percent of patients with TD1 have craniosynostosis; when present, it is usually mild and *not* universal.
  - TD2: Femora and other long bones are quite short but relatively straight.
    - Ninety-three percent or more of patients with TD2 have craniosynostosis; most are severely affected, with cloverleaf skull (kleebattschädel) common.
- Although craniosynostosis occurs in both subtypes, it is much more common (93% vs 27%) in TD2 than in TD1. Common to both TD1 and TD2 are:
  - Severe platyspondyly, which is usually more marked in TD1 than in TD2
  - Polymicrogyria and gray matter heterotopias
  - Both subtypes are associated with hydrocephalus.
  - Severe micromelia: Patients with TD1 demonstrate severe curving of the femora and humeri, whereas patients with TD2 have short but relatively straight long bones.
  - Severe shortening of the metacarpals, metatarsals, and phalanges of hands and feet
  - Marked rib shortening, with thorax of small caliber

Treatment

- Supportive, palliative care
- Genetic counseling

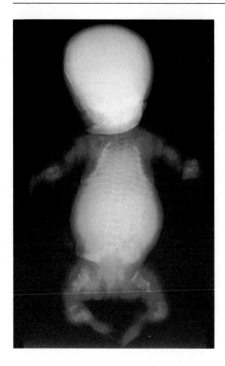

Figure 113D Osteogenesis imperfecta, type 2. Note the "crumpled" appearance of the markedly shortened long bones, due to innumerable antenatal fractures.

Prognosis

- Thanatophoric dysplasia is almost universally fatal. Most affected patients are stillborn, whereas live-born neonates usually succumb within the first week. Three patients with TD1 have been reported to survive until at least 9 years of age; all have been severely developmentally delayed, and all suffer from severe respiratory difficulties.

PEARLS

- TD is the most common lethal skeletal dysplasia, aside, perhaps, from osteogenesis imperfecta type 2, from which it is easily differentiated clinically and radiographically (**Fig. 113D**).
- Relatively large skull without craniosynostosis, with short and curved femora in a stillborn represents TD1.
- Cloverleaf or kleebattschädel skull (universal craniosynostosis) and short, relatively straight femora in a stillborn represent TD2.

PITFALLS

- Not all lethal skeletal dysplasias are TD or TD variants. Osteogenesis imperfecta type 2 is common and must be excluded.
- Some patients with TD1 may have a milder phenotype resembling achondroplasia. However, the latter patients thrive.

Suggested Readings

Baker KM, Olson DS, Harding CO, Pauli RM. Long-term survival in typical thanatophoric dysplasia type 1. Am J Med Genet 1997;70:427–436

Cohen MM. Some chondrodysplasias with short limbs: molecular perspectives. Am J Med Genet 2002;112:304–313

Nerlich AG, Freisinger P, Bonaventure J. Radiological and histological variants of thanatophoric dysplasia are associated with common mutations in FGFR-3. Am J Med Genet 1996;63:155–160

Tsai F-J, Tsai C-H, Chang J-G, Wu J-Y. Mutations in the fibroblast growth factor receptor 3 (FGFR3) cause achondroplasia, hypochondroplasia, and thanatophoric dysplasia: Taiwanese data. Am J Med Genet 1999;86:300–301

Wilcox WR, Tavorima PL, Krakow D, et al. Molecular, radiologic, and histopathologic correlations in thanatophoric dysplasia. Am J Med Genet 1998;78:274–281

CASE 114

Clinical Presentation

A young child presents with multiple bilateral painless, hard lumps adjacent to several joints. He also has mild limitation of wrist and elbow motion.

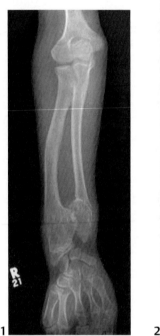 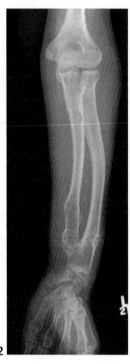

Figure 114A

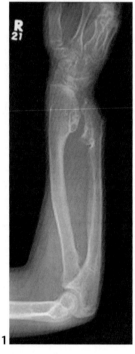 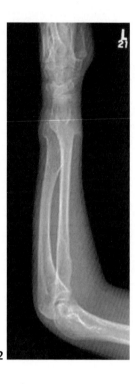

Figure 114B

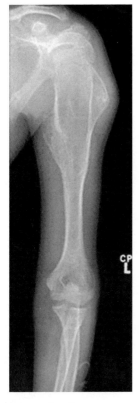

Figure 114C

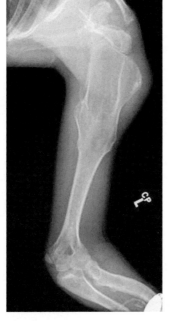

Figure 114D

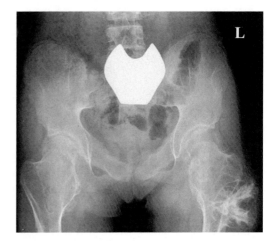

Figure 114E

Radiologic Findings

The tubular bone and modeling deformities shown in **Figs. 114A** to **114E** demonstrate metaphyseal broadening from multiple exostoses. Associated deformities of adjacent joints are present, including the distal radioulnar and radiocarpal joints. Note the variable appearance of the exostoses affecting the proximal humeri, femora, and ribs.

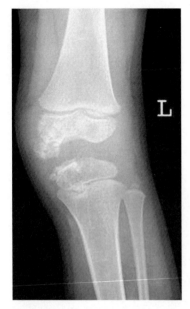

Figure 114F Frontal radiograph of the knee of a patient with Trevor disease showing enlargement of the distal femoral and proximal tibial epiphyses medially with irregularity in ossification.

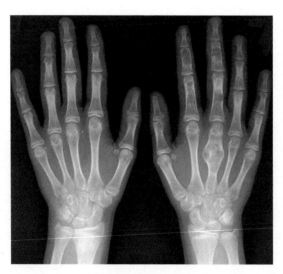

Figure 114G Hand radiograph of a patient with Ollier disease showing multiple enchondromatosis with expansion of the medullary space especially involving the left third metacarpal.

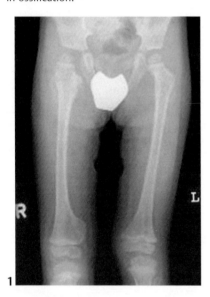

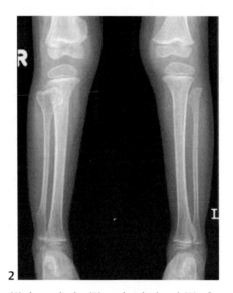

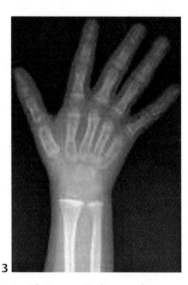

Figure 114H Radiographs of hip and femur (**1**), lower limbs (**2**), and right hand (**3**) of a patient with Langer-Giedion syndrome. Note the multiple exostoses of the right femur and fibula especially.

Diagnosis

Multiple hereditary exostoses (MHE) (osteochondromatosis, diaphyseal aclasis)

Differential Diagnosis

- Dysplasia epiphysealis hemimelica (Trevor disease) (**Fig. 114F**)
- Ollier disease (enchondromatosis) (**Fig. 114G**)
- Trichorhinophalangeal syndrome, type 2 (Langer-Giedion syndrome) (**Figs. 114H1** to **114H3**)

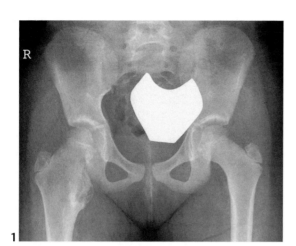
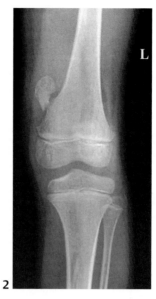

Figure 114I Two examples of isolated exostosis involving the right lesser trochanter (**1**) and distal femur (**2**).

- Sporadic, isolated osteochondromata (exostoses) (**Figs. 114I1** and **114I2**)
- Metachondromatosis

Discussion

Background

Multiple hereditary exostoses (MHE) is a common condition likely to be encountered in pediatric and adult radiology practices. Patients with MHE typically develop multiple painless juxta-articular masses in early childhood, often by the age of 2 years. These masses enlarge and become more numerous throughout childhood and typically cease growth with cessation of skeletal maturation (~16 years in females and 18 years in males). Patients with MHE experience symptoms due to the location, size, and growth of these masses, which consist of a cartilage cap of varying thickness overlying normal trabecular bone, with cortical continuity with adjacent normal bone.

Etiology

MHE consists of two subtypes, each of which demonstrates autosomal dominant transmission. Most cases are the result of spontaneous mutations. Point mutations in the gene *EXT1*, which encodes for exostosin-1, located on chromosome 8q24, produces the more phenotypically profound MHE subtype. Mutations in the *EXT2* gene, located on chromosome 11p11-p12, and which encodes for exostosin-2, produces a phenotypically milder subtype. Multiple point mutations for each subtype have been identified among different families.

Exostosin-1 and exostosin-2 are glycosyl transferases involved in the modulation of heparan sulfate biosynthesis and assembly, acting as suppressors. Defects in the *EXT1* and *EXT2* genes are "loss of function" mutations resulting in the development and growth of multiple exostoses (osteochondromata), due to the loss of this suppression activity. Improper assembly of heparan sulfate results in abnormal cartilage development and maturation.

Pathology/Histology

Exostoses are either sessile and broad-based or pedunculated and narrow-based. Both types may coexist within the same bone or the same area of an affected bone. The lesions consist of a cartilage cap of varying thickness overlying normal trabecular bone, which blend imperceptibly with surrounding trabeculae. The cortex and periosteum of the lesion also blend with surrounding cortical bone and periosteum. The lesions are typically located in a juxtaphyseal location in long bones and at variable locations within flat bones.

Clinical Findings

MHE is characterized by multiple painless, juxtaarticular masses that typically develop during early childhood. These lesions are bilateral and multifocal, and they may be symmetrical or asymmetrical in size and distribution. Some lesions produce limitation of joint motion and bursitis due to their juxtaarticular location. Growing lesions located in some areas (ribs, knees, wrists, vertebrae) may cause neurologic symptoms due to compression or deviation of adjacent neurovascular structures. Lesions in the popliteal fossa, ribs, and distal radius may cause pseudoaneurysms of adjacent arteries, with or without clinically symptomatic hemorrhage, due to abnormal friction. Males usually demonstrate a more severe phenotype than females.

Complications

- Short-term, intermediate-term, and long-term complications related to local orthopedic difficulties, such as limitation of joint motion, bursitis, and occasionally pseudoaneurysm formation, are nearly universal among patients with MHE.
- Significant long-term complications are related to malignant dedifferentiation of preexisting osteochondromas (almost exclusively into chondrosarcomas) as seen in 1 to 20% of patients.
- Common pseudo-Madelung deformity predisposes to wrist pain and limitation of motion.
- Vertebral involvement may produce pronounced scoliosis; focal osteochondromata may compress exiting nerve roots resulting in neuropathies.
- Local orthopedic complications due to lesion location (around large joints, within tubular bones of hand or flat bones of face/pelvis) are common.
- Pseudoaneurysm formation due to abnormal friction between an artery and adjacent exostosis may be seen in the popliteal fossa, axilla, wrist, and chest.
- Sarcomatous dedifferentiation of a preexisting osteochondroma into chondrosarcoma is seen in 1 to 20% of adult patients. The relative risk of each separate lesion is low, but as MHE patients have numerous exostoses, their overall risk is 1 to 20% over their life span. Any enlarging lesion in a patient who has achieved skeletal maturation, or the development of pain within a lesion, is suspicious for sarcomatous dedifferentiation. As many of these lesions are of low-grade, MRI is useful in assessing the thickness of the cartilaginous cap (usually >2 cm in chondrosarcomas) and the presence or absence of local invasion/spread.

Imaging Findings

RADIOGRAPHY

- Multiple metaphyseal sessile and/or pedunculated exostoses
- Asymmetric or symmetric
- Associated growth and joint deformity

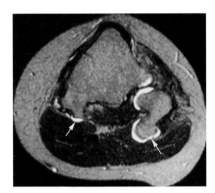

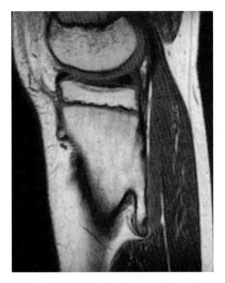

Figure 114J Axial gradient-echo sequence showing bright cartilage caps of exostoses involving the proximal tibia and fibula (arrows).

Figure 114K Parasagittal T1-weighted MRI showing large exostosis extending away from the knee in the posterior tibia.

ULTRASOUND

- Can show associated bursa and bursitis
- Can assess cartilaginous cap

CT

- Best for three-dimensional bony assessment
- Can evaluate complications, whether juxta-articular deformity, fracture, or malignant dedifferentiation

MRI

- Can visualize marrow extending into lesion (**Fig. 114J**)
- Best for associated soft tissue assessment including bursitis, compressive neuropathy, joint and physeal deformity, and pseudoaneurysm
- Can assess cartilaginous cap on cartilage sequence (**Fig. 114K**)

Treatment

- Orthopedic complications such as scoliosis and dislocations are often difficult to treat successfully, due to the progressive nature of the process during childhood and to lesion location.
- Large lesions, causing significant restriction of joint motion, and those causing pain may be resected.
- Scoliosis may be corrected using corrective bracing.

Prognosis

- Barring significant orthopedic complications in centrally located lesions, or malignant dedifferentiation of an exostosis, prognosis is for a normal life span.
- However, orthopedic complications, ranging from mild to significant, depending on the location and size of the lesions, are nearly universal.

- Long-term follow-up of these patients is mandatory, as 1 to 20% of patients will develop chondrosarcoma at the site of a preexisting exostosis.

PEARLS

- MHE is common; multiple painless, juxta-articular bony masses are most likely to represent MHE.
- Lesions grow throughout childhood, until physeal fusion.
- Lesions are common about the knees, shoulders, wrists, hips, and ankles.
- Both sessile and pedunculated lesions may be present within the same bone.
- Lesions point away from joints.

PITFALLS

- Simple isolated exostoses have identical radiographic appearance to those seen in MHE. It is the number and distribution that are suggestive of MHE.
- Not all patients with multiple exostoses have classic MHE. Patients with trichorhinophalangeal syndrome type 2 (TRP2) and patients with metachondromatosis manifest multiple exostoses; those in TRP2 point away from joints, whereas those in metachondromatosis generally point toward the joint.
- Occasionally, MHE may be mimicked by intraosseous expansile lesions in fibrous dysplasia, neurofibromatosis type 1, and proteus syndrome.

Suggested Readings

Taybi H. Lachman RS. Radiology of Syndromes, Metabolic Disorders and Skeletal Dysplasias. 4th ed. New York: Mosby-Year Book; 1996

MHE Coalition (online). Conference on Multiple Hereditary Exostoses. October 25–27, 2002. Phoenix, AZ

CASE 115

Clinical Presentation

A 16-month-old child presents with hypertelorism, an elongated, flattened forehead, and syndactyly of hands and feet.

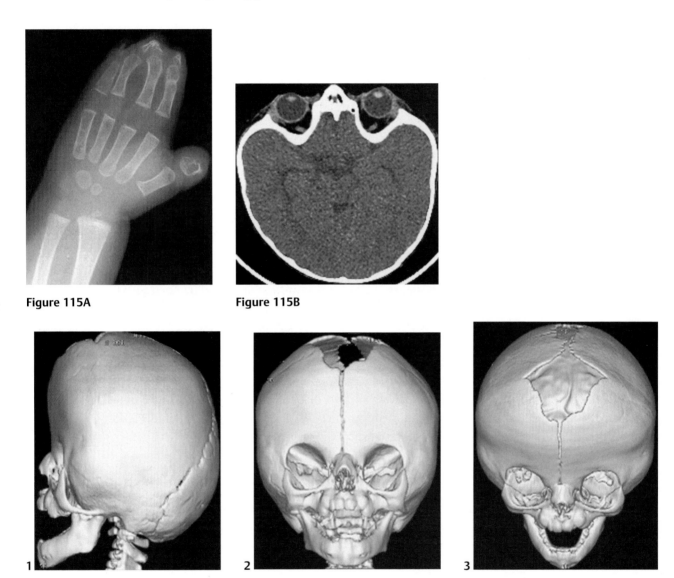

Figure 115A

Figure 115B

Figure 115C

Radiologic Findings

Radiograph of the left hand (**Fig. 115A**) demonstrates the characteristic "mitten hand" deformity, with hypoplasia of the first, third, and fourth metacarpals, abnormally short and wide first proximal "delta" phalanx, and symphalangism (i.e., syndactyly/ankylosis of the finger or toe joints) of second through fourth rays, with soft tissue syndactyly of the second through fifth rays. The right hand demonstrated an identical appearance. The anterior fontanelle is widely patent. There is synostosis of the coronal sutures, hypertelorism, and flattening and downward slanting of the shallow bony orbits (**Figs. 115B, and 115C**).

567

Diagnosis

Apert syndrome (acrocephalosyndactyly type 1)

Differential Diagnosis

- Carpenter syndrome
- Pfeiffer syndrome
- Saethre-Chotzen syndrome
- Crouzon syndrome
- Rubinstein-Taybi syndrome
- Amniotic band syndrome
- Isolated familial syndactyly syndromes

Discussion

Background

Many syndromes and conditions include abnormalities of both the craniofacial structures and the limbs. Patients with syndactyly, distal limb abnormalities, and craniosynotosis most often suffer from acrocephalosyndactyly. Of the specific entities within this grouping, Apert syndrome is the most common. The association between syndactyly and craniosynostosis was first described by Apert in 1906.

Etiology

Apert syndrome shows autosomal dominant heritance, but nearly all cases result from new gene mutations. The incidence of Apert syndrome in the general population is ~1 in 160,000 live births.

Apert syndrome appears to be caused by either of two distinct point mutations in fibroblast growth factor receptor 2 (FGFR2). Close phenotypic mimics are Crouzon syndrome and Pfeiffer syndrome, both of which are also caused by mutations in FGFR2.

Clinical Findings

Apert syndrome may be diagnosed prenatally and presents clinically at birth. Cranial findings seen in affected infants include a flattened, elongated forehead, turribrachycephaly, hypertelorism, exophthalmos, a bulbous nose, and a flattened nasal bridge. Nasopharyngeal obstruction is seen in 50%, due to midface hypoplasia. The orbits show downward slanting. Most patients demonstrate at least mild prognathism.

The hands are remarkable for bilaterally symmetric cutaneous syndactyly of the second through fifth rays (mitten hand). Nail fusion is common. The first ray is usually separate but abnormal, showing radial bowing of a shortened, widened thumb. The feet usually demonstrate complete simple syndactyly ("stocking foot"), often with fusion of the nails.

Older children usually demonstrate at least mild developmental delay. Variable ankylosis of large joints is common in older patients. Some patients may develop hydrocephalus and require ventriculoperitoneal shunting; however, no other systemic abnormalities are associated with this condition.

Complications

- Some patients develop progressive hydrocephalus, requiring ventriculoperitoneal shunting.

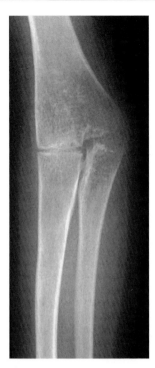 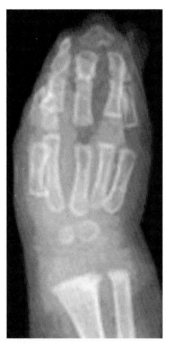 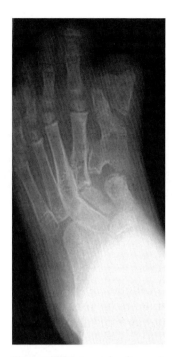

Figure 115D Frontal radiograph of right elbow demonstrating early ankylosis of radiocapitellar joint.

Figure 115E Frontal radiograph of right hand showing "mitten hand" deformity. The third proximal and middle phalanges are short and fused at the level of the obliterated proximal interphalangeal joint level (symphangilism). The fourth ray demonstrates a similar appearance.

Figure 115F Frontal radiograph of the left foot demonstrates a first proximal "delta" phalanx, with an obliquely oriented proximal physis. The first distal phalanx is radially angulated. Note bizarre partial duplication of first metatarsal and fusion of the second and third metatarsals to their corresponding cuneiforms.

Imaging Findings

RADIOGRAPHY

- Cranium:
  - Coronal sutural synostosis in 100%, lambdoid synostosis in 79%
  - Hypertelorism
  - High-arching palate, ± cleft
  - Widely patent metopic and sagittal sutures; large anterior fontanelle
  - Cervical vertebral fusions are common.
- Appendicular skeleton:
  - Shallow glenoid fossae
  - Variable ankylosis of large joints (**Fig. 115D**)
  - Hands show first proximal "delta" phalanx (short and wide, with an oblique to vertical physis), with resultant radial deviation of first distal phalanx.
  - Symphangilism (fusion of phalanges without demonstrable interphalangeal joints) of second through fifth rays of the hands and feet is common (**Fig. 115E**).
  - Cutaneous syndactyly of second through fifth rays of the hand (mitten hand)
  - Some patients demonstrate distal phalangeal bony synostosis.
  - Feet are remarkable for universal cutaneous syndactyly, symphangilism, and a first proximal delta phalanx (**Fig. 115F**).
  - Supernumerary tarsal bones are common, with older patients demonstrating variable hindfoot tarsal coalitions.

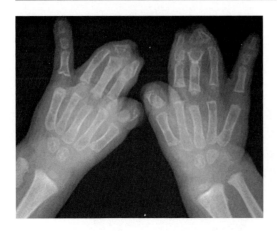

Figure 115G Frontal radiographs of both hands following first stage of phalangeal separation. The fifth ray has been separated from the fourth ray. Note persistent bony and soft tissue syndactyly of the second through fourth rays. Characteristic first proximal "delta" phalanx is present.

CT

- Dilatation of the lateral ventricles and prominence of extraaxial cerebrospinal fluid spaces are quite common; rarely require shunting prior to craniofacial surgery.
- Shallow anterior cranial fossa, with fusion of lesser wings of sphenoid creating a constricting "ring"
- Shallow, widened bony orbits with resultant proptosis.
- Hypertelorism.
- Coronal and often lambdoid synostosis, with delayed midline sutural fusion.
- Midface hypoplasia, usually with at least mild prognathism.
- High-arched hard palate.
- Tarsal coalitions are well evaluated with CT.

Treatment

- Some patients require tracheostomy due to nasopharyngeal obstruction secondary to midface hypoplasia.
- Digital separation procedures on the hands, to provide increased functionality, are best performed prior to age 3 (**Fig. 115G**).
- The feet are functional without digital separation, but they may require corrective surgery for symptomatic tarsal coalitions later in life.
- Craniofacial procedures to correct craniosynostosis and proptosis include sutural excision, cranial remodeling, and fronto-orbital advancement.

PEARL_____

- Constellation of distal appendicular fusion anomalies and craniosynostosis is highly suggestive of Apert syndrome.

PITFALLS_____

- Not all patients with acrocephalosyndactyly have Apert syndrome; however, Apert syndrome is the most common and severe condition in this category.
- Carpenter syndrome (acrocephalopolysyndactyly) is phenotypically quite similar, except for presence of supernumerary digits.

Suggested Readings

Apert ME. De l'acrocephalosyndactylie. Bull Mem Soc Med Hop Paris 1906;23:1310–1330

Cinalli G, Sainte-Rose C, Kollar EM, et al. Hydrocephalus and craniosynostosis. J Neurosurg 1998; 88:209–214

Cohen MM Jr. Short-limb skeletal dysplasias and craniosynostosis: what do they have in common? Pediatr Radiol 1997;27:442–446

Collins ED, Marsh JL, Vannier MW, Gilula LA. Spatial dysmorphology of the foot in Apert syndrome: three-dimensional computed tomography. Cleft Palate Craniofac J 1995;32:255–261

Gosain AK, Moore FO, Hemmy DC. The Kleebattschädl anomaly in Apert syndrome: intracranial anatomy, surgical correction, and subsequent cranial vault development. Plast Reconstr Surg 1997;100:1796–1802

Kreiborg S, Cohen MM Jr. The infant Apert skull. Neurosurg Clin N Am 1991;2:551–554

Marsh JL, Galic M, Vannier MW. The craniofacial anatomy of Apert syndrome. Clin Plast Surg 1991;18:237–249

Schauerte EW, St.-Aubin PM. Progressive synosteosis in Apert's syndrome (acrocephalosyndactyly) with a description of the roentgenographic changes in the feet. Am J Roentgenol Radium Ther Nucl Med 1966;97:67–73

CASE 116

Clinical Presentation

A 5-year-old female presents with right hip pain.

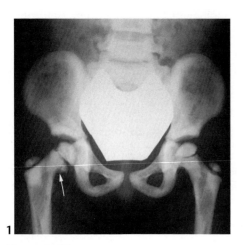
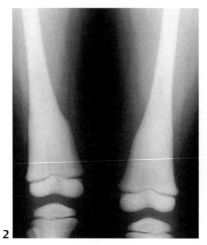

Figure 116A

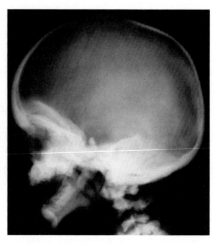

Figure 116B

Radiologic Findings

The frontal radiograph of the pelvis and femurs demonstrates a fracture of the proximal right femoral metaphysis (**Fig. 116A1**, arrow). There is underlying diffuse increased bone density and "Erlenmeyer flask" deformity of the distal femoral metaphyses (**Fig. 116A2**). The lateral x-ray of the skull shows diffuse thickening and increased density, which is most marked at the skull base (**Fig. 116B**).

Diagnosis

Osteopetrosis (Albers-Schönberg disease)

Differential Diagnosis

- Pyknodystostosis
  - Dense bones with Erlenmeyer flask deformity
  - Differentiating features include acrosteolysis, wormian bones, and loss of the normal antegonal angle of the mandible.
- Dysosteosclerosis
  - Short stature, osteosclerosis, and blindness due to compression of the optic nerve foramina
  - Differentiating features include platyspondyly and lucency of the metaphyses.
- Osteopathia striata
  - Cranial sclerosis and cranial nerve paralysis
  - Differentiating feature, osteosclerosis, has a vertically oriented striated appearance.
- Renal osteodystrophy
  - Dense bones with "rugger jersey" spine; may have rickets
  - Differentiating feature: absence of Erlenmeyer flask deformity

Discussion

Background and Classification

Osteopetrosis is a genetic disorder, which is characterized by generalized increased density of the bones. Osteopetrosis is commonly classified into three types by age of presentation. The *infantile malignant autosomal recessive form* presents as severe anemia with failure to thrive, and it is fatal within the first few years of life in the absence of effective treatment, that is, bone marrow transplant. The *intermediate autosomal recessive form* is milder, and it appears in the first decade of life. Clinical findings include short stature, anemia, and hepatomegaly. The *adult benign autosomal dominant form* is usually asymptomatic with full life expectancy and may have orthopedic complications such as fractures and osteomyelitis.

Etiology

Osteopetrosis is a sclerosing bone dysplasia due to failure of bone resorption as a consequence of dysfunctional osteoclasts. The osteoclasts do not respond normally to parathyroid hormone, and resorption of endochondral cartilage is markedly diminished, whereas bone formation occurs at a normal rate.

Some cases of osteopetrosis are caused by carbonic anhydrase II deficiency. This enzyme is present in bone cells and is activated by parathyroid hormone to promote bone resorption by facilitating the secretion of hydrogen ions. Therefore, a deficiency in carbonic anhydrase impairs bone resorption.

Clinical Findings

The major clinical features of osteopetrosis include anemia, thrombocytopenia, and hepatosplenomegaly due to extramedullary hematopoiesis. This is secondary to crowding of the bone marrow cavity from osteosclerosis. Pathologic fractures occur due to increased fragility of bone. This is secondary to unresorbed medullary bone and persistence of mechanically inferior calcified cartilage. Cranial

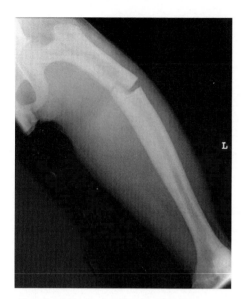

Figure 116C Frontal radiograph of left femur showing increased bone density with coxa vara deformity and femoral shaft fracture as a complication of osteopetrosis.

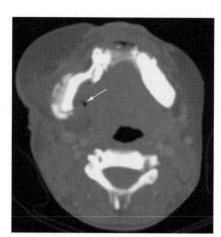

Figure 116D Axial CT shows destruction and periosteal reaction of the right mandible with associated soft tissue swelling and a small gas bubble (arrow) secondary to osteomyelitis.

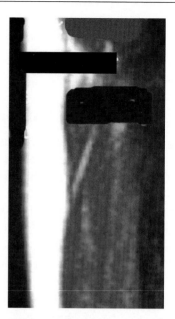

Figure 116E Frontal radiograph of hand shows diffuse, increased bone density with metaphyseal flaring and fraying in a patient with osteopetrosis complicated by rickets.

nerve palsies may result in blindness, deafness, and facial paralysis due to compression of the neural foramina.

Complications

- Fractures (**Fig. 116C**)
- Coxa vara deformity and bowing of long bones
- Pancytopenia with bleeding and infection
- Osteomyelitis: Most common site of osteomyelitis is the mandible, and it can be bilateral (**Fig. 116D**).
- Lymphoproliferative disease: leukemia, non-Hodgkin's lymphoma
- Rickets due to the inability of the osteoclasts to maintain a normal calcium–phosphorus balance (**Fig. 116E**)
- Hydrocephalus
- Narrowing of the neural foramina: may lead to optic atrophy and blindness

Gross Pathology and Biochemistry

Morphologic changes are most marked in the metaphyses. They include thickened primary trabeculae due to failure of resorption of primary spongiosa. There is narrowing and fibrosis of the marrow spaces with virtually no normal marrow tissue present. Biochemical abnormalities include elevated acid phosphatase levels.

Histology

Iliac crest bone biopsy is used to quantitate osteoclasts and assess bone marrow content by light microscopy. The size, number, and nucleation of osteoclasts are increased in osteopetrosis. On

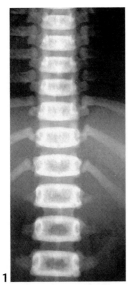 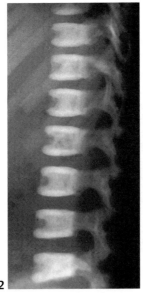

Figure 116F Frontal (**1**) and lateral (**2**) x-rays of thoracic lumbar spine show diffuse sclerosis of the vertebral bodies most marked along the end plates resulting in "sandwich" vertebrae.

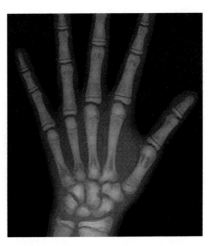

Figure 116G Frontal x-ray showing bone-in-bone appearance. These endobones are best seen in the small tubular bones of the hand.

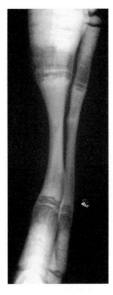

Figure 116H Frontal x-ray of tibia and fibula showing "Erlenmeyer flask" deformity with alternating horizontal and lucent bands of sclerosis.

electron microscopy, osteoclasts lack the normal ruffled border whereas the clear zone is markedly decreased or absent.

Imaging Findings

RADIOGRAPHY

- Generalized increased density of the skeleton (osteosclerosis)
- Lack of differentiation of bone cortex and medulla
- "Sandwich" vertebrae (**Figs. 116F1** and **116F2**)
- Bone in bone (**Fig. 116G**)
- Sclerotic horizontal striations of metaphyses
- Erlenmeyer flask deformity (**Fig. 116H**)
- Delayed skeletal maturation

PRENATAL ULTRASOUND

- Fractures
- Macrocephaly
- Hydrocephalus
- Increased echogenicity of bones

CT

- Bone sclerosis
- Hepatosplenomegaly
- Extramedullary hematopoiesis
- Narrowed cranial nerve foramina (**Fig. 116I**)
- Hydrocephalus

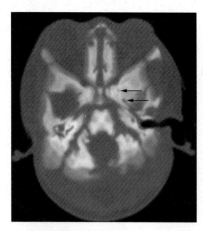

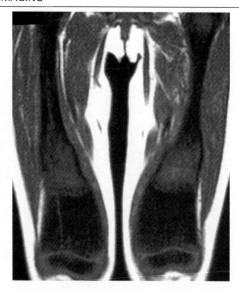

Figure 116I Axial CT of the head with bone windows. The skull base shows sclerosis with narrowing of the neural foramina (arrows).

Figure 116J Coronal T1-weighted MRI of both femurs showing bilateral diffuse low signal replacing the normal bone marrow signal due to osteosclerosis.

- Cortical atrophy
- Basal ganglia calcification with carbonic anhydrase deficiency

MRI

- Bone marrow is often low signal on all sequences due to sclerosis (**Fig. 116J**).
- Hyperintense regions on T1-weighted images in basal ganglia, thalami, and red nuclei.

BONE DENSITOMETRY

- Bone mineral density in osteopetrosis is 4 to 5 times higher than the mean for normal age and gender-matched controls.

Treatment

- Low calcium, high phosphate diet
- Steroids for hematologic complications
- High-dose calcitriol to stimulate osteoclasts and bone resorption
- Interferon increases bone resorption and hematopoiesis and improves leukocyte function.
- Bone marrow transplantation provides monocytes, which are osteoclast precursors. It is the only curative therapy and is utilized for the autosomal recessive forms of osteopetrosis. Bone marrow engraftment can be assessed with MRI.

Prognosis

- Depends on the type of osteopetrosis (see Discussion)

PEARLS

- Patients presenting with refractory or bilateral osteomyelitis of the jaw should be suspected of having osteopetrosis.
- Bone marrow transplantation results in resolution of sclerosis and skeletal deformities with normal bone mineral density within 3 years.

PITFALLS_____

- Despite the increased density of bones in osteopetrosis, there is increased bone fragility.
- Osteopetrosis complicated by rickets further increases bone fragility.

Suggested Readings

Greenspan A. Sclerosing bone dysplasias: a target-site approach. Skeletal Radiol 1991;20:561–583

Shapira F. Osteopetrosis: current clinical considerations. Clin Orthop & Rel Res 1993;294:34–44

Vanhoenacker FM, De Beuckeleer LH, Hul WV, et al. Sclerosing bone dysplasias: genetic and radio-clinical features. Eur Radiol 2000;10:1423–1433

CASE 117

Clinical Presentation

A newborn male presents with flattening of the nasal bridge, mild respiratory distress, and unusually short, broad distal phalanges of the hands and feet.

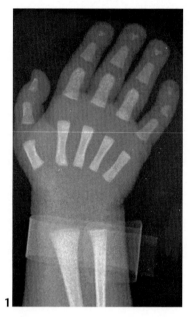

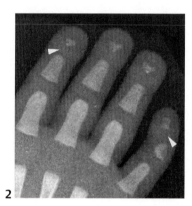

Figure 117A

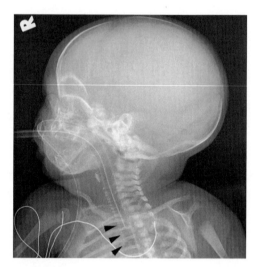

Figure 117B

Radiologic Findings

The AP radiograph of the hand shows abnormal morphology of the second through fourth distal phalanges, with distal broadening, proximal narrowing, and shortening of the tufts (**Fig. 117A1**), with puncta at the distal phalangeal epiphyses (**Fig. 117A2**, arrowheads). Dramatic calcification of the tracheal cartilaginous rings is seen on the oblique neck and upper chest radiograph (**Fig. 117B**, arrowheads).

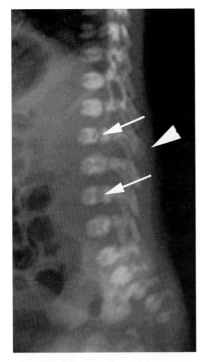

Figure 117C

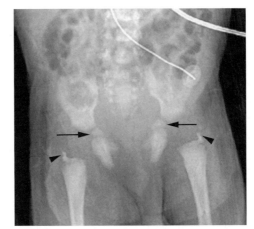

Figure 117D

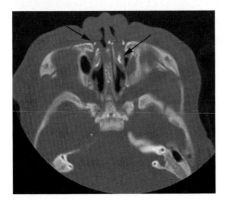

Figure 117E

The lateral view of the vertebral column shows several coronal clefts (**Fig. 117C,** arrows) and puncta at the tips of the spinous processes (**Fig. 117C,** arrowhead). The pelvic radiograph demonstrates characteristic calcific puncta within the triradiate cartilages (arrows) and greater trochanteric apophyses (arrowheads), as well as dramatic paraspinal puncta (**Fig. 117D**). CT of the nasal passage shows puncta within the nasal alae and septal cartilage (arrows), as well as severe choanal narrowing (**Fig. 117E**).

Diagnosis

Chondrodysplasia punctata (CDP), brachytelephalangic subtype (CDP-BT)

Differential Diagnosis

The most significant entities in the differential diagnosis for stippled epiphyses in the newborn are:

- Conradi-Hünermann syndrome (CDP–X-linked dominant, CDP–X-linked recessive) (**Fig. 117F**)
- Rhizomelic chondrodysplasia punctata (CDPR) (**Fig. 117G**)
- I-cell disease (shown in an older child, **Fig. 117H**)
- GM$_1$ gangliosidosis (**Fig. 117I**)
- Zellweger syndrome (**Figs. 117J** and **117K**)
- Antenatal warfarin exposure
- Brachytelephalangic chondrodysplasia punctata

Discussion

Background

For most radiologists, the differential diagnosis of punctate, stippled epiphyses is limited to a few entities, usually Conradi-Hünermann syndrome, Zellweger syndrome, and "chondrodysplasia punctata." However, to paraphrase Dr. Poznanski, CDP is a radiologic sign, not a distinct disease entity (Poznanski 1994). Indeed, the list of conditions associated with epiphyseal punctate calcifications is actually quite extensive and includes skeletal dysplasias, isolated single gene defects, inborn errors of metabolism, chromosomal trisomies/deletions, teratogenic exposures, infections, endocrinopathies, and maternal disorders (**Table 117A**).

Etiology

The pathogenesis of epiphyseal and extraskeletal cartilaginous calcific stippling has been best studied in a rat model of warfarin embryopathy. Rats administered warfarin produce offspring with premature punctate calcification of the nasal septum and snout, with resultant shortening and narrowing of the nasal passages. They also demonstrate abnormal calcific bridges within the physes of long bones and vertebrae. Within the nasal septum and epiphyses, chondrocytes are decreased in number and are abnormally clustered, demonstrating a disorganized pattern with premature punctate calcification within their surrounding matrix. These observations were confirmed by Barr and Burdi (1976) in their study of a human fetus with warfarin embryopathy.

Similar findings have been reported in histologic analysis of human patients with CDPR. These patients demonstrate clumps of disorganized epiphyseal chondrocytes separated by abnormal fibromuscular tissue containing punctate calcifications. Gaulier and colleagues (1987) reported similar findings in a patient with classic Conradi-Hünermann syndrome (CDP-XD); this patient also showed intramural calcification within epiphyseal vascular channels. Two reports of auricular biopsies in patients with Keutel syndrome (Keutel, 1972) describe multifocal, abnormal, progressive cartilaginous ossification. However, there has been no evidence to suggest that focal cartilaginous hemorrhage causes epiphyseal stippling in any of these disorders.

Matrix GLA protein (MGP) is produced by cartilage and is found in all noncalcified cartilaginous tissues. When properly carboxylated, its function is to inhibit hydroxyapatite formation

Table 117A Disorders Associated with Punctate Epiphyses

	Types
Single Gene Disorders and Skeletal Dysplasias	Acrodysostosis
	Adams-Oliver syndrome
	Astley-Kendall dysplasia
	Binder facies
	CDP-BT
	CDP-TM
	Conradi-Hünermann syndrome (CDP-XD, CDP-XR)
	Cerebrocostomandibular dysplasia
	Greenberg dysplasia
	CHILD syndrome (congential hemidysplasia with ichthyosiform erythroderma and limb defects)
	Dappled diaphyseal dysplasia
	Deafness, goiter, stippled epiphyses
	De Barsy syndrome
	de Lange syndrome
	Ichthyosis, hypogonadism
	Keutel syndrome
	Pacman dysplasia
Chromosomal Disorders	Trisomy 9
	Trisomy 13
	Trisomy 18
	Trisomy 21
	Various deletions
	X:Y translocation
	Triploidy 69XXX/XXY
	Turner syndrome (46XO)
Maternal Disorders	Vitamin K deficiency
	Systemic lupus erythematous (SLE)
Intrauterine Infections	Rubella
	Cytomegalovirus
	Listeria
Teratogens	Warfarin
	Ethanol
	Diphenylhydantoin
	Phenacetin
	Vitamin K antagonists
Inborn Errors of Metabolism	CDPR
	I-cell disease
	GM_1 gangliosidosis
	Galactosialidosis
	Niemann-Pick disease
	Vitamin K epoxide reductase deficiency
	Metachromatic leukodystrophy
	Smith-Lemli-Opitz syndrome
	Zellweger syndrome

within cartilage. Inactive, decarboxylated MGP is found in the nasal and epiphyseal cartilage of warfarin-treated rats; perhaps poor or absent MGP carboxylation represents the end result of numerous divergent metabolic pathways that produce the phenotype of chondrodysplasia punctata.

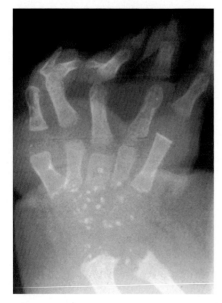

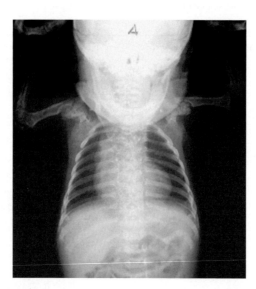

Figure 117F Right hand in a patient with CDP-XD Conradi-Hünermann syndrome, demonstrating carpal puncta and severe but variable metacarpal shortening due to punctate epiphyses. This is much more severe than the pattern seen in CDP-BT.

Figure 117G Radiographs showing severe rhizomelic shortening of the humeri, with dramatic proximal epiphyseal puncta. Such severe rhizomelic shortening is characteristic of CDPR and is not seen in CDP-BT.

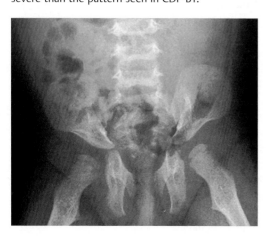

Figure 117H Pelvis in a patient with I-cell disease showing characteristic features of "dysostosis multiplex," with flaring of iliac wings and steep acetabular roofs. This is not a feature of CDP-BT.

Clinical Findings

- CDP-BT is relatively uncommon and is due to an X-linked recessive defect in arylsulfatase E (ARSE) synthesis; mapped to the Xp22.32 locus.
- Clinically present with nasal flattening and hypoplasia, as well as mild to severe respiratory distress
- Skeletal and extraskeletal calcific stippling is seen at birth, with no additional puncta forming postnatally.
- Patients demonstrate brachytelephalangy, with stippling at the epiphyses of most to all distal phalanges, with an "inverted triangle" appearance early; older children demonstrate shortened, broad distal phalanges due to early physeal fusion.
- Calcific puncta are commonly seen in vertebrae and paravertebral tissues, proximal and distal femora, triradiate cartilage of acetabula, proximal tibiae, tarsals, trachea, nasal septum, and nasal alae.

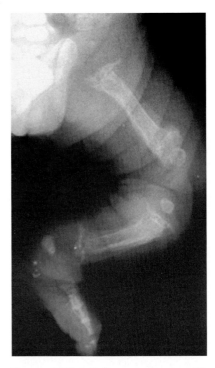

Figure 117I Left lower extremity with severe osteopenia, bowing, and tarsal puncta in a patient with GM$_1$ gangliosidosis. These findings are not seen in CDP-BT.

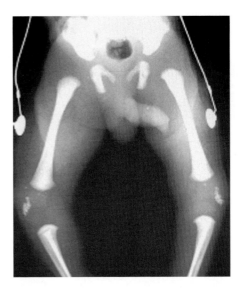

Figure 117J Lower extremities in a patient with Zellweger syndrome showing characteristic patellar puncta, not seen in CDP-BT.

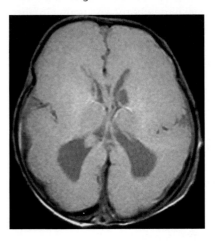

Figure 117K Zellweger syndrome. Proton density MRI shows subependymal cysts.

Complications

- Skeletal puncta are gradually incorporated into the surrounding, developing bone, usually becoming inapparent by 2 years of age. However, affected bones subsequently demonstrate slight alterations in morphology and in longitudinal growth.
- Vertebral and paravertebral puncta, as well as coronal and sagittal clefts, often result in scoliosis and/or kyphosis due to asymmetrical growth.
- Most patients with CDP-BT demonstrate at least mild short stature.
- Extraskeletal cartilaginous calcification also may produce significant long-term sequelae.
- Nasal hypoplasia and flattening may cause functionally appreciable nasal aperture and choanal stenosis, whereas dense tracheal calcification impairs circumferential growth, resulting in long-segment, fixed airway narrowing of potential clinical significance.

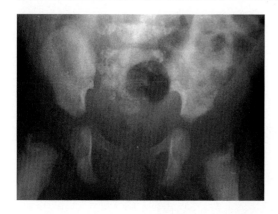

Figure 117L AP view of pelvis in an infant male with CDP-BT showing characteristic puncta involving greater trochanteric apophyses and triradiate cartilages.

Pathology

The pathologic aberration involved in CDP includes abnormal clumps of calcification within epiphyseal and extraskeletal cartilage, resulting in growth restriction.

Imaging Findings

RADIOGRAPHY

- Abnormal inverted triangle appearance of distal phalanges of hands and feet. Calcific puncta are seen at the distal phalangeal epiphyses in the newborn and young infant.
- Older children and adults show shortened, broadened distal phalanges, with early physeal fusion.
- Characteristic epiphyseal and apophyseal calcific stippling is seen only in newborns and young infants.
- Calcific puncta are seen at triradiate cartilage of pelvis, greater trochanterix apophyses, and in the paraspinal region.
- Coronal and sagittal vertebral clefts are seen in newborns and young infants.

CT

- Flattened nasal bridge
- Choanal narrowing
- Abnormal calcific stippling of cartilage of nasal alae and septum
- Abnormal calcification of tracheal cartilages

Treatment

- The most significant problem in affected infants is respiratory insufficiency.
- Severe choanal narrowing may require intervention.
- Tracheal cartilaginous calcifications result in poor growth of tracheal rings with resultant narrowing.
- Some patients have required tracheoplasty.

Prognosis

- Patients with CDP-BT have a normal life expectancy and suffer only from choanal narrowing.
- However, prognosis is variable for patients with other subtypes of CDP and depends on the specific entity.

PEARLS_____

- Universal brachytelephalangy is highly suggestive of CDP-BT; it may be seen in warfarin exposure and vitamin K epoxide reductase deficiency.
- Puncta of the triradiate cartilages and greater trochanters is characteristic of CDP-BT (**Fig. 117L**).
- CDP-BT is seen only in males (X-linked recessive).
- Long bones are not shortened in infancy.

PITFALLS_____

- The differential diagnosis is extensive (**Table 117A**).
- Nasal flattening may be seen in various ethnic groups; however, these individuals do not exhibit respiratory distress.
- Some patients may not demonstrate universal brachytelephalangy; in these patients, the differential diagnosis includes Keutel syndrome; CDP, tibial-metacarpal subtype (CDP-TM); and CDP-XD/XR.

Suggested Readings

Agamanolis DP, Novak RW. Rhizomelic chondrodysplasia punctata: report of a case with review of the literature and correlation with other peroxisomal disorders. Pediatr Pathol Lab Med 1995; 15:503–513

Barr M Jr, Burdi AR. Warfarin-associated embryopathy in a 17-week-old abortus. Teratology 1976; 14:129–134

Gaulier A, Chastagner C, Leloc'h H, Babin C. Lethal chondrodysplasia punctata, Conradi-Hunermann subtype A, one case. Pathol Res Pract 1987;182:72–79

Howe AM, Webster WS. The warfarin embryopathy: a rat model showing maxillonasal hypoplasia and other skeletal disturbances. Teratology 1992;46:379–390

International nomenclature of constitutional disorders of bone. International Skeletal Dysplasia Registry, 2001. ISDR is maintained Cedars-Sinai Hospital, Los Angeles, CA.

Keutel J, Jorgensen G, Gabriel P. A new autosomal recessive syndrome: peripheral pulmonary stenoses, brachytelephalangism, neural hearing loss and abnormal cartilage calcifications/ossification. Birth Defects 1972;5:60–68

Khosroshahi HE, Uluoglu O, Olgunturk R, Basaklar C. Keutel syndrome: a report of four cases. Eur J Pediatr 1989;149:188–191

Maroteaux P. Brachytelephalangic chondrodysplasia punctata: a possible X-linked recessive form. Hum Genet 1989;82:167–170

Patel M, Callahan J, Zhang S, et al. Early infantile galactosialidosis: prenatal presentation and post-natal follow-up. Am J Med Genet 1999;85:38–47

Poulos A, Sheffield L, Sharp P, et al. Rhizomelic chondrodysplasia punctata: clinical, pathologic, and biochemical findings in two patients. J Pediatr 1988;113:685–690

Poznanski AK. Punctate epiphyses: a radiological sign not a disease. Pediatr Radiol 1994;24:418–424

Taybi H, Lachman RS. Radiology of Syndromes, Metabolic Disorders, and Skeletal Dysplasias. 4th ed. St. Louis: Mosby; 1996.

CASE 118

Clinical Presentation

A young child presents with mild kyphosis, symmetrical short stature, coarsened facial features, and developmental delay.

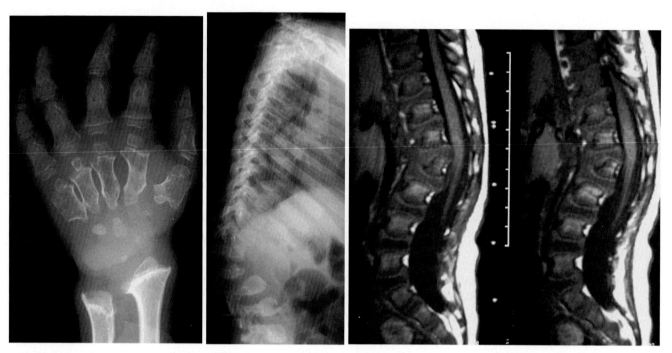

Figure 118A　　　　　　Figure 118B　　　　Figure 118C

Radiologic Findings

Frontal radiograph (**Fig. 118A**) of the hand demonstrates shortened metacarpals and phalanges. There is marked proximal tapering of metacarpals and distal phalangeal tapering. The distal radial and ulnar metaphyses are widened and irregular. All epiphyses demonstrate a bizarre, irregular appearance. Lateral view of the chest and spine (**Fig. 118B**) demonstrates broad, "oar"-shaped ribs, short and thick clavicles, rounded scapulae, and osteopenia. There is a gibbus (abnormal, abrupt kyphosis) deformity at the thoracolumbar junction, due to a pronounced anteroinferior beak at L2. Note the appearance of the gibbus with anterosuperior hypoplasia of L2 on sagittal T1-weighted MRI (**Fig. 118C**).

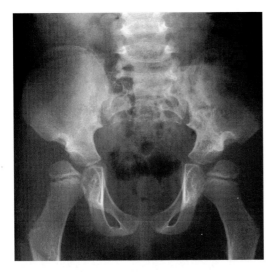

Figure 118D

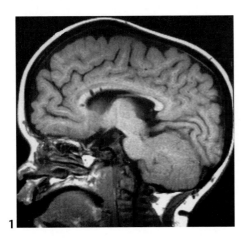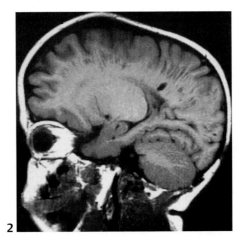

Figure 118E

Frontal radiograph of the pelvis shows abnormally steep acetabular roofs, flared, constricted iliac wings, and moderate bilateral coxa valga (**Fig. 118D**). Parasagittal and midline sagittal T1-weighted MR image of the brain demonstrate frontal bossing and abnormal soft tissue posterior to the dens, causing mild extradural impression on the thecal sac and cervical cord at C1 (**Fig. 118E**). Hypointense rounded foci are seen within the corpus callosum. The sella is J-shaped. Axial T2-weighted image (**Fig. 118F**) shows prominent perivascular Virchow-Robin spaces and delayed white matter myelination.

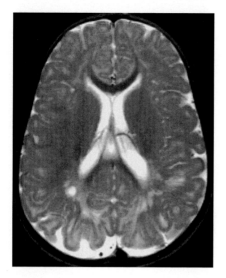

Figure 118F

Diagnosis

Hurler syndrome (mucopolysaccharidosis IH; MPS-IH)

Differential Diagnosis

- Hunter syndrome
- Scheie syndrome
- Morquio syndrome
- Other MPS subtypes
- Mucolipidoses

Discussion

Background

Hurler syndrome (MPS-IH) is but one of a group of phenotypically related conditions, often collectively termed *mucopolysaccharidoses*, that are caused by specific lysosomal enzymatic deficiencies. The enzymatic deficiencies render the lysosomes incapable of catabolizing particular subregions of complex intracellular glycosaminoglycans, resulting in intracellular and extracellular accumulation of these substances. The various entities in this broad disease category result in the intralysosomal accumulation of dermatan sulfate, chondroitin sulfate, heparan sulfate, and keratan sulfate, either specifically or in combination (**Table 118A**). Phenotypically, most of the entities in this category produce radiographically and clinically similar patterns, and are best diagnosed definitively via urinalysis and cultured leukocyte or fibroblast enzymatic assays. With the exception of Hunter syndrome, all demonstrate autosomal recessive inheritance.

The mucopolysaccharidoses produce a variable radiographic constellation of characteristic findings termed *dysostosis multiplex*. It is important to remember that this is a descriptive and generic term, not a diagnosis in and of itself. Dysostosis multiplex consists of variable proximal metacarpal tapering, anterior vertebral beaking, acetabular roof hypoplasia, diploic thickening, thoracolumbar gibbus formation, broadening of ribs, and short stature. The separate entities differ in the presence

Table 118A   Mucopolysaccharidoses

Type	Common Eponym	Enzymatic Defect
IH	Hurler syndrome	a-L-iduronidase
IHS	Hurler-Scheie syndrome	a-L-iduronidase
IS	Scheie syndrome	a-L-iduronidase
II	Hunter syndrome	Iduronidate sulfatase
IIIA	Sanfilippo syndrome, type A	Heparan sulfate sulfaminidase
IIIB	Sanfilippo syndrome, type B	a-N-acetyl-D glucosaminidase
IIIC	Sanfilippo syndrome, type C	Glucosamine-N-acetyl transferase
IIID	Sanfilippo syndrome, type D	N-acetyl glucosamine-6-sulfatase
IVA	Morquio syndrome, type A	N-acetyl glucosamine-6-sulfatase
IVB	Morquio syndrome, type B	Keratin sulfate galactosidase
VI	Maroteaux-Lamy syndrome	N-acetyl-galactosamine-4-sulfatase
VIII	Sly syndrome	a-glucuronidase

or absence of neurodevelopmental delay, severity of skeletal deformities, and associated extraskeletal comorbidities.

Etiology

Hurler syndrome (MPS-IH) is caused by the deficiency of α-L-iduronidase, an enzyme required for the degradation of dermatan sulfate and keratan sulfate. These compounds accumulate within intracellular lysosomes and are also found in extracellular tissues. These compounds are also excreted by the kidney and may be assayed for diagnostics.

Hurler syndrome is an autosomal recessive condition, as are all entities in the MPS category, with the exception of Hunter's syndrome, which is an X-linked recessive condition. Hurler syndrome is the most prevalent of the MPS subtypes, seen in 1 in 100,000 live births.

Clinical Findings

Although diagnosable in utero through amniocentesis, patients without a family history of Hurler syndrome are usually diagnosed in the late first or early second year of life. There are three clinically distinct subtypes of MPS-I: Hurler syndrome (MPS-IH), Scheie syndrome (MPS-IS), and Hurler-Scheie syndrome (MPS-HIS). All three are caused by deficient α-L-iduronidase, and all are radiographically similar. Patients with MPS-IH present with the most severe clinical symptoms, including progressive developmental delay; patients with MPS-IS have the typical skeletal manifestations but are developmentally normal; whereas patients with MPS-IHS present with intermediate developmental delay.

Clinical manifestations of Hurler syndrome include:

- Musculoskeletal:
  ○ Typical, coarsened facial features (formerly termed *gargoylism*)
  ○ Frontal bossing
  ○ Short stature
  ○ Progressive kyphosis or gibbus deformity
  ○ Joint contractures
- Cardiorespiratory:
  ○ Cardiac conduction defects
  ○ Hypertension
  ○ Cardiomyopathy
  ○ Progressive respiratory insufficiency, due to submucosal MPS deposition within trachea

- Neurological:
  - Progressive developmental delay
  - Progressive myelopathy, due to MPS deposition posterior to C1
- Other:
  - Hepatosplenomegaly
  - Cataracts
  - Recurrent otitis media
  - Progressive deafness
  - Macroglossia

Complications

- Without successful bone marrow transplantation (BMT), Hurler syndrome is invariably fatal, usually prior to age 20, due to respiratory failure, cardiac failure, or cervical cord compression.
- Progressive MPS deposition in the oropharyngeal and tracheal connective tissues eventually results in critical airway compromise; patients have been temporized via laser excision of tracheal and bronchial lesions.
- Critical hypertension due to intimal and medial MPS deposition within the large and medium-sized arteries, including the aorta, renal arteries, and coronary arteries, is common in untreated patients.
- Critical aortic and mitral stenosis, caused by MPS deposition within the valve leaflets, may be treated by valve replacement, with valves smaller than usual for patients of similar body mass.
- Sudden death may result from cord compression at the C1 level, caused by either C1–C2 subluxation, proliferative extradural soft tissue/MPS deposition posterior to the dens, or both. Cervical decompression and fusion may be life-prolonging in these patients.
- Progressive distal myelopathy due to gibbus formation and extradural MPS deposition may be treated by decompressive laminectomy.
- Hip subluxation/dislocation may be treated surgically, depending on the condition of the child.

Pathology

Intracellular and extracellular accumulation of dermatan sulfate and keratan sulfate

Imaging Findings

Hurler syndrome is the radiographic prototype for dysostosis multiplex, and it is the most common entity in this broad category. Imaging findings include:

RADIOGRAPHY

- Calvarial thickening, frontal bossing, J-shaped sella
- Platyspondyly, with marked anteroinferior beak or hook at L1 or L2, with resultant gibbus
- Odontoid hypoplasia
- Short, thick, broad clavicles
- Rounded scapulae
- Short, thick, oar-shaped ribs
- Undertubulated, shortened long bones
- Marked proximal metacarpal and metatarsal tapering
- Mild shortening of phalanges
- Steep acetabular roofs
- Flared, constricted iliac wings
- Calcified mitral anulus, with progressive cardiomegaly due to mitral stenosis/regurgitation

ULTRASOUND

- Hepatosplenomegaly, without focal lesions

MRI/CT

- Prominent, MPS-filled perivascular (Virchow-Robin) spaces
- Cyst-like foci within corpus callosum
- Delayed white matter myelination
- Frontal bossing
- J-shaped sella
- C1–C2 subluxation, with marked extraaxial soft tissue prominence posterior to dens, resulting in thecal sac/cord compression at C1 level, with possible myelopathic changes in the cervical spinal cord
- Proximal lumbar gibbus, with or without cord compression
- Mild to severe hydrocephalus

Treatment

- The only successful treatment for MPS-IH is BMT.
- BMT has been shown to slow or halt the progressive neurodevelopmental delay in patients with MPS-IH.
- In addition, corneal clouding also has improved in most patients after BMT. However, skeletal manifestations and spinal complications appear to progress despite successful engraftment.
- Cardiac valvular disease may be slowed or halted post-BMT.
- However, successful BMT is not guaranteed, and even successful BMT is associated with potential significant long-term complications.

PEARLS_____

- Classic radiologic constellation of dysostosis multiplex is suggestive of an MPS.
- Hurler syndrome is the most common of the MPS subtypes.
- MPS-IS mimics MPS-IH, with normal mentation.

PITFALLS_____

- Dysostosis multiplex is a descriptive term, not a diagnosis.
- Not all patients with dysostosis multiplex have MPS-IH.
- Mucolipidoses (e.g., I-cell disease) mimic mucopolysaccharidoses radiographically (**Fig. 118G**).
- Morquio syndrome types A and B have a distinctly different radiographic pattern from other MPS. These patients demonstrate characteristic anterior midbody vertebral beaking and generalized platyspondyly (**Fig. 118H**).
- The various entities causing the dysostosis multiplex radiographic constellation are best distinguished biochemically.
- J-shaped sella may be seen in many other entities.
- Prominent perivascular spaces may be normal variants.
- Anteroinferior beaking of L1 and L2 may be seen in some normal neonates.
- Anteroinferior beaking is common in achondroplasia (**Fig. 118I**). Skeletal survey will easily distinguish between the two entities.

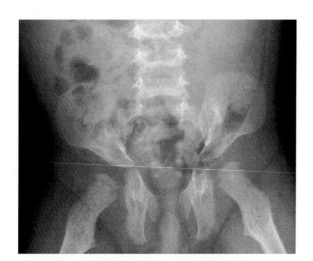

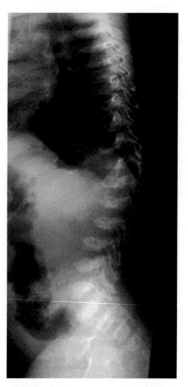

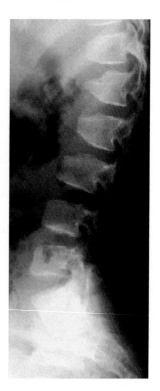

Figure 118G Frontal image of pelvis in a patient with mucolipidosis III (I-cell disease) demonstrates constriction and flaring of iliac wings, steep acetabulae, and coxa valga.

Figure 118H Lateral view of thoracolumbar vertebral column in a patient with Morquio syndrome, type A demonstrating characteristic midbody anterior beaking (arrowheads) and platyspondyly. Note the different appearance of the spine as compared with the patient with Hurler syndrome in **Fig. 118B**.

Figure 118I Lateral radiograph of thoracolumbar vertebral column of a patient with achondroplasia demonstrates short pedicles (arrowheads). Note the mild gibbus deformity and beaking deformity.

Suggested Readings

Adachi K, Chole RA. Management of tracheal lesions in Hurler syndrome. Arch Otolaryngol Head Neck Surg 1990;116:1205–1207

Eggli KD, Dorst JP. The mucopolysaccharidoses and related conditions. Semin Roentgenol 1986; 21:275–294

Fischer TA, Lehr H-A, Nixdorff U, Meyer J. Combined aortic and mitral stenosis in mucopolysaccharidosis type I-S (Ullrich-Scheie syndrome). Heart 1999;81:97–99

Lee C, Dineen TE, Brack M, Kirsch JE, Runge VM. The mucopolysaccharidoses: characterization by cranial MR imaging. AJNR Am J Neuroradiol 1993;14:1285–1292

Taccone A, Donati PT, Marzoli A, Dell'Acqua A, Gatti R, Leone D. Mucopolysaccharidosis: thickening of dura mater at the craniocervical junction and other CT/MRI findings. Pediatr Radiol 1993;23:349–352

Tandon V, Williamson JB, Cowie RA, Wraith JE. Spinal problems in mucopolysaccharidosis I (Hurler syndrome). J Bone Joint Surg Br 1996;78:938–944

Taybi H, Lachman RS. Radiology of Syndromes, Metabolic Disorders, and Skeletal Dysplasias. St. Louis: Mosby; 1996.

Taylor DB, Blaser SI, Burrows PE, Stringer DA, Clarke JTR, Thorner P. Arteriopathy and coarctation of the abdominal aorta in children with mucopolysaccharidosis: imaging findings. AJR Am J Roentgenol 1991;157:819–823

Vellodi A, Young EP, Cooper A, et al. Bone marrow transplantation for mucopolysaccharosisis type I: experience of two British centres. Arch Dis Child 1997;76:92–99

CASE 119

Clinical Presentation

A child presents with mild developmental delay and marked shortening of the fourth and fifth rays of hands and feet.

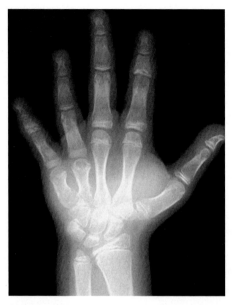

Figure 119A

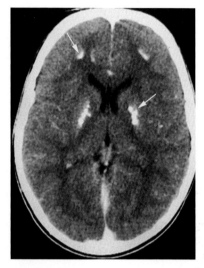

Figure 119B

Radiologic Findings

Anteroposterior radiograph of the left hand demonstrates marked shortening of the fourth and fifth metacarpals, with normal carpals and phalanges (**Fig. 119A**). Mineralization is normal. The axial non–contrast-enhanced CT of brain (**Fig. 119B**) demonstrates punctate calcifications within putamen bilaterally (arrows), as well as at the gray–white junction in a patchy but bilaterally symmetric fashion.

Diagnosis

Pseudohypoparathyroidism (PHP) (Albright hereditary osteodystrophy)

Differential Diagnosis

- Pseudopseudohypoparathyroidism (PPHP)
  - Phenotypically identical to PHP
  - Patients with PPHP are normocalcemic.
- Acrodysostosis
- Turner syndrome
- Sickle-cell disease
- Trauma
- Hypoparathyroidism
- Cranial radiation therapy
- Carbonic anhydrase type 2 deficiency

Discussion

Background

Metacarpal shortening can result from multiple diverse etiologies, including prior infection, trauma, infarction, inflammatory arthritis, skeletal dysplasia, or inborn error of metabolism. Intracranial calcifications may result from hypoxia, hypercalcemia, hypoparathyroidism, radiation therapy, and TORCH (Toxoplasmosis, Other, Rubella, Cytomegalovirus, Herpes) infections, among others. However, the combination of metacarpal shortening and intracranial calcifications is most consistent with the diagnosis of PHP or PPHP.

Etiology

PHP is a rare autosomal dominant condition that consists of refractory hypocalcemia and hyperphosphatemia, unresponsive to parathormone (PTH) therapy. The kidneys in patients with PHP and PPHP are resistant to PTH stimulation; therefore, these patients are hypocalcemic and hyperphosphatemic.

Phenotypic variability is common. There are several distinct subtypes, all due to heterozygous inactivating mutations of *GNAS1*, the gene that encodes the a chain of the Gs protein, a guanine nucleotide binding protein that functions as the signal transducer responsible for coupling neurotransmitter and hormone receptors to intracellular adenyl cyclase. Adenyl cyclase activation in turn is involved in PTH signal transduction. Maternally inherited mutations of *GNAS1* result in variable resistance to growth hormone (GH), parathyroid hormone (PTH), thyroid stimulating hormone (TSH), and luteinizing hormone (LH) and follicle stimulating hormone (FSH), a condition known as PHP 1a. Paternally transmitted *GNAS1* defects result in PPHP, which also is quite rare. These patients do not manifest the endocrinopathies seen in patients with PHP.

Clinical Findings

- Progressive short stature
- Mild developmental delay
- Patients with PHP 1a suffer from variable endocrinopathies, which may remain clinically silent.
- Brachydactyly

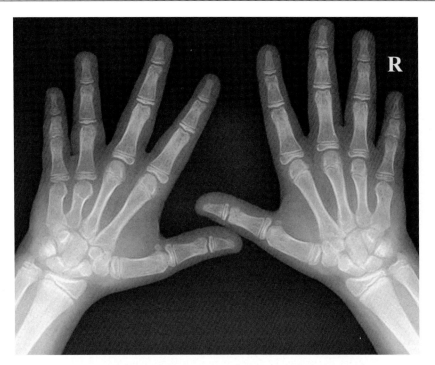

Figure 119C Radiographs of both hands demonstrate marked shortening of left fourth and fifth metacarpals, but only the right fifth metacarpal is affected.

- Dental hypoplasia
- Round "moon" face
- Retinopathy
- Tetany, seizures, and dystonia often manifest by 3 years of age.
- Spinal canal stenosis (rare)

Complications

- Spinal canal stenosis
- Variable endocrinopathies may become clinically symptomatic.

Pathology

- Ineffective Gs-mediated activity at the physis appears to result in premature physeal fusion. This accounts for brachydactyly and short stature.

Imaging Findings

RADIOGRAPHY

- Variable shortening of metacarpals and metatarsals, often isolated to the fourth ray; may be asymmetric (**Fig. 119C**)
- Young patients may demonstrate cone epiphyses of the distal phalanges.
- Some patients have universal brachymetaphalangia and brachymetatarsalia.
- Variable mild–moderate shortening of the long bones
- Premature physeal fusion results in variable shortening of phalanges and metatarsals/metacarpals (**Figs. 119D1, 119D2**, and **119E**).
- Progressive short stature

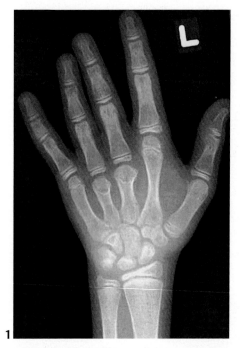
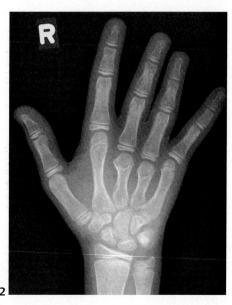

Figure 119D Radiographs of left (**1**) and right (**2**) hands showing bilaterally symmetric shortening of third and fourth metacarpals, with premature physeal fusion.

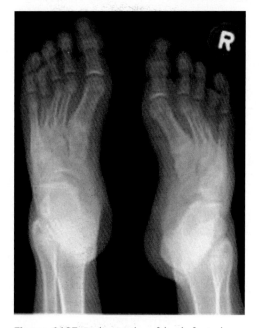
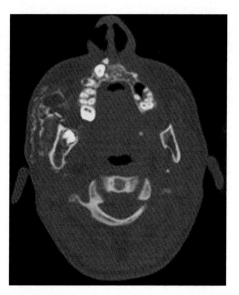

Figure 119E Radiographs of both feet showing bilaterally symmetric shortening of fourth metatarsals.

Figure 119F Axial CT depicting heterotopic calcification of soft tissues of the right face.

CT

- Calcifications of the thalamus, globus pallidus, caudate head, and putamen bilaterally (**Fig. 119B**)
- Focal calcifications of white matter at the gray-white junction
- Calcification of deep cerebellar nuclei
- Variable extracranial soft tissue calcifications (**Fig. 119F**)
- Flattened nasal bridge

Treatment

- Although believed to be metastatic in nature, the actual cause of intracranial and extracranial calcifications is unknown. These calcifications do not disappear under therapy.

PEARL_____

- The combination of isolated metacarpal shortening, short stature, mild developmental delay, and intracranial calcifications is quite suggestive of PHP or PPHP.

PITFALLS_____

- Isolated shortening of one or several metacarpals may be seen in Turner syndrome, sickle-cell disease, juvenile arthritis, prior meningococcemia, or remote trauma.
- Clinical correlation is required.
- Intracranial calcifications have an extensive differential diagnosis.

Suggested Readings

Ellie E, Julien J, Ferrer X, Riss I, Durquety MC. Extensive cerebral calcification and retinal changes in pseudohypoparathyroidism. J Neurol 1989;236:432–434

Germain-Lee EL, Groman J, Crane JL, Jan de Beur SM, Levine MA. Growth hormone deficiency in pseudohypoparathyroidism type 1a: another manifestation of multihormone resistance. J Clin Endocrinol Metab 2003;88:4059–4069

Illum F, Dupont E. Prevalences of CT-detected calcification in the basal ganglia in idiopathic hypoparathyroidism and pseudohypoparathyroidism. Neuroradiology 1985;27:32–37

Siejka SJ, Knezevic WV, Pullan PT. Dystonia and intracerebral calcification: pseudohypoparathyroidism presenting in an eleven-year-old girl. Aust N Z J Med 1988;18:607–609

van Dop C, Wang H, Mulaikal RM, Tolo VT, Rosenbaum AE. Pseudopseudohypoparathyroidism with spinal cord compression. Pediatr Radiol 1988;18:429–431

CASE 120

Clinical Presentation

A 13-month-old female infant presents with swelling of the left arm.

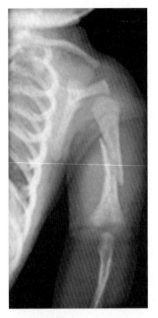

Figure 120A

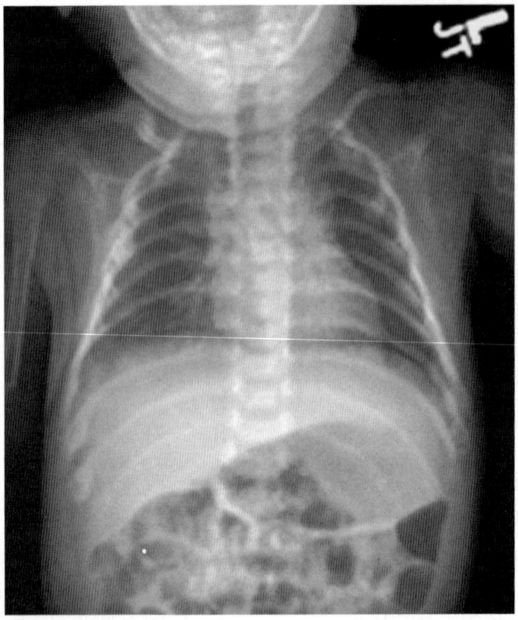

Figure 120B

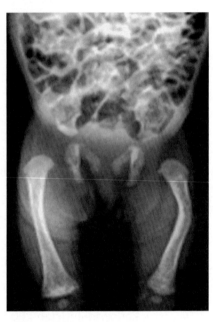

Figure 120C

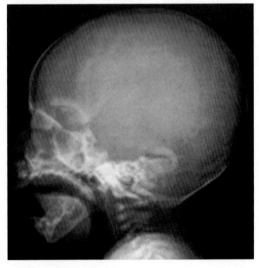

Figure 120D

Radiologic Findings

Frontal radiograph of the left humerus (**Fig. 120A**) shows an oblique fracture of the mid-shaft of the left humerus. Frontal view chest radiograph (**Fig. 120B**) demonstrates osteopenia and gracile ribs with multiple healing fractures. A fracture of the left humerus is also visualized. Radiograph of the lower extremities (**Fig. 120C**) demonstrates osteopenia and bowing of the femurs, greater on the left. Lateral view of the skull (**Fig. 120D**) demonstrates multiple wormian bones.

Diagnosis

Osteogenesis imperfecta (OI)

Differential Diagnosis

- Nonaccidental injury/child abuse
- Menkes (kinky hair) syndrome
- Hypophosphatasia
- Campomelic dysplasia

Discussion

Background

OI is one of the most common genetic disorders of connective tissue. OI is characterized by the following features: fragile bones, frequent fractures, limb bowing, spinal shortening, blue sclerae, deafness, poor dentition, ligamentous laxity, and easy bruising. Approximately 4 in 100,000 births present with OI.

Etiology

OI results from an abnormal quantity and/or quality of type I collagen. Mutations in the *COL1A1* gene on chromosome 17 or *COL1A2* gene on chromosome 7 alter the structure of the triple helix of collagen. This results in decreased synthesis of collagen or structurally abnormal collagen. Abnormalities in the collagen type I and collagen type III are detected in fibroblast cultures from skin extracts of patients with OI.

Clinical Findings

Variability in clinical features has led to the concept of heterogeneity based on a classification of four major types of OI, as shown in **Table 120A**.

Complications

- Nonunion of fractures
- Flail chest
- Osteomyelitis
- Osteosarcoma (rare)
- Basilar impression with brain stem compression
- Cardiomyopathy, mitral, or aortic valve disease

Pathology

Although information concerning the abnormal structure of collagen and intercellular substance in OI is available, the essential pathologic mechanism is frequently not detected. Characteristic to OI are numerous randomly distributed large osteocytes and osseous tissues lacking an organized trabecular pattern and more characteristic of woven or primitive bone.

Table 120A Classification of Osteogenesis Imperfecta

Classification	Genetics	Characteristics
Type I	Autosomal dominant	Mild (variable) bone fragility; most fractures occur early in childhood. Most common type and characterized by hearing loss, blue sclerae, dentinogenesis imperfecta, and easy bruising.
Type II	New dominant mutations(majority); <5% are autosomal recessive (especially group C)	Severe, lethal: Features include osteopenia, multiple fractures and deformity. Accordion-like crumpled long bones, beaded ribs. Poorly ossified skull and platyspondyly. Blue sclerae.
Type III	Autosomal recessive, rare disorder	Moderate to severe, nonlethal: Progressive fractures, bowing, and deformity. Markedly short stature and severe scoliosis. Popcorn calcifications
Type IV	Autosomal dominant	Mild to moderate (variable severity): Type IV is similar to type I, but usually there is greater bone deformity and normal sclerae (can be blue in childhood). Hearing impairment is less marked than in type I.

Imaging Findings

RADIOGRAPHY

- Long bones are frequently thin, bent, and osteopenic (**Fig. 120E**).
- Markedly deformed accordion-shaped femora in type II OI (**Fig. 120F**)
- Poorly ossified skull, wormian bones, and basilar impression (**Fig. 120G**)
- Scoliosis and multiple compression fractures of the vertebrae, with biconcave codfish vertebrae (**Fig. 120H**)
- Pelvis may be deformed.
- Gracile ribs
- Hyperplastic callus formation (**Fig. 120I**)
- Disruption of the normal physis with "popcorn calcification" due to repeated microfractures at the growth plate
- Enlarged and coned epiphyses

ULTRASOUND

Prenatal scan in second trimester

- Improved visualization of intracranial structures due to decreased skull mineralization
- Fractures of long bones and ribs
- Limb shortening and angulation deformity
- Platyspondyly

CT

- Narrow middle ear cavity with dysplastic bone proliferation, osteosclerosis

Treatment

- Growth hormone, calcitonin, and biphosphonate therapy to increase bone strength and reduce fractures
- Physical therapy muscle strengthening, which in turn improves bone density

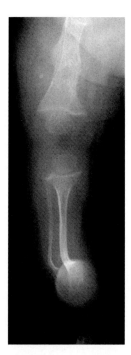

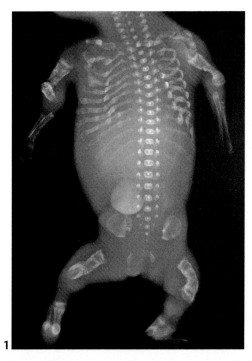

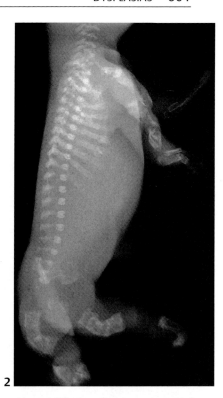

Figure120E Radiograph of lower extremity showing osteopenia and gracile tubular bones with bowing of the tibia and fibula. There is a fracture of the distal femoral shaft with callus formation.

Figure 120F Postnatal stillborn babygram frontal (**1**) and lateral (**2**) view of severe type II OI showing short ribs with multiple fractures. The long bones are micromelic with multiple fractures and are crumpled with accordion-shaped femora.

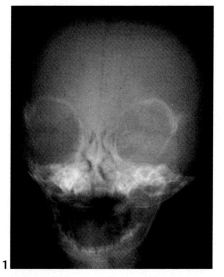

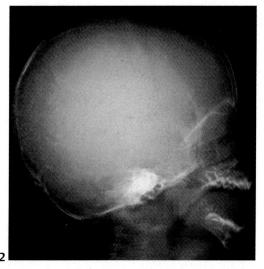

Figure 120G Frontal (**1**) and lateral (**2**) view of skull radiograph depicting osteopenia and multiple wormian bones.

- Bracing and splinting to support limbs, prevent fractures, and reduce the time of limb immobilization following fractures
- Surgery to straighten deformed bone and to decrease fractures

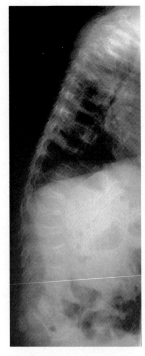

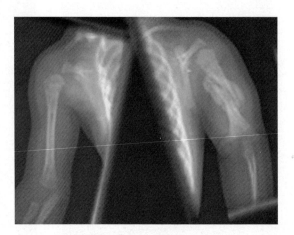

Figure 120H Radiograph of spine showing osteopenia and multiple compression fractures with biconcave vertebrae involving the thoracolumbar spine.

Figure 120I Radiograph of left humerus showing healing fracture with hyperplastic callus.

PEARLS

- Osteogenesis imperfecta is the most common second-trimester ultrasonographic diagnosis for fetus with short, bent limbs.
- Osteopenia and multiple wormian bones help distinguish OI from non-accidental injury.

PITFALLS

- Mild cases of OI type III or type IV, especially in patients with normal teeth, may be difficult to distinguish from child abuse.
- Metaphyseal corner fractures are uncommon in OI.

Suggested Readings

Ablin DS. Bone displasia series: osteogenesis imperfecta: a review. Can Assoc Radiol J 1998;49: 110–123

Root L. The treatment of osteogenesis imperfecta: symposium on metabolic bone disease. Orthop Clin North Am 1984;15:775–790

Taybi H, Lachman RS. Osteogenesis imperfecta. In: Taybi H, Lachman RS. Radiology of Syndromes, Metabolic Disorders, and Skeletal Dysplasias. 4th ed. St Louis: Mosby; 1996:876–882

CASE 121

Clinical Presentation

Stillborn with a small chest and mild limb shortening

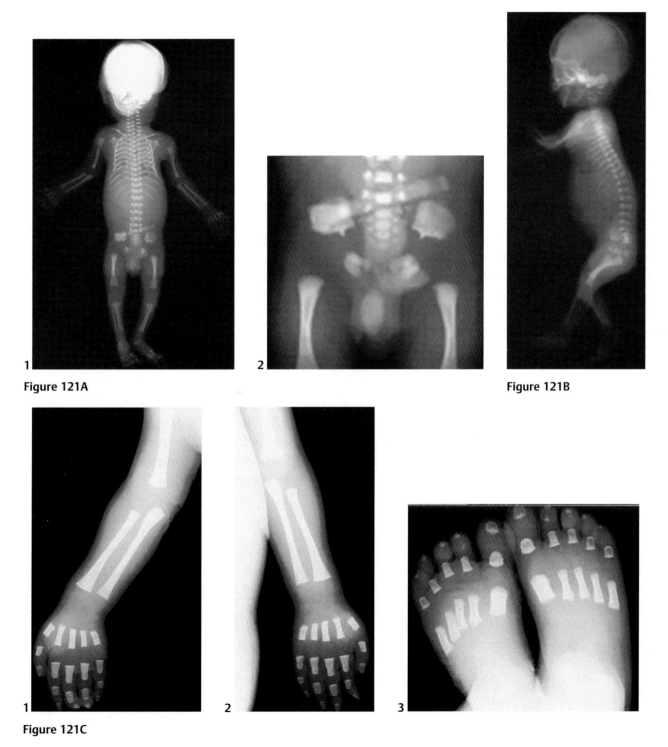

Figure 121A

Figure 121B

Figure 121C

Radiologic Findings

Anteroposterior (**Fig. 121A**) and lateral (**Fig. 121B**) chest radiographs demonstrate severe shortening of the ribs, with a resultant small thoracic cavity. The iliac wings are small and squared, with flattened acetabular roofs, narrow sacrosciatic notches, and prominent spikes at the medial and lateral acetabular margins. Proximal femoral metaphyses are irregular. There is mild limb shortening. The clavicles demonstrate a "handlebar" appearance. The hands (**Figs. 121C1** and **121C2**) and feet (**Fig. 121C3**) demonstrate mild shortening of metatcarpals, metatarsals, and phalanges.

Diagnosis

Asphyxiating thoracic dystrophy (ATD); Jeune syndrome

Differential Diagnosis

- Short rib polydactyly, type III (probably an allelic variant of ATD)
- Ellis-van Creveld syndrome (chondroectodermal dysplasia)
- Metaphyseal chondrodysplasia with exocrine pancreatic insufficiency (Schwachman-Diamond syndrome)

Discussion

Background

Several skeletal dysplasias manifest with respiratory insufficiency, small thoracic cavity, and shortening of ribs. The most common of these entities is ATD (Jeune syndrome), a fairly uncommon autosomal recessive condition first described in 1955 by Jeune, that demonstrates a spectrum of clinical severity. Severely affected newborns may die of respiratory insufficiency, whereas patients who survive the neonatal period often develop renal insufficiency later in life due to a concomitant cystic renal dysplasia. The incidence of ATD is 1 in 100,000 to 130,000 live births.

Etiology

ATD is an autosomal recessive condition in which the pathophysiologic mechanism is unknown. The defect is mapped to chromosome locus 15q13. Severe rib shortening results in a small thoracic cavity and pulmonary hypoplasia. The severity of pulmonary hypoplasia dictates neonatal survival. This entity is due to failure of proper enchondral ossification. Patients with ATD demonstrate inappropriate chondral column formation at the physes, with chondrocytes containing abnormal lipid vacuoles.

Clinical Findings

ATD demonstrates a spectrum of clinical severity, most likely due to allelic heterogeneity. Approximately 70 to 80% mortality is seen in the neonatal period, caused by severe pulmonary hypoplasia. Neonates present with respiratory distress due to decreased thoracic volume and a long, narrow thorax. Ventilation appears to be effected primarily by diaphragmatic contraction. Mild to moderate limb shortening is observed, involving proximal and distal segments, and patients occasionally demonstrate postaxial polydactyly of hands and feet. Patients who survive the neonatal period develop chronic renal insufficiency due to concomitant cystic renal disease, which may present by age 2 years. Retinal dystrophy is occasionally seen. Pancreatic cysts are seen in some patients. Hepatic fibrosis/cirrhosis may be severe.

Complications

- Some patients develop blindness due to retinal dysplasia.
- Some patients develop cirrhosis and hepatic failure.
- Most patients develop progressive renal failure due to concomitant cystic renal disease.

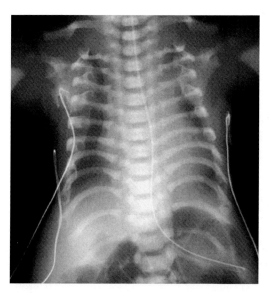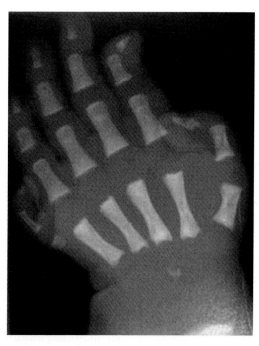

Figure 121D Frontal radiograph of the chest demonstrating horizontally oriented, short ribs and small scapulae.

Figure 121E Anteroposterior view of the hand showing postaxial polydactyly.

Imaging Findings

RADIOGRAPHY

- The ribs are severely shortened and horizontally oriented, resulting in a narrow, bell-shaped chest (**Fig. 121D**).
- The clavicles appear relatively elongated (handlebar appearance).
- The iliac wings are small, with narrowed sacrosciatic notches and prominent spikes or spurs at the medial and lateral acetabular margins.
- Flat, horizontal acetabulae
- Mild to moderate limb shortening, involving proximal and distal segments
- Mild to moderate shortening of the small tubular bones of the hands and feet, with occasional cone epiphyses
- ± postaxial polydactyly of hands (**Fig. 121E**) and/or feet
- Renal ultrasonography demonstrates numerous small cysts with increased cortical echogenicity.

Treatment

- Respiratory support in the neonatal period
- Progressive renal disease may require dialysis or renal transplantation.
- Lateral thoracic expansion has been utilized to increase the thoracic capacity in some children.

Prognosis

- Initial survival depends on the degree of pulmonary hypoplasia.
- Patients who survive the neonatal period tend to do well from a respiratory perspective.
- However, renal disease in many patients may require renal transplantation.

PEARLS_____

- This is the most common short rib dysplasia.
- Prominent spikes at medial and lateral acetabular margins are characteristic.
- Squared, small iliac wings are suggestive.
- Cystic renal disease in a patient with suggestive skeletal features supports the diagnosis of ATD.

PITFALLS_____

- Not all short limb dysplasias are ATD. Similar appearance of the chest and pelvis can be seen in patients with type III short-rib polydactyly (Verma-Naumoff) syndrome.
- Patients with achondroplasia often have mild rib shortening. However, the two conditions are clinically and radiographically distinctive.

Suggested Readings

Davis JT, Long FR, Adler BH, Castile RG, Weinstein S. Lateral thoracic expansion for Jeune syndrome: evidence of rib healing and new bone formation. Ann Thorac Surg 2004;77:445–448

Jeune M, Beraud C, Curron R. Dystrophic thoracique asphyxiante de caractere familial. Arch Franc Pediat 1955;12:886–891

Johnson CA, Gissen P, Sergi C. Molecular pathology and genetics of congenital hepatorenal fibrocystic syndromes. J Med Genet 2003;40:311–319

Ho NC, Francomano CA, van Allen M. Jeune asphyxiating thoracic dystrophy and short-rib polydactyly type III (Verma-Naumoff) are variants of the same disorder. Am J Med Genet 2000;90:310–314

Morgan NV, Baccheli C, Gissen P, Morton J, Ferrero GB, Silengo M, et al. A locus for asphyxiating thoracic dystrophy, ATD, maps to chromosome 15q13. J Med Genet 2003;40:431–435

CASE 122

Clinical Presentation

A 14-year-old boy presents with marked enlargement of the left fourth proximal and middle phalanges, left fifth middle phalanx, and ulnar aspect of the left hand.

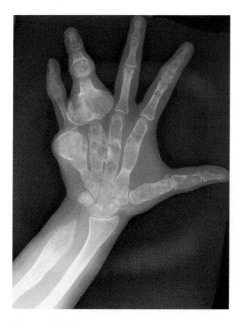

Figure 122A

Radiologic Findings

Hand radiograph (**Fig. 122A**) shows dramatic intramedullary expansion of the left fourth proximal and middle phalanges, as well as the distal aspect of the left fifth metacarpal. Similar, but less dramatic, foci of intramedullary expansion, with endosteal scalloping, involve the left first through fourth metacarpals, the left second and fifth middle phalanges, and the left fourth distal phalanx. In addition, the distal ulna is tapered and hypoplastic, with resultant ulnarization of the carpus (pseudo-Madelung deformity). Affected bones demonstrate an internal "ground-glass" matrix with endosteal scalloping and occasional punctate calcifications, without evidence of an extra-osseous soft tissue mass or sclerotic rim.

Diagnosis

Ollier disease (multiple enchondromas)

Differential Diagnosis

- Maffucci syndrome
- Multiple hereditary exostoses
- Klippel-Trénaunay-Weber syndrome
- Fibrous dysplasia
- Proteus syndrome
- Neurofibromatosis
- Macrodystrophia lipomatosa
- Primary bone cysts, including aneurysmal and unicameral bone cysts

Discussion

Background

Many conditions are associated with focal or diffuse osseous bowing and intraosseous expansile lesions. Patients with Ollier disease, or multiple enchondromas, first described in 1899, present with painless enlargement and deformity of short bones and long bones during childhood. This process is most commonly unilateral; when bilateral, it is usually asymmetrical. Affected long bones are often shortened, whereas affected short tubular bones may be grotesquely expanded and occasionally lengthened. This process is limited to the metaphyses and diaphyses.

This is a rare and sporadic entity. As is now recognized, ~20 to 50% of patients will develop malignant dedifferentiation of an intra-osseous lesion over the course of their lifetime; resultant tumors are usually chondrosarcomas. Astrocytomas of the central nervous system may develop in some patients.

Patients with Maffucci syndrome demonstrate numerous enchondromas as well as cutaneous and subcutaneous hemangiomas. These patients are also at high risk for osseous and CNS malignancies. Patients with neurofibromatosis may have focal bony expansion, but more commonly they demonstrate narrowing, elongation, and pseudoarthroses of affected long bones. Patients with multiple hereditary exostoses have exophytic expansile lesions; involvement of the distal radius and ulna may also characteristically produce the pseudo-Madelung deformity (**Fig. 122B**).

Etiology

Some patients demonstrate a mutation in PPR, the receptor for parathormone/parathormone-related peptide. This peptide is involved in maintaining chondrocytes in a nonhypertrophic proliferative state.

Pathology/Histology

The macroscopic features of Ollier syndrome include islands of benign resting cartilage within metaphyses and diaphyses, which subsequently proliferate. Microscopically, calcifications, ranging from punctate to "popcorn" in appearance may develop within the cartilaginous matrix.

Clinical Findings

Patients with Ollier syndrome commonly present with painless swelling of hands, wrists, and knees. Wrist and digital motion is often limited, and the long bones may be shortened. This process is

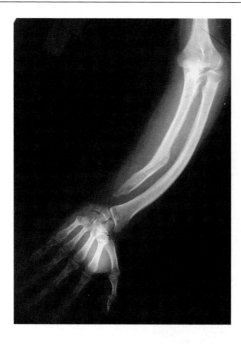

Figure 122B A child with multiple hereditary exostosis. Radiograph of the upper extremity shows exostosis of the proximal ulna causing partial radial head subluxation. Involvement of ulnar diaphysis produces pseudo-Madelung deformity similar to that shown in **Fig. 122A**.

usually unilateral; however, when bilateral it is often asymmetric but may also present in a bilateral, symmetric fashion. The pain may result from pathologic fracture or malignant dedifferentiation (usually later in life).

Complications

- Short-term and intermediate-term complications are related to local orthopedic limitations and to pathologic fractures.
- Pseudo-Madelung deformity may predispose to wrist pain and limitation of motion.
- Long-bone involvement may cause limitation of motion or dislocations about large joints.
- Vertebral involvement may produce pronounced scoliosis.
- Long-bone bowing deformities may occur.
- Local orthopedic complications due to lesion location (around large joints, within tubular bones of hand or flat bones of face/pelvis) are common.
- Involved bone is weaker than normal, predisposing to pathologic fracture.
- Significant long-term complications are related to orthopedic difficulties (deformity and pathologic fracture), to malignant dedifferentiation of preexisting enchondromas (almost exclusively into chondrosarcomas) as seen in 20 to 50% of patients, and to the development of CNS astrocytomas.
- Sarcomatous dedifferentiation of enchondromas is seen in 20 to 50% of adult patients and usually presents after age 40, although chondrosarcomas have been described as early as the second decade of life. Chondrosarcomas are of low to high histologic grade, and may be focal, multifocal, synchronous, or metachronous. Although usually seen in the metaphysis and diaphysis of long bones, chondrosarcomas have been reported in the pelvis, skull base, and within small tubular bones. As enchondromas should not grow after physeal closure, increase in size of an enchondroma associated with pain is suggestive of chondrosarcoma in an adult patient with Ollier disease. Periodic skeletal surveys thoroughout life are advocated to monitor the patient with Ollier disease.
- CNS malignancies are uncommon but may be seen occasionally in adults. These tumors range from low-grade gliomas to anaplastic astrocytomas. Chondromas occasionally are seen within the skull base (chondrocranium).

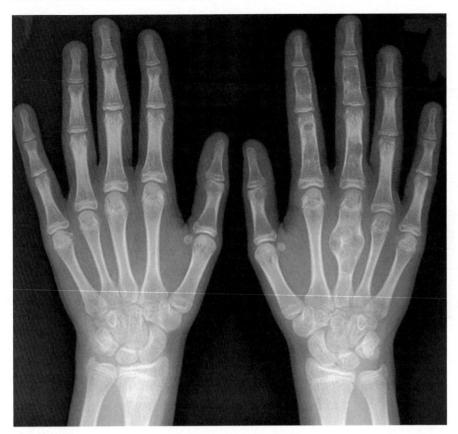

Figure 122C Older child with Ollier syndrome. Hand radiograph demonstrates unilateral expansile lesions of the right second and third rays.

Imaging Findings

RADIOGRAPHY

- In infancy or early childhood, round to oval lucent expansile foci are seen within the diametaphyses.
- Larger expansile, lucent lesions, often containing popcorn-type calcifications, causing endosteal cortical thinning are commonly seen in later childhood and adulthood.
- Occasionally, linear lucent streaks course from the physis through the metaphysis and into the diaphysis.
- Usually affects long bones and short tubular bones of hands and feet in a unilateral or asymmetric fashion (**Fig. 122C**)
- Occasionally may present with bilateral and symmetric involvement
- Vertebral involvement is uncommon.
- Affected long bones are classically expanded, often angulated, and almost universally shortened.
- Small tubular bones of the hands and feet are occasionally grotesquely enlarged and expanded, usually with marked cortical thinning and intralesional calcifications.

MRI

- MRI will demonstrate ectopic cartilage (high signal on T2-weighted and low on T1-weighted images) within metaphyses and diaphyses of affected bones.

Treatment and Prognosis

- Orthopedic complications such as scoliosis and dislocations are often difficult to treat successfully due to the progressive nature of the process during childhood and to lesion location.

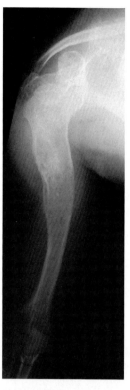

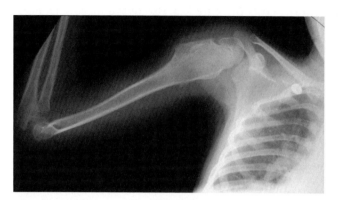

Figure 122D Radiograph depicting sessile exostosis of proximal humerus mimicking an enchondroma.

Figure 122E Radiograph showing fibrous dysplasia of proximal humerus causing expansion and angulation; again mimicking an enchondroma.

- Large lesions or those strategically located may be resected or, alternatively, curettaged and packed with bone chips.
- Long-bone bowing deformities may be treated by osteotomy, and scoliosis by corrective bracing. Limb-lengthening surgery may be utilized in some patients.
- Barring significant orthopedic complications in centrally located lesions, or malignant dedifferentiation of an intraosseous lesion or development of an astrocytoma, prognosis is for a normal life span. Orthopedic complications, ranging from mild to significant, depending on the location and size of the lesions, are nearly universal. However, 20 to 50% of patients will develop chondrosarcoma, and a smaller percentage will develop a CNS neoplasm, so long-term follow-up of these patients is mandatory.

PEARLS_____

- Long-bone/tubular-bone involvement is usually asymmetrical.
- Longitudinal lucent foci within metaphyses represent abnormal cartilage columns ("celery stalk" appearance).
- Lesions are intraosseous and expansile.
- Lesions often contain internal punctate, "popcorn" calcifications.

PITFALLS_____

- Identical bony lesions associated with soft tissue phleboliths are diagnostic of Maffucci syndrome. As in Ollier disease, patients with Maffucci syndrome have a significantly elevated risk for bony and CNS malignancy.
- Sessile osteochondromata may appear similar clinically and radiographically (**Fig. 122D**).

- Intraosseous lucent expansile lesions may be seen in fibrous dysplasia (**Fig. 122E**), neurofibromatosis type 1 (NF-1).
- Trilineage enlargement of an extremity in a dermatomal/sclerotomal distribution can be seen in macrodystrophia lipomatosa, NF-1, and in vascular syndromes such as Klippel-Trénaunay-Weber syndrome. In the latter, bony enlargement is diffuse and involves cortical and trabecular bone symmetrically, without intraosseous lucent lesions.

Suggested Readings

Azouz EM. Case report 418. Skeletal Radiol 1987;16:236–239

Jesus-Garcia R, Bongiovanni JC, Korukian M, Boatto H, Seixas MT, Laredo J. Use of the Ilizarov external fixator in the treatment of patients with Ollier disease. Clin Orthop Relat Res 2001;382:82–86

Kornak U, Mundlos S. Genetic disorders of the skeleton: a developmental approach. Am J Hum Genet 2003;73:447–474

Le A, Ball D, Pitman A, Fox R, King K. Chondrosarcoma of bone complicating Ollier disease: report of a favourable response to radiotherapy. Australas Radiol 2003;47:322–324

Liu J, Hudkins PG, Swee RG, Unni KK. Bone sarcomas associated with Ollier disease. Cancer 1987;59:1376–1385

Ly JQ, Beall DP. A rare case of infantile Ollier disease demonstrating bilaterally symmetric extremity involvement. Skeletal Radiol 2003;32:227–230

Miyawaki T, Kinoshita Y, Iizuka T. A case of Ollier disease of the hand. Ann Plast Surg 1997;38:77–80

Nguyen BD. Ollier disease with synchronous multicentric chondrosarcomas: scintigraphic and radiologic demonstration. Clin Nucl Med 2004;29:45–47

Omalu BI, Wiley CA, Hamilton RL. Case of the month. Brain Pathol 2003;13:419–420

Van Nielen KMB, de Jong BM. A case of Ollier disease associated with two intracerebral low-grade gliomas. Clin Neurol Neurosurg 1999;101:106–110

CASE 123

Clinical Presentation

A newborn infant presents with multiple dislocations of small and large joints, mild bowing of femora, bilateral clubfeet, and respiratory distress.

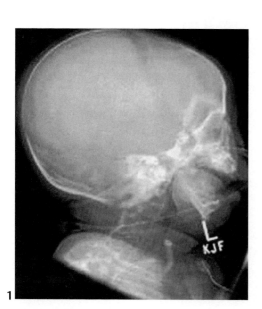
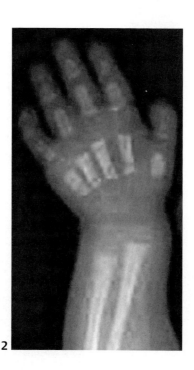

Figure 123A

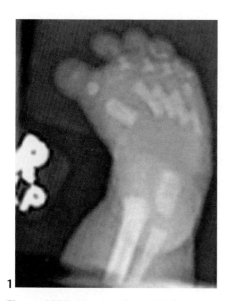
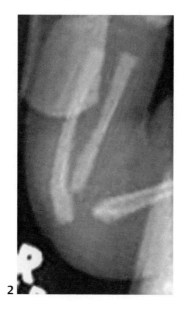
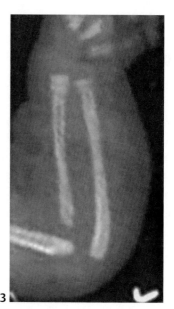

Figure 123B *(Continued on p. 614)*

613

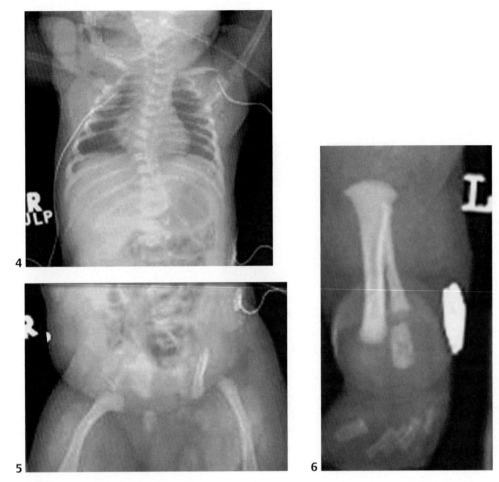

Figure 123B *(Continued)*

Radiologic Findings

Cervical platyspondyly with reversed lordosis and marked pedicular hypoplasia is present (**Fig. 123A1**). Moderate shortening of second through fifth metacarpals with severe shortening of first metacarpal (**Fig. 123A2**) and bilateral clubfeet (**Fig. 123B1**) with severe metatarsus adductus are observed. The elbow radiographs (**Figs. 123B2** and **123B3**) show bilateral radial head dislocation. The midthoracic vertebral column (**Fig. 123B4**) shows congenital dextroscoliosis. Severe hypoplasia of the distal scapulae with preservation of the glenoids is present. Mild lateral bowing of midfemoral diaphyses (**Fig. 123B5**) is noted. Congenital dislocation of left femoral head (**Fig. 123B5**) and hypoplasia of distal fibulae with vertical orientation of calcanei are also noted (**Fig. 123B6**).

Diagnosis

Campomelic dysplasia (campomelic syndrome)

Differential Diagnosis

- Diastrophic dysplasia
- Larsen syndrome
- Ehlers-Danlos syndrome
- Arthrogryposis
- Kyphomelic dysplasia
- Antley-Bixler syndrome

Discussion

Background

Campomelia means "bent bones," and campomelic dysplasia is a severe multisystem syndrome/dysplasia, usually manifesting bent (but not shortened) long bones. It is often fatal in the neonatal period. Long-term survivors usually demonstrate severe orthopedic, neurologic, and respiratory difficulties. The reported incidence is 0.5 per 100,000 live births.

Etiology

Campomelic dysplasia is an autosomal dominant defect in the *SOX-9* gene, located on chromosome 17. This defect results in haploinsufficiency of *SOX-9*, a transcription factor involved in both chondral development and sexual differentiation. For this reason, most patients with campomelic dysplasia, whether 46XY males or 46XX females, are phenotypically female.

The etiology for the bowing deformities is unknown. Theories include damage to the developing diaphyseal cartilage, with resultant fracture and repair, or possibly a primary defect in neural growth and differentiation, with the bony changes being secondary phenomena.

Clinical Findings

- Campomelic dysplasia presents at birth with:
  - Dolichocephaly, hypertelorism, low-set ears, hypotonia
  - Micrognathia, microstomia, cleft palate
  - Short neck, scoliosis, clubfeet
  - Protuberant abdomen
  - Bowing of long bones, usually lower extremities
  - Multiple dislocations of small and large joints
  - Severe respiratory insufficiency
- Survivors demonstrate:
  - Severe neurodevelopmental delay in many cases
  - Respiratory insufficiency
  - Scoliosis
  - Joint dislocations
  - Cardiac disease
  - Renal disease

Complications

- Often fatal in the neonatal period
- Respiratory insufficiency is common.

Imaging Findings

PLAIN RADIOGRAPHY

- Dramatic cervical vertebral hypoplasia (63%)
- Pedicular hypoplasia/aplasia of cervical and thoracic vertebrae, with resultant abnormal curvature of cervical vertebral column, often producing clinically significant cervical cord compression
- Bowing of the femora and other long bones is characteristic, although "acamptomelic" camptomelic dysplasia may occur.
- Although bowed or bent, the femora are of normal length.
- Mild-to-moderate brachymetacarpalia, especially first metacarpal, with mild brachydactyly
- Dramatic hypoplasia of the distal scapula, with sparing of the glenoid and scapular spine, is invariable and characteristic.
- Tracheal hypoplasia
- Small bowel malrotation
- Hydronephrosis (38%), renal hypoplasia
- Congenital heart disease (21%), usually patent ductus arterosus (PDA) and ventricular septal defect (VSD)
- Macrocephaly, hypertelorism, micrognathia, and cleft palate are common.
- Tibiae and fibulae are often hypoplastic and bowed.
- Scoliosis is common.
- Often have only 11 rib pairs
- Pelvic hypoplasia, with vertical iliac wings and ischia
- Dislocation of femoral heads
- Severe talipes equinovarus (clubfoot)
- CNS malformations, including polygyria, hydrocephalus, defects of corpus callosum, and absent olfactory bulbs
- Choanal atresia

Treatment

- Supportive only
- Most survivors are tracheostomy dependent.

Prognosis

- Camptomelic dysplasia carries a poor prognosis and is frequently fatal in utero or within the neonatal period.
- Long-term survivors exhibit severe orthopedic complications due to multiple small and large joint dislocations, as well as kyphoscoliosis. These patients are often tracheostomy-dependent and exhibit severe neurologic problems, including developmental delay and cervical myelopathy.

PEARL_____

- Extreme scapular hypoplasia is an invariable and diagnostic feature.

PITFALLS_____

- "Acampomelic" patients demonstrate the full range of abnormalities, especially the abnormal scapulae, without femoral bowing.
- Diastrophic dysplasia presents with cervical hypoplasia, clubfeet, scoliosis, and brachymetacarpalia/brachyphalangy. However, patients with diastrophic dysplasia have accelerated skeletal maturation about the hand and wrist.
- Extreme cervical hypoplasia, scoliosis, and multiple dislocations are seen in Larsen syndrome. However, patients with Larsen syndrome often demonstrate dual calcaneal ossification centers and have normal scapulae.
- Multiple large and small joint dislocations may be seen in arthrogryposis. These patients have normal scapulae and different clinical presentation.
- Shortened, bent femora are seen in kyphomelic dysplasia; the scapulae are normal in these patients.
- Antley-Bixler presents with multiple dislocations and bent femora; however, these patients also have radiohumeral synostoses and normal scapulae.

Suggested Readings

Houston CS, Opitz JM, Spranger JW, Macpherson RI, Reed MH, Gilbert EF, Herrmann J, Schinzel A. The campomelic syndrome: review, report of 17 cases, and follow-up on the currently 17-year-old boy first reported by Maroteaux et al in 1971. Am J Med Genet 1983;15:3–28

Huang B, Wang S, Ning Y, Lamb AN, Bartley J. Autosomal XX sex reversal caused by duplication of SOX9. Am J Med Genet 1999;87:349–353

Kornak U, Mundlos S. Genetic disorders of the skeleton: a developmental approach. Am J Hum Genet 2003;73:447–474

Macpherson RI, Skinner SA, Donnenfeld AE. Acampomelic campomelic dysplasia. Pediatr Radiol 1989;20:90–93

Mortier GR, Rimoin DL, Lachman RS. The scapula as a window to the diagnosis of skeletal dysplasias. Pediatr Radiol 1997;27:447–451

Pazzaglia UE, Beluffi G. Radiology and histopathology of the bent limbs in campomelic dysplasia: implications in the aetiology of the disease and review of theories. Pediatr Radiol 1987;17:50–55

Roth M. Campomelic syndrome: experimental models and pathomechanism. Pediatr Radiol 1991; 21:220–225

Taybi H, Lachman RS. Radiology of Syndromes, Metabolic Disorders, and Skeletal Dysplasias. 4th ed. St. Louis: Mosby; 1996

CASE 124

Clinical Presentation

A 7-year-old child presents with abnormal dentition, large anterior fontanelle, and hypermobile scapulae.

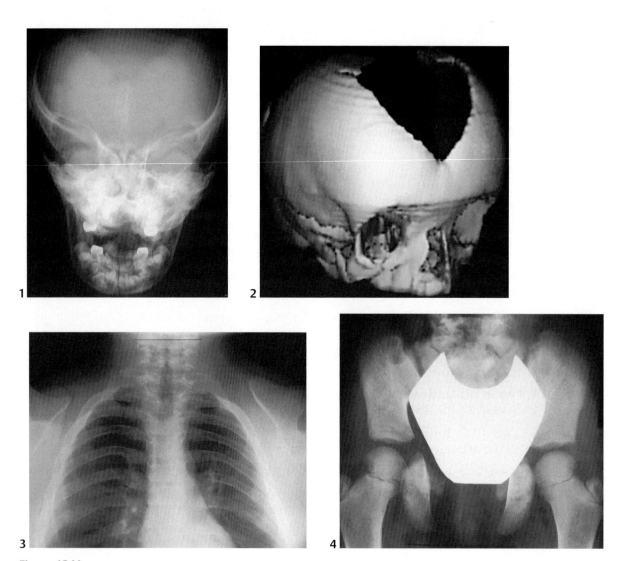

Figure 124A

Radiologic Findings

Anteroposterior radiograph (**Fig. 124A1**) of the cranium demonstrates a large, patent anterior fontanelle, along with a partially patent metopic suture. Three-dimensional CT (**Fig. 124A2**) confirms abnormally enlarged anterior fontanelle and partially patent metopic suture. Posteroanterior chest radiograph (**Fig. 124A3**) reveals extremely hypoplastic clavicles, with a slight proximomedial translation of the scapulae. Posteroanterior pelvis radiograph (**Fig. 124A4**) demonstrates hypoplastic ischia and pubic rami. The iliac wings are small and narrow. Acetabular roofs are horizontal, and the symphysis pubis is widened.

618

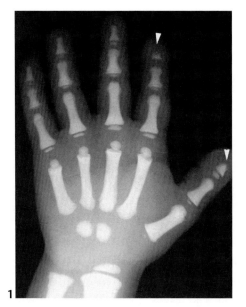 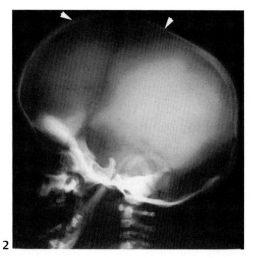

Figure 124B Patient with pyknodysostosis. Note marked osteosclerosis and distal tapering of tufts (acro-osteolysis; **1**, arrowheads). Lateral radiograph of calvarium shows large anterior fontanelle (**2**, arrowheads), osteosclerosis, and abnormal mandibular angle.

Diagnosis

Cleidocranial dysplasia

Differential Diagnosis

- Pyknodysostosis (**Figs. 124B1** and **124B2**)
- Hypophosphatasia
- Osteogenesis imperfecta
- Hydrocephalus
- Congenital pseudoarthrosis of the clavicle
- Birth-induced fracture

Discussion

Background

Formerly termed *cleidocranial dysostosis*, this entity is now more properly termed *cleidocranial dysplasia* to reflect the fact that this condition is a generalized skeletal dysplasia. Cleidocranial dysplasia is an autosomal dominant condition characterized by defective midline ossification, including abnormalities of the calvarium, dentition, clavicles, sternum, and pelvis. Incidence is 1 per 1,000,000 live births.

The clavicle functions as a strut to provide support and anchoring for the scapula during upper extremity motion. Embryologically, the clavicle is composed of several separate ossification centers that develop via intramembranous ossification. Although the clavicle is not infrequently fractured during normal vaginal delivery, congenital, nontraumatic abnormalities of the clavicles are uncommon and include pseudoarthroses and hypoplasia/aplasia due to cleidocranial dysostosis. When clavicular defects are associated with widely patent, bulging anterior fontanelle and hypoplasia/aplasia of ischial ossification centers, cleidocranial dysplasia is the diagnosis of choice.

Etiology

Cleidocranial dysplasia is caused by a defect in the gene encoding for the core binding factor A1 subunit, located on chromosome 6. This factor appears to modulate the relationship between osteoblastic differentiation and mechanical loading. This defect shows autosomal dominant heritance with complete penetrance and intrafamilial variability.

Clinical Findings

Patients demonstrate normal stature at birth, but exhibit short stature (height >2 SD below mean) by 4 to 8 years of age. Adult height for males is between the 5th and 50th percentile, whereas females are below the fifth percentile. Patients demonstrate disproportionate short stature, with limbs shorter than the trunk.

Patients with cleidocranial dysplasia demonstrate hypertelorism, frontal bossing, and brachycephaly. They also show persistent patency of cranial sutures, especially the metopic, with an enlarged, bulging anterior fontanelle. Dentition is often abnormal, with delayed tooth eruption and supernumerary teeth commonly seen. The nasal bridge is broad. The clavicles are abnormal, ranging from hypoplastic to aplastic, occasionally consisting of several ossification centers with apparent pseudoarthroses. Due to clavicular hypoplasia, the scapulae are abnormally opposable. The clavicular defect may be unilateral or asymmetrical. The ischial ossification centers are variably hypoplastic to aplastic, resulting in a widened symphysis pubis. The iliac wings are hypoplastic. In addition, there is a characteristic shortening (brachydactyly) of the second and fifth middle phalanges.

Complications

- Patency of anterior fontanelle theoretically subjects the brain to increased risk of penetrating trauma.
- Clavicular hypoplasia/aplasia results in lack of proper strut support for scapulae, limiting upper extremity strength.
- Defective dentition may require prosthetic/orthodontic treatment.
- Small pelvis may necessitate cesarean delivery for female patients.

Imaging Findings

- Calvarium:
  - Anterior fontanelle is enlarged in all patients and remains patent throughout life.
  - Cranial sutures also remain patent.
  - Defective dentition, including supernumerary teeth and delayed eruption
- Clavicles:
  - Hypoplastic to aplastic (10% are completely absent)
  - May consist of multiple ossification centers
  - Milder presentation may appear as pseudoarthrosis.
  - The defect may be bilateral and symmetric, bilateral but asymmetric, or unilateral (usually right).
- Chest:
  - Narrow upper chest, associated with mild respiratory difficulty
  - Poorly ossified or bifid sternum
- Pelvis:
  - Ischial ossification centers are variably hypoplastic to aplastic.
  - Widened symphysis pubis
  - Small, narrow iliac wings

- Elbows:
  ◦ Hypoplastic radial heads, often dislocated
- Digits:
  ◦ Hypoplasia of second and fifth middle phalanges, with cone epiphyses
  ◦ Variable tapering of distal phalanges

Treatment

- None, except for dental considerations

Prognosis

- No significant impact on long-term survival
- Clavicular hypoplasia may restrict patients from heavy overhead lifting or motion.
- Dental and obstetric complications may develop.

PEARL_____

- Excessively large anterior fontanelle in a younger child, or patent anterior fontanelle and/or cranial sutures in an older child or adult, is suggestive of this disorder. In such patients, evaluate the clavicles and pelvis for other stigmata of cleidocranial dysplasia.

PITFALLS_____

- Congenital pseudoarthroses or acute birth-related fractures may result in unusual appearance of clavicles, similar to mild presentations of cleidocranial dysplasia.
- Ischial ossification centers are not normally seen in markedly premature infants; however, clavicles should be present and normal.
- Anterior fontanelle may be large or bulging, and sutures may be widened in patients with hydrocephalus or other disorders (**Figs. 124B1** and **124B2**). If anterior fontanelle and sutures are prominent and clavicles/ischia are normal, suspect hydrocephalus.

Suggested Readings

Chitayat D, Hodgkinson KA, Azouz EM. Intrafamilial variability in cleidocranial dysplasia: a three generation family. Am J Med Genet 1992;42:298–303

Hall CM. International nosology and classification of constitutional disorders of bone (2001). Am J Med Genet 2002;113:65–77

Jensen BL. Somatic development in cleidocranial dysplasia. Am J Med Genet 1990;35:69–74

Ozonoff M. Pediatric Orthopedic Radiology. 2nd ed. Philadelphia: WB Saunders; 1992

Taybi H, Lachman RS. Radiology of Syndromes, Metabolic Diseases, and Skeletal Dysplasias. 4th ed. St. Louis: Mosby; 1996

CASE 125

Clinical Presentation

A newborn male presents with congenital heart disease, narrow chest, short extremities, and polydactyly of hands and feet. The nails are hypoplastic, and several primary teeth are present.

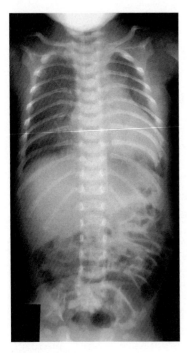

Figure 125A

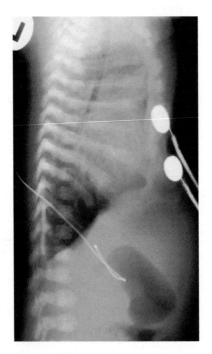

Figure 125B

Radiologic Findings

Frontal (**Fig. 125A**) and lateral (**Fig. 125B**) radiographs of chest and abdomen demonstrate cardiomegaly, with downshifted cardiac apex and increased pulmonary vascularity, suggesting ventricular septal defect, large atrial septal defect (ASD), or single atrium. The ribs are quite short, resulting in marked narrowing of the chest. The vertebrae are normal.

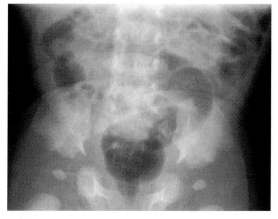

Figure 125C

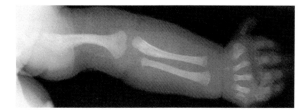

Figure 125D

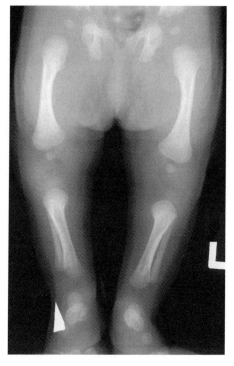

Figure 125E

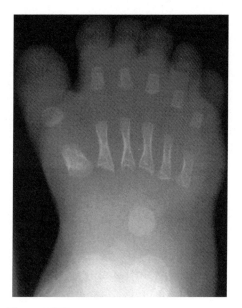

Figure 125F

The pelvis (**Fig. 125C**) demonstrates shortened, flattened iliac wings. The acetabulae show horizontal orientation, with pronounced medial and lateral "spikes." The proximal femoral ossification centers are prematurely visualized. The humerus, radius, and ulna are short and thick. The humerus and radius demonstrate proximal and distal metaphyseal flaring; the ulna is proximally widened. Postaxial hexadactyly is present, with distal duplication of the fifth metacarpal. The supernumerary sixth digit is well formed (**Fig. 125D**). The femora, tibiae, and fibulae are mildly shortened. The femora and tibiae are thick, with proximal and distal metaphyseal flaring (**Fig. 125E**). The feet demonstrate postaxial hexadactyly with a shortened first metatarsal and widening of the first proximal phalanx. The supernumerary sixth ray is well formed (**Fig. 125F**).

Diagnosis

Chondroectodermal dysplasia (Ellis-van Creveld syndrome)

Differential Diagnosis

- Asphyxiating thoracic dystrophy (ATD, Jeune syndrome)
- Short-rib polydactyly syndromes
- Familial polydactyly

Discussion

Background

The association of congenital heart disease, polydactyly, short stature, abnormal nails, and dental abnormalities was first described by Ellis and van Creveld in 1940 and further elucidated by McKusick in his study of 52 affected Amish patients published in 1964. Chondroectodermal dysplasia (Ellis-van Creveld syndrome) is a rare autosomal recessive condition, with an incidence in the general population of 0.9 per 100,000 live births. It is much more common in the Amish community of Lancaster County, Pennsylvania. Severity varies among affected families.

Etiology

The gene locus has been mapped to chromosome 4p16. Inheritance is autosomal recessive, with phenotypic variability.

Pathology

Histopathologic reports have often been somewhat contradictory. A recent report (Sergi et al, 2001) of a 25-week fetus demonstrated retarded maturation of physeal growth plates at all enchondral ossifi-cation centers, with disorganization of the physeal zones of proliferative and hypertrophic cartilage at the proximal aspect of the femur. Periosteal ossification appeared to overtake enchondral ossification, causing a "cupped" appearance at several sites. This fetus also demonstrated hepatic periportal fibrosis, pulmonary hypoplasia, and a ventricular septal defect.

Clinical Findings

Chondroectodermal dysplasia is usually evident at birth. Some patients may demonstrate situs inversus, Dandy-Walker malformation, cryptorchidism, and/or renal tubular dysplasia. Older patients may demonstrate delayed tooth eruption, small teeth, partial anodontia, and sparse hair. Adult height is usually less than the fifth percentile. Survival is dependent on the degree of respiratory insufficiency caused by thoracic hypoplasia and the severity of congenital heart disease. Some patients experience developmental delay. Relative hypoplasia of lateral tibial plateau may result in genu valgus deformity. Although autopsy reports describe periportal fibrosis and renal tubular dysplasia, this does not seem to be clinically evident in most patients.

The typical clinical features include:

- Abnormal frenulum (fusion of upper lip to underlying gingiva)
- Gingival cysts

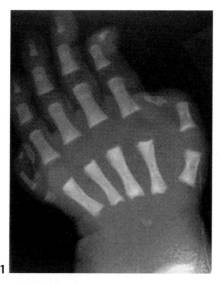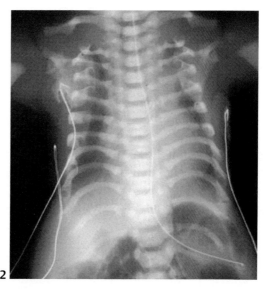

Figures 125G A patient with ATD demonstrating polydactyly (**1**), rib shortening, and a long, narrow thorax (**2**). However, long bones in these patients do not show the metaphyseal widening and rounding seen in chondroectodermal dysplasia.

- Neonatal tooth eruption; later, defective dentition is evident.
- Sparse hair
- Hypohidrosis
- Narrow chest
- Respiratory difficulty
- Congenital heart disease in ~60%, usually ASD or single atrium
- Short-limbed dwarfism, with shortened, bowed long bones
- Polydactyly of hands in all cases, polydactyly of feet in many
- Dysplastic nails

Complications

- Antenatal and neonatal mortality are due to the degree of respiratory insufficiency caused by thoracic hypoplasia (as in patients with ATD, **Figs. 125G**), and to the severity of underlying congenital heart disease.

Imaging Findings

- Chest:
  - Cardiomegaly, usually due to ASD or single atrium, with shunt vascularity
  - Marked narrowing of chest, with short, cupped ribs
- Pelvis:
  - "Trident" appearance of acetabulae, with medial and lateral spikes
  - Short, squared iliac wings
  - Narrow sacrosciatic notch
  - Premature ossification of femoral heads
- Long bones:
  - Short, thick, mildly bowed long bones
  - Widened, rounded metaphyses, especially of humeri, femora, and tibiae

- ◦ Short fibulae
- ◦ Genu valgum in some older patients due to hypoplasia of lateral tibial plateau
- Hands and feet:
  - ◦ Mild shortening of tubular bones of hands and feet
  - ◦ Postaxial polydactyly of hands in all patients, usually with partial duplication of fifth metacarpal and well-formed supernumerary sixth digit
  - ◦ Postaxial polydactyly of feet in many (25%) patients; often with a complete, well-formed supernumerary sixth ray
  - ◦ Older children and adults may demonstrate supernumerary postaxial carpal bones, often with postaxial carpal fusion anomalies (70%).
- Spine and calvarium:
  - ◦ Normal calvarium and spine

Treatment

- Treatment consists of correction of congenital heart disease and respiratory support.
- Defective dentition may require dental/orthodontic correction.
- Resection of supernumerary digits
- Corrective osteotomy for genu valgum

Prognosis

- Patients who survive the neonatal period and in whom congenital heart disease is corrected have normal life spans.

PEARL_____

- The combination of "trident" acetabulae, postaxial polydactyly, and shortened long bones with widened, rounded metaphyses is highly suggestive of chondroectodermal dysplasia.

PITFALLS_____

- Not all patients with short ribs and polydactyly have chondroectodermal dysplasia. Differential considerations include:
  - ◦ ATD: Some patients demonstrate polydactyly (**Fig. 125G1**), and all have short ribs (**Fig. 125G2**) and trident acetabulae. However, the metaphyses in ATD are not rounded and widened. Renal cystic disease is usually clinically evident and may be demonstrated ultrasonographically.
  - ◦ Short-rib polydactyly syndromes: In these conditions, the ribs are extremely short, with severe thoracic hypoplasia. These conditions are almost universally fatal.

Suggested Readings

Brueton LA, Dillon MJ, Winter RM. Ellis-van Creveld syndrome, Jeune syndrome, and renal-hepatic-pancreatic dysplasia: separate entities or disease spectrum? J Med Genet 1990;27:252–255

Ellis RWB, van Creveld S. A syndrome characterized by ectodermal dysplasia, polydactyly, chondrodystrophia, and congenital morbus cordis. Arch Dis Child 1940;15:65–84

McKusick VA, Egeland JA, Eldridge R, Krusen DE. Dwarfish in the Amish. I. The Ellis-van Creveld syndrome. Bull Johns Hopkins Hosp 1964;115:306–336

Qureshi F, Jacques SM, Evans MI, Johnson MP, Isada NB, Yang SS. Skeletal histopathology in fetuses with chondroectodermal dysplasia (Ellis-van Creveld syndrome). Am J Med Genet 1993;45:471–476

Sergi C, Voigtlander T, Zoubaa S, et al. Ellis-van Creveld syndrome: a generalized dysplasia of enchondral ossification. Pediatr Radiol 2001;31:289–293

Simon MW, Young LW. Radiological case of the month. Am J Dis Child 1986;140:665–666

Taybi H, Lachman RS. Radiology of Syndromes, Metabolic Disorders, and Skeletal Dysplasias. 4th ed. St. Louis: Mosby; 1996

INDEX